Sarcoma: Diagnosis and Management

Sarcoma:
Diagnosis and Management

Editor: Kath Hess

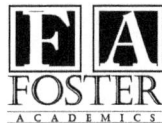

FA
FOSTER
ACADEMICS

www.fosteracademics.com

www.fosteracademics.com

FA
FOSTER
ACADEMICS

Cataloging-in-Publication Data

Sarcoma : diagnosis and management / edited by Kath Hess.
    p. cm.
Includes bibliographical references and index.
ISBN 978-1-63242-887-5
1. Sarcoma. 2. Sarcoma--Diagnosis. 3. Sarcoma--Treatment. 4. Cancer. 5. Tumors. I. Hess, Kath.
RC270 .S27 2020
616.994 075--dc23

Foster Academics,
118-35 Queens Blvd., Suite 400,
Forest Hills, NY 11375, USA

ISBN 978-1-63242-887-5 (Hardback)

Contents

Preface

Sarcomas are rare tumors arising from transformed cells of mesenchymal origin. These tumors occur more commonly in the bones and muscles, cartilage, tendons, nerves, fat and blood vessels of the limbs. These can however occur in other areas of the body as well. More than 50 types of sarcoma exist, which can be categorized under bone sarcoma (osteosarcoma) and soft tissue sarcoma. The susceptibility to sarcoma depends on a number of factors, such as family history of sarcoma, Paget's disease, genetic disorders such as Gardner syndrome, Li-Fraumeni syndrome, neurofibromatosis or retinoblastoma. Soft tissue sarcomas can grow anywhere in the body and may be difficult to detect. Osteosarcoma is comparatively easier to diagnose and presents symptoms such as swelling, pain in the affected bone and a limp. The treatment of sarcoma depends on the type of sarcoma, its location, and the extent of growth and metastasis. Surgery, chemotherapy, targeted therapies and radiation are the primary treatments for the management of sarcomas. This book is compiled in such a manner, that it will provide in-depth knowledge about the diagnosis and treatment of sarcoma. It is a valuable compilation of topics, ranging from the basic to the most complex advancements in oncology. It aims to serve as a resource guide for students and experts alike and contribute to the growth of the discipline.

This book is the end result of constructive efforts and intensive research done by experts in this field. The aim of this book is to enlighten the readers with recent information in this area of research. The information provided in this profound book would serve as a valuable reference to students and researchers in this field.

At the end, I would like to thank all the authors for devoting their precious time and providing their valuable contribution to this book. I would also like to express my gratitude to my fellow colleagues who encouraged me throughout the process.

Editor

Primary and secondary angiosarcomas: a comparative single-center analysis

Thorsten Hillenbrand, Franka Menge, Peter Hohenberger and Bernd Kasper[*]

Abstract

Background: Angiosarcomas (AS) are rare vascular malignancies. They are subdivided into primary (PAS) and secondary angiosarcomas (SAS). The objective was to compare the characteristics of AS subtypes.

Methods: Eighteen PAS and ten SAS patients treated at our institution between 2004 and 2012 were included in this study.

Results: Median age of PAS and SAS patients was 52.9 and 64.2 years, respectively (p = 0.1448). The percentage of women was 27.8% for PAS, but 80.0% for SAS (p = 0.0163). While PAS occurred throughout the body, the majority of SAS arose from the breast (p = 0.0012). All SAS were radiation-induced with a median latency of 7.7 years. The majority of patients with PAS and SAS underwent surgery as primary or recurrence treatment (p > 0.95). Local recurrence was developed by 27.8% of PAS and 50.0% of SAS (p = 0.4119). 61.1% of PAS metastasized, but only 40.0% of SAS (p = 0.4328). Median overall survival for PAS and SAS was 19 and 57 months, respectively (p = 0.2306).

Conclusion: Radical surgery remains the mainstay of both primary and recurrence treatment. SAS show a high local recurrence rate, while PAS tend towards developing early metastases. Overall, prognosis is poor for both groups.

Keywords: Primary angiosarcoma, Secondary angiosarcoma, Chemotherapy, Targeted therapy, Outcome

Background

Angiosarcomas (AS) are rare and aggressive malignancies representing about 2% of all adult soft tissue sarcomas [1]. They arise from endothelial cells of blood vessels or lymphatics either sporadically as primary neoplasms or secondary to chronic lymphedema or previous irradiation [2]. The latter constitutes an increasing complication following breast conserving surgery and radiotherapy in patients with breast cancer [3, 4]. Over 200 cases of radiation-induced AS of the breast are currently known in literature [5]. AS can occur throughout the body: most commonly in the head and neck area, followed by breasts and extremities. The remainder arise from different localizations like the liver, the heart and the bone [6]. The two conditions are similar in terms of histopathological features and immunohistochemical markers [7]. Secondary AS (SAS) differentiate from primary AS (PAS) in their pathogenesis by showing high level amplifications of MYC as well as FLT4 (VEGFR3) [8, 9]. Evidence-based recommendations are missing for the treatment of AS. Radical surgical en bloc resection with negative margins (R0) is the primary therapy for a potentially curable localized disease [10–12]. When indicated, surgery should be completed by adjuvant radiotherapy to prevent local recurrence [13, 14]. Inoperable, locally advanced or metastatic AS are treated by cytotoxic chemotherapy. Some clinical trials displayed that doxorubicin-based regimens and paclitaxel are two of the most active agents [15–17]. Furthermore, molecularly targeted therapy, in particular antiangiogenic therapy, constitutes a new option of treatment. Sorafenib was identified as an active agent against AS for instance [18]. Despite all therapeutic efforts, the patients' prognosis is still unfavorable [19, 20]. There is a relatively small amount of knowledge about the similarities and differences between the two subtypes of AS. As the objective of this retrospective study, the patient and tumor characteristics, treatment and outcome of the two different types of AS were analyzed.

*Correspondence: bernd.kasper@umm.de
Sarcoma Unit, Interdisciplinary Tumor Center Mannheim, Mannheim University Medical Center, University of Heidelberg, Theodor-Kutzer-Ufer 1-3, 68167 Mannheim, Germany

Methods

Patients

All adult patients with a confirmed pathohistological diagnosis of AS were identified from the Sarcoma Unit of the Interdisciplinary Tumor Center of the University Medical Center in Mannheim between 2004 and 2012. The study population consisted of 28 patients [13 women (46.4%), 15 men (53.6%)]. Acquisition of clinical data was obtained from the medical records. Patient and tumor characteristics including gender, age at diagnosis, subtype, tumor site, tumor-related symptoms, as well as metastasis at initial diagnosis, treatment, pattern of recurrence, occurrence of metastasis, date of last follow-up and survival were recorded and analyzed. In case of SAS, both type and age at diagnosis of pre-existing condition, latent time interval from radiotherapy to diagnosis of SAS and dosage of radiation were reviewed. This retrospective study was approved by the local ethics committee.

Statistical analysis

Progression-free survival (PFS) was defined as the time interval from the pathohistological diagnosis of AS until the time of first progression (local recurrence or metastasis) or the sarcoma-related death. Patients were censored at the last time of follow-up if they did not experience any disease progression or death. Overall survival (OS) was defined as the period of time from the pathohistological diagnosis until the patient's death. Patients were censored if they were still alive at the last follow-up. PFS and OS were calculated by using the method of Kaplan and Meier. Comparison of survival curves were performed by log-rank tests. Differences between the two AS subtypes were evaluated by t tests or Fisher's exact tests. StatXact 9.0 (Cytel Studios 2012, Cambridge, MA, USA) and SAS 9.2 (SAS Institute Inc. 2013, Cary, NC, USA) were used for the statistical analyses. Statistical level of significance was set at $\alpha = 0.05$.

Results

Patients and clinical presentation

Patient and tumor characteristics of PAS and SAS are shown in Table 1. From 2004 to 2012, a total of 28 patients with AS were identified. Of these, 18 patients were diagnosed with PAS (64.3%) and ten patients with SAS (35.7%). The majority of patients with PAS were represented by males (n = 13; 72.2%) while patients with SAS were dominated by females (n = 8; 80%). Fisher's exact test revealed statistical significance in gender distribution between the two groups (p = 0.0163). While PAS developed de novo, all patients with SAS had a previous history of radiotherapy with a median dose of 56 Gy (range 50.0–60.4 Gy). The most frequent condition for

which patients were irradiated was breast cancer (n = 8; 80%). Further conditions were chronic myeloid leukemia (n = 1; 10%) and thyroid gland autonomy (n = 1; 10%). The median age at the time of pre-existing diagnosis was 56.8 years (range 18.5–71.9 years). The median latent time interval from radiotherapy to diagnosis of SAS was 7.7 years (range 4.4–33.5 years). The majority of PAS occurred in deep soft tissue or internal organs (n = 12; 66.7%). Overall, the most common primary tumor sites were bone (n = 4; 22.2%), skin (n = 4; 22.2%), heart (n = 3; 16.7%) and breast (n = 2; 11.1%). In contrast, only 20% of SAS developed in internal organs [thyroid gland (n = 1), liver (n = 1)] and 80% (n = 8) in the breast or chest wall. The distribution of tumor localization showed a statistically significant difference (p = 0.0012).

Patients with cutaneous AS presented the following sites of origin: the scalp, the temple, the upper leg and presacral. AS of the bone caused painful restriction of mobility and were located in the thoracic vertebras 1–3, caput tibiae, os ilium and suprapatellar. All cardiac AS were located in the right atrium. AS of the mesentery of the small intestine (n = 1) and the adrenal gland (n = 1) were accompanied by spontaneous pain. AS of the thyroid gland appeared as a rapidly growing knotty swelling at the neck. One patient with AS of the deep soft tissue presented with a painful mass in the lower leg. AS of the breast (n = 2) arose from the parenchyma and presented with breast enlargement. In a single case, a bilateral localization was found. In contrast, SAS of the breast were located in the skin in each case and presented as blue-livid discoloration, erythematous plaques, bruise-like macules, blisters, nodules, indurations or exulcerations. The patient with AS of the liver reported about loss of weight, whereas the patient with AS of the thyroid gland presented with a painful mass causing swelling of the head, dyspnea and difficulties in swallowing. The most common metastatic sites at initial diagnosis were the lung (n = 2) and the bones (n = 2) in patients with PAS and the lung (n = 1) together with the skin (n = 1) in patients with SAS.

Primary therapy, recurrences and their treatment

Table 1 describes the initial treatment, the patterns of failure and their therapy. Surgical resection was the most common primary therapy for both patients with PAS (n = 11; 91.7%) and SAS (n = 7; 87.5%) presenting with localized disease (p > 0.95). Negative surgical margins were achieved in 72.7% of the patients with PAS (n = 8), while all patients with SAS (n = 7; 100%) were curatively resected (p = 0.2451). Among the ones with R0 resection, half of PAS patients (n = 4) received radiotherapy in adjuvant setting, but none of the SAS patients (p = 0.0769). Local recurrence was observed in 33.3%

Table 1 Patient, tumor, therapy and recurrence characteristics of PAS and SAS

Characteristic	Primary angiosarcomas		Secondary angiosarcomas		p value
	n	%	n	%	
Total number of patients	18	64.3	10	35.7	
Male	13	72.2	2	20	0.0163
Female	5	27.8	8	80	
Age at initial diagnosis, median	52.9 years		64.2 years		0.1448
Primary tumor site					0.0012
Superficial soft tissue or skin	4	22.2	0	0	
Deep soft tissue or internal organs	12	66.7	2	20	
Breast or chest wall	2	11.1	8	80	
At initial diagnosis					
Localized disease	12	66.7	8	80	0.6692
Metastatic disease	6	33.3	2	20	
Primary therapy					
Surgical resection					>0.95
Yes	16	88.9	9	90	
No	2	11.1	1	10	
R-status					0.2421
R0	8	50	8	88.9	
R1	3	18.8	0	0	
R2	1	6.2	0	0	
Unknown	4	25	1	11.1	
Radiotherapy					0.1282
Yes	5	27.8	0	0	
No	13	72.2	10	100	
Chemotherapy and targeted therapy					0.3642
Yes	6	33.3	1	10	
No	12	66.7	9	90	
Chemoradiotherapy					0.3571
Yes	0	0	1	10	
No	18	100	9	90	
Recurrence					0.2543
Yes	8	44.4	7	70	
No	10	55.6	3	30	
Local recurrence	5	27.8	5	50	0.4119
Recurrence therapy					
Surgical resection					>0.95
Yes	6	75	5	71.4	
No	2	25	2	28.6	
Radiotherapy					>0.95
Yes	1	12.5	0	0	
No	7	87.5	7	100	
Chemotherapy and targeted therapy					0.3147
Yes	3	37.5	5	71.4	
No	5	62.5	2	82.6	

of PAS patients (n = 4) and 50% of SAS patients (n = 4) with nonmetastatic disease at presentation (p = 0.6479). Overall, 61.1% of patients with PAS (n = 11) developed metastases, but only 40% of patients with SAS (n = 4) (p = 0.4328). In terms of metastatic sites, PAS metastasized most frequently into the lung (n = 4), followed by

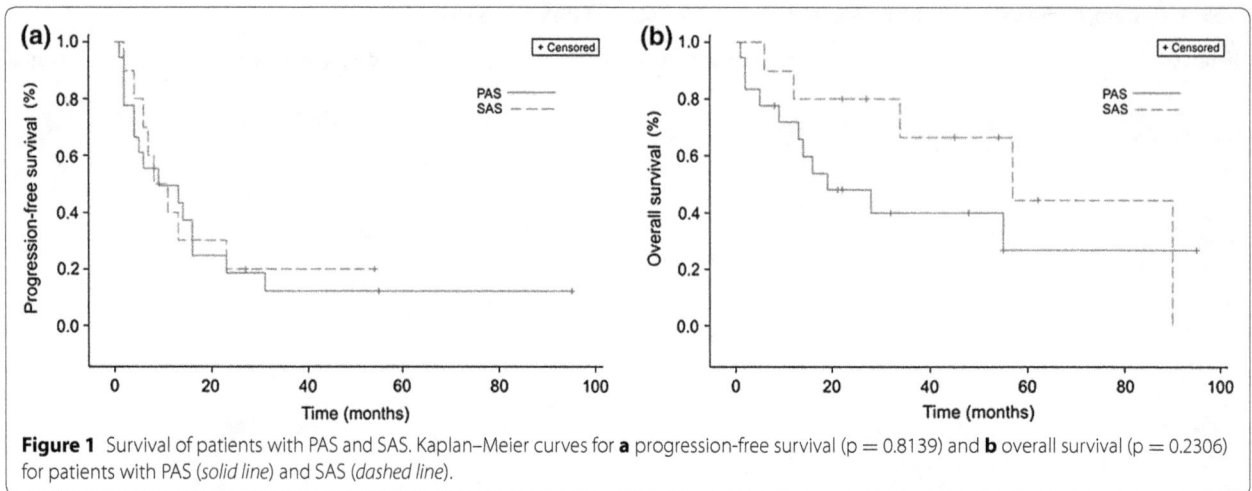

Figure 1 Survival of patients with PAS and SAS. Kaplan–Meier curves for **a** progression-free survival (p = 0.8139) and **b** overall survival (p = 0.2306) for patients with PAS (*solid line*) and SAS (*dashed line*).

the bones (n = 3) and the lymph nodes (n = 3). In the two latter sites, SAS did not develop metastases. In fact, the skin (n = 2) constituted the most common origin of metastases.

Chemotherapy and targeted therapy

The most commonly used chemotherapy regimen or targeted therapy agent was the combination of doxorubicin and ifosfamide for patients with PAS (n = 4) and single-agent sorafenib for patients with SAS (n = 5). Four patients with PAS underwent chemotherapy treatment with a combination of doxorubicin and ifosfamide: two had partial remission (PR) and two had progressive disease (PD). Only one patient with SAS receiving these two drugs had PR. Patients with PAS (n = 3) treated with sorafenib had PD, patients with SAS had stable disease (SD) (n = 3) and PD (n = 2). Two PAS patients had SD under the combination of doxorubicin and sorafenib, whereas SAS patients showed SD (n = 1) and PD (n = 1). Both patients with PAS (n = 1) and SAS (n = 1) had complete remission (CR) under treatment with pegylated-liposomal doxorubicin. In the paclitaxel group, one patient with PAS experienced SD, while one patient with SAS showed PD.

Survival

The median follow-up was 17.5 months (range 1–95 months) for PAS patients and 39.5 months (range 5–90 months) for SAS patients (p = 0.1235). Eleven patients with PAS (61.1%) have died during the study as opposed to five patients with SAS (50%). Patients with PAS had a median PFS of 9 months (range 1–31 months), whereas patients with SAS relapsed after a median duration of 9.5 months (range 2–23 months) (p = 0.8139) (Figure 1a). Median OS between patients with PAS

(19 months; range 1–55 months) and SAS (57 months; range 6–90 months) did not reach statistical significance (p = 0.2306) (Figure 1b). PAS and SAS 5-year OS rate was 6 and 20%, respectively.

Median PFS of PAS and SAS patients who presented with localized disease and were initially treated by surgery was 4 months (range 1–31 months) and 13 months (range 2–23 months), respectively (p = 0.5943). If negative surgical margins were achieved, median PFS was 10 months (range 2–31 months) and 13 months (range 2–23 months) for PAS and SAS patients, respectively (p = 0.6188). PAS and SAS patients presenting with nonmetastatic disease had a median survival from initial diagnosis to appearance of local recurrence of 19.5 months (range 2–31 months) and 10 months (range 2–23 months), respectively (p = 0.3045), whereas median PFS was 4.5 months (range 1–31 months) and 12 months (range 2–23 months), respectively (p = 0.5570).

Discussion

Primary and secondary AS are rare and aggressive neoplasms. The current analysis of 28 patients compared characteristics of these two subtypes demonstrating both similarities and differences. In this series, overrepresentation of SAS, female preponderance and the high percentage of breast SAS could be seen as a consequence of an increasing use of breast conserving therapy with postoperative radiotherapy in patients with breast carcinoma. That therapeutic procedure is associated with an about 3,200 times increased relative risk to develop SAS [21]. The median latency period from irradiation to diagnosis of SAS was 7.7 years. This fact was similar to findings in previous studies [7, 19]. Besides, the average latency tends to be shorter for breast SAS than for non-breast SAS (6.7 vs. 20.9 years; p = 0.148) [7]. In one case, breast SAS occurred after a latent time interval of 33.5 years being unusual for radiation-induced AS. Such a long period of time is rather reported for other radiation-induced sarcomas [22]. Postirradiation breast sarcomas (excluding AS) are generally diagnosed after a mean latency period of 14.3 years. In particular, radiation-induced breast malignant fibrous histiocytomas and fibroblastic sarcomas develop after a longer latency as opposed to postirradiation breast AS (p < 0.05) [23].

In this series, the percentage of surgery as initial therapy was higher than in previous reports (about 90 vs. 68–75%) [11, 19]. Negative microscopic margins were obtained in 88.9% of SAS patients, but only in half of PAS patients (p = 0.2421). This might be related to surgical methods depending on primary sites. In case of breast AS, R0 resection could be easily achieved through mastectomy (74% [24]). In opposition to that, resection of heart or cutaneous AS causes difficulties (0 and 21.3%, respectively [25, 26]) due to a potential tumor spread around vital structures. Furthermore, median PFS was increased by surgical resection in PAS patients presented with localized tumors when negative microscopic margins were achieved (4 to 10 months). SAS patients were not evaluated because all patients treated by surgery had R0 resection. Jallali et al. [27] found out that curatively resected patients with radiation-induced AS after breast conserving therapy had improved median survival compared to patients with incomplete excision (42 vs. 6 months). In general, surgical margin status has a major impact on patients' outcome since wide surgical resection with microscopically negative margins is accompanied by significantly prolonged OS and disease-specific survival (DSS), respectively [12, 20].

Radiotherapy constitutes another treatment option, preferably in the adjuvant setting. Mark et al. [13] observed statistically significant difference in 5-year OS between patients treated with and without additional radiotherapy, respectively (54 vs. 19%; p = 0.03). In our series, 27.8% of PAS patients received radiotherapy, but none of SAS patients (p = 0.1282). The latter have already received the maximum dose of radiotherapy in terms of predisposing disease. Nevertheless, in the Riad series, the risk of developing local recurrence was lower in patients with radiation-induced sarcomas, if they were reirradiated after surgical treatment (p = 0.043) [28]. Overall, Buehler et al. [19] analyzed AS patients with localized disease undergoing surgical resection and irradiation. They observed a decreased local recurrence rate (31 vs. 41%) and prolonged time to local recurrence (median 10 vs. 4 months).

In general, patients with inoperable, advanced or metastatic disease are treated by cytotoxic chemotherapy. However, the use is often hampered by the advanced age of patients, their co-morbidities and toxicities. The best outcome in our series was observed with pegylated-liposomal doxorubicin. Skubitz and colleagues [29] reported on six patients receiving this drug but none of them had CR. Three patients had PR, two had SD and one had PD. A study by Italiano evaluated efficacy of doxorubicin and weekly paclitaxel in 117 metastatic AS patients. They found out that response rate of both drugs was higher in patients with SAS as opposed to patients with PAS [16].

An alternative treatment option to conventional chemotherapy represents molecular targeted therapy in the form of angiogenesis inhibition, e.g. by sorafenib or bevacizumab. Maki et al. [18] assessed the efficacy of sorafenib in 145 patients with metastatic or recurrent sarcomas. These included 25 PAS patients (2 PR; response rate 8%) and 9 SAS patients (1 CR, 2 PR; response rate 33.3%). Sorafenib seems to be more active in patients with SAS as opposed to patients with PAS. In a phase II trial from the French Sarcoma Group (GSF/GETO) with 41 advanced AS patients, sorafenib showed a response rate of 23% in chemotherapeutical pretreated population whereas chemotherapy-naive patients had no response [30]. In contrast, no response could be observed in our series, irrespective if pretreated or not.

Our analysis is limited for various reasons. Firstly, the retrospective nature reduced the quality of data since there is no predefined therapeutic algorithm. In fact, AS represent rare and especially heterogeneous neoplasms why this single-center study is primarily descriptive. Furthermore, our small total number of patients was divided into more homogeneous subgroups to counteract limitations of outcome analysis. However, the impact of different treatment options, in particular the role of chemotherapy, targeted therapy and their combination, cannot be addressed adequately in this series and therefore has to be taken into account when interpreting the results. Accordingly, further evaluations with larger study populations are urgently needed.

Median survival from diagnosis to local recurrence tended to be longer in PAS patients compared to SAS patients with initially localized disease (19.5 vs. 10 months; p = 0.3045). According to Abraham et al. [10] the difference is clearly significant, resulting in a higher risk of local recurrence of SAS patients as opposed to PAS patients (p = 0.0001). While median PFS of all PAS and SAS patients showed similar results (9 vs. 9.5 months; p = 0.8139), it tends to be shorter in PAS patients presenting with nonmetastatic disease than in SAS patients (4.5 vs. 12 months; p = 0.5570). This observation might be caused by the more frequent occurrence of metastases in PAS patients during the course of the disease. OS analyses in different subgroups is hampered by both lack of endpoints and the small number of patients. However,

AS arising within irradiated tissue in patients with non-metastatic disease tended to have a shorter OS compared to patients with AS in other sites including lymphedematous fields in the Lindet series (26.5 vs. 45.9 months; p = 0.255). It must be taken into consideration that 22.4 and 62.6% of the entire cohort consist of patients with AS in pre-existing lymphedema and previously irradiated fields, respectively [31]. In particular, the outcome of PAS patients is significantly associated with longer DSS in comparison to SAS patients (p = 0.007) [10]. Different OS was observed between all patients with PAS and SAS in our series (19 vs. 57 months; p = 0.2306). Possible causes of the outcome are the diverse tumor biology, the primary site and the related therapy options. Hung et al. [7] also found no significant difference between PAS and SAS patients. Instead, shorter OS were observed in patients with breast SAS as opposed to patients with non-breast SAS. Moreover, Vorburger et al. [32] observed no statistically difference in terms of OS between patients with PAS and SAS of the breast. Overall, the prognosis remains poor for both PAS and SAS patients, but there seems to be a better perspective for the latter (5-year OS rate 6 and 20%, respectively). Furthermore, median OS of advanced soft-tissue sarcomas was 11.7 months in the Blay series [33]. In view of this fact, SAS belong to the circle of sarcoma entities with the best outcome.

Conclusion

In conclusion, we have demonstrated that primary and secondary AS constitute not only a rare and thoroughly aggressive, but also a heterogeneous disease. PAS occur at different localizations in the body while the majority of SAS arise from the breast of female patients. SAS show a high local recurrence rate, while PAS tend towards developing metastases. Radical surgical resection remains the mainstay of both primary and recurrence treatment. In future, multicenter prospective randomized trials should investigate new therapeutic strategies like the combination of molecular targeted therapy and cytotoxic chemotherapy. The prognosis is poor for both AS subtypes, but there seems to be a better outcome for SAS. While PFS shows similar results among the two groups, it tends to be shorter in PAS patients presenting with localized disease at initial diagnosis compared to SAS patients. However, subdivision of patients into more homogeneous subgroups is limited by our small number of patients. Also the study's retrospective nature and the rarity of the disease have an impact on the results which has to be considered. Hence, the relationship of primary and secondary AS has to be investigated, particularly in terms of molecular biology and clinicopathological features, in order to improve the specific treatment options and subsequently the survival.

Authors' contributions
All authors were involved in clinical data acquisition. TH analyzed and interpreted the data and drafted the manuscript. BK conceived the study. FM, PH and BK revised the article critically for important intellectual content. All authors read and approved the final manuscript.

Acknowledgments
We thank Lothar Pilz, Medical Faculty of Mannheim, for helping with statistical analysis. We also acknowledge financial support by Deutsche Forschungsgemeinschaft and Ruprecht-Karls-Universität Heidelberg within the funding programme Open Access Publishing.

Compliance with ethical guidelines

Competing interests
The authors declare that they have no competing interests.

References
1. Coindre JM, Terrier P, Guillou L, Le Doussal V, Collin F, Ranchere D et al (2001) Predictive value of grade for metastasis development in the main histologic types of adult soft tissue sarcomas: a study of 1240 patients from the French Federation of Cancer Centers Sarcoma Group. Cancer 91:1914–1926
2. Weiss SW, Goldblum JR (2001) Malignant vascular tumors. In: Weiss SW, Goldblum JR (eds) Enzinger and Weiss's soft tissue tumors, 4th edn. Mosby, St. Louis, pp 917–954
3. Nascimento AF, Raut CP, Fletcher CD (2008) Primary angiosarcoma of the breast: clinicopathologic analysis of 49 cases, suggesting that grade is not prognostic. Am J Surg Pathol 32:1896–1904
4. Torres KE, Ravi V, Kin K, Yi M, Guadagnolo BA, May CD et al (2013) Long-term outcomes in patients with radiation-associated angiosarcomas of the breast following surgery and radiotherapy for breast cancer. Ann Surg Oncol 20:1267–1274
5. Fraga-Guedes C, Gobbi H, Mastropasqua MG, Botteri E, Luini A, Viale G (2012) Primary and secondary angiosarcomas of the breast: a single institution experience. Breast Cancer Res Treat 132:1081–1088
6. Young RJ, Brown NJ, Reed MW, Hughes D, Woll PJ (2010) Angiosarcoma. Lancet Oncol 11:983–991
7. Hung J, Hiniker SM, Lucas DR, Griffith KA, McHugh JB, Meirovitz A et al (2013) Sporadic versus radiation-associated angiosarcoma: a comparative clinicopathologic and molecular analysis of 48 cases. Sarcoma. doi:10.1155/2013/798403
8. Guo T, Zhang L, Chang NE, Singer S, Maki RG, Antonescu CR (2011) Consistent MYC and FLT4 gene amplification in radiation-induced angiosarcoma but not in other radiation-associated atypical vascular lesions. Genes Chromosom Cancer 50:25–33
9. Manner J, Radlwimmer B, Hohenberger P, Mossinger K, Kuffer S, Sauer C et al (2010) MYC high level gene amplification is a distinctive feature of angiosarcomas after irradiation or chronic lymphedema. Am J Pathol 176:34–39
10. Abraham JA, Hornicek FJ, Kaufman AM, Harmon DC, Springfield DS, Raskin KA et al (2007) Treatment and outcome of 82 patients with angiosarcoma. Ann Surg Oncol 14:1953–1967
11. Fayette J, Martin E, Piperno-Neumann S, Le Cesne A, Robert C, Bonvalot S et al (2007) Angiosarcomas, a heterogeneous group of sarcomas with specific behavior depending on primary site: a retrospective study of 161 cases. Ann Oncol 18:2030–2036
12. Fury MG, Antonescu CR, Van Zee KJ, Brennan MF, Maki RG (2005) A 14-year retrospective review of angiosarcoma: clinical characteristics, prognostic factors, and treatment outcomes with surgery and chemotherapy. Cancer J 11:241–247
13. Mark RJ, Poen JC, Tran LM, Fu YS, Juillard GF (1996) Angiosarcoma. A report of 67 patients and a review of the literature. Cancer 77:2400–2406
14. Pawlik TM, Paulino AF, McGinn CJ, Baker LH, Cohen DS, Morris JS et al (2003) Cutaneous angiosarcoma of the scalp: a multidisciplinary approach. Cancer 98:1716–1726

15. Fata F, O'Reilly E, Ilson D, Pfister D, Leffel D, Kelsen DP et al (1999) Paclitaxel in the treatment of patients with angiosarcoma of the scalp or face. Cancer 86:2034–2037
16. Italiano A, Cioffi A, Penel N, Levra MG, Delcambre C, Kalbacher E et al (2012) Comparison of doxorubicin and weekly paclitaxel efficacy in metastatic angiosarcomas. Cancer 118:3330–3336
17. Penel N, Bui BN, Bay JO, Cupissol D, Ray-Coquard I, Piperno-Neumann S et al (2008) Phase II trial of weekly paclitaxel for unresectable angiosarcoma: the ANGIOTAX Study. J Clin Oncol 26:5269–5274
18. Maki RG, D'Adamo DR, Keohan ML, Saulle M, Schuetze SM, Undevia SD et al (2009) Phase II study of sorafenib in patients with metastatic or recurrent sarcomas. J Clin Oncol 27:3133–3140
19. Buehler D, Rice SR, Moody JS, Rush P, Hafez GR, Attia S et al (2014) Angiosarcoma outcomes and prognostic factors: a 25-year single institution experience. Am J Clin Oncol 37:473–479
20. Lahat G, Dhuka AR, Hallevi H, Xiao L, Zou C, Smith KD et al (2010) Angiosarcoma: clinical and molecular insights. Ann Surg 251:1098–1106
21. Strobbe LJ, Peterse HL, van Tinteren H, Wijnmaalen A A, Rutgers EJ (1998) Angiosarcoma of the breast after conservation therapy for invasive cancer, the incidence and outcome. An unforseen sequela. Breast Cancer Res Treat 47:101–109
22. De Smet S, Vandermeeren L, Christiaens MR, Samson I, Stas M, Van Limbergen E et al (2008) Radiation-induced sarcoma: analysis of 46 cases. Acta Chir Belg 108:574–579
23. Blanchard DK, Reynolds C, Grant CS, Farley DR, Donohue JH (2002) Radiation-induced breast sarcoma. Am J Surg 184:356–358
24. Seinen JM, Styring E, Verstappen V, Vult von Steyern F, Rydholm A, Suurmeijer AJ et al (2012) Radiation-associated angiosarcoma after breast cancer: high recurrence rate and poor survival despite surgical treatment with R0 resection. Ann Surg Oncol 19:2700–2706
25. Ge Y, Ro JY, Kim D, Kim CH, Reardon MJ, Blackmon S et al (2011) Clinicopathologic and immunohistochemical characteristics of adult primary cardiac angiosarcomas: analysis of 10 cases. Ann Diagn Pathol 15:262–267
26. Morgan MB, Swann M, Somach S, Eng W, Smoller B (2004) Cutaneous angiosarcoma: a case series with prognostic correlation. J Am Acad Dermatol 50:867–874
27. Jallali N, James S, Searle A, Ghattaura A, Hayes A, Harris P (2012) Surgical management of radiation-induced angiosarcoma after breast conservation therapy. Am J Surg 203:156–161
28. Riad S, Biau D, Holt GE, Werier J, Turcotte RE, Ferguson PC et al (2012) The clinical and functional outcome for patients with radiation-induced soft tissue sarcoma. Cancer 118:2682–2692
29. Skubitz KM, Haddad PA (2005) Paclitaxel and pegylated-liposomal doxorubicin are both active in angiosarcoma. Cancer 104:361–366
30. Ray-Coquard I, Italiano A, Bompas E, Le Cesne A, Robin YM, Chevreau C et al (2012) Sorafenib for patients with advanced angiosarcoma: a phase II trial from the French Sarcoma Group (GSF/GETO). Oncologist 17:260–266
31. Lindet C, Neuville A, Penel N, Lae M, Michels JJ, Trassard M et al (2013) Localised angiosarcomas: the identification of prognostic factors and analysis of treatment impact. A retrospective analysis from the French Sarcoma Group (GSF/GETO). Eur J Cancer 49:369–376
32. Vorburger SA, Xing Y, Hunt KK, Lakin GE, Benjamin RS, Feig BW et al (2005) Angiosarcoma of the breast. Cancer 104:2682–2688
33. Blay JY, van Glabbeke M, Verweij J, van Oosterom AT, Le Cesne A, Oosterhuis JW et al (2003) Advanced soft-tissue sarcoma: a disease that is potentially curable for a subset of patients treated with chemotherapy. Eur J Cancer 39:64–69

2

Osteosarcoma follow-up: chest X-ray or computed tomography?

Anna Paioli[1]* 📵, Michele Rocca[2], Luca Cevolani[3], Eugenio Rimondi[4], Daniel Vanel[4], Emanuela Palmerini[1], Marilena Cesari[1], Alessandra Longhi[1], Abate Massimo Eraldo[1], Emanuela Marchesi[1], Piero Picci[5] and Stefano Ferrari[1]

Abstract

Background: In patients with relapsed osteosarcoma, the surgical excision of all metastases, defined as second complete remission (CR-2), is the factor that mainly influences post-relapse survival (PRS). Currently a validated follow-up policy for osteosarcoma is not available, both chest X-ray and computed tomography (CT) are suggested for lung surveillance. The purpose of this study is to evaluate whether the type of imaging technique used for chest surveillance, chest X-ray or CT, influenced the rate of CR-2 and prognosis in patients with recurrent osteosarcoma.

Methods: Patients up to 40 years with extremity osteosarcoma enrolled in consecutive clinical trials and treated at the Rizzoli Institute from 1986 to 2009 were identified. Only patients who had lung metastases alone as first pattern of recurrence were considered for the analysis. The rate of CR-2, overall survival (OS) and PRS were the end-points of the study.

Results: The median follow-up was 47 months (1–300), 215 patients were eligible. Lung metastases were detected by chest X-ray in 100 (47%) patients, by CT in 112 (52%) and by symptoms in 3 (1%). CR-2 rate was 60% for patients followed by X-rays and 88% for those followed by CT (p < .0001). 5-year PRS was 30% (95% CI 21–39) in the X-ray group and 49% (95% CI 39–59) in the CT group (p = .0004). 5-year OS was 35% (95% CI 26–44) in the X-ray group and 60% (95% CI 51–70) in the CT group (p = .004).

Conclusions: A follow-up strategy with chest CT leads to a higher rate of CR-2 and significantly improves PRS and OS in osteosarcoma, compared to chest X-ray.

Keywords: Osteosarcoma, Follow-up, Chest X-ray, Chest computed tomography

Background

High-grade osteosarcoma is the most frequent primary bone tumor, with a peak of incidence in the second decade of life [1, 2]. The addition of multi-agent chemotherapy to surgery alone significantly improved survival rate, however, almost 40% of patients with localized disease relapse [3]. Recurrences usually occur within 3 years after the end of treatment, but late relapses, even after more than 10 years, are reported [4]. The most frequent site

of metastasis is the lung (more than 80% of cases), local recurrences occur in less than 10% of cases [5–7].

Post-relapse survival (PRS) after distant recurrence is poor [5–7]. The complete removal of all metastases, defined as a second complete surgical remission (CR-2), is the main prognostic factor for PRS and relate to long survival [8–16].

Other prognostic factors related to a better PRS are the site of relapse (lung vs others), the number of lung nodules (less than two) and a relapse free interval (RFI) of more than 2 years [5–7].

The role of chemotherapy in recurrent osteosarcoma is not yet well defined, but it has recently been emphasized in patients with a short relapse-free interval or in those who cannot achieve a complete surgical remission [3, 5, 6].

*Correspondence: anna.paioli@ior.it
[1] Chemotherapy Unit, Istituto Ortopedico Rizzoli, via Pupilli, 1, 40136 Bologna, Italy
Full list of author information is available at the end of the article

Osteosarcoma surveillance programs should be able to detect recurrence when complete removal of all known tumor sites is still feasible. Currently, an evidence-based follow-up policy is not available. International guidelines stress the importance of an intensive follow-up program focusing on the chest and on the primary tumor site, particularly for the first 4–5 years [3, 17]. A radiological follow-up is recommended for the chest, with X-ray or CT scan. Chest CT scan is more sensitive and sensible than chest X-ray in detecting lung metastases, but is burdened by higher radiation exposure and costs [18–20]. In clinical practice, follow-up programs vary in the different centers, both in terms of schedule and in terms of imaging techniques in use [21]. Whether the type of follow-up influences prognosis in patients with osteosarcoma is still debated.

In order to evaluate if the technique of chest surveillance (X-ray or CT) influence CR-2 rate and survival, we performed a retrospective cohort analysis of patients treated in a single Institution.

Patients and methods

Patients enrolled in clinical trials performed at the Rizzoli Institute between 1986 and 2006 were included in the analysis. Details of these studies have been published. IOR/OS-2 enrolled patients from 1986 to 1989 [22], IOR/OS-3 from 1990 to 1993 [23], IOR/OS-4 from 1993 to 1995 [24], Pilot ISG/OS from 1996 to 1997 [25], ISG/SSG-1 from 1997 to 2000 [26] and ISG/OS-1 from 2001 to 2006 [27].

Briefly, protocols included patients aged up to 40 years with localized high-grade osteosarcoma of the extremity. The strategy of treatment was based on delayed surgery after primary chemotherapy. The neo adjuvant schemes of treatment were mainly based on methotrexate, doxorubicin, cisplatin, ±ifosfamide. From our database we selected for the analysis the patients who relapsed and between these, those who had lung metastases alone at time of the first recurrence. Clinical charts were reviewed. Data collection was in accordance with the local ethical committee standards. A statement on consent to use the data for scientific purposes and publication was obtained from all patients. The imaging techniques used for chest surveillance changed over the study period. From 1986 to 1995 [22–24] follow-up was performed with chest X-ray, from 1996 to 2000 [25, 26] both chest X-ray and CT scan were used. Since 2001 patients were followed up only by CT [27]. When chest X-rays was used, follow-up schedule was every 2 months for the first 2 years, every 3 months the 3rd year, and then every 6 months. A confirmatory CT scan of the chest was performed in case of suspected nodules. Starting from 1996 all patients who completed chemotherapy underwent

CT of the chest, whereas those who were already followed up by X-rays continued with the same technique. When chest CT was used, follow-up schedule was every 3 months for the first 2 years, every 4 months in the 3rd and 4th year, and then every 6 months. All the patients were evaluated in a multidisciplinary team at the time of recurrence of the disease. The surgical approach foresaw lateral thoracotomy and manual palpation of the whole lung. In case of bilateral lesions, a contemporary surgery or two-staged surgery was performed. A wedge resection was performed when possible. Surgical staplers were used only in selected cases.

The rate of patients who achieved CR-2, overall survival (OS), and post relapse survival (PRS) were the end-points of the study. For each patient, date of the first surgical remission (CR-1), date of the first recurrence, pattern of recurrence, the imaging technique used for chest follow-up (X-ray or CT), relapse-free interval (RFI), number and size of lung nodules, laterality, treatment at recurrence were collected. Relapse free interval (RFI) was calculated from the date of CR-1 to first relapse. Post relapse survival (PRS) was calculated from the date of first relapse to date of death or last follow-up. Overall survival (OS) was calculated from the date of CR-1 to date of death or last follow-up. Survival curves were compared by Kaplan and Meier. Chi square and t test were used for comparison between groups when appropriate.

Results

Over the study period, 300 patients who recurred with lung metastases were identified. Lung metastases were associated with other recurrences in 63 patients, incomplete data were found in 22 patients. The remaining 215 patients were eligible for the analysis (Fig. 1). Median age at time of the first relapse was 15 years (range 6–43 years), 130 (60%) patients were male and 85 (40%) female.

Median RFI was 25 months (3–136 mos). Overall, 178 (83%) patients underwent surgery and 159 (74%) achieved a CR-2 status. All patients who did not reach CR-2 died. The 3- and 5-year PRS was 45% (95% CI 38–52) and 39% (95% CI 32–46) respectively, and the median PRS was 22 months (range 2–280 mos). With a median follow-up of 47 months (1–300 mos), OS was 64% (95% CI 58–71) at 3 years and 47% (95% CI 40–54) at 5 years.

Lung metastases were detected by chest X-ray in 100 (47%) patients, by CT scan in 112 (52%) and by symptoms in 3 (1%) patients. These last 3 patients, all followed-up by chest X-ray, were excluded from the analysis, none achieved a CR-2 and they all died of the disease.

Comparing the two groups of patients we observed no difference in terms of age, sex and site of the primary disease, while the rate of good responder patients was

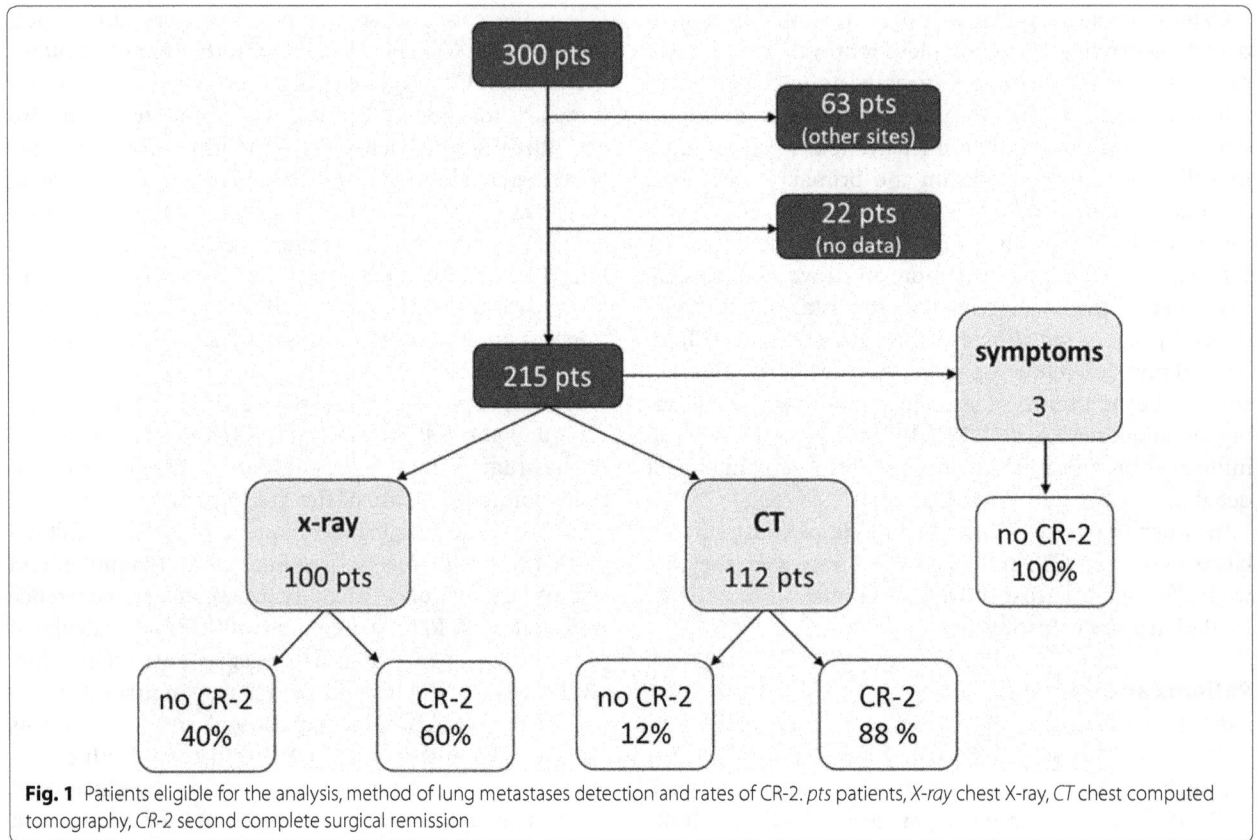

Fig. 1 Patients eligible for the analysis, method of lung metastases detection and rates of CR-2. *pts* patients, *X-ray* chest X-ray, *CT* chest computed tomography, *CR-2* second complete surgical remission

higher in the X-ray group compared to the CT group (Table 1). At first recurrence, the number of lung nodules did not differs among the two groups, while the incidence of bilateral lung metastases was higher and nodules were larger when lung relapses were detected by chest X-ray (Table 2). We observed a shorter median RFI and a higher rate of patients with a RFI of <2 years in the CT group.

At the time of recurrence, the use of chemotherapy was mainly based on high-dose ifosfamide. As reported in Table 3 the percentage of patients who received chemotherapy at recurrence did not differ in the chest-X-ray group compared with the CT group (p = .5). Most patients treated with chemotherapy underwent surgery, 24 in the X-ray group and 34 in the CT group. In both groups only 7 patients were treated preoperatively.

Patients were surgically treated in two Centers (Unit of General Surgery of the University of Modena and Unit of General Surgery of the Rizzoli Institute) by three surgeons B.A., M.R., C.S. All patients underwent lateral thoracotomy and manual palpation of the lung. In order to evaluate the whole lung, no patient was treated with video-assisted thoracoscopic resection. Up to 2000, bilateral wedge resection was performed in 22% of the patients, monolateral wedge resection in 57% of

Table 1 Patient and disease features according to imaging technique used for follow-up

	X-ray 100 pts	CT 112 pts	p
Age (years)			
Range	6–43	6–42	.7
Median	15	16	
Sex			
F	42 (42%)	42 (38%)	.5
M	58 (58%)	70 (62%)	
Site			
Femur	49 (49%)	56 (50%)	.9
Tibia	30 (30%)	32 (29%)	
Humerus	16 (16%)	19 (17%)	
Other	5 (5%)	5 (4%)	
Histological response	(90 pts)	(94 pts)	.02
Good	62 (69%)	49 (52%)	
Poor	28 (31%)	45 (48%)	

pts patients, *X-ray* chest X-ray, *CT* computed tomography

the patients, lobectomy with or without wedge resection in 21%. In the most recent years the percentage of monolateral wedge resection was 70%, bilateral wedge

Table 2 Pattern of lung relapse according to imaging technique used for follow-up

	X-ray 100 pts	CT 112 pts	p
RFI			
Median (months)	28.4	22.3	.01
<2 years (pts)	49 (49%)	72 (64%)	.02
Laterality			
Monolateral	63 (63%)	88 (79%)	.01
Bilateral	37 (37%)	24 (21%)	
n. nodules (162 pts)	84 pts	78 pts	.4
1	52 (62%)	47 (60%)	
2–5	23 (27%)	21 (27%)	
>5	9 (11%)	10 (13%)	
Size (112 pts) (cm)	54 pts	58 pts	.03
<2	20 (37%)	37 (64%)	
2–5	26 (48%)	19 (33%)	
≥5	8 (15%)	2 (3%)	

pts patients, *X-ray* chest X-ray, *CT* computed tomography, *RFI* relapse free interval

Table 3 Treatment and incidence of second complete surgical remission (CR-2) according to imaging technique used for follow-up

	X-ray 100 pts	CT 112 pts	p
Surgery			
Yes	73 (73%)	105 (94%)	<.0001
No	27 (27%)	7 (6%)	
1°line Chemo	(89 pts)	(104 pts)	.5
Yes	31 (35%)	41 (39%)	
No	58 (65%)	63 (61%)	
CR-2	60 (60%)	99 (88%)	<.0001

pts patients, *X-ray* chest X-ray, *CT* computed tomography, *Chemo* chemotherapy, *CR-2* second complete surgical remission

resection was 15%, lobectomy with or without wedge resection 15%.

Patients underwent surgery and achieved a CR-2 more frequently in the CT group as compared to the X-ray group (Table 3). CR-2 rate was 60% in patients followed up by X-ray, whereas it was 88% in those followed up by CT scan (p < .0001). We observed that the rate of patients who underwent surgery without achieving a CR-2 was higher in the chest X-ray group compared with CT group, 18 and 6% respectively (p = .01).

From 1996 to 2000 both X-ray and CT were used for chest surveillance. Seventy-five patients were included in this period, 19 were followed up by CT and 56 by X-ray. A CR-2 was obtained in all the patients followed with CT and in the 57% of patients followed by X-ray (p = .001).

The difference in terms of CR-2 translated in a significant difference in terms of PRS and OS between the two groups (Fig. 2). The 3- and 5- year PRS was 33% (95% CI 33–42) and 30% (95% CI 21–39) in the chest X-ray group and 58% (95% CI 49–68) and 49% (95% CI 39–59) in the CT scan group (p = .0004) (Table 3). Overall survival at 3 years was 58% (95% CI 48–68) in the X-ray group and 72% (95% CI 63–80) in the CT scan group, at 5-years it was 35% (95% CI 26–44) and 60% (95% CI 51–70) in the two groups, with a difference that was statistically significant. (p = .004) (Table 4).

Discussion

Results from our analysis show that the routinely use of chest CT scan, compared with X-ray, in the follow-up of osteosarcoma patients leads to a higher rate of second complete surgical remission (CR-2) and, consequently, to a significant benefit both in terms of PRS, and in terms of OS.

One of the main aim of oncology follow-up is early detection of recurrence, especially when effective strategy of treatment can be offered. We restricted the study population on patients who had metastases confined to the lung to emphasize better the potential benefit related to early diagnosis with regard to the follow-up programs. It is well known that this group of patients has a better probability of survival compared to that reported for those with multiple metastatic sites.

Relapse free interval of less than 2 years usually relate with a worse prognosis [5–7]. In our series we observed a higher rate of patients with RFI <2 years but a significantly better PRS and OS in the CT group compared with the X-ray group. The median RFI was shorter when patients were followed-up by CT, suggesting that the better prognosis observed in this group was probably due to the early diagnosis of recurrence, which led patients to be treated with surgery with radical intent more frequently, with a higher rate of CR-2.

The higher rates of necrosis after neo-adjuvant chemotherapy reported in the X-ray group compared with the CT group were probably related with the use of intraarterial infusion of cisplatin in most patients up to 1995 [22–24].

It is widely accepted that CT scan is superior to X-ray for the detection of lung nodules, but is under discussion whether the routine use of CT for chest surveillance can influence prognosis in patients with osteosarcoma. Data available in literature mainly comes from retrospective studies and only one prospective randomized study, which included both soft tissue and bone sarcomas.

It is interesting to note that in one study on soft tissue sarcomas where chest X-ray was used for follow-up, in 21 (37%) of 57 patients, lung metastases were detected

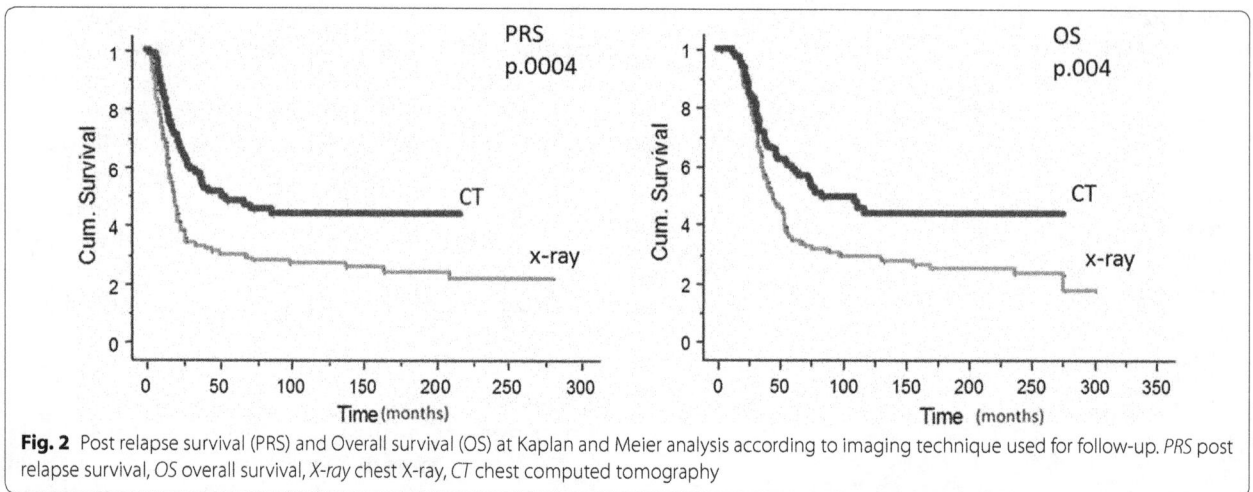

Fig. 2 Post relapse survival (PRS) and Overall survival (OS) at Kaplan and Meier analysis according to imaging technique used for follow-up. *PRS* post relapse survival, *OS* overall survival, *X-ray* chest X-ray, *CT* chest computed tomography

Table 4 Post relapse survival and overall survival at 3 and 5 years according to imaging technique used for follow-up

	X-ray 100 pts	CT 112 pts
PRS		
3-year PRS	33% (95% CI 33–42)	58% (95% CI 49–68)
5-year PRS	30% (95% CI 21–39)	49% (95% CI 39–59)
OS		
3-year OS	58% (95% CI 48–68)	72% (95% CI 63–80)
5-year OS	35% (95% CI 26–44)	60% (95% CI 51–70)

pts patients, *PRS* post relapse survival, *OS* overall survival, *CT* computed tomography, *95% CI* 95% confidence interval

when the patients had symptoms of lung involvement [28].

Similar results were reported in a more recent paper [29] where patients with high-grade primary bone or soft tissue sarcoma of the extremities followed-up by chest X-ray were included. Thirty-seven percent of the 90 patients with bone sarcomas who developed pulmonary metastases were detected outside the follow-up program, 13 were symptomatic. Overall, only nine (10%) patients survived after recurrence.

A retrospective analysis on a heterogeneous group of 174 patients with low and high grade soft tissue sarcomas has been reported [30]. Most were followed-up by chest X-ray. Only in 9 of 22 patients who developed isolated and asymptomatic lung metastases surgical resection was feasible whereas for the remaining patients the extent of the pulmonary disease did not allow metastasectomy.

A study that compared CT and X-ray of the chest in soft tissue sarcomass did not find any difference of survival related to the modalty of follow-up for the whole

study population [31]. Nevertheless, focusing on the 54 patients who recurred with lung metastases, the 4-year survival rate after detection of pulmonary metastasis was 0% in the chest X-ray cohort whereas it was 31.6% in the chest CT cohort (p < .05). Interestingly, as shown in our analysis, also in this study, unilateral lesions of smaller size were more frequently detected in CT group, leading to a higher rate of surgical complete remission.

The same group recently published results from a small retrospective study on high grade extremity osteosarcomas, both localized and metastatic [32]. The imagining technique recommended for chest surveillance was X-ray, CT scan was planned at the end of the treatment, in case of suspicious finding or in case of lung metastasis at diagnosis [32]. Twenty-two patients relapsed with lung metastases alone, 3 were detected by symptoms, 10 by X-ray and 9 by CT. The rate of patients surgically treated with curative intent was higher in the X-ray group (9/10) compared to CT group (6/9), as was number of patients remain relapse free, 5 in the X-ray group and 2 in the CT group. According to the authors, this difference is probably related to the higher baseline risk of relapse in patients followed with CT.

Only one randomized prospective trial on follow-up programs for patients with sarcoma of the extremities has been published [33]. Follow-up schedule (every 3 and 6 months) and chest imaging (chest X-ray and CT scan) were compared in a two-by-two factorial design. Authors reported that 3-year overall survival was 67% in the CT scan group and 66% in the X-ray group and concluded that the study demonstrated the non-inferiority of chest X-ray as compared to CT scan. Many criticisms can be addressed to this study. Firstly the heterogeneity of the sample, that included in the same analysis patients with soft tissue sarcomas and bone sarcomas, high and low grade and primary and recurrent sarcomas. Furthermore no data regarding histology of the bone sarcomas were given. It is well known that all these different entities have a different clinical behavior and a different response to treatments. For these reasons, the results obtained cannot be applicable to a single histotype and should not be considered conclusive. In our opinion, it is important to stress that the end point of the Indian study was the overall survival at 3 years. A rather short follow-up period considering that the available lines of chemotherapy treatment and the aggressive surgical approach can prolong post relapse survival in bone and soft tissue sarcomas [3, 4, 34, 35]. Also in our study if we considered overall survival, the difference was less apparent at 3 years (58 vs 72%), but at 5 years it reached a statistically significant (35 vs 60%).

We are aware of the radiation risks related to the routine use of CT for chest surveillance, particularly in children and young adults [36–39]. On the other hand, a 25% gain in terms of OS at 5 years as reported in our analysis indicated that the benefit related to the use of CT exceeded the risks of second malignancies associated [40].

A limit of our study is its retrospective design, and the long period of observation. A change in surgical techniques over the years could be a potential bias influencing results. However surgical procedures that allow the removal of metastases including a small amount of normal tissue around, like wedge resections, were available since early 1980s. The vast majority of the patients in our study, including patients who relapsed in the 1980s, were treated with wedge resections, monolateral or bilateral. It is important that the surgeon could evaluate the whole lung, in order to detect unrecognized nodules, for this reason no patient was treated with thoracoscopic resection [41]. Moreover, in the group of patients included when both X-ray and CT were used for chest surveillance, the higher rate of CR-2 related with the use of CT compared with X-ray was confirmed. The higher rate of patients who underwent surgery without achieving CR-2 reported in the X-ray group did not seem due to the availability of different surgical techniques, but rather to the delay of the diagnosis of recurrence and the higher incidence of large and bilateral lung metastases observed in this group.

Surgery was the treatment of choice at the time of first recurrence, however some patients in our series were treated with chemotherapy. The rate of patient treated with first line chemotherapy did not differ among the two group of patients. On the other hands, it is questionable whether chemotherapy at the time of recurrence has an impact on post relapse survival. In a previous paper including patients evaluated in the present analysis, we could not observe any benefit from chemotherapy in patients surgically free of disease [6]. A strength of our study is that we included a large and homogenous series of patients, treated and followed-up in a single Institution. All patients had high grade localized osteosarcoma at diagnosis and lung metastases alone at first recurrence. The surgical directions did not changed over the study period. At the time of recurrence all the patients were evaluated in a multi-disciplinary way together with the surgeon and, if indicated, they were treated by the same surgical team. In the group of patients followed-up with X-ray, in case of pathological findings, a confirmatory CT was performed. At the same way, in case of uncertain diagnosis when very small size nodules were detected in the CT group of patients, a new confirmatory CT was performed after 1 or 2 months, in order to evaluate the nodule growth. In the management of small lung nodules, when usually the resectability is not a problem, it is important to assess their behavior, in order to avoid overtreatment.

Conclusions

In conclusion, in patients with osteosarcoma of the extremity a follow-up strategy based on chest CT allows a higher rate of second complete remission and significantly improves prognosis with a higher probability of post relapse and overall survival when compared to surveillance based on chest X-ray.

Abbreviations

CR-2: second complete surgical remission; PRS: post relapse survival; OS: overall survival; CT: chest computed tomography; Chemo: chemotherapy; X-ray: chest X-ray; pts: patients; CR-1: first complete surgical remission; RFI: relapse free interval; 95% CI: 95% confidence interval; Mos: months; CR-1: first complete surgical remission.

Authors' contributions

AP, PP, DV, MR, SF: substantive intellectual contribution to conception and design of study, drafting and revision of manuscript, statistical analyses and interpretation of data. AP, EP, EM, ER, SF: final approval of the version to be published. AP, LC, MC, AL, MEA: patients selection/inclusion. All the authors declare that the work is original and has not been submitted or published elsewhere. All authors read and approved the final manuscript.

Author details

[1] Chemotherapy Unit, Istituto Ortopedico Rizzoli, via Pupilli, 1, 40136 Bologna, Italy. [2] General Surgery Unit, Istituto Ortopedico Rizzoli, via Pupilli, 1, 40136 Bologna, Italy. [3] Department of Orthopaedic Oncology, Istituto Ortopedico Rizzoli, via Pupilli, 1, 40136 Bologna, Italy. [4] Diagnostic and Interventional Radiology, Istituto Ortopedico Rizzoli, via Pupilli, 1, 40136 Bologna, Italy. [5] Department of Pathology, Istituto Ortopedico Rizzoli, via di Barbiano, 1/10, 40136 Bologna, Italy.

Acknowledgements

The authors thank Alba Balladelli for revision of the manuscript.

Competing interests

The authors declare that they have no competing interests.

Funding
This work was supported by: the Associazione Onlus "il Pensatore: Matteo Amitrano"; 5‰ donation (Italy).

References

1. Campanacci M. Bone and soft tissue tumors. Clinical features, imaging, pathology and treatment. 2nd ed. New York: Springer; 1999. p. 463–557.
2. Fletcher CDM, Bridge JA, Hogendoorn PCW, Mertens F. WHO classification of tumours of soft tissue and bone. 4th ed. Lyon: IARC Press; 2013.
3. Casali PG, Blay JY, Bertuzzi A, et al. Bone sarcomas: ESMO clinical practice guidelines for diagnosis, treatment and follow-up. Ann Oncol. 2014;25(Suppl):3.
4. Ferrari S, Bacci G, Picci P, Mercuri M, Briccoli A, Pinto D, Gasbarrini A, Tienghi A, Brach del Prever A. Long-term follow-up and post-relapse survival in patients with non-metastatic osteosarcoma of the extremity treated with neoadjuvant chemotherapy. Ann Oncol. 1997;8(8):765–71.
5. Kempf-Bielack B, Bielack SS, Jürgens H, Branscheid D, Berdel WE, Exner GU, Göbel U, Helmke K, Jundt G, Kabisch H, Kevric M, Klingebiel T, Kotz R, Maas R, Schwarz R, Semik M, Treuner J, Zoubek A, Winkler K. Osteosarcoma relapse after combined modality therapy: an analysis of unselected patients in the Cooperative Osteosarcoma Study Group (COSS). J Clin Oncol. 2005;23(3):559–68.
6. Ferrari S, Briccoli A, Bertoni F, Picci P, Tienghi A, Del Prever AB, Fagioli F, Comandone A, Bacci G. Postrelapse survival in osteosarcoma of the extremities: prognostic factors for long-term survival. J Clin Oncol. 2003;21(4):710–5.
7. Gelderblom H, Jinks RC, Sydes M, Bramwell VH, van Glabbeke M, Bramwell VH, Grimer RJ, Hogendoorn PC, McTiernan VH, Lewis IJ, Nooij MA, Taminiau AH, Whelan J. European Osteosarcoma Intergroup. Survival after recurrent osteosarcoma: data from 3 European Osteosarcoma Intergroup (EOI) randomized controlled trials. Eur J Cancer. 2011;47(6):895–902.
8. Saeter G, Høie J, Stenwig AE, Johansson AK, Hannisdal E, Solheim OP. Systemic relapse of patients with osteogenic sarcoma: prognostic factors for long term survival. Cancer. 1995;75:1084–93.
9. Putnam JB Jr, Roth JA, Wesley MN, Johnston MR, Rosenberg SA. Survival following aggressive resection of pulmonary metastases from osteogenic sarcoma: analysis of prognostic factors. Ann Thorac Surg. 1983;36:516–23.
10. Goorin AM, Delorey MJ, Lack EE, Gelber RD, Price K, Cassady JR, Levey R, Tapper D, Jaffe N, Link M, et al. Prognostic significance of complete surgical resection of pulmonary metastases in patients with osteogenic sarcoma: analysis of 32 patients. J Clin Oncol. 1984;2(5):425–31.
11. Leary SE, Wozniak AW, Billups CA, Wu J, McPherson V, Neel MD, Rao BN, Daw NC. Survival of pediatric patients after relapsed osteosarcoma: the St. Jude Children's Research Hospital experience. Cancer. 2013;119(14):2645–53. doi:10.1002/cncr.28111 **(Epub 2013 Apr 26)**.
12. Meyer WH, Schell MJ, Kumar AP, Rao BN, Green AA, Champion J, Pratt CB. Thoracotomy for pulmonary metastatic osteosarcoma: an analysis of prognostic indicators of survival. Cancer. 1987;59:374–9.
13. Huth JF, Eilber FR. Patterns of recurrence after resection of osteosarcoma of the extremity: strategies for treatment of metastases. Arch Surg. 1989;124:122–6.
14. Belli L, Scholl S, Livartowski A, Ashby M, Palangié T, Levasseur P, Pouillart P. Resection of pulmonary metastases in osteosarcoma: a retrospective analysis of 44 patients. Cancer. 1989;63:2546–50.
15. Skinner KA, Eilber FR, Holmes EC, Eckardt J, Rosen G. Surgical treatment and chemotherapy for pulmonary metastases from osteosarcoma. Arch Surg. 1992;127:1065–71.
16. Ward WG, Mikaelian K, Dorey F, Mirra JM, Sassoon A, Holmes EC, Eilber FR, Eckardt JJ. Pulmonary metastases of stage IIB extremity osteosarcoma and subsequent pulmonary metastases. J Clin Oncol. 1994;12(9):1849–58.
17. NCCN Clinical Practice Guidelines in Oncology (NCCN Guidelines®)—Bone Cancer Version 1.2016. In: NCCN guidelines for treatment of cancer by site. National Comprehensive Cancer Network. 2016 https://www.nccn.org/professionals/physician_gls/f_guidelines.asp. Accessed Jan 2016.
18. Vanel D, Henry-Amar M, Lumbroso J, Lemalet E, Couanet D, Piekarski JD, Masselot J, Boddaert A, Kalifa C, Le Chevalier T, Lemoine G. Pulmonary evaluation of patients with osteosarcoma: roles of standard radiography, tomography, CT, scintigraphy, and tomoscintigraphy. AJR Am J Roentgenol. 1984;143(3):519–23.
19. Goel A, Christy ME, Virgo KS, Kraybill WG, Johnson FE. Costs of follow-up after potentially curative treatment for extremity soft-tissue sarcoma. Int J Oncol. 2004;25(2):429–35.
20. Pass HI, Dwyer A, Makuch R, Roth JA. Detection of pulmonary metastases in patients with osteogenic and soft-tissue sarcomas: the superiority of CT scans compared with conventional linear tomograms using dynamic analysis. J Clin Oncol. 1985;3(9):1261–5.
21. Gerrand CH, Billingham LJ, Woll PJ, Grimer RJ. Follow up after primary treatment of soft tissue sarcoma: a survey of current practice in the United Kingdom. Sarcoma. 2007;2007:6. doi:10.1155/2007/34128
22. Bacci G, Picci P, Ferrari S, Ruggieri P, Casadei R, Tienghi A, Brach del Prever A, Gherlinzoni F, Mercuri M, Monti C. Primary chemotherapy and delayed surgery for non metastatic osteosarcoma of the extremity: results in 164 patients preoperatively treated with high doses of methotrexate, followed by cisplatin and doxorubicin. Cancer. 1993;72:1216–26.
23. Ferrari S, Mercuri M, Picci P, Bertoni F, Brach del Prever A, Tienghi A, Mancini A, Longhi A, Rimondini S, Donati D, Manfrini M, Ruggieri P, Biagini R, Bacci G. Nonmetastatic osteosarcoma of the extremity: results of a neoadjuvant chemotherapy protocol (IOR/OS-3) with high-dose methotrexate, intraarterial or intravenous cisplatin, doxorubicin, and salvage chemotherapy based on histologic tumor response. Tumori. 1999;85(6):458–64.
24. Bacci G, Ferrari S, Mercuri M, Longhi A, Capanna R, Tienghi A, Brach del Prever A, Comandone A, Cesari M, Bernini G, Picci P. Neoadjuvant chemotherapy for extremity osteosarcoma–preliminary results of the Rizzoli's 4th study. Acta Oncol. 1998;37(1):41–8.
25. Bacci G, Ferrari S, Longhi A, Picci P, Mercuri M, Alvegard TA, Saeter G, Donati D, Manfrini M, Lari S, Briccoli A, Forni C. Italian Sarcoma Group/Scandinavian Sarcoma Group. High dose ifosfamide in combination with high dose methotrexate, adriamycin and cisplatin in the neoadjuvant treatment of extremity osteosarcoma: preliminary results of an Italian Sarcoma Group/Scandinavian Sarcoma Group pilot study. J Chemother. 2002;14(2):198–206.
26. Ferrari S, Smeland S, Mercuri M, Bertoni F, Longhi A, Ruggieri P, Alvegard TA, Picci P, Capanna R, Bernini G, Müller C, Tienghi A, Wiebe T, Comandone A, Böhling T, Del Prever AB, Brosjö O, Bacci G. Saeter G; Italian and Scandinavian Sarcoma Groups. Neoadjuvant chemotherapy with high-dose Ifosfamide, high-dose methotrexate, cisplatin, and doxorubicin for patients with localized osteosarcoma of the extremity: a joint study by the Italian and Scandinavian Sarcoma Groups. J Clin Oncol. 2005;23(34):8845–52.
27. Ferrari S, Ruggieri P, Cefalo G, Tamburini A, Capanna R, Fagioli F, Comandone A, Bertulli R, Bisogno G, Palmerini E, Alberghini M, Parafioriti A, Linari A, Picci P, Bacci G. Neoadjuvant chemotherapy with methotrexate, cisplatin, and doxorubicin with or without ifosfamide in nonmetastatic osteosarcoma of the extremity: an Italian sarcoma group trial ISG/OS-1. J Clin Oncol. 2012;30(17):2112–8.
28. Whooley BP, Gibbs JF, Mooney MM, McGrath BE, Kraybill WG. Primary extremity sarcoma: what is the appropriate follow-up? Ann Surg Oncol. 2000;7:9–14.
29. Cool P, Grimer R, Rees R. Surveillance in patients with sarcoma of the extremities. Eur J Surg Oncol. 2005;31:1020–4.
30. Rothermundt C, Whelan JS, Dileo P, Strauss SJ, Coleman J, Briggs TW, Haile SR, Seddon BM. What is the role of routine follow-up for localised limb soft tissue sarcomas? A retrospective analysis of 174 patients. Br J Cancer. 2014;110(10):2420–6. doi:10.1038/bjc.2014.200 **(Epub 2014 Apr 15)**.
31. Cho HS, Park IH, Jeong WJ, Han I, Kim HS. Prognostic value of computed tomography for monitoring pulmonary metastases in soft tissue sarcoma patients after surgical management: a retrospective cohort study. Ann Surg Oncol. 2011;18(12):3392–8.
32. Rothermundt C, Seddon BM, Dileo P, Strauss SJ, Coleman J, Briggs TW, Haile SR, Whelan JS. Follow-up practices for high-grade extremity Osteosarcoma. BMC Cancer. 2016;6(16):301.
33. Puri A, Gulia A, Hawaldar R, Ranganathan P, Badwe RA. Does intensity of surveillance affect survival after surgery for sarcomas? Results of a randomized noninferiority trial. Clin Orthop Relat Res. 2014;472(5):1568–75.
34. Toulmonde M, Le Cesne A, Mendiboure J, Blay JY, Piperno-Neumann S, Chevreau C, Delcambre C, Penel N, Terrier P, Ranchère-Vince D, Lae M, Le Guellec S, Michels JJ, Robin YM, Bellera C, Italiano A. Long-term recurrence of soft tissue sarcomas: prognostic factors and implications for prolonged follow-up. Cancer. 2014;120(19):3003–6. doi:10.1002/cncr.28836 **(Epub 2014 Jun 18)**.

35. Bielack S, Kempf-Bielack B, Branscheid D, Carrle D, Friedel G, Helmke K, Kevric M, Jundt G, Jundt G, Kühne T, Maas R, Schwarz R, Zoubek A, Jürgens H. Second and subsequent recurrences of osteosarcoma: presentation, treatment, and outcomes of 249 consecutive cooperative osteosarcoma study group patients. J Clin Oncol. 2009;27(4):557–65.

36. Hall EJ, Brenner DJ. Cancer risks from diagnostic radiology: the impact of new epidemiological data. Br J Radiol. 2012;85(1020):e1316–7

37. Pearce MS, Salotti JA, Little MP, McHugh K, Lee C, Kim KP, Howe NL, Ronckers CM, Rajaraman P, Sir Craft AW, Parker L, Berrington de González A. Radiation exposure from CT scans in childhood and subsequent risk of leukaemia and brain tumours: a retrospective cohort study. Lancet. 2012;380(9840):499–505.

38. Fazel R, Krumholz HM, Wang Y, Ross JS, Chen J, Ting HH, Shah ND, Nasir K, Einstein AJ, Nallamothu BK. Exposure to low-dose ionizing radiation from medical imaging procedures. N Engl J Med. 2009;361(9):849–57. doi:10.1056/NEJMoa0901249.

39. Smith-Bindman R, Miglioretti DL, Johnson E, Lee C, Feigelson HS, Flynn M, Greenlee RT, Kruger RL, Hornbrook MC, Roblin D, Solberg LI, Vanneman N, Weinmann S, Williams AE. Use of diagnostic imaging studies and associated radiation exposure for patients enrolled in large integrated health care systems, 1996–2010. JAMA. 2012;307(22):2400–9.

40. Radiation Risks and Pediatric Computed Tomography (CT): A Guide for Health Care Providers. In: The causes and prevention of cancer. National Cancer Institute. 2012. https://www.cancer.gov/about-cancer/causes-prevention/risk/radiation/pediatric-ct-scans. Accessed 7 June 2016.

41. Ciccarese F, Bazzocchi A, Ciminari R, Righi A, Rocca M, Rimondi E, Picci P, Bacchi Reggiani ML, Albisinni U, Zompatori M, Vanel D. The many faces of pulmonary metastases of osteosarcoma: retrospective study on 283 lesions submitted to surgery. Eur J Radiol. 2015;84(12):2679–85.

3

Phosphorylated-insulin growth factor I receptor (p-IGF1R) and metalloproteinase-3 (MMP3) expression in advanced gastrointestinal stromal tumors (GIST)

Joan Maurel[1*†], Antonio López-Pousa[2], Silvia Calabuig[3], Silvia Bagué[4], Xavier Garcia del Muro[5], Xavier Sanjuan[6], Jordi Rubió-Casadevall[7], Miriam Cuatrecasas[8], Javier Martinez-Trufero[9], Carlos Horndler[10], Joaquin Fra[11], Claudia Valverde[12], Andrés Redondo[13], Andrés Poveda[14], Isabel Sevilla[15], Nuria Lainez[16], Michele Rubini[17], Xabier García-Albéniz[18], Javier Martín-Broto[19] and Enrique de Alava[20*†]

Abstract

Background: Most GISTs have mutations in KIT or PDGFRA. Patients with advanced GIST with KIT exon 9, PDGFRA mutation or WT for KIT and PDGFRA have a worse progression-free survival (PFS) compared to patients with KIT exon 11 mutated tumors. We evaluated the immunohistochemical (IHC) expression of p-IGF1R (Y1316) and MMP3 as predictors of PFS or overall survival (OS).

Methods: Ninety-two advanced GIST patients included in GEIS-16 study with KIT and PDGFRA mutational information were examined for p-IGF1R (Y1316) and MMP3 expression in a tissue micro-array. To study activation of the IGF1R system, we have used an antibody (anti-pY1316) that specifically recognizes the active phosphorylated form of the IGF1R. DNA was extracted from paraffin-embedded tissues and intronic PCR primers were used to amplify exons 9, 11, 13 and 17 of KIT, 12 and 18 of PDGFRA. Bidirectional sequencing with specific primers was performed on a ABI3100 sequencer using the Big Dye Terminator v3.1 kit. Multivariate model was built using a stepwise automated variable selection approach with criterion to enter the variable in the model of $p < 0.10$ and criterion to keep the variable in the model of $p < 0.05$. PFS was computed as the date of imatinib initiation to progression or death. Overall survival was defined as the time from imatinib initiation to death.

Results: Phospho-IGF1R was expressed only in 9 % (2/22) of cases without KIT mutation. MMP3 expression was detected in 2/5 patients (40 %) with PDGFRA mutation, 1/16 patients (6 %) with WT genotype and 7/71 patients (10 %) of KIT mutant patients. At univariate analysis KIT exon 11/13 mutation had better PFS than patients with exon 9 mutation, PDGFRA mutation or WT genotype ($p = 0.021$; HR: 0.46; 95 %CI (0.28–0.76). Less than 24 months disease free-interval (HR 24.2, 95 % CI 10.5–55.8), poor performance status (PS) (HR 6.3, 95 % CI 2.5–15.9), extension of disease; >1 organ (HR 1.89; 95 % CI 1.03–3.4) and genotype analysis (HR 0.57, 95 % CI 0.37–0.97) but not immunophenotype analysis (HR 1.53; 95 % CI 0.76–3.06) were the strongest prognostic factors for PFS in the multivariate analysis.

*Correspondence: jmaurel@clinic.ub.es; edealava@gmail.com
†Joan Maurel and Enrique de Alava contributed equally to this work
[1] Department of Medical Oncology, Hospital Clinic, CIBERehd, Translational Genomics and Targeted Therapeutics in Solid Tumors (IDIBAPS), Barcelona, Spain
[20] Pathology Department, Instituto de Biomedicina de Sevilla (IBiS), Hospital Universitario Virgen del Rocío/CSIC/Universidad de Sevilla, Seville, Spain
Full list of author information is available at the end of the article

Conclusions: Our results do not support p-IGF-1R and MMP3 evaluation in non-selected GIST patients but evaluation of this immunophenotype in WT and mutant PDGFR mutation in larger group of GIST patients, deserve merits.

Background

Gastrointestinal stromal tumour (GIST) is the most common sarcoma of the gastrointestinal tract. Imatinib mesylate (IM), a receptor tyrosine-kinase (RTK) inhibitor active against *KIT* and *PDGFRA*, is the standard treatment for advanced GIST patients [1, 2]. Mutations in the KIT and PDGFRA oncogenes are identified in 85–90 % of patients with advanced GIST. Most mutations in advanced GIST are located in *KIT* exon 11 (68–75 %) but also in exons 9 (8–15 %), 13 and 17 (1 %) and PDGFRA homologous exons (2–4 %) [2–4].

A small subgroup of GIST patients (10–15 %) shows primary IM resistance (i.e. disease progression in the first 6 months of IM treatment). Unfortunately, 70–80 % of IM-sensitive patients acquire secondary resistance due to new IM-resistant KIT or PDGFRA mutations and KIT amplification [5]. Mutational analysis of these genes affects prognosis and responsiveness to tyrosine kinase inhibitors [2]. D842V PDGFRA (1 %) and RAS and BRAF ($\leq$5 % of GIST) mutations, predicts primary IM resistance [6, 7].

Insulin-growth factor 1 receptor (IGF1R) is expressed in GIST patients [8, 9]. About 20–40 % of KIT/PDGFRA WT GIST patients show loss of function of the succinate dehydrogenase (SDH) including A, B, C, D complex which is associated to IGF1R expression [10, 11]. Although IGF1R expression is associated with a WT genotype, a very small subset of GIST SDHB-positive patients with mutations in KIT or PDGFRA (<1 % of all GIST) can also express IGF1R [11]. Recently IGF1R expression was found to be associated to lower response in advanced GIST but without affecting progression free survival or overall survival (OS) [12]. However, no previous studies have correlate IM efficacy and the activation of IGF1R (phospho-IGF1R). This aspect is important because phospho-IGF1R (p-IGF1R) expression does not correlate well with overall IGF1R expression [8]. MMP3 has been shown to be over-expressed (33-fold change) in a GIST-resistant (GIST882-R) cell line compared with the parental sensitive line [13].

Because p-IGF1R induce PI3K-AKT pathway activation and MMP3 can directly induce epithelial-mesenchymal transition [14], a widely known mechanisms of chemotherapy-resistance, we hypothesize that GIST patients with positive immunophenotype (either p-IGF-1R positive or MMP7 positive) can contribute to IM resistance. We selected patients with available tissue for biological analysis, from a cohort of advanced GIST patients treated with IM in 12 Spanish institutions included in the GEIS-16 study. The GEIS-16 study was a retrospective study to evaluate the role of metastatic surgical resection in GIST patients, sensitive to IM therapy [15].

Patients and methods

Study design

We selected patients from a cohort of advanced GIST patients treated with IM from January 2001 to December 2008 in 16 Spanish institutions included in the GEIS-16 study. Four institutions that participated in the GEIS-16 study did not participate in the GEIS-19 study. Only patients with available tissue for genotype and immunophenotype analysis were selected for the GEIS-19 study. Response rate was evaluated following RECIST criteria. The last patient status update was done in June 2015.

Mutational analysis

DNA was isolated from 3 to 20 μm FFPET sections. After deparaffinization, DNA was extracted using the QIAamp® DNA FFPE Tissue kit (Qiagen, Valencia, CA, USA) following the manufacturer's instructions. Amplification of exons 9, 11, 13 and 17 of KIT and exons 12 and 18 of PDGFRA was carried out as previously described [14, 15]. Ten microliters of PCR products were visualized in ethidium-bromide-stained 2 % UltraPure agarose gel (Life Technologies, Paisley, Scotland) and photographed. Negative controls were included in each set of amplifications. Bidirectional sequencing with specific primers was performed on an AB I3130xL sequencer using the Big Dye Terminator v3.1 kit (Applied Biosystems, Inc, Foster City, CA). Sequencing analysis, version 5.2 software (Applied Biosystems) and the National Center for Bioinformatics Information blast tool (http://www.ncbi.nlm.nih.gov/BLAST/) were used to confirm the mutation sequences for KIT (ENSG00000157404) and PDGFRA (ENSG00000134853).

Tissue microarray

Formalin-fixed paraffin embedded tissue samples of representative tumor regions from primary GISTs were collected for the preparation of 3 tissue microarrays. Briefly, three tissue cylinders with a diameter of 1.0 mm were punched out from morphologically representative areas of each donor tissue block and brought into a recipient paraffin block using a manual tissue arrayer.

Immunohistochemistry and scoring

To study activation of the IGF1R system, we have used a primary antibody (anti-pY1316) that specifically recognizes the phosphorylated (active) form of the IGF1R (Generous gift of Dr. Rubini, Ferrara, Italy). Briefly, paraffin-embedded sections were deparaffinized in xylene and rehydrated in downgraded alcohols and distilled water. Heat-induced epitope retrieval and a high-pH buffer (for anti-p-IGF1R) and citrate buffer pH6 (for anti-MMP3) (both buffers from Ventana Medical Systems, Tucson, AR) were applied for 30 min before the primary antibody. Then, tissue microarrays were incubated with anti-pY1316 antibody (dilution 1/50), and with an anti-MMP3 antibody (Abcam #ab137659; dilution 1/50), followed by a specific secondary antibody using the DAB Map detection kit (Ventana Medical Systems, Tucson, AR). Sections were counterstained with hematoxylin and analyzed by light microscopy. Cases were scored as positive or negative. Cases were scored as positive when at least 1 % of cells showed cytoplasmic expression of the molecule under study (either p-IGF1R, or MMP3).

Statistical analysis

Proportions are compared using Chi square test or Fisher's test when appropriate. Means are compared using t test. Survival analyses are done using Kaplan–Meier estimates and Cox proportional hazards model. Progression-free survival is defined as the time from the date Imatinib was started to the date of progression or death whichever occurred first. Overall survival is defined as the time from the date Imatinib was started to the date of death. Multivariate models are built using two approaches: (1) Entering all the variables in the model. (2) Using a stepwise automated variable selection approach with criterion to enter the variable in the model of $p < 0.10$ and criterion to keep the variable in the model of $p < 0.05$.

Results

Among 190 patients evaluated in the GEIS-16 study, 19 showed primary IM resistance (10 %). Paraffin-embedded tissue from primary tumours, were obtained from 92 untreated advanced GIST patients (46 % of the whole cohort of patients) for mutational analysis and tissue microarray construction (TMAs) in twelve Spanish Institutions. Eighty-eight patients were treated with 400 mg/day and 4 patients included in EORTC-ISG-AGITG phase III trial received 800 mg/day. Among 92 patients evaluated in GEIS-19 study 9 patients show primary IM resistance (10 %). Baseline characteristics of the patients according the immunophenotype are shown in Table 1. Seventy-one patients (78 %) had KIT mutations, 5 patients (5 %) had PDGFRA mutations and 16 patients (17 %) were WT for KIT and PDGFRA. Phospho-IGF1R

was expressed only in 9 % (2/21) of cases without KIT mutation. MMP3 was expressed in 10 % of cases. MMP3 expression was detected in 2/5 patients (40 %) with PDGFRA mutation, 1/16 patients (6 %) with WT genotype and 7/71 patients (10 %) of KIT mutant patients. Positive immunophenotype, was mostly observed in WT and PDGFR genotypes ($p = 0.006$). Representative cases of p-IGF1R and MMP3 expression are shown in Fig. 1.

Patients with mutations in KIT exon 11/13 showed higher response rate to IM (77 %) than patients with mutations in KIT exon 9 (25 %), PDGFRA (0 %) or wild-type (53 %) genotype ($p < 0.0001$). Response rate was observed in 4/11 (36 %) patients with MMP3 or p-IGF1R expression (1 patient was non-evaluable for response) vs 56/78 (71 %) in GIST patients without MMP3 or p-IGF1R expression (2 patients were non-evaluable for response) ($p = 0.025$). At univariate analysis KIT exons 11/13 had better PFS than patients with exon 9, PDGFRA mutation or WT genotype [$p = 0.037$; HR: 0.57; (95 % CI 0.33–0.97)]. Patients with MMP3 or p-IGF1R expression have non-significant poor PFS [14.1 months 95 % CI

Table 1 Patients characteristics according phenotype

Characteristic	Phenotype− (N = 80)	Phenotype+ (n = 12)	p value
Female	33 (41 %)	8 (66 %)	0.13
Mean age (SD)	60.7 (18.8)	65.1 (12.3)	0.20
Metastatic status			0.8
1 site	61 (76 %)	10 (83 %)	
>1 site	19 (24 %)	2 (17 %)	
Primary site			0.4
Stomach	30 (37)	5 (42)	
Small bowel	33 (41)	2 (16)	
Other	17 (22)	5 (42)	
KIT/PDGFR status			*0.006*
KIT mutation	64 (79 %)	7 (58 %)	
PDGFR	2 (3 %)	3 (25 %)	
WT	14 (18 %)	2 (17 %)	
ECOG PS			0.79
0–1	72 (90 %)	11 (92 %)	
2	8 (10 %)	1 (8 %)	
Liver metastasis	48 (60 %)	7 (58 %)	0.91
Surgery of primary	74 (92 %)	11 (92 %)	0.91
Disease free interval			
<24 months	20 (25 %)	4 (33 %)	0.5
>24 months	60 (75 %)	8 (67 %)	
Mean LDH (SD)	332.1 (160.8)	482.4 (429.8)	0.39
Mean leucocytes (SD)	7.1 (3)	8.1 (5.1)	0.56
Mean albumin (SD)	40.9 (7.1)	39.6 (6.1)	0.62

SD standard deviation

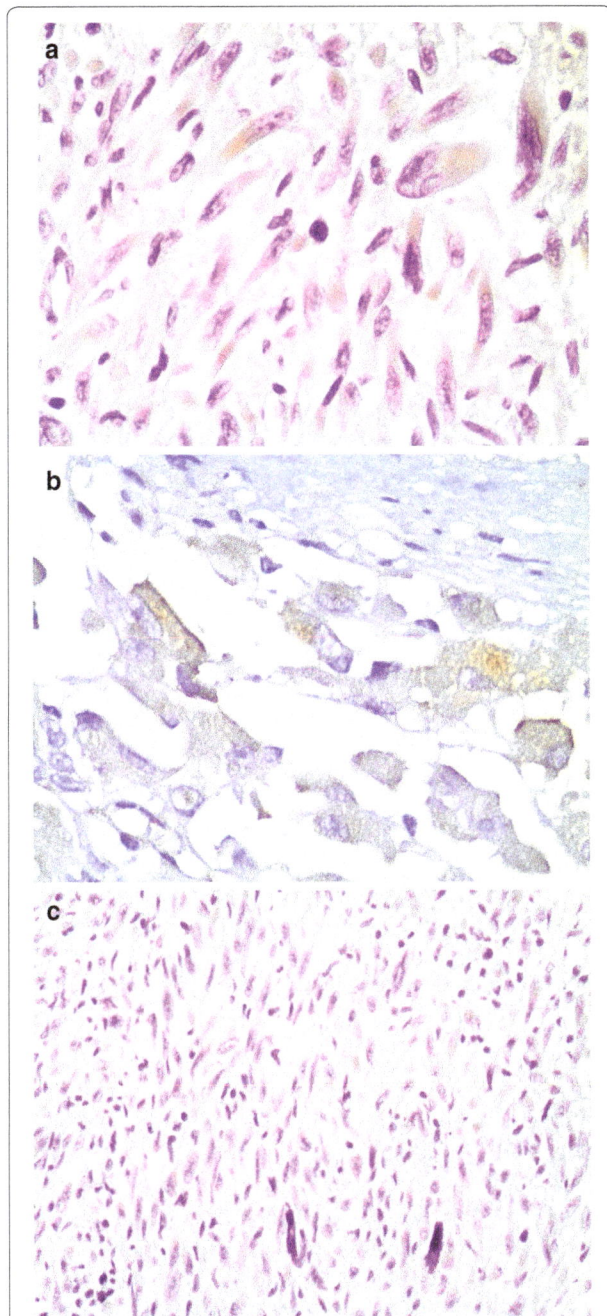

Fig. 1 a Mild expression of MMP-3 is present in the cytoplasm of tumor cells, especially those with a higher degree of anaplasia. (×200) **b** Expression of p-IGF1R was seen in tumoral cells. (×400) **c** Expression of p-IGF1R was seen in tumoral cells. (×200)

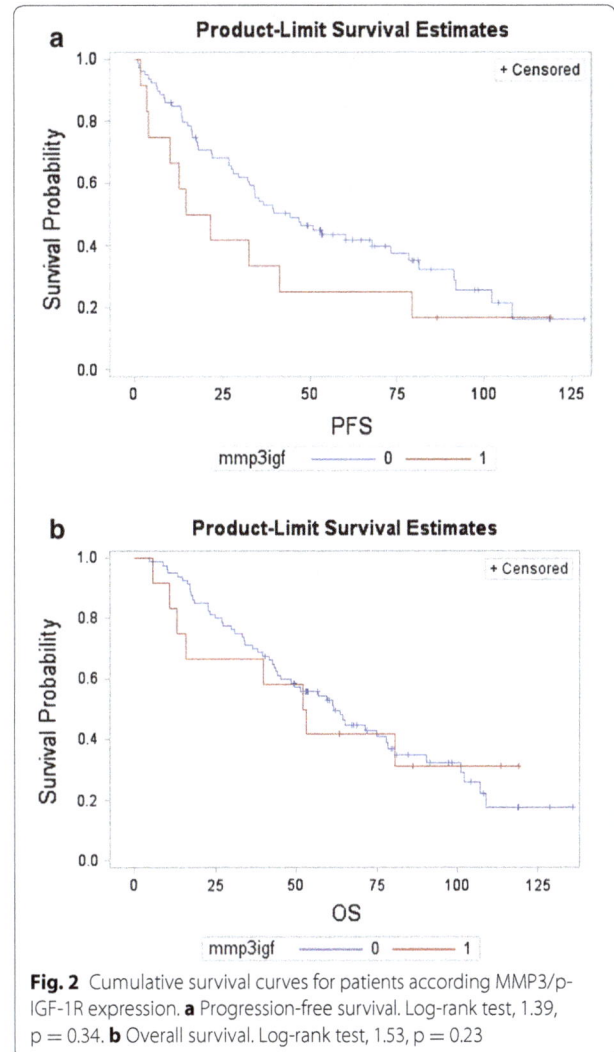

Fig. 2 Cumulative survival curves for patients according MMP3/p-IGF-1R expression. **a** Progression-free survival. Log-rank test, 1.39, p = 0.34. **b** Overall survival. Log-rank test, 1.53, p = 0.23

were also no differences in survival according MMP3 or p-IGF1R expression (Fig. 2b). For OS only performance status, disease free-interval, surgery of primary tumor and number of metastatic sites remain significant (Table 2).

Discussion

Our main findings reveal that, the proposed immunophenotype (p-IGF1R or MMP3 positive) correlates with poor response rate and a worse but statistically non-significant progression-free survival, after adjustment of all critical variables in the multivariate analysis.

IGF1R is expressed in a subset of GIST patients without KIT and PDGFRA mutations [10, 11]. We have confirmed that IGF1R activation is a rare event in KIT mutant patients but, although with a low frequency, this receptor is activated in GIST patients carrying PDGFRA mutations or WT genotype. MMP3 is expressed in less

(0–29.8)] than patients without either p-IGF1R or MMP3 expression [37.1 months 95 % CI (25.3–48.9)] (p = 0.33) (Fig. 2a. Disease free-interval, performance status (PS), extension of disease and genotype but not immunophenotype (p-IGF1R or MMP3) were the strongest prognostic factors for PFS in the multivariate analysis. There

Table 2 Univariate and multivariate analysis

	Univariate (PFS)		Univariate (OS)		Multivariate (PFS)		Multivariate (OS)	
	HR (95 % CI)	p value	HR (95 % CI)	p value	HR (95 % CI)	p value	HR (95 % CI)	p value
Group								
MMP3 and pIGF1R−	Reference		Reference		Reference		Reference	
MMP3 or pIGF1R+	1.39 (0.71–2.72)	0.34	1.10 (0.52–2.17)	0.95	1.53 (0.76–3.06)	0.23	1.67 (0.77–3.65)	0.20
Albumin >median	0.73 (0.44–1.23)	0.24	0.82 (0.47–1.44)	0.49				
Leucocytes >median	1.16 (0.73–1.85)	0.53	1.50 (0.90–2.49)	0.12				
LDH >median	1.36 (0.84–2.21)	0.21	1.50 (0.89–2.55)	0.13				
Age	0.99 (0.97–1.00)	0.33	0.99 (0.98–1.01)	0.51				
Kit mutation								
Exon 11/13	0.46 (0.28–0.76)	0.021	0.71 (0.41–1.21)	0.21	0.57 (0.33–0.97)	0.037		
Other	Reference		Reference					
ECOG								
PS 0	Reference		Reference		Reference		Reference	
PS 1	1.13 (0.67–1.8)	0.65	1.17 (0.66–2.07)	0.59	1.74 (0.99–3.07)	0.055	2.00 (1.08–3.67)	0.026
PS > 1	1.64 (0.73–3.68)	0.23	2.05 (0.88–4.76)	0.095	4.45 (1.85–10.76)	0.0009	5.25 (2.08–13.26)	0.0005
Female	1.02 (0.64–1.63)	0.92	1.01 (0.61–1.67)	0.96				
Primary site								
Stomach	1.61 (1.00–2.59)	0.050	1.36 (0.82–2.27)	0.24				
Others	Reference		Reference					
Extension of disease								Ta
1 metastatic organ	Reference		Reference		Reference		Reference	
2 or more metastatic organs	2.59 (1.52–4.42)	0.0005	2.56 (1.46–4.52)	0.0011	1.84 (1.03–3.27)	0.039	1.93 (1.03–3.62)	0.041
Surgery primary tumor								
Yes	Reference		Reference					
No	1.19 (0.51–2.75)		0.75 (0.27–2.08)	0.59			0.26 (0.09–0.76)	0.014
Disease-free interval		0.69						
<24 months	13.4 (6.93–25.77)	<0.0001	6.61 (3.72–11.79)	<0.0001	18.87 (8.54–41.73)	<0.0001	16.73 (7.97–35.13)	<0.0001
≥24 months	Reference		Reference		Reference		Reference	

than 10 % of KIT mutant and WT genotype in advanced GIST patients and in 40 % of PDGFRA mutant patients [16]. Although our data is limited to five patients, it could have clinical implications, because new drugs with potential activity in PDGFRA patients such as crenolanib [17] could be inactive in PDGFRA mutant patients that express MMP3.

We are tempted to speculate that in a small subset of patients with GIST with KIT mutations (10 %) and an important subset of WT genotype and PDGFRA mutations (21 %) our proposed immunophenotype bypass KIT signaling. It has been previously published that GIST patients with KIT mutation express p-STAT3 and p-AKT more intensely than patients with PDGFRA mutation [18]. Because MMP3 thought RAC1b can activate NF-kB and cyclin D1 but not AKT and STAT3 [19] and IGF1R not only activates AKT but also MEK/ERK pathway, our proposed immunophenotype may confer

KIT-independent IM resistance, specially, in the subset of WT or PDGFR mutant GIST patients.

Our study has several limitations. First the data comes from a retrospective cohort of patients and therefore PFS are more subject to investigator interpretation. Second, the phenotype implicates only 12 % of all the analyzed GIST patients. Third our cohort included a limited number of patients. Four, the percentage of WT KIT/PDGFR patients is slightly higher than in other published series. We cannot rule out that other more sensitive methods such as high-resolution melting analysis, could decrease the number of WT GIST patients. Finally, other RTK such as MET or FGFR3 that has been implicated recently in primary and secondary IM resistance, has not been evaluated [20, 21]. Despite of it, the multicenter nature of the study and the long follow-up (that include the genotype and all the important clinical variables) supports the strength of our conclusions.

Authors' contributions

JM and EA designed and wrote the manuscript. All authors revised the manuscript. JM and EA co-designed, reviewed, and revised the manuscript. All authors read and approved the final manuscript.

Author details

[1] Department of Medical Oncology, Hospital Clinic, CIBERehd, Translational Genomics and Targeted Therapeutics in Solid Tumors (IDIBAPS), Barcelona, Spain. [2] Department of Medical Oncology, Hospital Universitario Sant Pau, Barcelona, Spain. [3] Molecular Oncology Laboratory, Fundación de Investigación del Hospital General Universitario de Valencia, Valencia, Spain. [4] Pathology Department, Hospital Universitario Sant Pau, Barcelona, Spain. [5] Department of Medical Oncology, Institut Català d'Oncologia L'Hospitalet, Barcelona, Spain. [6] Pathology Department, Institut Català d'Oncologia L'Hospitalet, Barcelona, Spain. [7] Department of Medical Oncology, Institut Català d'Oncologia de Girona, Girona, Spain. [8] Pathology Department, Hospital Clínic, CIBERehd, IDIBAPS, Barcelona, Spain. [9] Department of Medical Oncology, Hospital Universitario Miguel Servet, Saragossa, Spain. [10] Pathology Department, Hospital Universitario Miguel Servet, Saragossa, Spain. [11] Department of Medical Oncology, Hospital Central de Asturias, Oviedo, Spain. [12] Department of Medical Oncology, Hospital Universitario Vall d'Hebron, Barcelona, Spain. [13] Hospital Universitario La Paz, Madrid, Spain. [14] Department of Medical Oncology, Fundación Instituto Valenciano de Oncología, Valencia, Spain. [15] Department of Medical Oncology, Hospital Universitario Virgen de la Victoria y Regional de Málaga, Málaga, Spain. [16] Department of Medical Oncology, Hospital de Navarra, Pamplona, Spain. [17] Department of Experimental and Diagnostic Medicine, Department of Epidemiology, University of Ferrara (UNIFE), Emilia-Romagna, Italy. [18] Harvard T.H. Chan School of Public Health, Boston, MA, USA. [19] Instituto de Biomedicina de Sevilla (IBiS), Hospital Universitario Virgen del Rocío/CSIC/Universidad de Sevilla, Seville, Spain. [20] Pathology Department, Instituto de Biomedicina de Sevilla (IBiS), Hospital Universitario Virgen del Rocío/CSIC/Universidad de Sevilla, Seville, Spain.

Acknowledgements

The authors thank Teresa Hernandez and Susana Fraile for their excellent technical support. This work was supported by a Jose Maria Buesa Grant (to J. Maurel).

Competing interests

The authors declare that they have no competing interests.

References

1. Verweij J, Casali PG, Zalcberg J, LeCesne A, Reichardt P, Blay JY, et al. Progression-free survival in gastrointestinal stromal tumours with high-dose imatinib: randomised trial. Lancet. 2004;364:1127–34.
2. Heinrich MC, Corless CL, Demetri GD, Blanke CD, von Mehren M, Joensuu H, et al. Kinase mutations and imatinib response in patients with metastatic gastrointestinal stromal tumor. J Clin Oncol. 2003;21:4342–9.
3. Heinrich MC, Owzar K, Corles CL, et al. Correlation of kinase genotype and clinical outcome in the north American intergroup phase III trial of imatinib mesylate for treatment of advanced gastrointestinal stromal tumor: CALGB 150105 study by cancer and leukemia group B and Southwest oncology group. J Clin Oncol. 2008;26:5360–7.
4. Debiec-Rychter M, Sciot R, Le Cesne A, Schlemmer M, Hohenberger P, van Oosterom AT, EORTC Soft Tissue and Bone Sarcoma Group, Italian Sarcoma Group, Australasian Gastrolntestinal Trials Group, et al. KIT mutations and dose selection for imatinib in patients with advanced gastrointestinal stromal tumours. Eur J Cancer. 2006;42:1093–103.
5. Heinrich MC, Corless CL, Blanke CD, Demetri GD, Joensuu H, Roberts PJ, Eisenberg BL, von Mehren M, Fletcher CD, Sandau K, McDougall K, Ou WB, Chen CJ, Fletcher JA. Molecular correlates of imatinib resistance in gastrointestinal stromal tumors. J Clin Oncol. 2006;24:4764–74.
6. Cassier PA, Fumagalli E, Rutkowski P, Schöffski P, Van Glabbeke M, Debiec-Rychter M, et al. Outcome of patients with platelet-derived growth factor receptor alpha-mutated gastrointestinal stromal tumors in the tyrosine kinase inhibitor era. Clin Cancer Res. 2012;18:4458–64.
7. Miranda C, Nucifora M, Molinari F, Conca E, Anania MC, Bordoni A, et al. KRAS and BRAF mutations predict primary resistance to imatinib in gastrointestinal stromal tumors. Clin Cancer Res. 2012;18:1769–77.
8. Tarn C, Rink L, Merkel E, Flieder D, Pathak H, Koumbi D, et al. Insulin-like growth factor 1 receptor is a potential therapeutic target for gastrointestinal stromal tumors. Proc Natl Acad Sci USA. 2008;105:8387–92.
9. Pantaleo MA, Astolfi A, Di Battista M, Heinrich MC, Paterini P, Scotlandi K, et al. Insulin-like growth factor 1 receptor expression in wild-type GISTs: a potential novel therapeutic target. Int J Cancer. 2009;125:2991–4.
10. Belinsky MG, Rink L, Flieder DB, Jahromi MS, Schiffman JD, Godwin AK, Mehren MV. Overexpression of insulin-like growth factor 1 receptor and frequent mutational inactivation of SDHA in wild-type SDHB-negative gastrointestinal stromal tumors. Genes Chromosom Cancer. 2013;52:214–24.
11. Lasota J, Wang Z, Kim SY, Helman L, Miettinen M. Expression of the receptor for type I insulin-like growth factor (IGF1R) in gastrointestinal stromal tumors: an immunohistochemical study of 1078 cases with diagnostic and therapeutic implications. Am J Surg Pathol. 2013;37:114–9.
12. Valadão M, Braggio D, Santos AF, Pimenta-Inada HK, Linhares E, Gonçalves R, et al. Involvement of signaling molecules in the prediction of response to imatinib treatment in metastatic GIST patients. J Surg Res. 2012;178:288–93.
13. Mahadevan D, Cooke L, Riley C, Swart R, Simons B, Della Croce K, et al. A novel tyrosine kinase switch is a mechanism of imatinib resistance in gastrointestinal stromal tumors. Oncogene. 2007;26:3909–19.
14. Nelson CM, Khauv D, Bissell MJ, Radisky DC. Change in cell shape is required for matrix metalloproteinase-induced epithelial-mesenchymal transition of mammary epithelial cells. J Cell Biochem. 2008;105:25–33.
15. Rubió-Casadevall J, Martinez-Trufero J, Garcia-Albeniz X, Calabuig S, Lopez-Pousa A, Del Muro JG, et al; the Spanish Group for Research on Sarcoma (GEIS). Role of Surgery in Patients with Recurrent, Metastatic, or Unresectable Locally Advanced Gastrointestinal Stromal Tumors Sensitive to Imatinib: A Retrospective Analysis of the Spanish Group for Research on Sarcoma (GEIS). Ann Surg Oncol.2015;22:2948-57.
16. Nannini M, Biasco G, Astolfi A, Pantaleo MA. An overview on molecular biology of KIT/PDGFRA wild type (WT) gastrointestinal stromal tumours (GIST). J Med Genet. 2013;50:653–6.
17. Heinrich MC, Griffith D, McKinley A, Patterson J, Presnell A, Ramachandran A, Debiec-Rychter M. Crenolanib inhibits the drug-resistant PDGFRA D842V mutation associated with imatinib-resistant gastrointestinal stromal tumors. Clin Cancer Res. 2012;18:4375–8.
18. Kang HJ, Nam SW, Kim H, Rhee H, Kim NG, Kim H, et al. Correlation of KIT and platelet-derived growth factor receptor alpha mutations with gene activation and expression profiles in gastrointestinal stromal tumors. Oncogene. 2005;24:1066–74.
19. Matos P, Jordan P. Increased Rac1b expression sustains colorectal tumor cell survival. Mol Cancer Res. 2008;6:1178–84.
20. Javidi-Sharifi N, Traer E, Martinez J, Gupta A, Taguchi T, Dunlap J, et al. Crosstalk between KIT and FGFR3 promotes gastrointestinal stromal tumor cell growth and drug resistance. Cancer Res. 2015;75:880–91.
21. Cohen NA, Zeng S, Seifert AM, Kim TS, Sorenson EC, Greer JB, et al. Pharmacological inhibition of KIT Activates MET signaling in gastrointestinal stromal tumors. Cancer Res. 2015;75:2061–70.

4

UK guidelines for the management of soft tissue sarcomas

Adam Dangoor[1]* , Beatrice Seddon[2], Craig Gerrand[3], Robert Grimer[4], Jeremy Whelan[2] and Ian Judson[5]

Abstract

Soft tissue sarcomas (STS) are rare tumours arising in mesenchymal tissues, and can occur almost anywhere in the body. Their rarity, and the heterogeneity of subtype and location means that developing evidence-based guidelines is complicated by the limitations of the data available. However, this makes it more important that STS are managed by teams, expert in such cases, to ensure consistent and optimal treatment, as well as recruitment to clinical trials, and the ongoing accumulation of further data and knowledge. The development of appropriate guidance, by an experienced panel referring to the evidence available, is therefore a useful foundation on which to build progress in the field. These guidelines are an update of the previous version published in 2010 (Grimer et al. in Sarcoma 2010:506182, 2010). The original guidelines were drawn up following a consensus meeting of UK sarcoma specialists convened under the auspices of the British Sarcoma Group (BSG) and were intended to provide a framework for the multidisciplinary care of patients with soft tissue sarcomas. This current version has been updated and amended with reference to other European and US guidance. There are specific recommendations for the management of selected subtypes of disease including retroperitoneal and uterine sarcomas, as well as aggressive fibromatosis (desmoid tumours) and other borderline tumours commonly managed by sarcoma services. An important aim in sarcoma management is early diagnosis and prompt referral. In the UK, any patient with a suspected soft tissue sarcoma should be referred to one of the specialist regional soft tissues sarcoma services, to be managed by a specialist sarcoma multidisciplinary team. Once the diagnosis has been confirmed using appropriate imaging, plus a biopsy, the main modality of management is usually surgical excision performed by a specialist surgeon. In tumours at higher risk of recurrence or metastasis pre- or post-operative radiotherapy should be considered. Systemic anti-cancer therapy (SACT) may be utilized in some cases where the histological subtype is considered more sensitive to systemic treatment. Regular follow-up is recommended to assess local control, development of metastatic disease, and any late-effects of treatment. For local recurrence, and more rarely in selected cases of metastatic disease, surgical resection would be considered. Treatment for metastases may include radiotherapy, or systemic therapy guided by the sarcoma subtype. In some cases, symptom control and palliative care support alone will be appropriate.

Background

Rationale and objective of guidelines

Soft tissue sarcomas (STS) are a relatively uncommon group of malignancies. On average a general practitioner may only see one sarcoma in their career. To improve diagnosis and treatment of these tumours, management was rationalized to peer-reviewed regional soft-tissue sarcoma services, and a smaller number of specialist units which also treat primary bone tumours [1]. An outline of best practice was set out in the National Institute for Health and Clinical Excellence Improving Outcomes Guidance for people with sarcoma (NICE-IOG) [2] published in 2006.

These guidelines are an attempt to review current evidence concerning soft-tissue sarcoma diagnosis and treatment, and provide recommendations to support best practice. They are not intended to be prescriptive, but aim to improve the quality of care for patients with STS by helping identify and inform the key decisions involved in their management. They will hopefully provide a

*Correspondence: adam.dangoor@uhbristol.nhs.uk
[1] Bristol Cancer Institute, Bristol Haematology & Oncology Centre, University Hospitals Bristol NHS Trust, Bristol BS2 8ED, UK
Full list of author information is available at the end of the article

useful resource for sarcoma services to help guide multidisciplinary team (MDT) case discussions, and patient management.

Methods

This updated guideline has been authored and reviewed by specialists from the UK involved in diagnosing and treating patients with sarcoma. They include members of the British Sarcoma Group (BSG), and NHS England Sarcoma Clinical Reference Group (CRG). As with the previous version, current NICE, NCCN (National Comprehensive Cancer Network, US), and ESMO (European Society for Medical Oncology) guidance were referenced, tailoring the recommendations for UK practice. It provides a brief review of the current state of established knowledge in sarcoma diagnosis and management, with guidance on what is considered current best practice in the UK. It has been derived by a consensus of expert opinion based on their interpretation of currently available data, and their own clinical experience.

Scope of guidelines

These recommendations apply principally to soft tissue sarcomas arising from limbs and trunk and although, where appropriate, specific guidance is given according to histological subtype it is recognised that some tumours, for example, Ewing sarcoma, and embryonal and alveolar rhabdomyosarcoma, require a different approach to management, and are excluded from this guidance [3]. These rare subtypes are relatively more common in paediatric and young adult patients. Ewing sarcoma arising in soft tissue are managed in accordance with guidelines for Ewing sarcoma of bone (see UK bone sarcoma guidelines [4]). Rhabdomyosarcoma is the commonest sarcoma in children and appropriately managed by children's cancer multidisciplinary teams (MDTs), often within international clinical trials such as EpSSG RMS 2005 [5, 6] which include comprehensive treatment guidance. For other histologies arising in children and young people (often referred to as non-rhabdomyosarcoma, soft tissue sarcomas, NRSTS) much less evidence exists for optimal management, in particular the application of chemotherapy and radiotherapy. Close working between children's cancer MDTs and sarcoma MDTs should be regarded as best practice.

Specific recommendations on the management of retroperitoneal and uterine sarcomas, as well as aggressive fibromatosis (desmoid tumours), plus some other conditions referred commonly to sarcoma MDTs, are included separately within this guideline. Bone sarcomas and gastrointestinal stromal tumours (GISTs) are subject to their own specific BSG guidelines. The latest bone sarcoma guidelines have recently been published [4] and the GIST guidelines are currently being updated.

These guidelines focus on clinical effectiveness, giving a picture of what treatments a specialist sarcoma multidisciplinary team should have access to within the UK, subject to some flexibility to allow for evolving practice, but they do not employ the same detailed analysis of cost effectiveness as NICE. In rare situations, treatment options may be suggested where NHS funding is not established. Unfortunately, with rare tumours such as sarcoma, NICE, and the Cancer Drugs Fund (CDF), may be less likely to evaluate potential treatments. These guidelines can be considered to represent a broad consensus in 2016. They will require updating as knowledge and treatment evolve.

Specialised soft-tissue sarcoma services

Following the publication of the National Institute for Health and Clinical Excellence Improving Outcomes Guidance for people with sarcoma (NICE-IOG) [2] in 2006, the services for patients with sarcoma in England and Wales were centralised. There are currently five centres providing both bone and soft-tissue sarcoma services, and an additional ten centres who diagnose and treat only soft-tissue sarcoma, passing on referrals of suspected bone sarcomas to their regional bone sarcoma centre [7] and collaborating on aspects of management. In England, services are commissioned and delivered in accordance with the current NHS England service specification [8]. In Scotland, the Scottish Sarcoma Network coordinates care of patients at five centres, and in Northern Ireland all bone sarcomas are managed at Musgrave Park Hospital with soft-tissue sarcomas also seen at four other centres.

Each specialist service must have a multidisciplinary team (MDT) made up of radiologists, surgeons, medical and clinical oncologists, pathologists, specialist nurses, and an MDT co-ordinator. The surgical team will include specialist plastic, general, or orthopaedic surgeons, with an extended team available, which may include retroperitoneal, thoracic, vascular, and other surgical disciplines, plus allied health professionals such as physiotherapists and occupational therapists. Supportive and palliative care services also contribute. The MDT will hold weekly meetings to discuss new suspected, and proven cases of sarcoma. The MDT meeting outcomes should be provided promptly to referring clinicians.

Epidemiology

Sarcomas are relatively uncommon tumours accounting for approximately 1% of all adult cancers [9]. They constitute a heterogeneous group of tumours of mesenchymal cell origin, often with a distinct age distribution, site of presentation, natural biological behaviour and prognosis. There are more than 50 subtypes divided into two broad categories: soft tissue sarcomas and sarcomas of bone [10].

Historically, because of the heterogeneity of this group of tumours, the true incidence has generally been under-reported. In 2010 around 3300 people were diagnosed with soft tissue sarcoma in the UK, with around 90 cases in children under 15. In the Teenage and Young Adult (TYA) age range (17–25 years) around 80 cases were recorded [11]. The National Cancer Intelligence Network (NCIN) reports that the incidence of STS is approximately 45/million population per year (NCIN) [12]. Bone sarcomas are rarer with an incidence around a fifth that of STS; 559 new cases were recorded in 2011 [11]. However, they represent a significant proportion of the cancer burden in young people under the age of 20 years.

Soft tissue sarcomas may occur at any age, most often in middle aged and older adults; however, as a proportion of paediatric malignancies they are relatively common comprising 7–10% of all childhood cancers. They are an important cause of death in the 14–29 years' age group [13–16].

Approximately half of all STS patients with intermediate or high-grade tumours develop metastatic disease requiring systemic treatment [17]; the overall survival is approximately 55% at 5 years [12, 18].

Aetiology

For the vast majority of cases, the aetiology is unknown, although there are certain genetic associations, such as the 10% lifetime risk of malignant peripheral nerve sheath tumour (MPNST) in individuals with familial neurofibromatosis, caused by mutations in the *NF1* gene [19, 20]. There is an increased risk of sarcomas, both bone and soft tissue, in patients who have had a familial retinoblastoma, caused by inherited mutations in the *RB* gene [21]. Similarly, there is an increased risk of sarcomas, and other cancers in families with Li-Fraumeni syndrome who have inherited mutations in the *TP53* tumour suppressor gene [22]. There is also a small risk of sarcoma in areas of the body previously treated using radiotherapy, for example angiosarcoma following treatment for breast cancer.

Clinical presentation

Due to the heterogeneous sites of origin of STS, it is difficult to clearly define the clinical features of the disease. However, a soft tissue lump exhibiting any of the following three clinical features should be considered to be malignant until proved otherwise [23]:

1. Increasing in size.
2. Size more than 5 cm.
3. Painful.

The more of these clinical features present, the greater the risk of malignancy with increasing size being the best individual indicator. In addition, deeper lying masses are more likely to be sarcomas.

Soft tissue masses are not uncommon and most will turn out to be benign, often lipomata. NICE produced updated guidelines in 2015, aimed at primary care, for early diagnosis of soft tissue sarcomas [24]. They suggest that the criteria for urgent referral should be adhered to even if the risk of malignancy is only 3%.

• Consider an urgent direct access ultrasound scan (to be performed within 2 weeks) to assess for soft tissue sarcoma in adults with an unexplained lump that is increasing in size.
• Consider a suspected cancer pathway referral (for an appointment within 2 weeks) for adults if they have ultrasound findings that are suggestive of soft tissue sarcoma or if ultrasound findings are uncertain and clinical concern persists.

If there is a particularly high suspicion of malignancy, and requesting an ultrasound in the primary care setting might introduce delay, then direct urgent referral to the regional sarcoma service should be considered. Regional services should provide referral advice on their websites or urgent referral forms. Any lesions previously thought to be benign that increase in size or develop other suspicious features should be considered for further investigation. Other diagnoses to consider in the case of palpable masses include metastases and lymphoma.

Any retroperitoneal or intra-abdominal mass with imaging appearances suggestive of a soft tissue sarcoma should be referred to a specialist centre before biopsy or surgical treatment.

Key recommendations

1. Any patient with a soft tissue mass that is increasing in size, or has a size more than 5 cm, whether or not it is painful, should either be referred for an urgent ultrasound scan, or referred directly to a sarcoma diagnostic centre.
2. If the ultrasound scan does not confidently confirm a benign diagnosis, then the patient should be referred for further investigation on an urgent suspected cancer pathway referral.
3. Any retroperitoneal or intra-abdominal mass with imaging appearances suggestive of a soft tissue sarcoma should be referred to a specialist centre before biopsy or surgical treatment.

Referral and assessment

Regional diagnostic services

The regional sarcoma services should support the development of efficient pathways for the investigation of suspected sarcomas. This may include providing information to local primary care or radiology services on the initial investigation and onward referral of patients with soft-tissue masses, and effective pathways to make direct suspected-cancer referrals when required.

Carcinosarcomas are generally viewed as epithelial tumours exhibiting sarcomatous differentiation. Although new biological insights are emerging [25], currently management would usually be as for epithelial tumours, and guided by the relevant cancer MDT.

Imaging

Diagnostic

Any patient with a suspected STS should be referred for an initial ultrasound scan, or direct to a diagnostic centre for triple assessment with clinical history, imaging, and biopsy [24]. An initial ultrasound is often useful in lower-risk cases to confirm benign conditions such as simple lipomata. In the hands of a non musculo-skeletal ultrasonographer however errors may arise and so there should be a low threshold for referral for further investigation. A more definitive ultrasound may be performed by a musculoskeletal radiologist who ideally is a member of the sarcoma MDT. Any patients with suspicious ultrasound or clinical features should usually have an MRI scan of the region affected. Plain X-ray may be used to identify bone involvement and risk of fracture, or to detect calcification. For retroperitoneal tumours CT is often more convenient, and as useful as MRI.

Staging

Patients with a confirmed STS should be staged with a CT chest to exclude pulmonary metastases prior to definitive treatment, although plain chest X-ray may be acceptable in a minority of cases (e.g. the frail elderly and those with small, low grade lesions). In most cases CT abdomen/pelvis and isotope bone scan are not routine staging investigations, but CT may be considered, particularly in lower extremity tumours [26]. Depending on the histological type and other clinical features [26], further staging assessments may be advised as below:

- CT or MRI scan for regional lymph node assessment for synovial sarcoma, clear cell sarcoma, or epithelioid sarcoma due to a higher risk of nodal involvement.
- Atypical lipomatous tumours (ALT) of the extremities have a very low risk of metastatic spread and so chest X-ray may be considered adequate staging (see "Lipomas and atypical lipomatous tumours" section).
- In cases of myxoid liposarcoma soft-tissue metastases are more common and so abdominal and pelvic CT scan should be performed. Alternatively,

although not yet established as routine practice, whole-body MRI has been shown to have potential utility in identifying occult metastatic disease and can be considered [27].
- Brain CT or MRI can be considered in cases of alveolar soft part sarcoma and clear cell sarcoma due to a higher incidence of brain metastases [28].
- Positron emission tomography (PET-CT) scanning is not yet proven as a routine investigation in sarcoma although may be considered before performing radical surgery, such as amputation for primary or recurrent disease [29]. It also provides a single investigation which can replace a separate CT and bone scan, and is being applied more commonly in sarcomas of younger patients such as Ewing sarcoma and rhabdomyosarcoma [30, 31]. Although some work has been done assessing tumour response to systemic treatment using PET; this is currently still investigational. PET-CT might have some utility in diagnosing neurofibromatosis 1 (NF1) associated malignant peripheral nerve sheath tumours (MPNST) [32, 33].

Biopsy

The standard approach to diagnosis of a suspicious mass is percutaneous core needle biopsy—several cores should be taken to maximise diagnostic yield. However, an incisional biopsy may be necessary on rare occasions, and excision biopsy may be the most practical option for small superficial lesions (<2 cm diameter). Biopsies of large lipomatous lesions with concerning features, should aim to sample areas appearing more heterogeneous on imaging, and need to be interpreted with caution as areas of dedifferentiation may be missed. The biopsy should be planned in such a way that the biopsy tract can be safely removed at the time of definitive surgery to reduce the risk of seeding, and should be performed at a diagnostic clinic by, or in conjunction with, a specialist radiologist or sarcoma surgeon. Fine needle aspiration (FNA) is not recommended as a primary diagnostic modality, although it may be considered for confirming disease recurrence, or nodal metastases.

Histology—diagnosis

Histological diagnosis should be made according to the 2013 WHO Classification [10] to determine the grade and stage of the tumour. The grade should be provided in all cases where possible based on a recognised system. In Europe, the Fédération Nationale des Centres de Lutte Contre le Cancer (FNCLCC) grading system is generally used, which distinguishes three grades (Table 1) [34, 35]. The mitotic rate should be recorded. Because of tumour heterogeneity, a core biopsy may not provide accurate information about grade [36]. In addition, certain translocation-driven sarcomas have a relatively uniform cellular morphology and,

Table 1 FNCLCC histological grading criteria [34, 35]

Tumour differentiation	Necrosis	Mitotic count (n per 10 high power fields)
1. Well	0: Absent	1: n < 10
2. Moderate	1: <50%	2: 10–19
3. Poor (anaplastic)	2: ≥50%	3: n ≥ 20

The sum of the scores of the three criteria determines the grade of malignancy. Grade 1 = 2 or 3; Grade 2 = 4 or 5; Grade 3 = 6

as such, can be misleadingly scored as intermediate, rather than high grade. This is especially true for myxoid/round cell liposarcomas, for which a different grading system based on the percentage of round cells is often used. Additional information may be provided by radiological imaging, and histology may be modified following assessment of the complete surgical resection specimen.

Pathologic diagnosis relies on morphology and immunohistochemistry. Increasingly it should be complemented by molecular pathology to confirm those diagnoses characterised by a specific genetic abnormality, such as an activating mutation, chromosomal translocation, or chromosomal amplification, using for example fluorescent in situ hybridisation (FISH), or reverse transcription polymerase chain reaction (RT-PCR) [37]. It may have particular utility when the clinical pathologic presentation is unusual, or the histological diagnosis is doubtful. Molecular testing is now routine to confirm diagnoses such as Ewing sarcoma, rhabdomyosarcoma, synovial sarcoma, and to differentiate lipomas from atypical lipomatous tumours/well-differentiated liposarcomas.

Histology—resection

The report on the resected specimen should comply with the recommendations for reporting of STS produced by the Royal College of Pathologists [37]. The pathology report should include an appropriate description of tumour depth (in relation to the superficial fascia) and margins (whether they are intralesional, marginal, or wide, and include distance from surrounding tissues, or the presence of an anatomical barrier). The pathologic assessment of margins should be made in collaboration with the surgeon, and confirmation obtained as to whether the tumour was excised intact. Tumour size and grade should be documented noting that the latter cannot be reliably assessed after pre-operative treatment with radiotherapy or systemic therapy. In this setting the tumour may be assessed for histological response to treatment although the prognostic implications are not well established, in contrast to their utility in osteosarcoma or Ewing sarcoma of bone.

If feasible, it is recommended that tumour samples should be collected and frozen, both for future research and because new molecular pathological assessment

techniques may become available later that could yield new information of direct value to the individual patient. Any tissue thus obtained is governed by the Human Tissue Authority; hence appropriate informed consent will need to be obtained from the patient.

Classification of margins

Historically, four categories of surgical margin have been described histologically: intralesional, marginal, wide and radical [38]. Whilst still included in the most recent ESMO guidance, they are summarised below.

Intralesional Margin runs through tumour and therefore tumour remains.

Marginal Surgical plane runs through pseudocapsule (reactive zone). The local recurrence rate is high because of tumour satellites in the reactive tissue. There are however prognostic differences between a planned and unplanned marginal excision.

Wide Surgical plane is in normal tissue but in the same compartment as the tumour. The recurrence rate is low and is related only to skip lesions in the affected compartment.

Radical The tumour is removed including affected compartments and there is a minimal risk of local recurrence.

However, the recent dataset from the Royal College of Pathologists [37] focuses more simply on the clearance in millimetres of the closest surgical margin, the type of tissue at the margin (e.g. fascia, fat, muscle or skin), whether the invasive margin is infiltrative or pushing, and presence or otherwise of vascular invasion. It is recognised that there is likely to be wide variation in the use of these descriptions and a more pragmatic approach, used in other cancer types, may be to simply classify the margins according to whether there is tumour at the cut edge or not:

R0—no tumour at the cut edge.

R1—tumour extends to cut edge.

R2—macroscopic residual tumour.

Margin assessment is complex and must take into account both the histological subtype of the resected sarcoma and the nature of the R1 resection margin. A positive resection margin at an intentionally preserved critical structure (planned margin) may have quite different prognostic significance to a multifocal R1 margin on the muscular surface of a resected specimen [39].

Staging

The most commonly used staging system for soft-tissue sarcoma, produced by the American Joint Committee on Cancer [40], includes information on both the grade

(Table 1) and stage of the tumour (Table 2). The 8th edition of the staging system will be published shortly and include consideration of anatomical location.

The final stage groupings are not altered whether the tumour is superficial or deep, and are thus as follows:

Stage I

- IA = low grade, small (G1/X, T1a/b, N0, M0).
- IB = low grade, large (G1/X, T2a/b, N0, M0).

Stage II

- IIA = intermediate or high grade, small (G2/3, T1a/b, N0, M0).
- IIB = intermediate grade, large (G2, T2a/b, N0, M0).

Stage III

- High grade, large, (G3, T2a/b, N0, M0).
- Regional node involvement, with any size and grade of primary tumour (G1-3, T1-2, N1, M0).

Stage IV

- Metastasis identified (G1-3, T1-2, N0-1, M1).

Table 2 AJCC TNM Classification for STS [40]

Classification	Description
Primary tumour (T)	
TX	Primary tumour cannot be assessed
T0	No evidence of primary tumour
T1	Tumour ≤5 cm in greatest dimension
	T1a Superficial tumour
	T1b Deep tumour
T2	Tumour >5 cm in greatest dimension
	T2a Superficial tumour
	T2b Deep tumour
Regional lymph nodes (N)	
NX	Regional lymph nodes cannot be assessed
N0	No regional lymph node metastasis
N1	Regional lymph node metastasis
Distant metastasis (M)	
M0	No distant metastasis
M1	Distant metastasis
Histologic grade (G)	
GX	Grade cannot be assessed
G1	Well-differentiated
G2	Moderately differentiated
G3	Poorly differentiated

Physical examination, diagnostic radiology and biopsy provide the AJCC criteria input data needed to stage STS

Key recommendations

1. All patients with a suspected STS should be managed by a specialist Sarcoma MDT as specified in the NICE guidance.
2. Ultrasound scan by a musculoskeletal radiologist should be considered as the first-line investigation, and may be supplemented by ultrasound-guided core biopsy.
3. Magnetic resonance imaging and core needle biopsy are recommended prior to definitive surgery.
4. Imaging of the thorax by CT scan for lung metastases should be done prior to radical treatment. Further staging may be considered depending on subtype and location of the sarcoma.

Management of localised disease

Soft tissue sarcomas are a diverse group of tumours and, as our understanding of the differing natural history and response to treatment improves, it is increasingly possible to tailor treatment according to the individual histology. The major therapeutic goals are long-term survival, avoidance of local recurrence, maximising function, and minimising morbidity.

All patients should have their care managed by a formally constituted sarcoma MDT. Decisions about surgery, chemotherapy, radiotherapy and the timing of all these modalities should be made by the Sarcoma MDT. For site specific STS (e.g. gynaecological, head and neck) there should be a formal relationship between the sarcoma MDT and the site-specific MDT. In organising services in England reference should be made to the NICE quality standard for sarcoma [41] and the current NHS England sarcoma Service Specification [8]. The devolved nations may use these documents as reference but will have their own recommendations. Coordination with the sarcoma MDT helps to ensure optimal management of the sarcoma subtypes, recruitment to clinical trials, and enhances accurate data collection on sarcoma diagnoses and outcomes. In all cases the treatment options will be discussed with the patient, who should be supported by a specialist nurse.

For most limb and truncal tumours conservative surgery, in selected cases, combined with pre- or post-operative radiotherapy is standard treatment, and achieves high rates of local control whilst maintaining optimal function. Radiotherapy may be avoided in patients with low-grade tumours that have been completely resected, or those with small, superficial high-grade tumours resected with wide margins.

Surgery
Surgery for localised disease
Surgery is the standard treatment for all patients with adult-type, localised soft tissue sarcomas, and should

be performed by a surgeon who has appropriate training in the treatment of sarcoma. Evaluation of the resectability of a tumour is determined by the surgeon in consultation with the Sarcoma MDT, and depends on the tumour stage, the anatomical location, and the patient's comorbidities. The primary aim of surgery is to completely excise the tumour with a margin of normal tissue. What constitutes an acceptable margin of normal tissue is not universally agreed but is commonly accepted as 1 cm soft tissue, or equivalent (e.g. a layer of fascia). However, on occasion, anatomical constraints mean that a true wide resection is not possible without the sacrifice of critical anatomical structures (such as major nerves, or blood vessels) and in this situation, it may be acceptable to leave a planned microscopic positive surgical margin, having considered the risks of recurrence and morbidity of more radical surgery and having discussed these fully with the patient [42]. It is recognised that there is a group of low-grade tumours, which have a low risk of local recurrence and metastasis (e.g. atypical lipomatous tumours, see "Lipomas and atypical lipomatous tumours" section), and it may be appropriate to treat these by planned marginal excision. In some situations, amputation may be the most appropriate surgical option to obtain local control and offer the best chance of cure.

For cases where a compartmentectomy or significant muscle resection to obtain clear margins will be required, reconstruction with free-functioning, or pedicled, muscle transfer may be considered at the time of primary surgery. This has the advantage of a single operative episode for the patient, but risks performing a definitive reconstructive procedure before clear margins have been histologically confirmed.

For patients who have undergone surgery and have an unplanned positive margin, re-excision should be undertaken if adequate margins can be achieved with acceptable morbidity. Macroscopic residual disease imparts a poor prognosis and local control is unlikely to be achieved even with addition of post-operative radiotherapy [43].

Patients with tumours that, because of size or position, are considered borderline resectable should be considered for neo-adjuvant treatment with chemotherapy (systemic or regional), or radiotherapy [44]. This decision will be guided by the histology of the tumour, likely sensitivity to systemic treatment, and the performance status of the patient (see below). Pre-operative radiotherapy should always be considered for myxoid liposarcoma due to the high response rate [45]. For other subtypes however, a significant reduction in size of the tumour is less likely so the aim may instead be to devitalise the margins of an anticipated marginal excision.

Surgery in the presence of metastatic disease

Surgical resection of the primary tumour remains an option as a palliative procedure in patients with metastatic disease. However, radiotherapy or chemotherapy may be more appropriate and the decision must take into account factors such as the patient's likely prognosis, symptoms (e.g. pain or ulceration), co-morbidity, the expected morbidity of surgery, histological sub-type and the extent of metastases.

Isolated limb perfusion

Where available, isolated limb perfusion (ILP) may be a useful pre-operative technique for reducing the size of difficult, but potentially resectable, tumours in an extremity where limb preservation may not otherwise be possible. ILP employs local high-dose chemotherapy (melphalan) plus tumour necrosis alpha (TNFα), and hyperthermia, restricted to the affected limb using arterial and venous cannulation and a tourniquet. ILP has been shown to shrink peripheral tumours, thus rendering them operable, and should be considered in selected cases [46, 47]. It is also of particular importance as an adjunct to surgical resection for local recurrence in the post-radiotherapy setting where further radiotherapy cannot be delivered and close margins are likely. In addition, ILP may be considered for palliation of unresectable sarcomas that would otherwise require an amputation, although if the tumour subsequently remains inoperable the durability of response is limited. Currently there is only limited availability of this service for STS, at the Royal Marsden Hospital in London, and the Beatson Cancer Centre in Glasgow.

Radiotherapy
Adjuvant radiotherapy

Both pre- and post-operative radiotherapy are considered to be standard approaches for most intermediate or high-grade soft tissue sarcomas. The addition of radiotherapy to surgery allows preservation of function with similar local control rates, and survival, to radical resection (i.e. compartmental excision/amputation) [48]. The majority of patients with low-grade tumours will not require radiotherapy. However, it should be considered for those with large, deep tumours with close or incomplete margins of excision, in whom re-excision is not possible, especially if adjacent to vital structures that could limit further surgery in the future. Patients who have undergone a compartmental resection or amputation do not require adjuvant radiotherapy assuming that the margins are clear.

The recommended post-operative radiation dose is 60–66 in 1.8–2 Gy fractions [49]. A two-phase technique using a shrinking field is commonly employed for limb sarcomas; 50 Gy to the initial larger volume followed by 10–16 Gy to a smaller volume [49]. This dose may need to be reduced if the field includes critical structures (for example the brachial plexus). Intensity-modulated radiation therapy (IMRT) should be considered to optimise the treatment volume, improve dose conformity, and reduce toxicity [50]. A phase II study of IMRT for sarcoma is underway in the UK, and ideally patients should be treated within the trial setting (IMRiS. Health Research Authority) [51].

The VORTEX clinical trial of post-operative radiotherapy for extremity soft-tissue sarcomas has completed recruiting in the UK [52]. This randomised clinical trial is comparing the standard post-operative two-phase, shrinking field, radiotherapy technique, with a single phase applied to a smaller treatment volume. The aim is to potentially spare normal tissue, and hence improve subsequent limb function, without compromising local control. The preliminary results of the study should be available in 2016 and may influence standard practice.

Pre-operative radiotherapy in limb sarcoma utilises a lower dose of 50 Gy as well as a smaller treatment volume covering the pre-operative tumour volume rather than the post-operative tumour bed. It has been shown to be associated with increased acute, post-operative complications compared to the standard post-operative treatment, but less late toxicity, with equivalent tumour control [53, 54]. In the UK, pre-operative radiotherapy has become routine in some centres. It may be preferred particularly where the size of the radiation field required for post-operative treatment is likely to be associated with significant late morbidity, or when the tumour is of borderline operability and pre-operative radiotherapy might render the tumour operable [44], or devitalise the margins of an anticipated marginal excision. If pre-operative radiotherapy is used there is a slightly higher incidence of post-operative morbidity including acute wound healing problems. Approaches which include the use of local or free flaps might be advantageous to avoid wound complications. Free flaps may reduce the risk of post-operative wound breakdown, minimise the dead space, and reconstruct the defect. A two team surgical approach (resection and reconstruction) reduces the operative time. Pre-operative radiotherapy may be less appropriate in cases where wound healing is more likely to be problematic, such as proximal thigh/groin or axillary locations. In addition, if a patient has a rapidly growing, painful tumour early surgery may be preferred. For certain radiosensitive histological subtypes, such as myxoid liposarcoma, pre-operative radiotherapy may be particularly advantageous, given the degree of tumour shrinkage that can be achieved [44, 45]. The standard regimen for pre-operative radiotherapy is 50 Gy, over 5 weeks,

followed by surgery approximately 4–6 weeks after completion of radiotherapy. A further 10–16 Gy may be given post-operatively if tumour margins are positive, after careful consideration, although recent evidence suggests this is unlikely to be beneficial and may result in excess late toxicity [55].

Definitive radiotherapy

The use of radiotherapy alone is unusual in the treatment of sarcoma. However, in a small number of cases the sarcoma may be considered unresectable due to location, local invasion, or because resection would lead to unacceptable morbidity or a poor functional outcome. In these cases, radiotherapy can occasionally provide a durable remission although local recurrence rates are high. Outcomes appear related to tumour size, grade, and radiation dose [56–59]; doses of over 60 Gy may be employed. In patients with significant life-limiting comorbidities lower dose, palliative radiotherapy is an option.

Proton therapy

Proton therapy is a highly specialised method of delivering high-dose radiotherapy to a target volume, whilst minimising dose to surrounding normal tissue. It is considered for a number of defined indications which may include spinal or paraspinal soft-tissue sarcomas in both adults and children [60]. It is commissioned by NHS England where applications for treatment are considered by a "Proton Panel". Currently patients are sent overseas for treatment, but two new facilities are under construction at The Christie NHS Foundation Trust in Manchester and University College Hospital (UCLH) NHS Foundation Trust. The services in these centres are due to commence in 2018 and 2019 [61].

Chemotherapy
Adjuvant chemotherapy

The role of adjuvant chemotherapy for most STS remains unproven. Although currently not regarded as standard treatment in the UK, there is conflicting evidence, and it may be considered for individual patients with higher risk tumours and potentially chemo-sensitive subtypes on the basis that benefit cannot be excluded. Table 3 provides a general guide as to likely relative chemosensitivity. Due to a lack of published comparative data the table is based on the referenced paper [62], modified in light of the clinical experience of the authors and reviewers of these guidelines. In most cases treatment of relapsed disease is palliative and the best chance of obtaining cure is therefore with primary treatment. In those subtypes with particularly poor prognosis, such as cardiac sarcoma, where salvage treatment for relapse would be difficult, the threshold for using adjuvant chemotherapy

Table 3 Soft tissue sarcomas grouped by chemosensitivity

Relative chemosensitivity	Examples of soft tissue sarcomas
Chemotherapy integral to management	Ewing's sarcoma family tumours
	Embryonal and alveolar rhabdo-myosarcoma
Chemosensitive	Desmoplastic small round cell tumour
	Synovial sarcoma
	Myxoid/round cell liposarcoma
	Uterine leiomyosarcoma
Moderately chemosensitive	Pleomorphic liposarcoma
	Epithelioid sarcoma
	Pleomorphic rhabdomyosarcoma
	Leiomyosarcoma
	Angiosarcoma
Relatively chemo-insensitive	Malignant peripheral nerve sheath tumour
	Myxofibrosarcoma
	Dedifferentiated liposarcoma
	Clear cell sarcoma
	Endometrial stromal sarcoma
Chemoinsensitive	Alveolar soft part sarcoma
	Extraskeletal myxoid chondrosarcoma

Modified from R. Salgado and E. van Marck [62] by a consensus view of the authors and other guideline contributors

may be lower. It may also be considered in other situations where local relapse would be untreatable or where adequate radiotherapy could not be administered owing to the sensitivity of adjacent structures, for example spinal cord. A meta-analysis published in 1997 reported an improvement in local control and progression free survival; however, although there was a trend towards an overall survival benefit this was not statistically significant [63]. These data have been supported by two more recent overviews [64, 65]. The latter did not use original trial data and included a large Italian trial which, when published in 2001, reported a significant survival benefit for adjuvant chemotherapy; although this has not been maintained with long-term follow-up [66]. The final data from EORTC 62,931 [67], the largest trial of adjuvant chemotherapy for STS, have failed to demonstrate any clear benefit from chemotherapy in local control, relapse-free survival or overall survival in patients treated with adjuvant chemotherapy. Interestingly however, it did demonstrate improved survival in both study arms compared with previous trials, perhaps due to improved surgical techniques and increased use of adjuvant radiotherapy.

One of the issues with trials of adjuvant treatment up until now is the blanket approach of a standard chemotherapy combination for all sarcomas. It is hoped that as more effective treatments are developed for specific sarcoma subtypes, these could be tested in the adjuvant setting with a greater chance of benefit.

Neo-adjuvant chemotherapy

The data to support neo-adjuvant chemotherapy for STS is mainly limited to retrospective series, and phase 2 trials [68]. However pre-operative chemotherapy, or chemoradiotherapy, may be considered for those patients with large high-grade tumours that are considered borderline resectable by the sarcoma MDT [69]. The age, and any comorbidity of the patient, together with the histology of the tumour need to be taken into account. There is a wide variation in chemosensitivity between different histological subtypes (Table 3). If the tumour is chemosensitive and adjacent to critical organs, then chemotherapy may potentially render the tumour suitable for conservative surgery whereas otherwise more radical surgery would be necessary. For example, for synovial sarcoma response rates of 28% [70] in a recent review of European trials, to over 50% in a single-centre series, have been reported [71, 72]. Similarly, myxoid liposarcomas are considered to be significantly more responsive than the majority of STS [72, 73], although radiotherapy alone may be sufficient [44]. With variable response of individual tumours to chemotherapy, the tumour should be monitored closely due to the risk of progression on treatment, in which case surgery can be expedited.

Key recommendations

1. Surgery is the standard treatment for most patients with localised STS.
2. For those patients with resectable disease, a wide excision through normal uninvolved tissues is the surgical procedure of choice.
3. Defining a "wide" margin is controversial, but with the addition of effective adjuvant therapy (e.g. radiotherapy) a tumour free margin (R0) may be adequate.
4. Where a wide excision is not possible due to anatomical constraints, a planned marginal or microscopically positive margin against a critical structure, plus radiotherapy, for intermediate and high grade tumours, may be an appropriate means of achieving tumour control while maintaining physical function.
5. Occasionally, amputation should be undertaken as the only surgical option to achieve adequate margins.
6. For patients with borderline resectable tumours, pre-operative treatment with chemotherapy and/or radiotherapy should be considered depending on histology.
7. Pre- or post-operative radiotherapy is recommended along with surgical resection of the primary tumour for the majority of patients with high-grade tumours,

and for selected patients with large or marginally excised, low-grade tumours.

8. The recommended dose for post-operative radiotherapy is 60–66 Gy.
9. Pre-operative radiotherapy is advantageous in terms of better long-term functional outcome, with equivalent rates of disease control, when compared with post-operative radiotherapy. There is however an increased risk of acute post-operative wound complications.
10. The recommended dose for pre-operative radiotherapy is 50 Gy.
11. Adjuvant chemotherapy is not routinely recommended but could be considered in situations where achieving local control is likely to be compromised, or the risk of metastatic disease is particularly high, with a lower threshold for its use in the more chemosensitive sarcoma subtypes.

Prognosis and follow-up for primary disease

Prognosis following primary treatment can be estimated by well-established nomograms based on grade, depth, size, and diagnosis as well as patient age [74]; some specialist centres have made online calculators available [75]. It appears that outcomes may have improved over the past 20 years [76], although NCIN data are less convincing [12]. Local recurrence is related to grade, margins of excision, and use of radiotherapy. Whilst most events will arise in the first 5 years following diagnosis late relapses may occur, according to this French Sarcoma Group study, particularly in retroperitoneal or very large STS [77].

In common with other tumour sites, there are few published data supporting specific follow-up protocols for STS patients, and there is an urgent need for research. Patients may be reassured by follow-up, and early detection of local relapse or pulmonary metastases may improve prognosis in some patients. Follow-up should be discussed with the patient and the rationale and limitations explained.

A survey on follow-up illustrated how varied the approach is at different centres, with no agreement on imaging, follow-up intervals, or total duration of follow-up [78]. Practices such as discharging patients treated for low-grade tumours at 5 years, when evidence suggests they recur late, require review. A recently reported trial comparing standard follow-up, with greater intensity follow-up and more imaging, failed to show any difference in outcome [79]. Furthermore, a recent retrospective study of follow-up for detection of local recurrence, demonstrated that most are detected clinically, casting doubt on the utility of routine surveillance MRI scanning [80].

It is recommended that standard follow-up consists of:

1. Clinical history,
2. Clinical examination to focus on local recurrence, with imaging using ultrasound or MRI where indicated by clinical suspicion, or if the primary site is difficult to examine clinically (e.g. pelvic tumours),
3. Chest X-ray, with subsequent CT used for investigating abnormalities.
4. Monitoring for late-effects of treatment.

In certain cases, this standard follow-up can be extended or adapted according to individual risk or local practice. If a patient were deemed unfit either for pulmonary metastasectomy or systemic treatment, then diagnosing metastases when the patient is asymptomatic has little purpose, so for example, the chest X-ray could be dispensed with; indeed, referral back to primary care might be most appropriate.

As per the ESMO guidelines [28], it is recommended that patients with intermediate/high grade tumours, which most commonly relapse within 2–3 years, should be followed every 3–4 months in the first 2–3 years, then twice a year up to the fifth year, and once a year thereafter for a minimum of 8–10 years. It is recommended that patients with low-grade tumours should be followed up every 4–6 months for 3–5 years, then annually thereafter, for at least 10 years. In low-grade sarcoma where the risk of local recurrence is the main reason for follow-up, suitably educated patients, with tumours resected from easily examined regions can be considered for discharge from formal follow-up, with an option to self-refer back to the service if any abnormality is identified.

A further value of follow-up is to monitor for adverse, late effects of treatment. Patients who have received radiotherapy may, for example be at risk of second malignancies or accelerated atherosclerosis in the radiotherapy field. Following chemotherapy there may be deterioration of renal function, and reduced fertility. In women, early menopause may require interventions for issues such as bone health. Investigations for late-effects of treatment should be considered such as full blood count, renal profile, hormone profile, and echocardiography. Patients treated in childhood for paediatric sarcomas may be handed on to adult services, and it is important that suitable follow-up continues. Survivorship is an area of cancer management on which there has been more focus in recent times. Physical disability is a major feature of the survivorship experience of patients treated for soft tissue sarcoma [81], and follow-up should support the patient in trying to minimise the impact of their treatment. Low activity levels put sarcoma survivors at further cardiovascular risk, which should be considered when constructing a follow-up regimen.

Key recommendations

1. It is recommended that patients with intermediate or high-grade sarcoma are followed up every 3–4 months for the first 2–3 years, then twice a year for up to 5 years, and annually thereafter for a total of 8–10 years.
2. Patients with low-grade sarcoma should be followed up every 4–6 months for 3–5 years, then annually.
3. Standard follow-up practice should consist of:

    a. Review of any new symptoms reported by the patient,
    b. Clinical examination to focus on local recurrence, with imaging follow-up where indicated by clinical suspicion,
    c. Routine chest X-ray to exclude pulmonary metastases,
    d. Monitoring for late-effects of treatment.
4. New models of follow-up warrant further investigation.

Prognosis and treatment of advanced disease

In almost all cases, the treatment intention for metastatic disease is palliation. Approximately 50% of patients with high-grade sarcoma develop distant metastases and eventually die of disseminated disease, with a median survival of approximately 12 months from diagnosis of metastases [82–84]. There are more recent data suggesting that this survival figure may be rather conservative with some improvement in outcomes over time to a median of around 18 months [85, 86].

The management of advanced disease is complex; the approach to palliative treatment depends to some extent on whether or not symptoms are present, and the potential toxicities of treatment. In order to achieve control of symptoms such as pain, or dyspnoea, it is often necessary to achieve some degree of tumour shrinkage. Clearly however in the absence of significant symptoms, disease stabilisation is an equally valid aim, to prolong good quality of life. A consistent finding in studies of soft tissue sarcoma is that overall survival, as in GIST [87, 88], is defined by absence of disease progression, not degree of response.

The treatment of advanced disease may involve a combination of various strategies, often used in a stepwise fashion, particularly for those patients with a prolonged disease course. The options will take into account the disease histology, distribution, volume, plus likely sensitivity to systemic treatment. Along with systemic treatment, surgery and radiotherapy may be considered to target symptomatic metastases or in an attempt to prolong the remission period. Other techniques, such as microwave or radiofrequency ablation, may have a role. Medications for pain or other complications such as bone metastases may be considered. Bisphosphonates or denosumab may be useful in reducing fracture risk or bone pain, based on data from other cancers, although radiotherapy or surgery may also be indicated. In some patients, metastases may behave fairly indolently and periods without active treatment are often appropriate. Other areas to focus on are good supportive care, potentially involving specialist palliative care services, in coordination with primary care.

For a number of patients, particularly those with poor performance status or significant comorbidities, standard supportive care with symptom control alone, is often the most appropriate option. Early involvement of community palliative care teams should be considered in all patients with advanced disease.

Systemic anti-cancer therapy (SACT) for sarcoma

The development of optimal treatment protocols is hampered by the rarity and heterogeneity of sarcoma. The incidence of many of the individual sub-types of soft tissue sarcoma is too small to permit large-scale prospective randomised controlled trials. Accordingly, data are gathered from a range of studies which include single-site and multisite phase 2 trials, retrospective case series, sub-analyses of trials for which a range of histological sub-types are included and, for the rarer sub-types, individual case reports.

A national algorithm produced by the NHS England Sarcoma Clinical Reference Group (CRG) has been proposed to guide the systemic treatment of sarcoma in England; a draft is under review. This is likely to be endorsed by the British Sarcoma Group and should therefore be used alongside this guideline.

The published response rates for chemotherapy in STS vary enormously, from 10 to 50% depending on the drugs used, patient selection, and histological subtype (Table 3). It has been established that good performance status, young age, and absence of liver metastases predict a good response to chemotherapy and improved survival time [83]. It is increasingly understood that response rate is only one measure of treatment efficacy with many of the newer therapies leading to a clinical benefit through disease stabilisation. A differential response to chemotherapy according to histological subtype has been noted, and as knowledge increases it is expected that it will become increasingly possible to individualise treatment. For example; synovial sarcoma, leiomyosarcoma and myxoid liposarcoma are recognised as having higher response rates to chemotherapy. Conversely, alveolar soft part sarcoma, extraskeletal myxoid chondrosarcoma and solitary fibrous tumour are generally regarded as insensitive to chemotherapy, and there are only occasional reports of responses in clear cell sarcoma. However, in the era of targeted therapies merely looking at response rates to standard chemotherapy is starting to be superseded by more specific relationships between histology and therapeutics.

Current and future trials are focusing on targeting new therapies more specifically, utilising genomic profiling, a better understanding of tumourogenesis, and the mechanisms of drug activity. In addition, a better understanding of the immune system has led to the development of new agents such as the immune-checkpoint inhibitors which are showing great promise in other tumour types. A significant challenge in sarcoma management is that given the rarity of the disease, and the numerous subtypes, it is difficult to perform large enough trials to gain the gold-standard, randomised evidence, that is preferred when developing treatment recommendations. It therefore means that, in contrast to other cancers, treatment may be given on the basis of phase II trials, small randomised phase III trials, and even for the very rare subtypes, case series. It is important therefore, where possible to develop multicentre clinical trials and recruit patients into them. Increasingly it is clear that rather than treating sarcoma as one condition, systemic treatment should be tailored to the histology or genetics of the individual subtype [89–91].

Selection of SACT

As noted above, in the UK the proposed national SACT Algorithm should guide systemic treatment of sarcoma. In addition, treatment of advanced disease may involve other modalities such as radiotherapy or surgery, and so multidisciplinary team review is important. Systemic treatment should ideally be guided by established protocols, preferably shared nationally. There is potential variability in dosing and administration, particularly in the use of agents such as ifosfamide, and care should be taken to use treatment protocols that maximise benefit whilst ensuring optimal management, and minimisation, of potential toxicities. Techniques such as the use of ambulatory infusions can be used to enhance patient convenience, and free-up valuable inpatient resources [92].

In a cost-constrained health system there is a challenge to fund all active agents, particularly in rare diseases. Some of the treatments considered may fall outside current standard NHS funding, and this will have to be taken into account when discussing the options with patients.

In most cases of metastatic soft-tissue sarcoma the choice of first-line chemotherapy will be between single-agent doxorubicin, or combined doxorubicin and ifosfamide. The latter combination has not been shown to improve survival, although delivers a higher response rate at a cost of increased toxicity [84, 93]. This may be an important consideration if the patient is symptomatic due to tumour size, or a reduction in tumour volume might facilitate other treatment options. The performance status of the patient and comorbidities will play an important role in treatment selection particularly in view of potential cardiac toxicity of doxorubicin and renal toxicity seen with ifosfamide. Treatment dose is also a consideration with higher doses shown to potentially improve efficacy [94].

Standard second-line treatment is ifosfamide, which is also used first-line where anthracyclines are contraindicated, for example in patients at high risk of cardiac complications, or patients pre-treated with anthracyclines. Clinical trials have indicated a dose–response relationship, and a dose of 9–10 g/m^2 is recommended [95]. In unselected sarcomas the response rate is in the region of 8%, although higher response rates have been observed with high-dose (>12 g/m^2) and continuous infusion ifosfamide regimens [28, 96, 97]. Responses may be higher in certain subtypes such as synovial sarcoma, whilst leiomyosarcoma is arguably less responsive and alternative agents may be more appropriate [98]. Ifosfamide is usually given over two to three days as an inpatient, but more recently infusional regimens administering treatment via a pump over two weeks have been utilised [99]. Treatment given in this way is usually better tolerated, but so far is most established in retroperitoneal liposarcoma, and is not yet a standard of care. Renal toxicity of ifosfamide can be significant and close monitoring is required. More rarely neurotoxicity is seen; more often in debilitated patients with low albumin levels.

An alternative second-line option is the combination of gemcitabine and docetaxel. The evidence for gemcitabine and docetaxel is greatest for uterine leiomyosarcoma. However, subsequent studies have demonstrated activity in soft tissue leiomyosarcoma and other tumour types including undifferentiated pleomorphic sarcoma [100, 101]. The GeDDiS trial in which this regimen was compared with doxorubicin in the first-line setting for all sarcoma subtypes, showed it to be non-inferior, but more toxic [102].

Trabectedin, licensed as second-line treatment for all soft tissue sarcomas, was approved by the European Medicines Agency (EMA) on the basis of a randomised trial comparing two different treatment regimens in patients with predominantly leiomyosarcoma and liposarcoma [103]. A recently completed trial in patients with leiomyosarcoma and liposarcoma comparing trabectedin with dacarbazine demonstrated significant superiority for trabectedin resulting in the drug being licensed in the USA [104]. Other tumours, such as synovial sarcoma, and particularly myxoid liposarcoma, may also be sensitive. It appears to be active in sarcomas related to chromosomal translocations [105, 106]. When assessing clinical benefit, it should be noted that a period of disease stabilisation may often occur for some time before response is seen. Trabectedin is currently approved by NICE and treatment can continue until disease progression. It exhibits less haematological toxicity than doxorubicin or ifosfamide but prescribers need to be aware of rare, but potentially serious rhabdomyolysis, and hepatic toxicity.

Beyond doxorubicin, ifosfamide, gemcitabine/docetaxel, and trabectedin, there are no standard chemotherapy options and decisions will be made based on patient fitness, and a balance of likely benefit and toxicities. Consideration of previous clinical benefit from chemotherapy, and more chemo-sensitive subtypes of sarcoma may support further treatment. Below are a number of options included in the proposed Sarcoma Chemotherapy Algorithm:

- Liposomal doxorubicin (Caelyx): could be considered at any line for vascular intimal sarcomas, angiosarcomas [107], cardiac sarcomas, and patients who have received previous anthracyclines, or have impaired cardiac function [108]. It can be combined with ifosfamide. It also has activity in fibromatosis (see "Desmoid-type fibromatosis" section).
- Paclitaxel: may be used as first or second line treatment of angiosarcomas [109].
- Oral cyclophosphamide and prednisolone: a low toxicity combination suitable for elderly patients unlikely to tolerate more toxic chemotherapy [110].
- Pazopanib: has data supporting its use in metastatic STS (not liposarcoma). A placebo controlled study demonstrated a 3-month improvement in progression-free survival in STS, with no particular superiority in any individual subtype. [111, 112]. Of note, activity was also seen in refractory desmoplastic small round cell tumour. This class of VEGFR inhibitor (including sunitinib) has also demonstrated activity in haemangiopericytoma/malignant solitary fibrous tumour [113], which is relatively resistant to chemotherapy (although see dacarbazine below), and in refractory desmoid tumours/fibromatosis [114].
- Dacarbazine: in the past used more commonly in STS, it has come to be used primarily for leiomyosarcoma, either as a single agent or in combination with gemcitabine [115]. Activity has also been reported against solitary fibrous tumour/haemangiopericytoma [116].

It should be noted that not all active agents mentioned above are currently funded by the NHS in the UK for the indications described. Funding varies across the devolved nations and is regularly under review.

Although not yet appraised by NICE, or commonly used in the UK, in April 2016 eribulin received marketing authorisation from the European Medicines Agency (EMA) for the treatment of unresectable liposarcoma following prior anthracycline-containing therapy. This followed subgroup analysis of a study comparing eribulin with dacarbazine for previously treated patients with liposarcoma or leiomyosarcoma [117].

Management of local recurrence

Local recurrences are often accompanied by metastatic disease and patients should be carefully staged for this. In the absence of overt metastatic disease every attempt should be made to regain local control by further surgery with adequate margins (wide or radical), and radiotherapy (if not used previously). Amputation may be needed in selected cases.

Management of lung metastases

Following a diagnosis of lung metastases, the decision regarding metastasectomy should be based on disease-free period following primary surgery, absence of other metastases, number of lesions per lung, tumour growth, and evolution of disease (ESMO 2014) [28]. In the absence of a significant disease-free interval, the CT scan (or PET-CT scan to complete staging) should be repeated at a three-month interval, and if no new lesions have appeared and the disease is operable, surgery is usually recommended. The practice of performing an interval scan and delaying surgery can be difficult to explain to patients, but the risk of immediate surgery is that further multiple metastases appear rapidly, rendering the morbidity of surgery pointless, and potentially delaying systemic treatment. Other approaches can also be considered such as radiofrequency or microwave ablation. More recently stereotactic ablative radiotherapy (SABR), a very targeted form of high-dose hypo-fractionated radiotherapy, has become another potential option. While there are few data from prospective studies reporting survival of STS patients surgically treated for thoracic metastases, there are many long-term survivors (reported variously at 20–40% of all patients undergoing lung surgery) who have had the procedure [118]. It however remains unproven that metasectomy improves long term survival.

Management of extrapulmonary oligometastases

In most cases extrapulmonary metastases will be treated with systemic treatment. In selected cases surgery, radiofrequency ablation (RFA), cryotherapy, or radiotherapy may be considered for limited metastatic disease to prolong remission or reduce symptoms.

Electrochemotherapy (ECT) is an emerging technique that may be useful in the management of refractory dermal and subcutaneous metastases in certain tumour subtypes, for example angiosarcoma [119, 120].

Best Supportive Care

Supportive and palliative care should always be considered in cases of advanced disease. For many patients, systemic therapy, radiotherapy, or surgery may not be appropriate, and an early and honest conversation about treatment options, potential toxicities and quality of life is important. Involvement of a sarcoma specialist nurse to support the patient through the diagnostic process and discussion of options can be invaluable. Early referral to specialist palliative care services in the community should be considered. Although prognostication can be difficult and inexact, most patients and their families will want some idea of likely outcomes and this should be explored with them. Discussions concerning end-of-life care preferences may also be appropriate.

Key recommendations

1. Systemic treatments for the majority of advanced STS are not curative; median survival time is 12–18 months. Published chemotherapy response rates vary enormously; from 10–50% depending on the drugs used, patient selection, and tumour grade and histological subtype.
2. Treatment recommendations should be guided by patient performance status, disease extent, rate of progression, and potential sensitivity to treatment.
3. Standard first-line treatment is single-agent doxorubicin.
4. Ifosfamide may be used first-line if anthracyclines are contraindicated, and is a standard option for second-line therapy.
5. Although the combination of doxorubicin and ifosfamide has not been demonstrated to improve survival in comparison to single agent doxorubicin first-line, response rates are higher and it may be considered in individual patients where a response would improve symptoms or facilitate other treatment modalities.
6. Additional second-line agents include trabectedin, and the combination of gemcitabine and docetaxel. The choice of agent depends on histology, toxicity profile and patient preference.
7. A number of other agents such as dacarbazine and pazopanib can be considered beyond second-line depending on patient fitness and funding constraints.
8. Surgical resection of locally recurrent disease should be considered where feasible. For patients with oligometastatic disease surgery, radiotherapy, or ablative therapies (RFA, SABR, cryotherapy, microwave, ECT) should be considered in individual cases, although there are limited data on survival benefit.

Uterine and retroperitoneal sarcomas

Given the heterogeneity of sarcoma presentations many patients are managed in collaboration with other multidisciplinary teams. For England, reference should be made to the NICE Quality Standard, QS78 [41] and National Sarcoma Service Specification [8]. The MDTs should combine expertise to ensure optimal management taking into consideration tumour location, and subtype. Uterine sarcomas in the UK are usually managed primarily by regional gynaecological cancer MDTs, but strong links to the sarcoma MDT should be maintained to ensure that patients are appropriately registered, managed, considered for clinical trials, and referred for systemic treatment if required for metastatic disease. Retroperitoneal sarcomas should be managed by surgeons who are members of the sarcoma MDT although not every UK STS centre will have this service available and cross-referral may be required. Gastrointestinal stromal tumours (GIST) are usually managed in collaboration with GI surgical services, and are discussed in separate BSG guidance.

Uterine sarcomas

This group includes uterine leiomyosarcomas (LMS), endometrial stromal sarcomas (ESS), and undifferentiated endometrial sarcoma (UES). Standard treatment for all localised tumours is total abdominal hysterectomy (TAH), with some differences between the tumour types as described below [28]. Carcinosarcomas (malignant mixed Mullerian tumours, MMMT) are considered as epithelial tumours and, although new biological insights are emerging [25], should be treated accordingly, unless the sarcomatous element predominates.

Uterine leiomyosarcoma

Uterine LMS, a cancer of the smooth muscle, accounts for 35–40% of all uterine sarcomas; LMS can affect young women in their mid-20 s, although most patients will be aged 50–60 years. Pre-operatively it is difficult to differentiate benign leiomyomas from malignant LMS and so the surgical approach should be planned accordingly; laparoscopic morcellation is contraindicated for uterine sarcoma due to higher risk of recurrence and metastasis [121–123]. The risk of inadvertent morcellation of a uterine sarcoma increases significantly with age [124], and the US Food and Drug Administration (FDA) released a safety communication concerning the procedure in 2014 [125]. Standard surgical management for non-metastatic disease is total abdominal hysterectomy

(TAH) with, or without bilateral salpingo-oophorectomy (BSO). Retention of the ovaries can be considered in premenopausal women. Lymphadenectomy is not routinely required as incidence of lymph node involvement is less than 5%. Adjuvant pelvic radiotherapy for FIGO stage I and II disease is not recommended routinely [126]. Adjuvant pelvic radiotherapy may be considered for selected high-risk cases, for example after tumour rupture, where local relapse may be reduced, although a survival benefit has not been demonstrated [127]. Adjuvant chemotherapy is not routinely recommended but, as for other STS, can be considered in high-risk disease where there is some limited evidence [128, 129]. Chemotherapy for advanced/metastatic disease is as for STS at other sites, with doxorubicin as first line, although ifosfamide may be relatively less effective in LMS [98]. The combination of gemcitabine and docetaxel has demonstrated activity in the second-line setting in leiomyosarcoma. Trabectedin also seems to have useful activity [130].

Oestrogen receptor (ER) and progesterone receptor (PgR) expression is seen in approximately 50% of patients with uterine LMS. Some low and intermediate grade tumours may be sensitive to oestrogen deprivation, e.g. using aromatase inhibitors, although there are very few published data on this situation [131]. It is however reasonable to look for receptor expression in those with relatively indolent tumours for which treatment with an aromatase inhibitor or a progestogen might be appropriate. However, receptor expression does not guarantee response to oestrogen-lowering therapy, and use of oestrogen-lowering therapies should be used with particular caution in patients with high-grade rapidly progressing tumours.

Endometrial stromal sarcoma

Although a rare uterine malignancy, this is the second most prevalent uterine sarcoma, and a generally indolent disease with a long natural history. It was formally known as "low grade ESS", on the basis of a mitotic count of less than 10 mitoses per 10 high powered fields, but is now termed simply ESS, with no distinction between "grade" (mitotic count is now recognised not to be prognostic). There is a high incidence of oestrogen (ER) and progesterone receptor (PR) expression, and evidence that these tumours are hormonally responsive. Standard surgical treatment is therefore total abdominal hysterectomy, with bilateral salpingo-oophorectomy in pre-menopausal women; hormone replacement therapy (HRT) is contraindicated postoperatively [132]. A single small study has suggested that adjuvant progestogens after surgery may improve outcome; routine use is not indicated but could be considered in high risk patients [133]. The role of adjuvant pelvic radiotherapy is uncertain given

the paucity of published data. Recurrent or metastatic disease may respond to anti-oestrogen therapy, with an aromatase inhibitor, or a progestogen. Tamoxifen is not recommended since its action may be pro-oestrogenic in this setting. Chemotherapy is an option if hormonal therapy fails. Given the indolent nature of the condition, surgery for metastatic disease should be considered.

Undifferentiated endometrial sarcoma

This disease entity was formally known as "high grade ESS", but is now termed undifferentiated endometrial sarcoma (UES). It is a highly aggressive anaplastic malignancy that does not express ER and PR, with a poor prognosis even for early stage disease, and uncertain response to systemic treatment. Surgical management is TAH with or without BSO, and the option of adjuvant pelvic radiotherapy [126]. Follow-up protocols and systemic treatment for advanced disease parallel those for adult-type soft tissue sarcomas [28]. Oestrogen-lowering therapies are generally not used.

There has been some reported success with cisplatin in treating uterine sarcomas but figures are distorted because of high numbers of carcinosarcoma/malignant mixed Mullerian tumour (MMMT) patients in the only large trial. No subset analysis has been offered, therefore this drug is not recommended.

Key recommendations

1. Standard treatment for all localised uterine sarcomas is TAH. Lymphadenectomy is not routinely indicated.
2. Total abdominal hysterectomy, with bilateral oophorectomy is indicated for endometrial stromal sarcoma. These patients should not have post-operative hormone replacement therapy, and tamoxifen is contraindicated. Use of adjuvant oestrogen deprivation therapy is not routinely indicated.
3. Adjuvant pelvic radiotherapy has not been shown to improve survival, and is not routinely indicated in FIGO stage I and II disease. However, it could be considered for selected high-risk cases.
4. Advanced/metastatic LMS and undifferentiated endometrial sarcoma are treated systemically with the same drugs as STS at other sites. There is retrospective evidence that ifosfamide may be less effective in leiomyosarcoma.
5. Advanced/metastatic ESS can be treated with oestrogen deprivation therapy, with an aromatase inhibitor or progestogen.

Retroperitoneal sarcomas

Although the principles of management of retroperitoneal sarcomas are similar to those for extremity tumours, there are some important differences. Surgical management should be by surgeons specialised in the management of retroperitoneal sarcoma who are members of the sarcoma MDT.

Contrast-enhanced CT of the chest, abdomen, and pelvis is used for staging and may be a valuable aid to diagnosis of well-differentiated/dedifferentiated liposarcoma, and in helping to plan surgery. In most cases biopsy will be required to confirm the diagnosis, although may be considered unnecessary if the radiological appearances are typical for retroperitoneal liposarcoma. The biopsy track should be planned to reduce any risk of tumour seeding or complications.

Complete primary macroscopic resection gives the best chance of long-term cure and so the importance of surgical planning is paramount. Surgical margins are often more difficult to define as transcoelomic spread with distant contamination within the abdomen may occur. The goal of 'wide excision' is unlikely to be achievable in most cases. Here, the objective is "planned marginal excision", achieving appropriate margins that balance tumour control with minimising operative morbidity and retaining function. However, multi-visceral resection may be appropriate if necessary to permit "*en bloc*" resection of tumour, organs frequently sacrificed include kidney and spleen, and partial organ resection and vascular reconstructions may occasionally be required. Pre-operative assessment of contralateral renal function should be considered. Resection of tumour leaving behind gross macroscopic disease is of limited benefit and may cause unnecessary morbidity. Studies have shown the importance of adherence to proper surgical guidelines in the management of this disease, with a direct impact on survival [134].

The role of pre or post-operative radiotherapy is less well defined, and although it may be of value in individual patients, it is not considered routine. It is often difficult to define the radiation volume and dose is limited due to the risk of small bowel and other organ toxicity. In cases where it is possible to define "high-risk margins" postoperative radiotherapy to a dose of 45–50 in 1.8 Gy fractions should be considered [135]. In certain situations, for example, low pelvic tumours, higher doses of radiation may be given as normal tissue tolerance is greater. Pre-operative radiotherapy is increasingly becoming a preferred option as the treatment volume is smaller and better defined and the tumour acts as its own "spacer" [136]. Currently the STRASS trial, randomising patients with RPS to surgery or surgery plus pre-operative radiotherapy, is recruiting patients [137].

There is currently no evidence to support the use of neo-adjuvant or adjuvant chemotherapy in the management of retroperitoneal sarcomas, although as in other STS is may be considered in more sensitive histologies such as synovial sarcoma.

Routine CT scanning for asymptomatic relapse is controversial due to the relative ineffectiveness of salvage surgery. However, surgery for local recurrence may be considered in cases where there has been a reasonable disease-free interval (over 12 months) particularly in low-grade disease, or disease demonstrating a good response to systemic treatment.

Palliative chemotherapy should be considered for the same indications as limb sarcomas but well-differentiated/de-differentiated liposarcoma is relatively chemoresistant. Options usually include doxorubicin, infusional ifosfamide, or trabectedin any of which might be considered in the first-line setting. Early data suggests that eribulin may have a role [117] although it has not yet been appraised by NICE.

For many patients with advanced disease, aggressive therapy may not be appropriate, and good symptomatic management, and palliative care support are required.

Key recommendations

1. Standard treatment is *en bloc* complete resection with macroscopically clear margins.
2. Treatments for relapse are relatively ineffective; symptomatic management and palliative support of the patient should be offered where appropriate.

Borderline tumours

This group of soft tissue tumours are not considered typical sarcomas. They tend to remain localised, and whilst local recurrence following surgery can occur, they do not generally metastasise.

Lipomas and atypical lipomatous tumours

The most common differential diagnosis seen by the sarcoma MDT is that between lipoma and atypical lipomatous tumours (ALT), also known as well-differentiated liposarcoma (WDL). Essentially ALT and WDL are synonymous, as described in the WHO classification [10]. The latter term is more commonly applied to tumours in sites such as the retroperitoneum and mediastinum where surgical excision with a wide margin is unlikely, and therefore local recurrence almost inevitable; progressive dedifferentiation with each recurrence is often observed (see "Retroperitoneal sarcomas" section). ALT/WDL of the extremities is distinct from lipoma in that it has the propensity for local recurrence, however dedifferentiation into a more aggressive disease is extremely rare.

Differentiating lipoma and ALT radiologically is not reliable but certain features seen on MRI can be helpful such as size and intratumoural septation [138, 139]. Histological and cytogenetic analysis of tumour allows confirmation of diagnosis, although small pre-operative biopsies may be misleading [140, 141].

Surgical resection is the usual treatment for ALT, and the prognosis is usually excellent [142–144]. However, particularly in older patients, if surgery is likely to be morbid, or the patient has significant comorbidities then radiological surveillance can be considered. In larger tumours, or those where clear margins are difficult to achieve, adjuvant radiotherapy may very occasionally be considered [145].

Key recommendations
1. Atypical lipomatous tumours and well differentiated liposarcomas are essentially synonymous. Surgical resection with a clear margin is standard treatment and prognosis is usually excellent.

Desmoid-type fibromatosis
Fibromatosis is a benign, clonal tumour, which although sometimes locally aggressive (even fatal on occasion), has not been reported to metastasise. Although usually sporadic it may occur in association with familial adenomatous polyposis (FAP), or Gardner syndrome caused by germline mutations in the APC gene. Cases of sporadic fibromatosis usually harbour mutations in CTNNB1, the gene for beta-catenin.

Diagnostic investigation follows the standard process for STS. The disease may occur at the sites of previous scars and can be related to hormonal changes in women, for example surrounding pregnancy. Pregnancy related fibromatosis tends to have a good outcome and progression during pregnancy is common but manageable. It is not generally a contraindication to future pregnancy [146]. In cases where a link to FAP may be more likely (e.g. young male, abdominal disease, CTNNB1 mutation negative) then it is important to exclude a family history of bowel cancer, and it may be appropriate to screen for germline APC mutations or consider investigations such as colonoscopy.

The natural history of the disease is unpredictable and optimal management is not fully established, although a European Consensus has recently been published and provides useful guidance [147]. Following initial diagnosis, the tumour may continue to grow, stabilise, or even regress spontaneously [148]. The 5-year progression-free survival may be up to 50%. In addition, surgical resection even with apparently clear margins results in relatively high rates of local recurrence in up to half of cases. Increasingly, watchful waiting is considered the standard first-line option. Interval review with MRI scans is recommended and treatment initiated on significant disease progression.

Standard treatment in cases where surveillance is not selected, or progression has occurred, is complete surgical excision. Unlike the general situation with STS the finding of positive margins is less closely related to risk of relapse; long-term remission may be seen despite positive margins, and conversely relapse is not uncommon in clearly resected disease. The exception to this is fibromatosis arising in the abdominal wall of young females, where relapse rates following surgery are low; in one series under 10% at 5 years [149].

Radiotherapy may be effective treatment for patients with unresectable tumours or may be given as adjuvant therapy following surgery for recurrent disease, especially if further surgery would result in significant morbidity and functional deficit. A dose of 50–56 Gy is usually employed [150, 151].

Systemic treatment is recommended in selected cases with unresectable disease and is another option following progression during watchful waiting. Hormone therapies such as tamoxifen have been reported to be beneficial but, because of the unpredictable natural history of this disease, their true value remains unproven due to the lack of appropriate clinical trial data. Nonsteroidal anti-inflammatory drugs (NSAIDs) have been reported to improve the response to tamoxifen. The precise choice of NSAID is uncertain and although selective COX2 inhibitors have been used, the evidence that they are superior is lacking. NSAIDS have an impact on the beta-catenin signalling pathway.

Chemotherapy is usually reserved for patients with significant symptoms who have failed to respond to more benign interventions such as the use of NSAIDs and tamoxifen. Weekly administration of methotrexate and vinblastine or vinorelbine has reasonable activity and is generally well tolerated. More recently pegylated liposomal doxorubicin (Caelyx) has been reported to have significant activity with acceptable toxicity, and currently is considered treatment of choice by many investigators [152]. Targeted therapies such as imatinib and pazopanib have also been investigated, and both objective remissions and disease stabilisation have been reported [114, 153, 154]. Another option for limb tumours is isolated limb perfusion (ILP) with tumour necrosis factor alpha and melphalan.

Key recommendations
1. A diagnosis of familial adenomatous polyposis (FAP) needs to be considered in some fibromatosis cases.
2. Initial standard treatment for fibromatosis is watchful waiting.
3. Systemic treatments such as tamoxifen, NSAIDS or chemotherapy may be used definitively, or neoadjuvantly before surgery.
4. Surgery can be considered if progression occurs.
5. Radiotherapy can be used in the adjuvant setting, or for inoperable disease.

Peripheral nerve tumours

Peripheral nerve tumours are often referred to, or managed by, sarcoma services, and include several subtypes including neurofibromas, schwannomas, and malignant peripheral nerve sheath tumours (MPNST). They may be benign or malignant, and sporadic, or in a significant minority of cases, associated with the genetic conditions neurofibromatosis type 1 or 2. The latter conditions will not be discussed in detail in this guideline but overall management is likely to be in collaboration with regional genetic medicine or specialist neurofibromatosis services.

Presentation may be as a mass, but pain, or focal neurological symptoms may also be a feature. Rapid progression of symptoms or signs may indicate a higher likelihood of malignancy [155]. Ultrasound, and in particular MRI scans can suggest the diagnosis with features such as direct continuity with a nerve or location along a typical nerve distribution [156]. PET-CT may assist in differentiating benign from malignant tumours [32, 33].

In many cases a biopsy will be appropriate to confirm the diagnosis. However, this can be painful for the patient, or rarely associated with neurological injury. Therefore, some lesions with characteristic appearances on MRI scan may be considered for excision biopsy under general anaesthetic. Expert pathological assessment will be required as nerve tumours can be diagnostically challenging [157].

Treatment is usually surgical resection, although in some cases management can be conservative with observation alone. Surveillance may be considered in asymptomatic schwannomas, or other neural tumours with no malignant features [158]. For benign tumours resection with minimisation of residual neurological deficit is the aim, and in many cases can result in improvement in peripheral nerve function [159]. Malignant peripheral nerve sheath tumours (MPNST) are aggressive tumours with a relatively poor prognosis [160]. In general management is as for malignant soft-tissue sarcomas as described earlier in this guideline.

Key recommendations

1. In the presence of a peripheral nerve tumour a diagnosis of neurofibromatosis should be considered.
2. Treatment is usually surgical excision although surveillance can be considered in clearly benign cases.
3. Malignant peripheral nerve sheath tumours are aggressive malignancies treated in the same way as other high-grade sarcomas.

Dermatofibrosarcoma protuberans (DFSP)

DFSP is a rare neoplasm of the dermal layer of the skin. This is best considered a borderline malignancy that rarely metastasises but is locally aggressive, may produce significant morbidity, and occasionally proves fatal. Local recurrence following surgery is common and wide excision is essential except in situations where wide excision would result in significant morbidity or functional loss. In this instance, Mohs surgery can provide an alternative to initial wide excision and may be delivered through collaboration with a skin cancer MDT.

Radiotherapy should be considered for inoperable disease, and can result in durable remissions. Adjuvant radiotherapy may also be used if the margins are involved and re-excision is not possible [161].

Systemic treatment is appropriate in selected cases with unresectable or metastatic disease. DFSP is driven by a t(17;22) translocation that results in over-expression of platelet derived growth factor beta (PDGFβ). Therefore, the PDGFβ receptor may be inhibited by imatinib, which is licensed for the treatment of unresectable DFSP [162].The challenges with using targeted agents such as this for benign conditions are balancing the toxicity with benefit, the financial cost, and also defining an appropriate end-point, and optimum duration of treatment.

Key recommendations

1. Treatment of DFSP is wide surgical excision, Mohs surgery may be appropriate in selected cases to reduce functional loss.
2. Adjuvant radiotherapy may be considered if surgical resection is incomplete, and re-excision not possible.
3. Imatinib may provide an option for neo-adjuvant treatment in borderline resectable disease, or effective palliation for patients with unresectable DFSP.

Atypical fibroxanthoma (AFX)

AFX is a low-grade cutaneous spindle cell tumour considered a superficial variant of malignant fibrous histiocytoma (MFH). It may be mistaken clinically or histologically for other spindle cell tumours. It is usually cured by surgical excision although local recurrence is fairly common and metastases are seen in less than 1% of cases. AFX greater than 2 cm in size and with other adverse pathological features may be regarded as pleomorphic dermal sarcomas [163]; they appear to share similar oncogene expression and mutations [164].

Key recommendation

1. AFX is usually cured by surgical excision, although larger tumours with adverse pathological features may be regarded as pleomorphic dermal sarcomas.

Tenosynovial giant cell tumour (TGCT)

This family of benign neoplastic conditions presents as two forms, reclassified by the WHO in 2013 [10], as either a single nodule (localised, L-TGCT; previously GCT of tendon sheath or nodular tenosynovitis) or multiple nodules (diffuse-type, D-TGCT; previously pigmented villonodular synovitis, PVNS), generally affecting the synovium in young adults. It is usually treated by surgery alone but local relapses can occur [165]. Arthroscopic or open synovectomy may have a role in diffuse disease. In nodular intraarticular disease, the aim is complete removal, and doing this without morsellisation may be advantageous.

The role of radiotherapy is unclear but may be considered for symptomatic residual or recurrent disease when further excision is not possible. Yttrium synovectomy has been used in the adjuvant setting in diffuse intraarticular disease [166]. Due to a translocation involving the macrophage colony-stimulating factor (*M-CSF* or *CSF1*) gene seen in a proportion of cells, imatinib has demonstrated activity in its treatment [167]. It may be considered for a 3-month course prior to surgery in borderline operable cases, although will require approval for funding. Its use in the palliative setting can also be considered although the treatment endpoints and duration are not clear [168]. New targeted drugs are currently undergoing investigation.

Key recommendation
1. Tenosynovial giant cell tumour is generally treated by surgery alone, although rarely radiotherapy or imatinib may have a role.

Inflammatory myofibroblastic tumour (IMT)
IMT is a neoplasm consisting of a spindle-cell proliferation and inflammatory infiltrate. It most commonly occurs in the lungs but can be seen in the abdomen and pelvis or maxillofacial region. Treatment is usually surgical excision although local recurrences and very rarely metastases can occur. It may respond to steroids, but in around 50% of cases rearrangements in the *ALK* locus on chromosome 2p23 have been detected. In these cases, treatment with an *ALK* targeting drug such as crizotinib may be useful [169] and is currently being investigated in the CREATE study [170].

Key recommendation
1. Inflammatory myofibroblastic tumour is treated with surgery, although may be responsive to steroids or crizotinib.

Summary of key recommendations
Clinical presentation
1. Any patient with a soft tissue mass that is increasing in size, or has a size more than 5 cm, whether or not it is painful, should either be referred for an urgent ultrasound scan, or referred directly to a sarcoma diagnostic centre.

2. If the ultrasound scan does not definitely confirm benign pathology, then the patient should be referred for further investigation on an urgent suspected cancer referral pathway.
3. Any retroperitoneal or intra-abdominal mass with imaging appearances suggestive of a soft tissue sarcoma should be referred to a specialist centre before biopsy or surgical treatment.

Referral and assessment
1. All patients with a suspected STS should be managed by a specialist Sarcoma MDT as specified in the NICE guidance.
2. Ultrasound scan by a musculoskeletal radiologist should be considered as the first-line investigation, and may be supplemented by ultrasound-guided core biopsy.
3. Magnetic resonance imaging and core needle biopsy are recommended prior to definitive surgery.
4. Imaging of the thorax by CT scan for lung metastases should be done prior to radical treatment. Further staging may be considered depending on subtype and location of the sarcoma.

Management of localised disease
1. Surgery is the standard treatment for most patients with localised STS.
2. For those patients with resectable disease, a wide excision through normal uninvolved tissues is the surgical procedure of choice.
3. Defining a "wide" margin is controversial, but with the addition of effective adjuvant therapy (e.g. radiotherapy) a tumour free margin (R0) may be adequate.
4. Where a wide excision is not possible due to anatomical constraints, a planned marginal or microscopically positive margin against a critical structure, plus radiotherapy, for intermediate and high grade tumours, may be an appropriate means of achieving tumour control while maintaining physical function.
5. Occasionally amputation should be undertaken as the only surgical option to achieve adequate margins.
6. For patients with borderline resectable tumours, preoperative treatment with chemotherapy and/or radiotherapy should be considered depending on histology.
7. Pre- or post-operative radiotherapy is recommended along with surgical resection of the primary tumour for the majority of patients with high-grade tumours, and for selected patients with large or marginally excised, low-grade tumours.
8. The recommended dose for post-operative radiotherapy is 60–66 Gy.

9. Pre-operative radiotherapy is advantageous in terms of better long-term functional outcome, with equivalent rates of disease control, when compared with post-operative radiotherapy. There is however an increased risk of acute post-operative wound complications.

10. The recommended dose for pre-operative radiotherapy is 50 Gy.

11. Adjuvant chemotherapy is not routinely recommended but could be considered in situations where achieving local control is likely to be compromised, or the risk of metastatic disease is particularly high, with a lower threshold for its use in the more chemosensitive sarcoma subtypes.

Prognosis and follow-up for primary disease

1. It is recommended that patients with intermediate or high-grade sarcoma are followed up every 3–4 months for the first 2–3 years, then twice a year for up to 5 years, and annually thereafter for a total of 8–10 years.

2. Patients with low-grade sarcoma should be followed up every 4–6 months for 3–5 years, then annually.

3. Standard follow-up practice should consist of:

   a. Review of any new symptoms reported by the patient,
   b. Clinical examination to focus on local recurrence, with imaging follow-up where indicated by clinical suspicion,
   c. Routine chest X-ray to exclude pulmonary metastases.
   d. Monitoring for late-effects of treatment.

4. New models of follow-up warrant further investigation.

Prognosis and treatment of advanced disease

1. Systemic treatments (SACT) for the majority of advanced STS are not curative; median survival time is 12–18 months. Published chemotherapy response rates vary enormously; from 10–50% depending on the drugs used, patient selection, and tumour grade and histological subtype.

2. Treatment recommendations should be guided by patient performance status, disease extent, rate of progression, and potential sensitivity to treatment.

3. Standard first-line treatment is single-agent doxorubicin.

4. Ifosfamide may be used first-line if anthracyclines are contraindicated, and is a standard option for second-line therapy.

5. Although the combination of doxorubicin and ifosfamide has not been demonstrated to improve survival in comparison to single agent doxorubicin first-line, response rates are higher and it may be considered in individual patients where a response would improve symptoms or facilitate other treatment modalities.

6. Additional second-line agents include trabectedin, and the combination of gemcitabine and docetaxel. The choice of agent depends on histology, toxicity profile and patient preference.

7. A number of other agents such as dacarbazine and pazopanib can be considered beyond second-line depending on patient fitness and funding constraints.

8. Surgical resection of locally recurrent disease should be considered where feasible. For patients with oligometastatic disease surgery, radiotherapy, or ablative therapies (RFA, SABR, cryotherapy, microwave, ECT) should be considered in individual cases, although there are limited data on survival benefit.

Uterine sarcomas

1. Standard treatment for all localised uterine sarcomas is TAH. Lymphadenectomy is not routinely indicated.

2. Total abdominal hysterectomy with bilateral oophorectomy is indicated for endometrial stromal sarcoma. These patients should not have post-operative hormone replacement therapy and tamoxifen is contraindicated. Use of adjuvant oestrogen deprivation therapy is not routinely indicated.

3. Adjuvant pelvic radiotherapy has not been shown to improve survival, and is not routinely indicated in FIGO stage I and II disease. However, it could be considered for selected high-risk cases.

4. Advanced/metastatic LMS and undifferentiated endometrial sarcoma are treated systemically with the same drugs as STS at other sites. There is retrospective evidence that ifosfamide may be less effective in leiomyosarcoma.

5. Advanced/metastatic ESS can be treated with oestrogen deprivation therapy, with an aromatase inhibitor or progestogen.

Retroperitoneal sarcomas

1. Standard treatment is en bloc complete resection with macroscopically clear margins.

2. Treatments for relapse are relatively ineffective; symptomatic management and palliative support of the patient should be offered where appropriate.

Lipomas and atypical lipomatous tumours

1. Atypical lipomatous tumours and well differentiated liposarcomas are essentially synonymous. Surgical resection with a clear margin is standard treatment and prognosis is usually excellent.

Desmoid-type fibromatosis

1. A diagnosis of familial adenomatous polyposis (FAP) needs to be considered in some fibromatosis cases.
2. Initial standard treatment for fibromatosis is watchful waiting.
3. Systemic treatments such as tamoxifen, NSAIDS or chemotherapy may be used definitively, or neoadajuvantly before surgery for fibromatosis.
4. Surgery can be considered for fibromatosis if progression occurs.
5. Radiotherapy can be used in the adjuvant setting, or for inoperable fibromatosis.

Peripheral nerve tumours

1. In the presence of a peripheral nerve tumour a diagnosis of neurofibromatosis should be considered.
2. Treatment of peripheral nerve tumours is usually surgical excision although surveillance can be considered in clearly benign cases.
3. Malignant peripheral nerve sheath tumours are aggressive malignancies treated in the same way as other high-grade sarcomas.

Dermatofibrosarcoma protruberans (DFSP)

1. Treatment of DFSP is wide surgical excision, Mohs surgery may be appropriate in selected cases to reduce functional loss.
2. Adjuvant radiotherapy may be considered for DFSP if surgical resection is incomplete, and re-excision not possible.
3. Imatinib may provide an option for neo-adjuvant treatment in borderline resectable disease, or effective palliation for patients with unresectable DFSP.

Atypical fibroxanthoma (AFX)

1. AFX is usually cured by surgical excision, although larger tumours with adverse pathological features may be regarded as pleomorphic dermal sarcomas.

Tenosynovial giant cell tumour (TGCT)

1. Tenosynovial giant cell tumour is generally treated by surgery alone, although rarely radiotherapy or imatinib may have a role.

Inflammatory myofibroblastic tumour (IMT)

1. Inflammatory myofibroblastic tumour is treated with surgery, although may be responsive to steroids or crizotinib.

Authors' contributions

All authors contributed to the content of the manuscript. AD updated the guideline text from the previous version published in 2010, with amendments and suggestions from the co-authors. British Sarcoma Group members were circulated the draft text for review, with those acknowledged below providing significant contributions. All authors read and approved the final manuscript.

Author details

[1] Bristol Cancer Institute, Bristol Haematology & Oncology Centre, University Hospitals Bristol NHS Trust, Bristol BS2 8ED, UK. [2] Department of Oncology, University College London Hospital NHS Trust, London NW1 2PG, UK. [3] The Newcastle upon Tyne Hospitals NHS Foundation Trust, Freeman Hospital, Newcastle-upon-Tyne NE7 7DN, UK. [4] Royal Orthopaedic Hospital NHS Trust, Birmingham B31 2AP, UK. [5] Royal Marsden NHS Foundation Trust, London SW3 6JJ, UK.

Acknowledgements

The authors would like to thank the following for valuable review, suggestions and amendments: Dr. David Peake (Consultant Clinical Oncologist, Queen Elizabeth Hospital, Birmingham), Mr. Andrew Hayes (Consultant Sarcoma Surgeon, Royal Marsden, London), Dr. Rick Haas (Consultant Radiation Oncologist, Netherlands Cancer Institute, Amsterdam), The East Midlands Sarcoma Service (Nottingham University Hospital & Leicester Royal Infirmary), Dr. CR Chandrasekar (Consultant Orthopaedic Oncology Surgeon, Royal Liverpool University Hospital), Mr. Paul Wilson (Consultant Plastic and Sarcoma Surgeon, North Bristol NHS Trust), Dr. Robin Jones (Medical Oncologist, Royal Marsden Hospital), Sam Hackett (Sarcoma Specialist Nurse, Sarcoma UK, London).

Adam Dangoor, Beatrice Seddon, Craig Gerrand, Robert Grimer, Jeremy Whelan and Ian Judson—On Behalf of the British Sarcoma Group.

Competing interests

AD has received support for conference attendance from Pharma Mar and served as an advisory board member for Lilly and GSK. BS also received support for conference attendance from Pharma Mar and served as an advisory board member for Lilly, Ariad, Clinigen, and Novartis. IJ has received honoraria for advisory boards or speaking engagements from GSK, Amgen, Clinigen, Nektar, Ariad, and Lilly. The remaining authors declare that they have no competing interests.

References

1. Grimer R, Judson I, Peake D, Seddon B. Guidelines for the management of soft tissue sarcomas. Sarcoma. 2010;2010:506182. doi:10.1155/2010/506182.
2. NICE Guidance on Cancer Studies, Improving Outcomes for People with Sarcoma, National Institute for Health and Clinical Excellence, CSG9 March 2006. https://www.nice.org.uk/guidance/csg9. Accessed 25 Jan 2016.
3. National Institute for Health and Clinical Excellence (NICE), Improving outcomes with children and young people with cancer, CSG7 August 2005. https://www.nice.org.uk/guidance/csg7. Accessed 25 Jan 2016.
4. Gerrand C, Athanasou N, Brennan B, Grimer R, Judson I, Morland B, Peake D, Seddon B, Whelan J, British Sarcoma Group. UK guidelines for the management of bone sarcomas. Clin Sarcoma Res. 2016;6:7.
5. Euro Ewing 2012. International Randomised Trial for the Treatment of newly diagnosed Ewing's sarcoma family of tumours. http://public. ukcrn.org.uk/Search/StudyDetail.aspx?StudyID=13804. Accessed 20 Jan 2016.
6. A protocol for non metastatic rhabdomyosarcoma (European Paediatric Soft Tissue Sarcoma Study Group STS 2006 04 RMS 2005 (ESSG1). http://public.ukcrn.org.uk/search/StudyDetail.aspx?StudyID=2247. Accessed 20 Jan 2016.
7. Sarcoma Specialist Centres. http://sarcoma.org.uk/health-professionals/sarcoma-specialist-centres. Accessed 22 Apr 2016.
8. National Health Service (NHS) Highly Specialised Commissioning Group. http://www.england.nhs.uk/commissioning/spec-services/npc-crg/group-b/b12/. Accessed 22 Apr 2016.
9. Jemal A, Siegel R, Ward E, Murray T, Xu J, Thun MJ. Cancer statistics, 2007. CA Cancer J Clin. 2007;57(1):43–66.
10. Fletcher CDM, Sundaram M, Rydholm A, Coindre JM, Singer S. WHO classification of tumours of soft tissue and bone. 4th edn, Lyon: IARC Press; 2013. https://www.iarc.fr/en/publications/pdfs-online/pat-gen/bb5/bb5-classifsofttissue.pdf. Accessed 26 Apr 2016.

11. Soft tissue sarcoma statistics. Cancer Research UK. http://www.cancer-researchuk.org/health-professional/cancer-statistics/statistics-by-cancer-type/soft-tissue-sarcoma#heading-Zero. Accessed 22 Apr 2016.

12. NCIN Bone and soft tissue sarcomas. UK incidence and survival. 1996–2010. 2nd edn; 2013. p. 1–17. http://www.ncin.org.uk/cancer_type_and_topic_specific_work/cancer_type_specific_work/sarcomas/. Accessed 22 Apr 2016.

13. Albritton K, Bleyer WA. The management of cancer in the older adolescent. Eur J Cancer. 2003;39(18):2584–99.

14. Birch JM, Alston RD, Quinn M, Kelsey AM. Incidence of malignant disease by morphological type, in young persons aged 12–24 years in England, 1979–1997. Eur J Cancer. 2003;39(18):2622–31.

15. Geraci M, Birch JM, Alston RD, Moran A, Eden TOB. Cancer mortality in 13 to 29-year-olds in England and Wales, 1981–2005. Br J Cancer. 2007;97(11):1588–94.

16. Ferrari A, Bleyer A. Participation of adolescents with cancer in clinical trials. Cancer Treat Rev. 2007;33(7):603–8.

17. Coindre J-M, Terrier P, Guillou L, et al. Predictive value of grade for metastasis development in the main histologic types of adult soft tissue sarcomas: a study of 1240 patients from the French Federation of Cancer Centers sarcoma group. Cancer. 2001;91(10):1914–26.

18. Kotilingam D, Lev DC, Lazar AJF, Pollock RE. Staging soft tissue sarcoma: evolution and change. CA Cancer J Clin. 2006;56(5):282–91.

19. Rasmussen SA, Friedman JM. NF1 gene and neurofibromatosis 1. Am J Epidemiol. 2000;151(1):33–40.

20. Uusitalo E, Rantanen M, Kallionpää RA, Pöyhönen M, Leppävirta J, Ylä-Outinen H, Riccardi VM, Pukkala E, Pitkäniemi J, Peltonen S, Peltonen J. Distinctive Cancer Associations in patients with neurofibromatosis type 1. J Clin Oncol. 2016;34(17):1978–86.

21. Chen CS, Suthers G, Carroll J, Rudzki Z, Muecke J. Sarcoma and familial retinoblastoma. Clin Exp Ophthal. 2003;31(5):392–6.

22. Bell DW, Varley JM, Szydlo TE, Kanf DH, Wahrer DC, Shannon KE, Lubratovich M, Verselis SJ, Isselbacher KJ, Fraumeni JF, et al. Heterozygous germ line hCHK2 mutations in Li-Fraumeni syndrome. Science. 1999;286(5449):2528–31.

23. Johnson CJD, Pynsent PB, Grimer RJ. Clinical features of soft tissue sarcomas. Ann R Coll Surg Engl. 2001;83(3):203–5.

24. Suspected cancer: recognition and referral NICE Guidance NG12 June 2015, Section 1.11. http://www.nice.org.uk/guidance/ng12. Accessed 25 Jan 2016.

25. Matsuo K, Takazawa Y, Ross MS, Elishaev E, Podzielinski I, Yunokawa M, Sheridan TB, Bush SH, Klobocista MM, Blake EA, et al. Significance of histologic pattern of carcinoma and sarcoma components on survival outcomes of uterine carcinosarcoma. Ann Oncol. 2016;27(7):1257–66.

26. King DM, Hackbarth DA, Kilian CM, Guillermo F, Carrera MD. Soft-tissue sarcoma metastases identified on abdomen and pelvis CT imaging. Clin Orthop Relat Res. 2009;467(11):2832–44.

27. Seo SW, Kwon JW, Jang SW, Jang SP, Park YS. Feasibility of whole-body MRI for detecting metastatic myxoid liposarcoma: a case series. Orthopedics. 2011;34(11):e748–54.

28. ESMO/European Sarcoma Networking Group. Soft tissue and visceral sarcomas: ESMO clinical practice guidelines for diagnosis, treatment and follow-up. Ann Oncol. 2014;25(Suppl 3):iii102–12.

29. Roberge D, Vakilian S, Alabed YZ, Turcotte RE, Freeman CR, Hickeson M. FDG PET/CT in initial staging of adult soft-tissue sarcoma. Sarcoma. 2012;2012:960194. doi:10.1155/2012/960194.

30. Federico SM, Spunt SL, Krasin MJ, Billup CA, Wu J, Shulkin B, Mandell G, McCarville MB. Comparison of PET-CT and conventional imaging in staging pediatric rhabdomyosarcoma. Pediatr Blood Cancer. 2013;60(7):1128–34.

31. Quartuccio N, Fox J, Kuk D, Wexler LH, Baldari S, Cistaro A, Schöder H. Pediatric bone sarcoma: diagnostic performance of ^{18}F-FDG PET/CT versus conventional imaging for initial staging and follow-up. AJR Am J Roentgenol. 2015;204(1):153–60.

32. Ferner RE, Golding JF, Smith M, Calonje E, Jan W, Sanjayanathan V, O'Doherty M. [18F] 2-fluoro-2-deoxy-D-glucose as a diagnostic tool for neurofibromatosis 1 (NF 1) associated malignant peripheral nerve sheath tumours (MPNSTs): a long-term clinical study. Ann Oncol. 2008;19(2):390–4.

33. Brahmi M, Thiesse P, Ranchere D, Mognetti T, Pinson S, Renard C, Decouvelaere AV, Blay JY, Combemale P. Diagnostic accuracy of PET/CT-guided percutaneous biopsies for malignant peripheral nerve sheath tumors in neurofibromatosis type 1 patients. PLoS ONE. 2015;10(10):e0138386. doi:10.1371/journal.pone.0138386 (eCollection 2015).

34. Guillou L, Coindre JM, Bonichon F, Nguyen BB, Terrier P, Collin F, Vilain MO, Mandard AM, Le Doussal V, Leroux A, et al. Comparative study of the National Cancer Institute and French Federation of Cancer Centers Sarcoma Group grading systems in a population of 410 adult patients with soft tissue sarcoma. J Clin Oncol. 1997;15:350–62.

35. Trojani M, Contesso G, Coindre JM, Rouesse J, Bui NB, de Mascarel A, Goussot JF, David M, Bonichon F, Lagarde C. Soft-tissue sarcomas of adults; study of pathological prognostic variables and definition of a histopathological grading system. Int J Cancer. 1984;33:37–42.

36. Lin X, Davion S, Bertsch EC, Omar I, Nayar R, Laskin WB. FNCLCC grading of soft tissue sarcomas on needle core biopsies using surrogate markers. Hum Pathol. 2016;56:147.

37. Royal College of Pathologists Dataset for cancer histopathology reports on soft tissue sarcomas (3rd edition). https://www.rcpath.org/resourceLibrary/g094_datasetsofttissue_mar14-pdf.html. Accessed 20 Jan 2016.

38. Enneking WF, Spanier SS, Goodman M. A system for the surgical staging of musculoskeletal sarcoma. Clinical Orthop Rel Res. 1980;153:106–20.

39. O'Donnell PW, Griffin AM, Eward WC, Sternheim A, Catton CN, Chung PW, O'Sullivan B, Ferguson PC, Wunder JS. The effect of the setting of a positive surgical margin in soft tissue sarcoma. Cancer. 2014;120(18):2866–75. doi:10.1002/cncr.28793.

40. Edge SB, Byrd DR, Compton CC, et al. (editors). AJCC Cancer Staging Manual. 7th ed. New York: Springer; 2010, p. 291–298.

41. Sarcoma NICE quality standard QS78 January 2015. https://www.nice.org.uk/guidance/qs78. Accessed 25 Jan 2016.

42. Gerrand CH, Wunder JS, Kandel RA, O'Sullivan B, Catton CN, Bell RS, Griffin AM, Davis AM. Classification of positive margins after resection of soft-tissue sarcoma of the limb predicts the risk of local recurrence. J Bone Joint Surg Br. 2001;83(8):1149–55.

43. Alektiar KM, Velasco J, Zelefsky MJ, Woodruff JM, Lewis JJ, Brennan MF. Adjuvant radiotherapy for margin-positive high-grade soft tissue sarcoma of the extremity. Int J Radiat Oncol Biol Phys. 2000;48(4):1051–8.

44. Le Grange F, Cassoni AM, Seddon BM. Tumour volume changes following pre-operative radiotherapy in borderline resectable limb and trunk soft tissue sarcoma. Eur J Surg Oncol. 2014;40(4):394–401.

45. Roberge D, Skamene T, Nahal A, Turcotte RE, Powell T, Freeman C. Radiological and pathological response following pre-operative radiotherapy for soft-tissue sarcoma. Radiother Oncol. 2010;97(3):404–7. doi:10.1016/j.radonc.2010.10.007.

46. Eggermont AMM, de Wilt JHW, ten Hagen TLM. Current uses of isolated limb perfusion in the clinic and a model system for new strategies. Lancet Oncol. 2003;4(7):429–37.

47. Smith HG, Cartwright J, Wilkinson MJ, Strauss DC, Thomas JM, Hayes AJ. Isolated limb perfusion with melphalan and tumour necrosis factor α for in-transit melanoma and soft tissue sarcoma. Ann Surg Oncol. 2015;2015(22 Suppl 3):356–61. doi:10.1245/s10434-015-4856-x.

48. Yang JC, Chang AE, Baker AR, Sindelar WF, Danforth DN, Topalian SL, DeLaney T, Glatstein E, Steinberg SM, Merino MJ, et al. Randomized prospective study of the benefit of adjuvant radiation therapy in the treatment of soft tissue sarcomas of the extremity. J Clin Oncol. 1998;16(1):197–203.

49. Haas RL, Delaney TF, O'Sullivan B, Keus RB, Le Pechoux C, Olmi P, Poulson JP, Seddon B, Wang D. Radiotherapy for management of extremity soft tissue sarcomas: why, when, and where? Int J Radiat Oncol Biol Phys. 2012;84(3):572–80.

50. O'Sullivan B, Griffin AM, Dickie CI, Sharpe MB, Chung PWM, Catton CN, Ferguson PC, Wunder JS, Deheshi BM, White LM, et al. Phase 2 study of preoperative image-guided intensity-modulated radiation therapy to reduce wound and combined modality morbidities in lower extremity soft tissue sarcoma. Cancer. 2013;119(10):1878–84.

51. NHS Health Research Authority. IMRiS - A phase II study of intensity modulated 2158 radiotherapy (IMRT) in primary bone and soft tissue sarcoma. http://www.hra.nhs.uk/news/research-summaries/imris/. Accessed 4 Aug 2016

52. University of Birmingham. Vortex Trial - A randomised phase III trial concerning post-operative radiotherapy given to adult patients with

extremity soft tissue sarcoma. http://www.birmingham.ac.uk/research/activity/mds/trials/crctu/trials/vortex/index.aspx. Accessed 4 Aug 2016

53. O'Sullivan B, Davis AM, Turcotte R, Bell R, Catton C, Chabot P, Wunder J, Kandel R, Goddard K, Sadura A, et al. Preoperative versus postoperative radiotherapy in soft-tissue sarcoma of the limbs: a randomised trial. Lancet. 2002;359(9325):2235–41.

54. Davis AM, O'Sullivan B, Turcotte R, Bell R, Catton C, Chabot P, Wunder J, Hammond A, Bwenk V, Kandel R, et al. Late radiation morbidity following randomization to preoperative versus postoperative radiotherapy in extremity soft tissue sarcoma. Radiother Oncol. 2005;75(1):48–53.

55. Al Yami A, Griffin AM, Ferguson PC, Catton CN, Chung PW, Bell RS, Wunder JS, O'Sullivan B. Positive surgical margins in soft tissue sarcoma treated with preoperative radiation: is a positive boost necessary? Int J Radiat Biol Phys. 2010;77(4):1191–7.

56. Kepka L, DeLaney TF, Suit HD, Goldberg SI. Results of radiation therapy for unresected soft-tissue sarcomas. Int J Radiat Oncol Biol Phys. 2005;63(3):852–9.

57. Slater JD, McNeese MD, Peters LJ. Radiation therapy for unresectable soft tissue sarcomas. Int J Radiat Oncol Biol Phys. 1986;12(10):1729–34.

58. Smith KB, Indelicato DJ, Knapik JA, Morris C, Kirwan J, Zlotecki RA, Scarborough MT, Gibbs CP, Marcus RB. Definitive radiotherapy for unresectable pediatric and young adult nonrhabdomyosarcoma soft tissue sarcoma. Pediatr Blood Cancer. 2011;57(2):247–51. doi:10.1002/pbc.22961.

59. Andrä C, Rauch J, Li M, Ganswindt U, Belka C, Saleh-Ebrahimi L, Ballhausen H, Nachbichler SB, Roeder F. Excellent local control and survival after postoperative or definitive radiation therapy for sarcomas of the head and neck. Radiat Oncol. 2015;10(10):140. doi:10.1186/s13014-015-0449-x.

60. DeLaney TF, Haas RL. Innovative radiotherapy of sarcoma: Proton beam radiation. Eur J Cancer. 2016;62:112–23. doi:10.1016/j.ejca.2016.04.015.

61. NHS Commissioning, Highly Specialised services. Proton Beam Therapy. https://www.england.nhs.uk/commissioning/spec-services/highly-spec-services/pbt/. Accessed 05 Aug 2016.

62. Salgado R, van Marck E. Soft tissue tumours: the surgical pathologist's perspective, In: De Schepper AM, Vanhoemacker F, Gielen J, Parizel PM, editors. Imaging of soft tissue tumors, 3rd edn. Berlin: Springer; 2006. p. 107–16.

63. Tierney JF. Adjuvant chemotherapy for localised resectable soft-tissue sarcoma of adults: meta-analysis of individual data. Lancet. 1997;350(9092):1647–54.

64. Sarcoma Meta-analysis Collaboration (SMAC). Adjuvant chemotherapy for localised resectable soft tissue sarcoma in adults. Cochrane Database Syst Rev. 2000;(4):CD001419. doi:10.1002/14651858.CD001419.

65. Pervaiz N, Colterjohn N, Farrokhyar F, Tozer R, Figueredo A, Ghert M. A systematic meta-analysis of randomized controlled trials of adjuvant chemotherapy for localized resectable soft-tissue sarcoma. Cancer. 2008;113(3):573–81.

66. Frustaci S, Gherlinzoni F, De Paoli A, Bonetti M, Azzarelli A, Comandone A, Olmi P, Buonadonna A, Pignatti G, Barberi E, et al. Adjuvant chemotherapy for adult soft tissue sarcomas of the extremities and girdles: results of the Italian randomized cooperative trial. J Clin Oncol. 2001;19(5):1238–47.

67. Woll PJ, Reichardt P, Le Cesne A, Bonvalot S, Azzarelli A, Hoekstra HJ, Leahy M, Van Coevorden F, Verweij J, Hogendoorn PC, et al. EORTC Soft Tissue and Bone Sarcoma Group and the NCIC Clinical Trials Group Sarcoma Disease Site Committee. Adjuvant chemotherapy with doxorubicin, ifosfamide, and lenograstim for resected soft-tissue sarcoma (EORTC 62931): a multicentre randomised controlled trial. Lancet Oncol. 2012;13(10):1045–54. doi:10.1016/S1470-2045(12)70346-7.

68. Nathenson MJ, Sausville E. Looking for answers: the current status of neoadjuvant treatment in localized soft tissue sarcomas. Cancer Chemother Pharmacol. 2016;78(5):895–919 (**Review**).

69. Palassini E, Ferrari S, Verderio P, De Paoli A, Martin-Broto J, Quagliuolo V, Comandone A, Sangalli C, Palmerini E, Lopez-Pousa A, et al. Feasibility of preoperative chemotherapy with or without radiation therapy in localized soft tissue sarcomas of limbs and superficial trunk in the Italian sarcoma Group/Grupo Espanol de Investigacion en Sarcomas Randomized Clinical Trial: three versus five cycles of full-dose epirubicin plus ifosfamide. J Clin Oncol. 2015;33(31):3628–34.

70. Vlenterie M, Litière S, Rizzo E, Marrèaud S, Judson I, Gelderblom H, Le Cesne A, Wardelmann E, Messiois C, Gronchi A, van der Graaf WT. Outcome of chemotherapy in advanced synovial sarcoma patients: review of 15 clinical trials form the European Organisation for Research and Treatment of Cancer Soft Tissue and Bone Sarcoma Group; setting a new landmark for studies in this entity. Eur J Cancer. 2016;58:62–72.

71. Spurrell EL, Fisher C, Thomas JM, Judson IR. Prognostic factors in advanced synovial sarcoma: an analysis of 104 patients treated at the Royal Marsden Hospital. Annal Oncol. 2005;16(3):437–44.

72. Karavasilis V, Seddon B, Ashley S, Al-Muderis O, Fisher C, Judson I. Significant clinical benefit of first-line palliative chemotherapy in advanced soft-tissue sarcoma. J Clin Oncol. 2006;24:18S (**abstract 9520**).

73. Jones RL, Fisher C, Al-Muderis O, Judson IR. Differential sensitivity of liposarcoma subtypes to chemotherapy. Eur J Cancer. 2005;41(18):2853–60.

74. Grobmyer SR, Brennan MF. Predictive variables detailing the recurrence rate of soft tissue sarcomas. Curr Opin Oncol. 2003;15(4):319–26.

75. Memorial Sloan Kettering Cancer Centre. Prediction tools. https://www.mskcc.org/cancer-care/types/soft-tissue-sarcoma/prediction-tools. Accessed 27 Apr 2016.

76. Jacobs AJ, Michels R, Stein J, Levin AS. Improvement in overall survival from extremity soft tissue sarcoma over twenty years. Sarcoma. 2015;2015(2015):279601. doi:10.1155/2015/279601.

77. Toulmonde M, Le Cesne A, Mendiboure J, Blay JY, Piperno-Neumann S, Chevreau C, Delcambre C, Penel N, Terrier P, Ranchère-Vince D, et al. Long-term recurrence of soft tissue sarcomas: prognostic factors and implications for prolonged follow-up. Cancer. 2014;120(19):3003–6. doi:10.1002/cncr.28836.

78. Gerrand CH, Billingham LJ, Woll PJ, Grimer RJ. Follow up after primary treatment of soft tissue sarcoma: a survey of current practice in the United Kingdom. Sarcoma. 2007;. doi:10.1155/2007/34128.

79. Puri A, Gulia A, Hawaldar R, Ranganathan P, Badwe RA. Does intensity of surveillance affect survival after surgery for sarcomas? Results of a randomized noninferiority trial. Clin Orthop Relat Res. 2014;472(5):1568–75. doi:10.1007/s11999-013-3385-9.

80. Rothermundt C, Whelan JS, Dileo P, Strauss SJ, Coleman J, Briggs TW, Haile SR, Seddon BM. What is the role of routine follow-up for localised limb soft tissue sarcomas? A retrospective analysis of 174 patients. Br J Cancer. 2014;110(10):2420–6. doi:10.1038/bjc.2014.200.

81. Kwong TN, Furtado S, Gerrand C. What do we know about survivorship after treatment for extremity sarcoma? A systematic review. Eur J Surg Oncol. 2014;40(9):1109–24. doi:10.1016/j.ejso.2014.03.015.

82. Blay J-Y, van Glabbeke M, Verweij J, van Oosterom AT, Le Cesne A, Oosterhuis JW, Judson I, Nielsen OS. Advanced soft-tissue sarcoma: a disease that is potentially curable for a subset of patients treated with chemotherapy. Eur J Cancer. 2003;39(1):64–9.

83. van Glabbeke M, van Oosterom AT, Oosterhuis JW, Mouridsen H, Crowther D, Somers R, Verweij J, Santoro A, Buesa J, Tursz T. Prognostic factors for the outcome of chemotherapy in advanced soft tissue sarcoma: an analysis of 2185 patients treated with anthracyclines containing first-line regimens—an European organization for research and treatment of cancer soft tissue and bone sarcoma group study. J Clin Oncol. 1999;17(1):150–7.

84. Judson I, Verweij J, Gelderblom H, Hartmann JT, Schoffski P, Blay JY, Kerst JM, Sufliarsky J, Whelan J, Hohenberger P, et al. Doxorubicin alone versus intensified doxorubicin plus ifosfamide for first-line treatment of advanced metastatic soft-tissue sarcoma: a randomised controlled phase 3 trial. Lancet Oncol. 2014;15(4):415–23. doi:10.1016/S1470-2045(14)70063-4.

85. SEER Stat Fact Sheets: Soft Tissue including Heart Cancer. http://SEER.cacner.gov/statfaccts/html/soft.html. Accessed 25 Jan 2016.

86. Harris SJ, Maruzzo M, Thway K, Al-Muderis O, Jones RL, Miah A, Benson C, Judson IR. Metastatic soft tissue sarcoma, an analysis of systemic therapy and impact on survival. J Clin Oncol. 2015;33:(suppl; abstr 10545). http://meetinglibrary.asco.org/content/145234-156. Accessed 25 Jan 2016.

87. Grünwald V, Litière S, Young R, Messiou C, Lia M, Wardelmann E, van der Graaf W, Gronchi A, Judson I, EORTC STBSG. Absence of progression, not extent of tumour shrinkage, defines prognosis in soft-tissue

sarcoma—an analysis of the EORTC 62012 study of the EORTC STBSG. Eur J Cancer. 2016;17(64):44–51.

88. Le Cesne A, Van Glabbeke M, Verweij J, Casali PG, Findlay M, Reichardt P, Issels R, Judson I, Schoffski P, Leyvraz S, et al. Absence of progression as assessed by response evaluation criteria in solid tumors predicts survival in advanced GI stromal tumors treated with imatinib mesylate: the intergroup EORTC-ISG-AGITG phase III trial. J Clin Oncol. 2009;27(24):3969–74. doi:10.1200/JCO.2008.21.3330.

89. Radaelli S, Stacchiotti S, Casali PG, Gronchi A. Emerging therapies for adult soft tissue sarcoma. Expert Rev Anticancer Ther. 2014;14(6):689–704.

90. Linch M, Miah AB, Thway K, Judson IR, Benson C. Systemic treatment of soft-tissue sarcoma—gold standard and novel therapies. Nat Rev Clin Oncol. 2014;11(4):187–202.

91. Noujaim J, Thway K, Sheri A, Keller C, Jones RL. Histology-driven therapy: the importance of diagnostic accuracy in guiding systemic therapy of soft tissue tumors. Int J Surg Pathol. 2016;24(1):5–15. doi:10.1177/1066896915606971.

92. Newston C, Ingram B. Ambulatory chemotherapy for teenagers and young adults. Br J Nurs. 2014;23(4):S36–S38–42.

93. Bramwell VH, Anderson D, Charette ML. Doxorubicin-based chemotherapy for the palliative treatment of adult patients with locally advanced or metastatic soft tissue sarcoma. Cochrane Database of Systematic Reviews, No 3, Article ID CD003293; 2003.

94. O'Bryan RM, Baker LH, Gottlieb JE, Rivkin SE, Balcerzak SP, Grumet GN, Salmon SE, Moon TE, Hoogstraten B. Dose response evaluation of adriamycin in human neoplasia. Cancer. 1977;39:1940–8.

95. van Oosterom AT, Mouridsen HT, Nielsen OS, Dombernowsky P, Krzemieniecki K, Judson I, Svancarova L, Spooner D, Hermans C, Van Glabbeke M, et al. Results of randomised studies of the EORTC Soft Tissue and Bone Sarcoma Group (STBSG) with two different ifosfamide regimens in first- and second-line chemotherapy in advanced soft tissue sarcoma patients. Eur J Cancer. 2002;38(18):2397–406.

96. Palumbo R, Palmeri S, Antimi M, et al. Phase II study of continuous-infusion high-dose ifosfamide in advanced and/or metastatic pretreated soft tissue sarcomas. Ann Oncol. 1997;8(11):1159–62.

97. Buesa JM, López-Pousa A, Martín J, Anton A, Garcia del Muro J, Bellmunt J, Arranz F, Valenti V, Escudero P, Menendez D, et al. Phase II trial of first-line high-dose ifosfamide in advanced soft tissue sarcomas of the adult: a study of the Spanish Group for Research on Sarcomas (GEIS). Ann Oncol. 1998;9(8):871–6.

98. Sleijfer S, Ouali M, van Glabbeke M, Krarup-Hansen A, Rodenhuis S, Le Cesne A, Hogendoorn PC, Verweij J, Blay JY. Prognostic and predictive factors for outcome to first-line ifosfamide-containing chemotherapy for adult patients with advanced soft tissue sarcomas: an exploratory, retrospective analysis on large series from the European Organization for Research and Treatment of Cancer-Soft Tissue and Bone Sarcoma Group (EORTC-STBSG). Eur J Cancer. 2010;46(1):72–83. doi:10.1016/j.ejca.2009.09.022.

99. Martin-Liberal J, Alam S, Constantinidou A, Fisher C, Khabra K, Messiou C, Olmos D, Mitchell S, Al-Muderis O, Miah A, et al. Clinical activity and tolerability of a 14-day infusional Ifosfamide schedule in soft-tissue sarcoma. Sarcoma. 2013;2013(1):868973–6.

100. Leu KM, Ostruszka LJ, Shewach D, Zalupski M, Sondak V, Biermann JS, Lee JS, Couwlier C, Palazzolo K, Baker LH. Laboratory and clinical evidence of synergistic cytotoxicity of sequential treatment with gemcitabine followed by docetaxel in the treatment of sarcoma. J Clin Oncol. 2004;22(9):1706–12.

101. Maki RG, Wathen JK, Patel SR, Priebat DA, Okuno SH, Samuels B, Fanucchi M, Harmon DC, Schuetze SM, Reinke D, et al. Randomized phase II study of gemcitabine and docetaxel compared with gemcitabine alone in patients with metastatic soft tissue sarcomas: results of sarcoma alliance for research through collaboration study. J Clin Oncol. 2007;25(19):2755–63.

102. Seddon BM, Whelan J, Strauss, SJ, Leahy MG, Woll, PJ, Cowie F, Rothermundt CA, Wood Z, Forsyth S, Khan I, Nash S, Patterson P, Beare S. GeDDiS: A prospective randomised controlled phase III trial of gemcitabine and docetaxel compared with doxorubicin as first-line treatment in previously untreated advanced unresectable or metastatic soft tissue sarcomas (EudraCT 2009-014907-29). J Clin Oncol. 2015;33(suppl; abstr 10500)

103. Demetri GD, Chawla SP, von Mehren M, Ritch P, Baker LH, Blay JY, Hande KR, Keohan ML, Samuels BL, Schuetze S, et al. Efficacy and safety of trabectedin in patients with advanced or metastatic liposarcoma or leiomyosarcoma after failure of prior anthracyclines and ifosfamide: results of a randomized phase II study of two different schedules. J Clin Oncol. 2009;27(25):4188–96.

104. Demetri GD, von Mehren M, Jones RL, Hensley ML, Schuetze SM, Staddon A, Milhem M, Elias A, Ganjoo K, Tawbi H, et al. Efficacy and safety of trabectedin or dacarbazine for metastatic liposarcoma or leiomyosarcoma after failure of conventional chemotherapy: results of a phase III randomized multicentre clinical trial. J Clin Oncol. 2016;34(80):786–93.

105. Le Cesne A, Cresta S, Maki RG, Blay JY, Verweij J, Poveda A, Casali PG, Balaña C, Schöffski P, Grosso F, et al. A retrospective analysis of antitumour activity with trabectedin in translocation-related sarcomas. Eur J Cancer. 2012;48(16):3036–44. doi:10.1016/j.ejca.2012.05.012.

106. Kawai A, Araki N, Sugiura H, Ueda T, Yonemoto T, Takahashi M, Morioka H, Hiraga H, Hiruma T, Kunisada T, et al. Trabectedin monotherapy after standard chemotherapy versus best supportive care in patients with advanced, translocation-related sarcoma: a randomised, open-label, phase 2 study. Lancet Oncol. 2015;16(4):406–16. doi:10.1016/S1470-2045(15)70098-7.

107. Skubitz KM, Haddad PA. Paclitaxel and pegylated-liposomal doxorubicin are both active in angiosarcoma. Cancer. 2005;104(2):361–6.

108. Barrett-Lee PJ, Dixon JM, Farrell C, Jones A, Leonard R, Murray N, Palmieri C, Plummer CJ, Stanley A, Verrill MW. Expert opinion on the use of anthracyclines in patients with advanced breast cancer at cardiac risk. Ann Oncol. 2009;20(5):816–27. doi:10.1093/annonc/mdn728.

109. Schlemmer M, Reichardt P, Verweij J, Hartmann JT, Judson I, Thyss A, Hogendoorn PC, Marreaud S, Van Glabbeke M, Blay JY. Paclitaxel in patients with advanced angiosarcomas of soft tissue: a retrospective study of the EORTC soft tissue and bone sarcoma group. Eur J Cancer. 2008;44:2433–6.

110. Mir O, Domont J, Cioffi A, Bonvalot S, Boulet B, Le Pechoux C, Terrier P, Spielmann M, Le Cesne A. Feasibility of metronomic oral cyclophosphamide plus prednisolone in elderly patients with inoperable or metastatic soft tissue sarcoma. Eur J Cancer. 2011;47(4):515–9.

111. van der Graaf WT, Blay JY, Chawla SP, Kim DW, Bui-Nguyen B, Casali PG, Schoffski P, Aglietta M, Staddon AP, Beppu Y, et al. Pazopanib for metastatic soft-tissue sarcoma (PALETTE): a randomised, double-blind, placebo-controlled phase 3 trial. Lancet. 2012;379(9829):1879–86. doi:10.1016/S0140-6736(12)60651-5.

112. Frezza AM, Benson C, Judson IR, Litiere S, Marreaud S, Sleijfer S, Blay JY, Dewji R, Fisher C, van der Graaf W et al. Pazopanib in advanced desmoplastic small round cell tumours: a multi-institutional experience. Clin Sarcoma Res. 2014;4:7. doi: 10.1186/2045-3329-4-7. eCollection 2014. http://clinicalsarcomaresearch.biomedcentral.com/articles/10.1186/2045-3329-4-7. Accessed 25 Jan 2016.

113. Maruzzo M, Martin-Liberal J, Messiou C, Miah A, Thway K, Alvarado R, Judson I, Benson C. Pazopanib as first line treatment for solitary fibrous tumours: the Royal Marsden Hospital experience. Clin Sarcoma Res. 2015;5:5. doi:10.1186/s13569-015-0022-2.

114. Martin-Liberal J, Benson C, McCarty H, Thway K, Messiou C, Judson I. Pazopanib is an active treatment in desmoid tumour/aggressive fibromatosis. Clin Sarcoma Res. 2013;3(1):13. doi:10.1186/2045-3329-3-13.

115. Garcia del Muro X, Lopez-Pousa A, Maurel J, Martin J, Martinez-Trufero J, Casado A, Gomez-Espana A, Fra J, Cruz J, Poveda A, et al. Randomized phase II study comparing gemcitabine plus dacarbazine versus dacarbazine alone in patients with previously treated soft tissue sarcoma: a Spanish Group for Research on sarcoma study. J Clin Oncol. 2011;29(18):2528–33. doi:10.1200/JCO.2010.33.6107.

116. Stacchiotti S, Tortoreto M, Bozzi F, Tamborini E, Morosi C, Messina A, Libertini M, Palassini E, Cominetti D, Negri T, et al. Dacarbazine in solitary fibrousa tumour: a case series analysis and preclinical evidence vis-à-vis temozolomide and antiangiogenics. Clin Cancer Res. 2013;19(18):5192–201. doi:10.1158/1078-0432.CCR-13-0776.

117. Schöffski P, Chawla S, Maki RG, Italiano A, Gelderblom H, Choy E, Grignani G, Camargo V, Bauer S, Rha SY, et al. Eribulin versus dacarbazine in previously treated patients with advanced liposarcoma or leiomyosarcoma: a randomized, open-label, multicentre, phase 3 trial. Lancet. 2016;387(10028):1629–37.

118. Treasure T, Fiorentino F, Scarci M, Moller H, Utley M. Pulmonary metasta-sectomy for sarcoma: a systematic review of reported outcomes in the context of Thames Cancer Registry data. BMJ Open. 2012;2:e001736. doi:10.1136/bmjopen-2012-001736.

119. Campana LG, Bianchi G, Mocellin S, Valpione S, Campanacci L, Brunello A, Donati D, Sieni E, Rossi CR. Electrochemotherapy treatment of locally advanced and metastatic soft tissue sarcomas: results of a non-com-parative phase II study. World J Surg. 2014;38(4):813–22. doi:10.1007/s00268-013-2321-1.

120. Benevento R, Carafa F, Di Nardo D, Pellino G, Letizia A, Taddeo M, Gambardella A, Canonico S, Santoriello A. Angiosarcoma of the breast: a new therapeutic approach? Int J Surg Case Rep. 2015;2015(13):30–2. doi:10.1016/j.ijscr.2015.06.004.

121. Park J-Y, Park S-K, Kim D-Y, Kim J-H, Kim Y-M, Kim Y-T, Nam J-H. The impact of tumour morcellation during surgery on the prognosis of patients with apparently early uterine leiomyosarcoma. Gynecologic Oncol. 2011;122(2):255–9.

122. Morice P, Rodriguez A, Rey A, Pautier P, Attallah D, Genestie C, Pomel C, Lhomme C, Haie-Meder C, Duvillard P, et al. Prognostic value of initial surgical procedure for patients with uterine sarcoma: analysis of 123 patients. Eur J Gynecologic Oncol. 2003;24(3–4):237–40.

123. Seidman MA, Oduyebo T, Muto MG, Crum CP, Nucci MR, Quade BJ. Peritoneal dissemination complicating morcellation of uterine mesen-chymal neoplasms. PLoS ONE. 2012;7(11):e50058.

124. Brohl AS, Li L, Andikyan V, Običan SG, Cioffi A, Hao K, Dudley JT, Ascher-Walsh C, Kasarskis A, Maki RG. Age-stratified risk of unexpected uterine sarcoma following surgery for presumed benign leiomyoma. Oncol. 2015;20:433–9.

125. US FDA UPDATED Laparoscopic Uterine Power Morcellation in Hyster-ectomy and Myomectomy: FDA Safety Communication. http://www.fda.gov/MedicalDevices/Safety/AlertsandNotices/ucm424443.htm. Accessed 31 Jul 2016.

126. Seddon BM, Davda R. Uterine sarcomas—recent progress and future challenges. Eur J Radiol. 2011;78(1):30–40.

127. Reed NS, Mangioni C, Malmström H, Scarfone G, Poveda A, Pecorelli S, Tateo S, Franchi M, Jobsen JJ, Coens C, Teodorovic I, et al. European Organisation for Research and Treatment of Cancer Gynaecological Cancer Group. Phase III randomised study to evaluate the role of adju-vant pelvic radiotherapy in the treatment of uterine sarcomas stages I and II: an European Organisation for Research and Treatment of Cancer Gynaecological Cancer Group Study (protocol 55874). Eur J Cancer. 2008;44:808–18.

128. Hensley ML, Ishill N, Soslow R, Larkin J, Abu-Rustum N, Sabbatini P, Konner J, Tew W, Spriggs D, Aghajanian CA. Adjuvant gemcitabine plus docetaxel for completely resected stages I–IV high grade uterine leiomyosarcoma: results of a prospective study. Gynecol Oncol. 2009;112:563–7.

129. Hensley ML, Wathen JK, Maki RG, Araujo DM, Sutton G, Priebat DA, George S, Soslow RA, Baker LH. Adjuvant therapy for high-grade, uterus- limited leiomyosarcoma: results of a phase 2 trial (SARC 005). Cancer. 2013;119:1555–61.

130. Samuels BL, Chawla S, Patel S, von Mehren M, Hamm J, Kaiser PE, Schuetze S, Li J, Aymes A, Demetri GD. Clinical outcomes and safety with trabectedin therapy in patients with advanced soft tissue sarco-mas following failure of prior chemotherapy: results of a worldwide expanded access program study. Ann Oncol. 2013;24(6):1703–9. doi:10.1093/annonc/mds659.

131. George S, Feng Y, Manola J, Nucci MR, Butrynski JE, Morgan JA, Ramaiya N, Quek R, Penson RT, Wagner AJ, et al. Phase 2 trial of aromatase inhibi-tion with letrozole in patients with uterine leiomyosarcomas expressing estrogen and/or progesterone receptors. Cancer. 2014;120(5):738–43.

132. Amant F, Floquet A, Friedlander M, Kristensen G, Mahner S, Nam EJ, Powell MA, Ray-Coquard I, Siddiqui N, Sykes P, Westermann AM, Sed-don B. Gynecologic Cancer InterGroup (GCIG) consensus review for endometrial stromal sarcoma. Int J Gynecol Cancer. 2014;24(9 Suppl 3):S67–72.

133. Chu MC, Mor G, Lim C, Zheng W, Parkash V, Schwartz PE. Low-grade endometrial stromal sarcoma: hormonal aspects. Gyn Oncol. 2003;90(1):170–6.

134. Toulmonde M, Bonvalot S, Meeus P, Stoeckle E, Riou O, Isambert N, Bompas E, Jafari M, Delcambre-Lair C, Saada E, et al. Retroperitonel

sarcomas: patterns of care at diagnosis, prognostic factors and focus on main histological subtypes: a multicentre analysis of the French Sarcoma Group. Ann Oncol. 2014;25(3):735–42.

135. Feng M, Murphy J, Griffith KA, Baker LH, Sondak VK, Lucas DR, McGinn CJ, Ray ME. Long term outcomes after radiotherapy for retrop-eritoneal and deep truncal sarcoma. Int J Radiat Oncol Biol Phys. 2007;69(1):103–10.

136. Tzeng CW, Fiveash JB, Popple RA, Amoletti JP, Russo SM, Urist MM, Bland KI, Heslin MJ. Preoperative radiation therapy with selective dose escalation to the margin at risk for retroperitoneal sarcoma. Cancer. 2006;107(2):371–9.

137. A phase III randomized study of preoperative radiotherapy plus surgery versus surgery alone for patients with Retroperitoneal sarcomas (RPS)—STRASS. http://www.eortc.be/protoc/details.asp?protocol=62092. Accessed 26 Apr 2016.

138. Nagano S, Yokouchi M, Setoguchi T, Ishidou Y, Sasaki H, Shimada H, Komiya S. Differentiation of lipoma and atypical lipomatous tumor by a scoring system: implication of increased vascularity on pathogenesis of liposarcoma. BMC Musculoskelet Disord. 2015;16:36. doi:10.1186/s12891-015-0491-8.

139. Fisher SB, Baxter KJ, Staley CA 3rd, Fisher KE, Monson DK, Murray DR, Oskouei SV, Weiss SW, Kooby DA, Maithel SK, Delman KA. The General Surgeon's quandary: atypical lipomatous tumor vs lipoma, who needs a surgical oncologist? J Am Coll Surg. 2013;217(5):881–8. doi:10.1016/j.jamcollsurg.2013.06.003.

140. Nishio J. Contributions of cytogenetics and molecular cytogenet-ics to the diagnosis of adipocytic tumors. J Biomed Biotechnol. 2011;2011:524067. doi:10.1155/2011/524067.

141. Dei Tos AP. Liposarcomas: diagnostic pitfalls and new insights. Histopa-thology. 2014;64(1):38–52. doi:10.1111/his.12311.

142. Sommerville SM, Patton JT, Luscombe JC, Mangham DC, Grimer RJ. Clinical outcomes of deep atypical lipomas (well-differentiated lipoma-like liposarcomas) of the extremities. ANZ J Surg. 2005;75(9):803–6.

143. Kito M, Yoshimura Y, Isobe K, Aoki K, Momose T, Suzuki S, Tanaka A, Sano K, Akahane T, Kato H. Clinical outcome of deep-seated atypical lipomatous tumor of the extremities with median-term follow-up study. Eur J Surg Oncol. 2015;41(3):400–6. doi:10.1016/j.ejso.2014.11.044.

144. Mussi CE, Daolio P, Cimino M, Giardina F, De Sanctis R, Morenghi E, Parafioriti A, Bartoli MS, Bastoni S, Cozzaglio L, et al. Atypical lipomatous tumors: should they be treated like other sarcoma or not? Surgical consideration from a bi-institutional experience. Ann Surg Oncol. 2014;21(13):4090–7. doi:10.1245/s10434-014-3855-7.

145. Cassier PA, Kantor G, Bonvalot S, Lavergne E, Stoeckle E, Le Péchoux C, Meeus P, Sunyach MP, Vaz G, Coindre JM, et al. Adjuvant radiotherapy for extremity and trunk wall atypical lipomatous tumor/well-differen-tiated LPS (ALT/WD-LPS): a French Sarcoma Group (GSF-GETO) study. Ann Oncol. 2014;25(9):1854–60.

146. Fiore M, Coppola S, Cannell AJ, Colombo C, Bertagnolli MM, George S, Le Cesne A, Gladdy RA, Casali PG, Swallow CJ, et al. Desmoid-type fibromatosis and fibromatosis and pregnancy: a multi-institutional analysis of recurrence and obstetric risk. Ann Surg. 2014;259:973–8.

147. Kasper B, Baumgarten C, Bonvalot S, Haas R, Haller F, Hohenberger P, Moreau G, van der Graaf WTA, Gronchi A. Desmoid Working Group. Management of sporadic desmoid-type fibromatosis: a European consensus approach based on patients' and professionals' expertise—a sarcoma patients EuroNet and European Organisation for Research and Treatment of Cancer/Soft Tissue and Bone Sarcoma Group initiative. Eur J Cancer. 2015;51(2):127–36.

148. Phillips SR, A'Hern R, Thomas JM. Aggressive fibromatosis of the abdom inal wall, limbs and limb girdles. B J Surg. 2004;91(12):1624–9.

149. Wilkinson MJ, Chan KE, Hayes AJ, Strauss DC. Surgical outcomes follow-ing resection for sporadic abdominal wall fibromatosis. Ann Surg Oncol. 2014;21(7):2144–9.

150. Guadagnolo BA, Zagars GK, Ballo MT. Long-term outcomes for desmoid tumors treated with radiation therapy. Int J Radiat Oncol Biol Phys. 2008;71(2):441–7.

151. Keus RB, Nout RA, Blay JY, de Jong JM, Hennig I, Saran F, Hartmann JT, Sunyach MP, Gwyther SJ, Ouali M, Kirkpatrick A, Poortmans PM, Hogen-doorn PC, van der Graaf WT. Results of a phase II pilot study of moder-ate dose radiotherapy for inoperable desmoid-type fibromatosis–an

EORTC STBSG and ROG study (EORTC 62991-22998). Ann Oncol. 2013;24(10):2672–6.

152. Constantinidou A, Scurr M, Jones R, Al-Muderis O, Judson I. Treatment of aggressive fibromatosis with pegylated liposomal doxorubicin; the Royal Marsden Hospital experience, J Clin Oncol. 2009;27(15S), abstract10519.

153. Dufresne A, Penel S, Salas S, Le Cesne A, Perol D, Bui B, Brain E, Ray-Coquard I, Jimenez M, Blay J. Updated outcome with long-term follow-up of imatinib for the treatment of progressive or recurrent aggressive ibromatosis (desmoids tumor): a FNCLCC/French Sarcoma Group phase II trial. J Clin Oncol. 2009;27:15S, 10518

154. Chugh R, Wathen JK, Patel SR, Maki RG, Meyers PA, Schuetze SM, Priebat DA, Thomas DG, Jacobson JA, Samuels BL, Benjamin RS, Baker LH. Sarcoma Alliance for Research through Collaboration (SARC). Efficacy of imatinib in aggressive fibromatosis: results of a phase II multicenter Sarcoma Alliance for Research through Collaboration (SARC) trial. Clin Cancer Res. 2010;16(19):4884–91.

155. Valeyrie-Allanore L, Ismaïli N, Bastuji-Garin S, Zeller J, Wechsler J, Revuz J, Wolkenstein P. Symptoms associated with malignancy of peripheral nerve sheath tumours: a retrospective study of 69 patients with neurofibromatosis 1. Br J Dermatol. 2005;153(1):79–82.

156. Woertler K. Tumors and tumor-like lesions of peripheral nerves. Semin Musculoskelet Radiol. 2010;14(5):547–8.

157. Rodriguez FJ, Folpe AL, Giannini C, Perry A. Pathology of peripheral nerve sheath tumors: diagnostic overview and update on selected diagnostic problems. Acta Neuropathol. 2012;123(3):295–319.

158. Golan JD, Jacques L. Nonneoplastic peripheral nerve tumors. Neurosurg Clin N Am. 2004;15(2):223–30.

159. Gosk J, Gutkowska O, Urban M, Wnukiewicz W, Reichert P, Ziółkowski P. Results of surgical treatment of schwannomas arising from extremities. Biomed Res Int. 2015;2015:547926. doi:10.1155/2015/547926.

160. Valentin T, Le Cesne A, Ray-Coquard I, Italiano A, Decanter G, Bompas E, Isambert N, Thariat J, Linassier C, Bertucci F, Bay JO, Bellesoeur A, Penel N, Le Guellec S, Filleron T, Chevreau C. Management and prognosis of malignant peripheral nerve sheath tumors: the experience of the French Sarcoma Group (GSF-GETO). Eur J Cancer. 2016;56:77–84.

161. Rutkowski P, Debiec-Rychter M. Current treatment options for denatofibrosarcoma protruberans. Expert Rev Anticancer Ther. 2015;15(8):901–9.

162. Rutkowski P, Dębiec-Rychter M, Nowecki Z, Michej W, Symonides M, Ptaszynski K, Ruka W. Treatment of advanced dermatofibrosarcoma protuberans with imatinib mesylate with or without surgical resection. J Eur Acad Dermatol Venereol. 2011;25(3):264–70. doi:10.1111/j.1468-3083.2010.03774.x.

163. Miller K, Goodlad JR, Brenn T. Pleiomorphic dermal sarcoma: adverse histologic features predict aggressive behavior and allow distinction from atypical fibroxanthoma. Am J Surg Pathol. 2012;36(9):1317–26. doi:10.1097/PAS.0b013e31825359e1.

164. Helbig D, Ihle MA, Pütz K, Tantcheva-Poor I, Mauch C, Büttner R, Quaas A. Oncogene and therapeutic target analyses in atypical fibroxanthomas and pleomorphic dermal sarcomas. Oncotarget. 2016;7(16):21763–74.

165. Van der Heijden L, Gibbons CL, Dijkstra PD, Kroep JR, van Rijswijk CS, Nout RA, Bradley KM, Athanasou NA, Hogendoorn PC, van de Sande MA. The management of diffuse-type giant cell tumour (pigmented villonodular synovitis) and giant cell tumour of tendon sheath (nodular tenosynovitis). J Bone Joint Surg Br. 2012;94(7):882–8.

166. Staals EL, Ferrari S, Donati DM, Palmerini E. Diffuse-type tenosynovial giant cell tumour: current treatment concepts and future perspectives. Eur J Cancer. 2016;4(63):34–40.

167. Cassier PA, Gelderblom H, Stacchiotti S, Thomas D, Maki RG, Kroep JR, van der Graaf WT, Italiano A, Seddon B, Dômont J, Bompas E, Wagner AJ, Blay JY. Efficacy of imatinib mesylate for the treatment of locally advanced and/or metastatic tenosynovial giant cell tumor/pigmented villonodular synovitis. Cancer. 2012;118(6):1649–55. doi:10.1002/cncr.26409.

168. Blay JY, El Sayadi H, Thiesse P, Garret J, Ray-Coquard I. Complete response to imatinib in relapsing pigmented villonodular synovitis/tenosynovial giant cell tumor (PVNS/TGCT). Ann Oncol. 2008;19(4):821–2.

169. Butrynski JE, D'Adamo DR, Hornick JL, Dal Cin P, Antonescu CR, Jhanwar SC, Ladanyi M, Capelletti M, Rodig SJ, Ramaiya N, et al. Crizotinib in ALK-rearranged inflammatory myofibroblastic tumor. N Eng J Med. 2010;363(18):1727–33.

170. CREATE: Cross-tumoral Phase 2 With Crizotinib (CREATE). https://clinical-trials.gov/ct2/show/NCT01524926. Accessed 25 Apr 2016.

5

Response to anti-PD1 therapy with nivolumab in metastatic sarcomas

L. Paoluzzi[1]*⊙, A. Cacavio[1], M. Ghesani[2], A. Karambelkar[2], A. Rapkiewicz[3], J. Weber[1] and G. Rosen[1]

Abstract

Background: Manipulation of immune checkpoints such as CTLA4 or PD-1 with targeted antibodies has recently emerged as an effective anticancer strategy in multiple malignancies. Sarcomas are a heterogeneous group of diseases in need of more effective treatments. Different subtypes of soft tissue and bone sarcomas have been shown to express PD-1 ligand.

Methods: We retrospectively analyzed a cohort of patients (pts) with relapsed metastatic/unresectable sarcomas, who were treated with nivolumab provided under a patient assistance program from the manufacturer. Pts underwent CT or PET/CT imaging at baseline and after at least four doses of nivolumab; RECIST 1.1 criteria were used for response assessment.

Results: Twenty-eight pts with soft tissue (STS, N = 24) or bone sarcoma (N = 4), received IV nivolumab 3 mg/kg every 2 weeks from July 2015. Median age was 57 (24–78), male:female ratio was 14:14; the median number of nivolumab cycles was eight. Eighteen pts concomitantly received pazopanib at 400–800 mg daily. The most common side effect was grade 1–2 LFT elevations; grade 3–4 toxicity occurred in five patients (colitis, LFT elevations, pneumonitis). Twenty-four pts received at least four cycles. We observed three partial responses: one dedifferentiated chondrosarcoma, one epithelioid sarcoma and one maxillary osteosarcoma (last two patients on pazopanib); nine patients had stable disease including three leiomyosarcomas; 12 patients had progression of disease including 4 leiomyosarcoma. Clinical benefit (response + stability) was observed in 50% of the evaluable patients.

Conclusions: These data provide a rationale for further exploring the efficacy of nivolumab and other checkpoint inhibitors in soft tissue and bone sarcoma.

Keywords: Sarcoma, Immunotherapy, Nivolumab, PD-1, Check point inhibitors

Background

Soft tissue (STS) and bone sarcomas are a heterogeneous group of diseases with an estimated 15,000 new cases in the US in 2016, and more than 50 different subtypes [1, 2]. Given their rarity and diversity, enrollment into prospective clinical trials has been very challenging, even in the context of cooperative groups. Despite new studies elucidating the genomic basis and the sensitivity to chemotherapy of specific subtypes, the overall prognosis of patients with metastatic sarcoma remains poor in most cases. Since 2012, new drugs such as pazopanib,

and for more specific subtypes, trabectedin and eribulin, have been approved for patients who have relapsed after front line chemotherapy, but the response rates for these agents remains suboptimal [3]. Immunotherapy has recently provoked great interest in oncology after phase III clinical trials have shown significant efficacy in chemotherapy-resistant malignancies such as metastatic melanoma or renal cell carcinoma, and activity in chemotherapy-sensitive histologies including non-small cell lung cancer, head and neck cancer, MSI-high colon cancer and Hodgkin's lymphoma.

Programmed death 1 (PD-1) is a surface receptor expressed on activated and exhausted T cells, which mediates inhibition of activation, cytokine secretion and lytic activity upon binding with its ligands (PD-L1 and

*Correspondence: luca.paoluzzi@nyumc.org
[1] Department of Medicine, NYU Langone Medical Center, New York, NY, USA
Full list of author information is available at the end of the article

PD-L2). The role of the PD-1/PDL-1 axis in suppression of T cell activation and its targeting through specific monoclonal antibodies, has been the basis for the success achieved in a number of clinical trials [4]. Tumor PD-L1 expression has been reported in up to 65% of different subtypes of sarcomas [5]. The degree of PD-1 positivity in tumor-infiltrating lymphocytes (TILs) and PD-L1 expression in tumor specimens from 105 cases of soft tissue sarcomas, has been correlated with a poorer prognosis and more aggressive disease [6]. While preclinical studies and retrospective analyses of clinical data may provide a rationale for immune-mediated strategies against sarcoma, there are currently very limited clinical data to support the use of anti-PD-1 antibodies in this setting. We report herein a retrospective series of twenty-eight patients with metastatic or locally advanced soft tissue or bone sarcoma who received the PD-1 antibody nivolumab under a patient assistant program off protocol, with or without pazopanib. We describe for the first time clinical benefit in different subtypes, as shown by disease regression or stabilization.

Patients and methods

Between July 2015 and August 2016, twenty-eight patients with a diagnosis of soft tissue or bone sarcoma were treated with nivolumab. All patients but two, previously received one line of systemic treatment; patients receiving pazopanib before starting nivolumab were continued on this treatment given concern for disease flare after discontinuation, as described for other tyrosine kinase inhibitors [7]. The following data were recorded for all patients: gender, age, location of the primary sarcoma, stage, median number of prior therapies, ECOG performance status, number of cycles of nivolumab administered. Nivolumab was given at the standard dose of 3 mg/kg IV every 2 weeks; the drug was provided by the manufacturer under a patient assistant program. Complete blood count, electrolytes, liver and kidney function tests were performed before each cycle of treatment, more often if clinically indicated; all toxicities were recorded at each visit (at least every 2 weeks), as per NCI CTCAE v.4.0. Baseline scans consisted of PET/CT or CT scans with IVC, imaging was repeated every two or three months. Next generation sequencing to determine the presence of specific mutations in a panel of 50 genes was performed in one patient with a dedifferentiated chondrosarcoma responding to nivolumab alone; the polymerase chain reaction (PCR) product for specific mutations was sequenced on an Ion Torrent PGM instrument (Thermo Fisher Scientific, Waltham, MA). PD-L1 expression was assessed in selected patients who had evaluable tissue for testing (N = 10) and performed at Esoterix Genetic Laboratories (Integrated Oncology,

New York, NY). PD-L1 positive was defined as a tumor proportion score (% of at least 100 viable tumor cells with complete or partial 1 + membrane staining) of 50% for at least 100 viable tumor cells exhibiting membrane staining. For PD-L1 detection, we used the PD-L1 IHC 28-8 pharmDx assay (Dako North America Inc, CA, USA).

Results

Patients and treatment

The clinical characteristics of the patients are shown in Table 1. A total of 28 patients with a diagnosis of metastatic (n = 26) or unresectable (n = 2) soft tissue or bone sarcoma received IV nivolumab every 2 weeks; median age was 57 years, female to male ratio was 14:14, ECOG performance status was 0–1 for 24 patients, and 2 for the remaining 4 patients. Eighteen patients received concomitant pazopanib. The median number of prior systemic

Table 1 Patient baseline characteristics

Factor	No
Age	
Median	57
Range	24–78
Sex	
Female	14
Male	14
Soft tissue sarcoma	24
Bone sarcoma	4
Location	
Extremity	6
Abdomen/pelvis	12
Axial	2
Head/neck	5
Chest	3
Stage	
IV	26
Unresectable	2
ECOG PS	
0–1	24
2	4
Nivolumab	
Cycles (median)	8
Range	1–26
On Pazopanib	18
Prior treatments (including neoadjuvant/adjuvant)	
Median	2
Range	0–6
Anthracycline	15
Ifosfamide	10
Gemcitabine	9
Docetaxel	7

treatments, including neoadjuvant and adjuvant chemo-therapy was 2 (range 0–6). Sarcoma subtypes are listed in Additional file 1: Table S1; twenty-four patients had a diagnosis of a soft tissue sarcoma with leiomyosarcoma (LMS) being the most common subtype (n = 7); four patients had conventional osteosarcoma (OS).

Safety

Table 2 shows all the adverse events (AE); most side effects were grade 1–2 with a predominance of LFT abnormalities (8 out of 10 patients on pazopanib). Grade 3–4 AE were experienced by four patients, all on pazo-panib. One patient experienced grade 3 elevation of AST/ALT/alkaline phosphatase and grade 4 bilirubin elevation after two cycles of nivolumab; liver biopsy was consistent with drug related hepatitis; she discontinued treatment with normalization of bilirubin, and improve-ment of ALT/AST to grade 1. A second patient experi-enced grade 3 ALT elevation that improved to grade 1 once both nivolumab and pazopanib were discontinued and high dose steroids (prednisone 1 mg/kg/daily) were administered with a slow taper over about 2 months; she subsequently restarted treatment with both drugs. A third patient had grade 4 AST/grade 3 ALT/alkaline phosphatase elevations with grade 3 pneumonitis that required intubation; he recovered after high dose ster-oids and he was able to restart pazopanib only, after LFTs normalized. A fourth patient experienced grade 3 colitis that significantly improved with high dose steroids; she was restarted on treatment with both pazopanib and nivolumab until she progressed.

Efficacy outcomes

Twenty-four patients were evaluable for response (Fig. 1). Four patients were not evaluable for the following

reasons: liver toxicity after 2 cycles (n = 1); patients lost at follow up (n = 2), concomitant radiation therapy (n = 1). We observed three partial responses (PR) and they included: a 74 year-old patient with a dedifferenti-ated chondrosarcoma (DC), after six cycles of nivolumab alone with PR maintained after 26 cycles (Fig. 2a; Addi-tional file 1: Figure S1). The NGS-tumor 50 panel only showed non-synonymous variants of unknown signifi-cance for the PIK3CA and TP53 genes; PD-L1 staining was 20%. A second PR was observed in a 46 year-old female with a relapsed, OS of the left maxilla. She had a minimal clinical response to nivolumab given for four cycles; pazopanib was then added and it was given for only one month (Fig. 2b). The rationale to add pazo-panib after 4 cycles of nivolumab alone, relied on the following considerations: (1) the original lesion showed abundant vascularization; (2) pazopanib targets the vas-cular endothelial growth receptors VEGF-1, VEGFR-2, VEGF-3; (3) nivolumab alone was tolerated very well; (4) a resection of this challenging lesion could potentially give the best chance for a long progression free survival in this young patient. After one month of pazopanib, her facial lesion significantly regressed and the patient had major clinical benefit in terms of improved eating hab-its and pain control. At that point we thought it was in the patient's best interest to undergo surgery. At the time of resection, the tumor showed extensive necrosis and margins were negative. PD-L1 in this patient was <5%. A third PR was observed in a 24 year-old man with a proxi-mal type epithelioid sarcoma (EpS) metastatic to the lung progressing on pazopanib. We decided to continue paz-opanib given the concern for disease flare after discon-tinuation as described for other tyrosine kinase inhibitors [7]. This patient had a PR after four cycles of nivolumab, progression (PD) due to a new lesion in the left lung after

Table 2 Safety

	Grade 1–2			Grade 3–4		
	On Pz (No.)	NO Pz (No.)	Total (No.)	On Pz (No.)	NO Pz (No.)	Total (No.)
Hematologic						
Anemia	3	1	4	–	–	–
Neutropenia	1	–	1	–	–	–
Thrombocytopenia	1	1	2	–	–	–
Non-hematologic						
Diarrhea	3		3	1		1
Pneumonitis	1		1	1		1
Rash	3	1	4	–	–	–
Hypothyroidism	6	2	8	–	–	–
LFTs	8	2	10	3		3

Toxicity was graded as per NCI CTCAE v4.0

Pz pazopanib, 400–800 mg po daily; *LFTs* liver function tests abnormalities

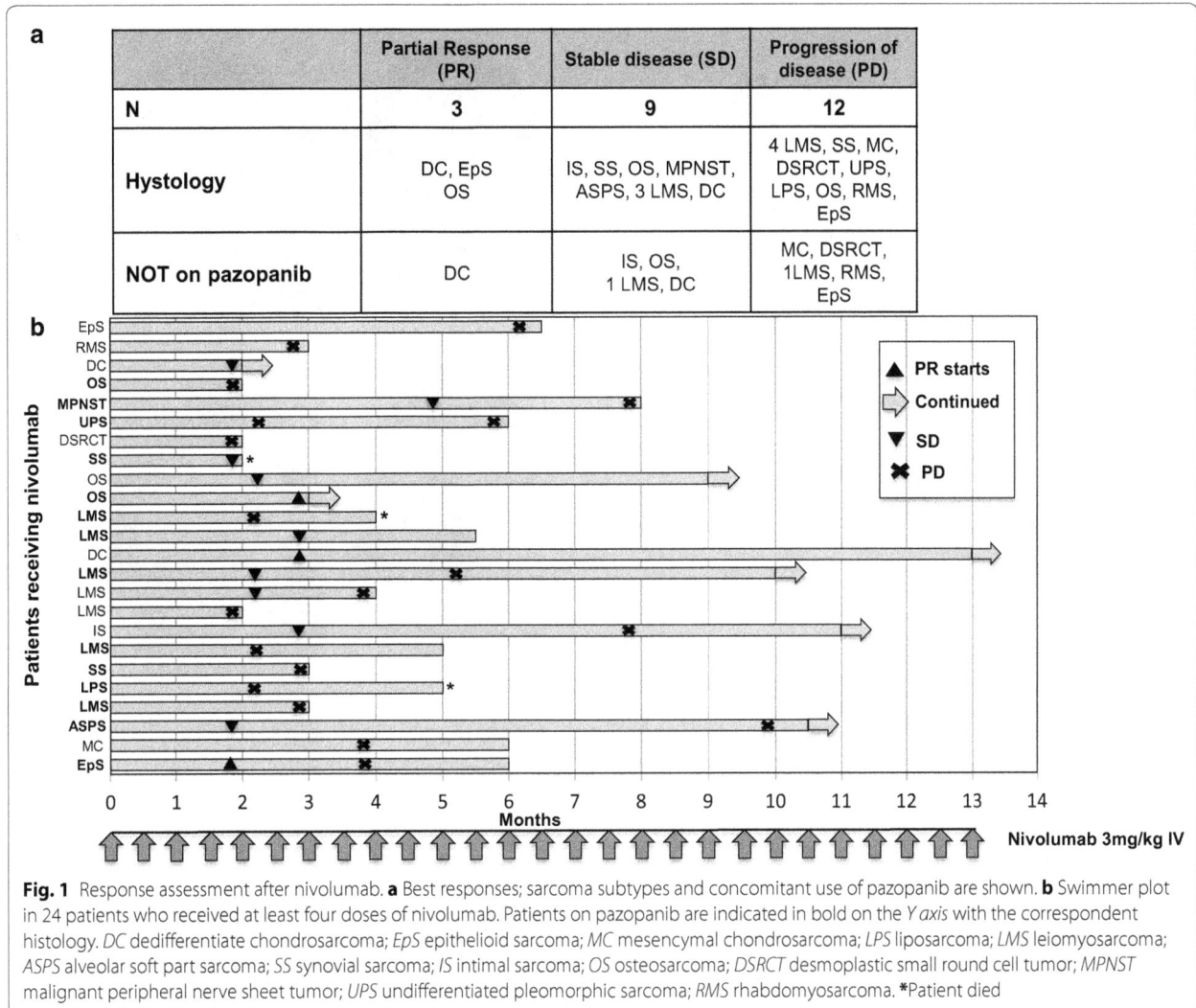

Fig. 1 Response assessment after nivolumab. **a** Best responses; sarcoma subtypes and concomitant use of pazopanib are shown. **b** Swimmer plot in 24 patients who received at least four doses of nivolumab. Patients on pazopanib are indicated in bold on the Y axis with the correspondent histology. *DC* dedifferentiate chondrosarcoma; *EpS* epithelioid sarcoma; *MC* mesencymal chondrosarcoma; *LPS* liposarcoma; *LMS* leiomyosarcoma; *ASPS* alveolar soft part sarcoma; *SS* synovial sarcoma; *IS* intimal sarcoma; *OS* osteosarcoma; *DSRCT* desmoplastic small round cell tumor; *MPNST* malignant peripheral nerve sheet tumor; *UPS* undifferentiated pleomorphic sarcoma; *RMS* rhabdomyosarcoma. *Patient died

four additional cycles; he had further PD in the lung after four more cycles and nivolumab was stopped.

Nine patients had stable disease (SD): five patients received pazopanib plus nivolumab while four patients received nivolumab alone (one dedifferentiated chondrosarcoma, one leiomyosarcoma, one intimal sarcoma and one osteosarcoma).

A patient with an alveolar soft part sarcoma (ASPS) progressing on pazopanib, with a slight PD (~25% increase per RECIST criteria) after nine cycles of nivolumab, he is overall asymptomatic and continues treatment with both drugs; two patients with uterine LMS, both progressing on pazopanib alone, one had SD after five cycles (PD after 6 more) and the other SD after six cycles (nivolumab stopped after five more cycles because of pneumonitis); a patient with a LMS of the vulva had SD after five cycles of nivolumab alone but a

PD after three additional cycles; a patient with an intimal sarcoma (IS) of the right pulmonary artery metastatic to both lungs, experienced a SD after six cycles of nivolumab alone (the primary site was not evaluable because previously irradiated); he had PD after six additional cycles but continues nivolumab because he is asymptomatic; a patient with a synovial sarcoma (SS) had a SD after four cycles, but died from complications during surgery for repair of a pulmonary artery pseudo-aneurysm; a patient with a maxillary OS had SD after five cycles of nivolumab alone (confirmed after a total of 16 cycles); a patient with a malignant peripheral sheet tumor (MPNST), on pazopanib, had stability after four cycles but progressed after six additional cycles of nivolumab; a patient with a dedifferentiated myxoid chondrosarcoma (MC) had SD after four cycles of nivolumab.

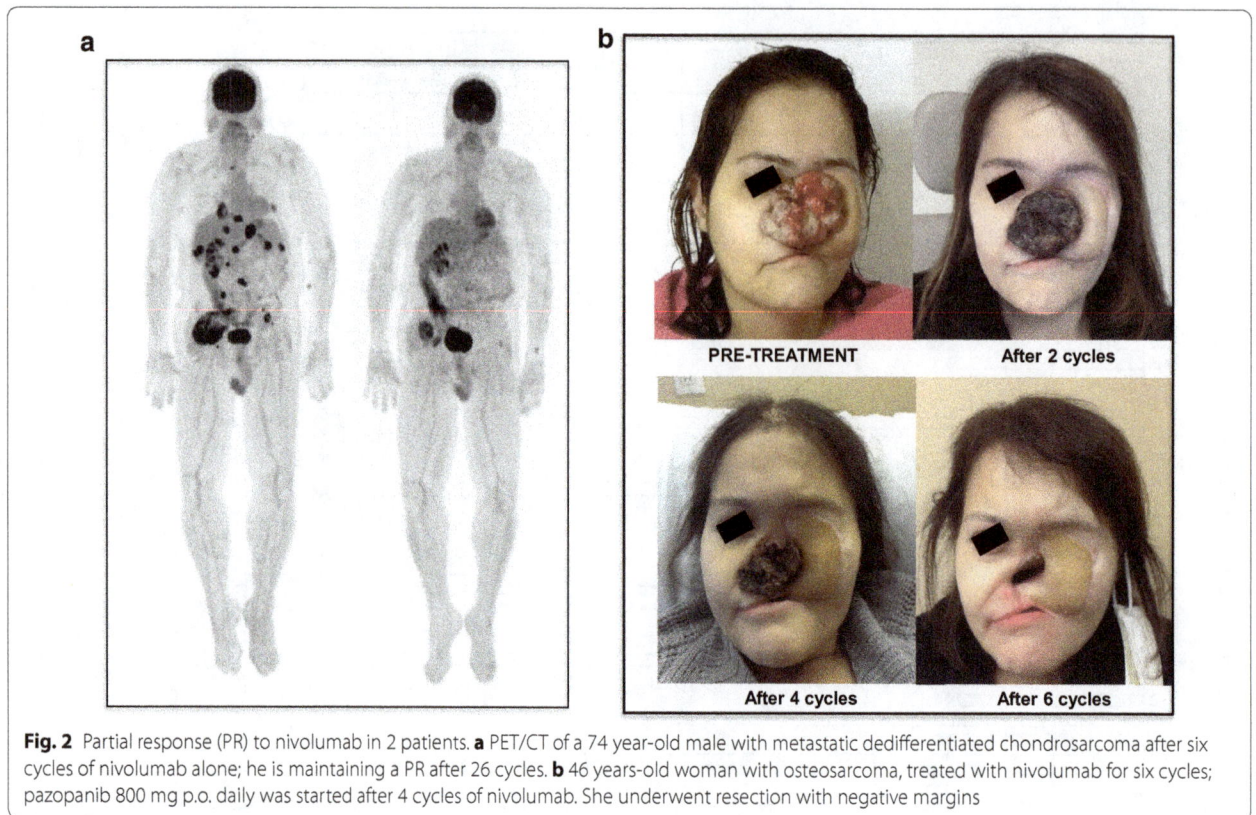

Fig. 2 Partial response (PR) to nivolumab in 2 patients. **a** PET/CT of a 74 year-old male with metastatic dedifferentiated chondrosarcoma after six cycles of nivolumab alone; he is maintaining a PR after 26 cycles. **b** 46 years-old woman with osteosarcoma, treated with nivolumab for six cycles; pazopanib 800 mg p.o. daily was started after 4 cycles of nivolumab. She underwent resection with negative margins

Overall, 12 out of 24 evaluable patients had clinical benefit (PR + SD). Twelve patients had PD: four patients with LMS (three on pazopanib): one transferred care to another hospital after six cycles, one had PD after five cycles, confirmed after five more, and switched to another treatment, one received five cycles and died after an accidental fall, a last one had a PD after four cycles on nivolumab alone. Additional PD in patients on pazopanib included: one with a MC after four cycles (confirmed after 4 more), one with a liposarcoma (LPS) after five cycles (confirmed after 6 more), one with an OS after four cycles; a patient with a SS after six cycles complicated by severe pneumonitis; one patient with an undifferentiated pleomorphic sarcoma (UPS) of the right upper extremity after five cycles (confirmed after 7 more). Patient with PD on nivolumab alone included: one with a desmoplastic small round cell tumor (DSRCT) after four cycles; one patient with a rhabdomyosarcoma (RMS) after six cycles; one with an EpS after 13 cycles.

Discussion

Patients with metastatic soft tissue sarcomas generally have a poor prognosis, with low response rates after first line chemotherapy [3]. Of note, the tyrosine kinase inhibitor pazopanib was approved by the FDA in 2012 on the basis of a phase III randomized trial showing improved

PFS in the second line setting; the overall response rate was only 6% [8].

Multiple recent genomic studies have provided better insight into sarcoma biology through a more accurate classification by molecular subtype, identification of recurrent mutations in oncogenic pathways and evidence of epigenetic dysregulation [9]. Barretina et al. [10] for example, recently provided a comprehensive database of sarcoma genome alterations in 207 samples of STS; despite their elucidation of genes and signaling pathways not previously associated with STS, we still lack appropriate pharmacologic tools for targeting specific genomic alterations.

Several subtypes of STS are characterized by specific chromosomal translocations which result in unique fusion proteins; while many of them function as transcription factors, making their therapeutic targeting quite challenging, these proteins may represent attractive targets from an immunotherapy standpoint [11]. Immunogenicity of sarcoma is supported by several preclinical studies and some clinical data with human sarcoma specimens.

Immunotherapeutic strategies in sarcoma have included cytokine-based immunotherapies, treatment with muramyl tripeptide phosphatidyl ethanolamine in osteosarcoma, vaccines and adoptive immunotherapy to cite a few examples, although none have appeared promising to date [12]. Our retrospective analysis shows the potential clinical benefit from treatment of soft tissue and bone sarcomas with the anti-PD1 antibody nivolumab.

This is not a prospective study, and given the retrospective nature of this series, it has several limitations; data on patients who received either nivolumab alone (N = 10) or nivolumab + pazopanib (N = 18), were pulled together in order to capture a possible signal of activity from immunotherapy (alone or in combination) that may be helpful for a following prospective study. Additionally, this is small study with multiple hystologies included: the largest group of patient had a diagnosis of leiomyosarcoma (N = 7), but most subtypes are represented by only 1 or 2 patients.

In our series we showed disease improvement or stabilization in 12/24 patients evaluable for response. Eighteen out of twenty-eight patients concomitantly received pazopanib, however 1 partial response was observed in a dedifferentiated chondrosarcoma on nivolumab alone. Another response was seen in a patient with an unresectable maxillary OS who received four cycles of nivolumab and only one month of pazopanib that was started after the 4 cycles of nivolumab. A third patient with an epithelioid sarcoma, progressing on pazopanib, had a partial response after only four cycles of nivolumab; unfortunately he progressed after four additional cycles. Of note, overall responses were observed in some subtypes that are generally resistant to traditional chemotherapy such as dedifferentiated chondrosarcoma and epithelioid sarcoma. Interestingly, all the three aforementioned patients received adjuvant radiation therapy up to 20 years before, bringing up the possibility of a distant abscopal effect as hypothesized for other diseases such as melanoma [13].

At least three prospective phase II studies are exploring the role of the checkpoint inhibitors pembrolizumab and nivolumab in metastatic STS/bone sarcomas and/or uterine LMS; preliminary data were recently presented at the ASCO 2016 conference for two studies. Pembrolizumab showed some interesting responses in undifferentiated pleomorphic sarcoma (4/9), liposarcoma (2/9), synovial (1/9), chondrosarcoma (1/6) and osteosarcoma (1/19); no responses were seen in LMS (0/10) and Ewing sarcoma (1/13) [14]. Interestingly in our series, we also observed a partial response in one patient with a dedifferentiated chondrosarcoma and a PD-L1 expression that was higher compared to all other tested patients (20% versus less than 5%); additionally, Kostine et al. [15] recently showed that this specific subtype of bone sarcoma expresses PD-L1 in association with immune-infiltrating cells and HLA class I in nearly 50% of cells. Immunotherapy with check-point inhibitors seems a particularly promising

approach for the treatment of this rare and challenging histology but more data is needed.

A second prospective study is exploring nivolumab in 12 patients with uterine LMS and showed no responses [16]. In our series, among seven patients with LMS we observed 4 PD and 3 SD. LMS is characterized by a significant degree of morphologic and molecular heterogeneity and different molecular subtypes may respond differently to immunotherapy [17].

The combination of nivolumab and pazopanib is interesting but needs dose optimization to prevent, in particular, excessive liver toxicity. Nivolumab at 2 mg/kg every 3 weeks has been combined with pazopanib at 800 mg po daily in patients with renal cell carcinoma; about 70% of patients experienced grade 3–4 side effects, mainly LFT abnormalities, fatigue and diarrhea [18].

Conclusion

We describe a cohort of 28 sarcoma patients with metastatic or unresectable soft tissue or bone sarcomas who were treated with the anti-PD-1 antibody nivolumab with or without the tyrosine kinase inhibitor pazopanib; we found evidence of clinical benefit with a half of the evaluable patients experiencing a partial response or a stabilization of disease after at least 4 cycles of nivolumab. Given the potential activity of nivolumab alone and promising data when combined with pazopanib, we are planning a prospective, phase II randomized study of nivolumab alone versus nivolumab with pazopanib, in metastatic soft tissue and bone sarcomas; correlative studies will include tumor and serum sampling for correlation with the clinical endpoints of response and progression-free survival.

Additional file

Additional file 1. Table S1. Sarcoma subtypes. Primary site and concomitant treatment with pazopanib given at 400-800 mg po daily, are indicated. DC = dedifferentiate chondrosarcoma; MC = mesenchymal chondrosarcoma; LPS-DD = dedifferentiated liposarcoma; LMS = leiomyosarcoma; ASPS = alveolar soft part sarcoma; SS = synovial sarcoma; EpS = epithelioid sarcoma; IS = intimal sarcoma; UPS = undifferentiated pleomorphic sarcoma; DFSP = dermatofibrosarcoma protuberans; OS = osteosarcoma: MPNST = malignant peripheral nerve sheet tumor; DSRCT = desmoplastic small round cell tumor; RP = retroperitoneum; UE = upper extremity; LE = lower extremity. **Figure S1.** Partial response (PR) to nivolumab in a 74 year-old male with metastatic dedifferentiated chondrosarcoma. This patient received 6 cycles of IV nivolumab 3 mg/kg every 2 weeks; he is maintaining a PR after 26 cycles.

Abbreviations

pts: patients; STS: soft tissue sarcoma; PD-1: programmed death 1; PDL-1: programmed death ligand 1; PCR: polymerase chain reaction; TILs: tumor infiltrating lymphocytes; LFT: liver function tests; AST: aspartate transaminase; ALT: alanine transaminase; LMS: leiomyosarcoma; OS: osteosarcoma; DC: dedifferentiated chondrosarcoma; EpS: epithelioid sarcoma; IS: intimal sarcoma; SS: synovial sarcoma; MPNST: malignant peripheral nerve sheet tumor; MC:

mesenchymal chondrosarcoma; LPS: liposarcoma; UPS: undifferentiated pleomorphic sarcoma; DSRCT: desmoplastic small round cell tumor; RMS: rhabdomyosarcoma; ASPS: alveolar soft part sarcoma; AE: adverse event; PD: progression of disease; SD: stable disease; PR: partial response; PFS: progression free survival; CTLs: cytotoxic T-lymphocytes.

Authors' contributions
LP and GR conceived the study and the design. LP and AC carried out data collection. LP and JW drafted the manuscript. AR performed pathologic review and immunohistochemical analysis. MG and AK interpreted the radiographic data. All authors read and approved the final manuscript.

Author details
[1] Department of Medicine, NYU Langone Medical Center, New York, NY, USA.
[2] Department of Radiology, NYU Langone Medical Center, New York, NY, USA.
[3] Department of Pathology, New York University School of Medicine, Laura and Isaac Perlmutter Cancer Center, 10th floor, Room 1041, 160 East 34th street, New York, NY, USA.

Acknowledgements
We thank Bristol-Myers Squibb for providing nivolumab under a patient assistance program.

Competing interests
Dr. Jeffrey Weber accepts honoraria for advisory boards, and consulting fees. He is named on a patent filed by Moffitt Cancer center for an Ipilimumab biomarker. All remaining authors declared that they have no competing interests.

References
1. Siegel RL, Miller KD, Jemal A. Cancer statistics, 2016. Cancer J Clin. 2016;66(1):7–30.
2. Jo VY, Fletcher CD. WHO classification of soft tissue tumors: an update based on the 2013 (4th) edition. Pathology. 2014;46(2):95–104.
3. Pang A, Carbini M, Maki RG. Contemporary therapy for advanced soft-tissue sarcomas in adults: a review. JAMA Oncol. 2016;2(7):941-47.
4. Choudhury N, Nakamura Y. The importance of immunopharmacogenomics in cancer treatment: patient selection and monitoring for immune checkpoint antibodies. Cancer Sci. 2016;107(2):107–15.
5. D'Angelo SP, Shoushtari AN, Agaram NP, Kuk D, Qin LX, Carvajal RD, Dickson MA, Gounder M, Keohan ML, Schwartz GK, Tap WD. Prevalence of tumor-infiltrating lymphocytes and PD-L1 expression in the soft tissue sarcoma microenvironment. Hum Pathol. 2015;46(3):357–65.
6. Kim JR, Moon YJ, Kwon KS, Bae JS, Wagle S, Kim KM, Park HS, Lee H, Moon WS, Chung MJ, Kang MJ, Jang KY. Tumor infiltrating PD1-positive lymphocytes and the expression of PD-L1 predict poor prognosis of soft tissue sarcomas. PLoS ONE. 2013;8(12):e82870.
7. Griffioen AW, Mans LA, de Graaf AM, Nowak-Sliwinska P, de Hoog CL, de Jong TA, Vyth-Dreese FA, van Beijnum JR, Bex A, Jonasch E. Rapid angiogenesis onset after discontinuation of sunitinib treatment of renal cell carcinoma patients. Clin Cancer Res. 2012;18(14):3961–71.
8. van der Graaf WT, Blay JY, Chawla SP, Kim DW, Bui-Nguyen B, Casali PG, Schöffski P, Aglietta M, Staddon AP, Beppu Y, Le Cesne A, Gelderblom H, Judson IR, Araki N, Ouali M, Marreaud S, Hodge R, Dewji MR, Coens C, Demetri GD, Fletcher CD, Dei Tos AP, Hohenberger P, EORTC Soft Tissue and Bone Sarcoma Group, PALETTE study group. Pazopanib for metastatic soft-tissue sarcoma (PALETTE): a randomised, double-blind, placebo-controlled phase 3 trial. Lancet. 2012;379(9829):1879–86.
9. Lim J, Poulin NM, Nielsen TO. New strategies in sarcoma: linking genomic and immunotherapy approaches to molecular subtype. Clin Cancer Res. 2015;21(21):4753–9.
10. Barretina J, Taylor BS, Banerji S, Ramos AH, Lagos-Quintana M, Decarolis PL, Shah K, Socci ND, Weir BA, Ho A, Chiang DY, Reva B, Mermel CH, Getz G, Antipin Y, Beroukhim R, Major JE, Hatton C, Nicoletti R, Hanna M, Sharpe T, Fennell TJ, Cibulskis K, Onofrio RC, Saito T, Shukla N, Lau C, Nelander S, Silver SJ, Sougnez C, Viale A, Winckler W, Maki RG, Garraway LA, Lash A, Greulich H, Root DE, Sellers WR, Schwartz GK, Antonescu CR, Lander ES, Varmus HE, Ladanyi M, Sander C, Meyerson M, Singer S. Subtype-specific genomic alterations define new targets for soft-tissue sarcoma therapy. Nat Genet. 2010;42(8):715–21.
11. Tseng WW, Malu S, Zhang M, Chen J, Sim GC, Wei W, Ingram D, Somaiah N, Lev DC, Pollock RE, Lizée G, Radvanyi L, Hwu P. Analysis of the intratumoral adaptive immune response in well differentiated and dedifferentiated retroperitoneal liposarcoma. Sarcoma. 2015;2015:547460.
12. Burgess M, Tawbi H. Immunotherapeutic approaches to sarcoma. Curr Treat Options Oncol. 2015;16(6):26.
13 Chandra RA, Wilhite TJ, Balboni TA, Alexander BM, Spektor A, Ott PA, Ng AK, Hodi FS, Schoenfeld JD. A systematic evaluation of abscopal responses following radiotherapy in patients with metastatic melanoma treated with ipilimumab. Oncoimmunology. 2015;4(11):1046028.
14 Tawbi HA-H, Burgess MA, Crowley J, van Tine BA, Hu J, Schuetze S, D'Angelo SP, Attia S, Priebat DA, Okuno SH, Riedel RF, Davis LE, Movva S, Reed DR, Baker LH, Reinke DK, Maki RG, Patel S, for SARC028 Investigators. Safety and efficacy of PD-1 blockage using pembrolizumab in patients with advanced soft tissue (STS) and bone sarcomas (BS): results of SARC028-a multicenter phase II study. J Clin Onc. 2016;34(15):11006.
15 Kostine M, Cleven AH, de Miranda NF, Italiano A, Cleton-Jansen AM, Bovée JV. Analysis of PD-L1, T-cell infiltrate and HLA expression in chondrosarcoma indicates potential for response to immunotherapy specifically in the dedifferentiated subtype. Mod Pathol. 2016;29(9):1028–37.
16 George S, Barysauskas CM, Solomon S, Tahlil K, Malley R, Hohos M, Polson K, Loucks M, Wagner AJ, Merriam P, Morgan JA, Rodig SJ, Hodi FS, Shapiro G, Demetri GD. Phase II study of nivolumab in metastatic leiomyosarcoma of the uterus. J Clin Oncol. 34, 2016 **(supplemental abstract 11007)**.
17 Beck AH, Lee CH, Witten DM, Gleason BC, Edris B, Espinosa I, Zhu S, Li R, Montgomery KD, Marinelli RJ, Tibshirani R, Hastie T, Jablons DM, Rubin BP, Fletcher CD, West RB, van de Rijn M. Discovery of molecular subtypes in leiomyosarcoma through integrative molecular profiling. Oncogene. 2010;29(6):845–54.
18 Amin A, Plimack ER, Infante JR, Ernstoff MS, Rini BI, McDermott DF, Knox JJ, Pal SK, Voss MH, Sharma P, Kollmannsberger CK, Chin Heng DY, Spratlin JL, Shen Y, Kurland JF, Gagnier P, Hammer HJ. Nivolumab (anti-PD-1; BMS-936558, ONO-4538) in combination with sunitinib or pazopanib in patients (pts) with metastatic renal cell carcinoma (mRCC). ASCO. J Clin Oncol. 2014;32(5) **(supplemental abstract 5010)**.

6

Fifteen years of irinotecan therapy for pediatric sarcoma: where to next?

Lars M. Wagner* 🆔

Abstract

Over the past 15 years, irinotecan has emerged as an important agent for treating pediatric sarcoma patients. This review summarizes the activity noted in previous studies, and outlines current issues regarding scheduling, route of administration, and amelioration of side effects. Also discussed are new pegylated and nanoliposomal formulations of irinotecan and its active metabolite, SN-38, as well as future plans for how irinotecan may be used in combination with other conventional cytotoxic as well as targeted agents.

Keywords: Irinotecan, Sarcoma, Ewing sarcoma, Rhabdomyosarcoma

Background

Irinotecan is a camptothecin analogue that has taken on growing importance in the treatment of pediatric sarcomas such as Ewing sarcoma and rhabdomyosarcoma. Irinotecan is a prodrug that is spontaneously converted by endogenous carboxylesterases to its active metabolite, SN-38. Like other camptothecins such as topotecan, SN-38 mediates cytotoxicity by stabilizing the DNA-topoisomerase I complex created during replication. This stabilization prevents religation of DNA, and so "poisons" the activity of the topoisomerase I enzyme.

Irinotecan was initially approved by the US Food and Drug Administration for the treatment of colon cancer in 1996. Three years later, Furman et al. reported the first pediatric phase I clinical trial of irinotecan [1]. This landmark study was based on the preclinical observation of improved efficacy when using a protracted multi-day schedule, as opposed to a single dose given every 3 weeks [2]. Such protracted scheduling provides greater exposure of this S phase-specific drug, especially when given for 5 consecutive days 2 weeks in a row (d × 5 × 2 schedule). The objective responses observed in three patients with relapsed rhabdomyosarcoma were consistent with the enhanced preclinical activity seen in pediatric sarcoma xenografts using this schedule, and this trial was

followed by subsequent studies designed to: (1) explore various schedules of administration, (2) reduce toxicity, (3) improve convenience and maximize SN-38 exposures, and (4) define the activity of irinotecan as a single agent and in combination with other drugs. In this review, we will identify key findings from these past studies, and also discuss new formulations and potentially synergistic therapeutic partners for irinotecan.

Schedules of irinotecan administration

Several schedules of irinotecan administration have been studied in children, ranging from one large dose every 3 weeks as used in adults [3, 4], to once weekly [5], daily × 3 [6], daily × 5 [7], and the original d × 5 × 2 schedule first studied by Furman et al. [1, 8, 9]. All schedules have been tolerable, although notably the pattern of toxicity is schedule-dependent. For example, when using larger but infrequent dosages, the principal toxicity is myelosuppression. In contrast, diarrhea and abdominal pain are more prominent with the protracted lower-dose schedule.

Only one pediatric study has directly compared the efficacy of different schedules of irinotecan. In that trial, 89 evaluable patients with recurrent rhabdomyosarcoma were randomized to receive vincristine combined with irinotecan given either on a d × 5 or a d × 5 × 2 schedule [10]. The overall incidence of grade 3–4 adverse events was similar. As expected, patients on the shorter schedule experienced more myelosuppression, while

*Correspondence: lars.wagner@uky.edu
Division of Pediatric Hematology/Oncology, Kentucky Clinic Suite, University of Kentucky, J-457, Lexington, KY 40536, USA

those on the longer schedule had more gastrointestinal toxicity. Importantly, because there was no significant difference in efficacy, and since the shorter schedule is more convenient and less expensive, the d × 5 schedule has emerged as the most popular schedule for newer regimens.

Ameliorating toxicity

In most pediatric studies of irinotecan, myelosuppression is mild and growth factor is rarely required. Instead, diarrhea and abdominal pain are the usual dose-limiting toxicities. Early-onset diarrhea may occur during or immediately after irinotecan administration, and is usually manageable with atropine. More common and problematic is the late-onset diarrhea noted about 1 week after starting therapy. While prompt administration of loperamide may help with mild gastrointestinal toxicity, some patients experience severe diarrhea and abdominal pain, and this morbidity can impact compliance even when the tumor is responding to treatment [7, 8].

The mechanism of late-onset diarrhea is complex. Local accumulation of the active metabolite SN-38 in the gut results in direct cytotoxicity and secretory diarrhea [11]. SN-38 is usually inactivated through hepatic glucuronidation and then excreted in the bile into the intestine. However, reactivation of SN-38 can occur as a result of glucuronidases which are produced by enteric bacteria [reviewed in 12]. Therefore, one approach for reducing irinotecan-associated diarrhea is to use antibiotics to eradicate the Gram negative aerobic bacteria that produce these glucuronidases, thereby reducing the reactivation of local SN-38 in the gut. That strategy proved efficacious in a phase I trial of orally administered irinotecan in which the daily use of the oral cephalosporin cefixime reduced the incidence of grade 3–4 diarrhea such that the maximum tolerated dose was 50 % higher than what could be achieved without antibiotic support [13]. A 50 % increase in the tolerable dose was also noted in patients receiving intravenous irinotecan in a similar trial [14]. This practice of using cephalosporins before, during, and after the irinotecan course has now been universally employed in all pediatric trials of orally administered irinotecan, given that the poor bioavailability requires higher drug doses to achieve acceptable SN-38 exposures. One common approach when using the d × 5 schedule of irinotecan is to administer cephalosporins (either cefixime or cefpodoxime) starting 2 days before chemotherapy and continuing until 3 days after finishing chemotherapy, which makes for a 10-day course of antibiotics and avoids the continuous administration that may lead to antibiotic resistance or *C difficile* infections. In contrast to orally administered irinotecan, cephalosporin prophylaxis is not routinely done when standard doses of irinotecan are given intravenously, as the incidence of ≥grade 3 diarrhea is under 10 % [7]. Instead, antibiotic prophylaxis is usually only used in patients experiencing significant toxicity during the previous course, as a way to maintain dose intensity [15].

The detoxification of SN-38 through hepatic glucuronidaiton is mediated by *UGT1A1*. In adult studies, patients with the *UGT1A1*28* polymorphism have increased toxicity from irinotecan [16]. However, in pediatric studies this genotype/phenotype relationship has not been observed. For example, in the largest series of 74 patients taken from 5 pediatric studies in patients receiving protracted irinotecan, there was no increase in either hematologic or gastrointestinal toxicity in patients homozygous for *UGT1A1*28* [17]. Based on this and similar reports [18], prospective genotyping of pediatric patients receiving protracted irinotecan is not routinely performed.

Maximizing convenience: oral administration

The protracted administration schedule of intravenous irinotecan is inconvenient for patients and costly to administer, prompting interest in oral administration. There is no commercially available tablet or capsule formulation of irinotecan, and so the intravenous preparation has been given orally. Because of the bitter taste, it is usually masked in cran-grape juice to improve palatability [13]. The oral bioavailability is less than 20 %, requiring higher dose of oral irinotecan are necessary to achieve SN-38 exposures similar to intravenous administration. However, metabolism of orally administered irinotecan is more efficient, given that the intestinal tract contains high levels of carboxylesterases, which may presystemically metabolize irinotecan to SN-38 and increase the SN-38/irinotecan ratio by threefold or more [19].

Pediatric clinical trials have shown the dose of 60 mg/m^2/dose on a d × 5 × 2 schedule was tolerable and produced SN-38 exposures that were similar to those seen with intravenous doses of 20 mg/m^2, when accounting for the wide intrapatient variability in irinotecan metabolism [13, 18]. However, the relationship between oral and intravenous dosing is not exactly linear. For example, the daily oral dose of 90 mg/m^2 appears comparable to the intravenous dose of 50 mg/m^2 when using similar pharmacokinetic assays [20]. To date there have been over 200 pediatric patients treated on trials of oral irinotecan [13, 18, 20–22]. Although there have been no studies directly comparing the efficacy of oral vs. intravenous administration, the roughly similar SN-38 exposures, response rates, and toxicity profiles suggest they are fairly equivalent when using the dose conversions noted above.

The benefits of oral administration include greater patient convenience and time away from the clinic, as well as up to five-fold reduction in cost [23]. The strategy is generally feasible, and because of the considerable benefits could be considered in most situations. However, there are occasional patients who have difficulty taking the medication orally, no matter what methods are used to mask the flavor. Also, for patients with ongoing nausea or chronic gastrointestinal complaints, oral absorption may be limited and make this strategy inappropriate.

Improving SN-38 exposure

Efforts to increase SN-38 exposure are based on the assumption of a dose–response relationship for irinotecan therapy for pediatric sarcoma, which is intuitive but not yet proven clinically. Given gastrointestinal toxicity is the usual limiting toxicity, one strategy for dose escalation is to reduce irinotecan-associated diarrhea with cefixime as described above. McGreggor et al. have shown in a phase I trial this approach allows for an increase in intravenous irinotecan dosing from 20 to 30 mg/m^2/day on the d $\times$ 5 $\times$ 2 schedule [14], although the efficacy of higher doses has not been formally assessed.

Another strategy to increase drug exposure is to reduce efflux of irinotecan out of cells by using the small molecule gefitinib to inhibit the ABCG2 drug transporter. Through this mechanism gefitinib can reverse irinotecan resistance in vitro even in cell lines that lack amplification of the epidermal growth factor receptor [24], which is the usual therapeutic target for this agent. ABCG2 is expressed in the small intestine, and co-administration of gefitinib can increase the bioavailability of oral irinotecan by four-fold [25]. Dose-finding studies of gefitinib in combination with both intravenous and oral irinotecan have been reported [22, 25], but there has not yet been efficacy assessment in a phase II trial.

Activity of single-agent irinotecan

Single-agent irinotecan has been studied in a variety of pediatric trials. As predicted from mouse xenograft models [2, 26], responses have consistently been seen in patients with rhabdomyosarcoma and Ewing sarcoma. Response rates as high as 38 % for Ewing sarcoma/primitive neuroectodermal tumor and 16 % for rhabdomyosarcoma have been reported [9]. However, activity of single-agent irinotecan in larger multi-institutional phase II studies has been disappointing. For example, in a Children's Oncology Group (COG) phase II trial using intravenous administration on a d $\times$ 5 schedule, response rates in relapsed patients were under 10 % for both rhabdomyosarcoma and Ewing sarcoma [7]. These results have led to the current practice of partnering irinotecan with another agent, such as vincristine or temozolomide, as described below. There is less experience using irinotecan for treatment of osteosarcoma or

non-rhabdomyosarcoma soft tissue sarcoma, with only rare responses noted [20, 27].

Identifying potential therapeutic partners

Preclinical experience shows camptothecins can synergize with microtubule inhibitors such as vincristine [28]. This combination has been most thoroughly evaluated in rhabdomyosarcoma, a disease in which vincristine is an established active agent. In newly-diagnosed patients with metastatic rhabdomyosarcoma, Pappo et al. reported a response rate of 42 % with single-agent irinotecan, which increased to 70 % when combined with vincristine [15]. The vincristine + irinotecan (VI) combination is tolerable, and a recent phase III trial for newly-diagnosed intermediate-risk rhabdomyosarcoma showed that incorporating cassettes of VI alternating with vincristine, dactinomycin, and cyclophosphamide (VAC) is as effective as using VAC alone, which had historically been the standard treatment for these patients [29]. As expected, febrile neutropenia and thrombocytopenia were less in patients receiving the VI cassettes, although there was more diarrhea. Moving forward, the COG is planning to use the VAC + VI regimen because it reduces the overall exposure to alkylating agents that may cause secondary malignancies and infertility.

Irinotecan has also been paired with the methylating agent temozolomide, given that modest myelosuppression seen from irinotecan allows for combination with drugs having more hematologic toxicity. Houghton et al. demonstrated schedule-dependent synergy with these two drugs against rhabdomyosarcoma xenografts [30], with maximum activity seen when temozolomide is given at least 1 h before irinotecan [31]. This is consistent with the proposed mechanism in which temozolomide-induced methylation of DNA causes localization of topoisomerase I-DNA complexes that are more susceptible to the cytotoxic effects of irinotecan [32]. This temozolomide + irinotecan (TI) combination has been particularly active in Ewing sarcoma, with reported response rates between 29 and 63 % [33–35]. The dose-limiting toxicities of irinotecan (diarrhea) and temozolomide (myelosuppression) are non-overlapping, and the combination is well-suited for oral administration. Because of the tolerability of this regimen, investigators have used TI as a backbone on which to add other drugs such as vincristine [20, 36, 37], as well as biologic agents discussed below.

A variety of other conventional chemotherapy agents have been combined with irinotecan to treat pediatric sarcoma, including carboplatin [38], oxaliplatin and/or gemcitabine [39–41], ifosfamide [42], and docetaxel [43]. None have achieved the response rates reported with VI or TI, and in some cases unexpected toxicities

Table 1 Key phase II and III studies using irinotecan in pediatric sarcoma patients

Reference	Lead author	Phase	Other agents given with irinotecan	Population	Comments
[30]	Hawkins	III	Vincristine	Newly-diagnosed intermediate-risk RMS	VI alternating with VAC is as efficacious as VAC alone, and may reduce long-term toxicity
[15]	Pappo	II	Vincristine	Newly-diagnosed metastatic RMS	Response rate to induction rose from 46–70 % after addition of vincristine
[38]	Dharmajan	II	Carboplatin, radiation	Newly-diagnosed intermediate or high-risk RMS	Local control rate of 89 %; reduced mucositis compared to historical controls
[10]	Mascarenhas	II	Vincristine	Relapsed RMS	Similar rates of response and grade 3–4 toxicity between d × 5 vs d × 5 × 2 schedule
[37]	Mixon	II	Temozolomide, vincristine	Relapsed RMS	One complete response in 4 patients
[33]	Kurucu	II	Temozolomide	Relapsed ES	Response rate 55 %
[34]	Wagner	II	Temozolomide	Relapsed ES	Response rate 29 %
[35]	Casey	II	Temozolomide	Relapsed ES	Response rate 63 %
[36]	Raciborska	II	Temozolomide, vincristine	Relapsed ES	Response rate 68 %
[43]	Yoon	II	Docetaxel	Relapsed ES	Response rate 33 %
[42]	Crews	II	Ifosfamide	Newly-diagnosed high-risk osteosarcoma	Ifosfamide reduced SN-38 exposures

RMS rhabdomyosarcoma, *ES* Ewing sarcoma

or pharmacokinetic interactions were seen. For example, although intermittent dosing of oxaliplatin and irinotecan was well tolerated in adults with colon cancer, severe pancreatic inflammation was seen when oxaliplatin was used together with protracted irinotecan in children [39]. Further, in a combination trial of ifosfamide and irinotecan for osteosarcoma patients, markedly reduced concentrations of SN-38 were noted, suggesting a major drug interaction that could compromise efficacy [42]. These findings demonstrate the importance of performing dose-finding and pharmacokinetic studies for novel combinations. A summary of published combination phase II and III studies of irinotecan-based regimens for pediatric sarcoma is provided in Table 1.

Future combinations to be explored

One focus in sarcoma therapeutics has been the addition of targeted agents onto conventional chemotherapy backbones. This strategy is particularly attractive if the targeted agent has either single-agent activity, or if it potentiates the cytotoxicity of standard chemotherapy drugs. An example is the addition of mTOR inhibitors such as temsirolimus to the TI regimen [21]. Responses in rhabdomyosarcoma patients to single-agent temsirolimus have been limited [44], but its combination with cyclophosphamide and vinorelbine showed promising activity in a recent COG trial [45]. Results from this study provided the rationale for the next upcoming COG phase III trial for intermediate-risk rhabdomyosarcoma, which will study the VAC/VI backbone with or without temsirolimus.

Another example is the combination of irinotecan-based regimens with a monoclonal antibody against the insulin growth factor receptor type I receptor (IGF-1R). Although the single-agent response rates to IGF-1R antibodies in phase II trials have been generally disappointing [reviewed in 46], there have been occasional patients with impressive and durable responses in patients with Ewing sarcoma and rhabdomyosarcoma [47, 48]. The COG has recently completed a phase II trial of the IGF-1R antibody cixutumumab together with multi-agent conventional chemotherapy for patients with newly-diagnosed metastatic rhabdomyosarcoma (ClinicalTrials.gov identifier NCT01055314). Interestingly, in the comparator arm of the study temozolomide was added on to the same chemotherapy backbone, which included irinotecan. Final results of this study are not yet available.

A third example is the use of inhibitors against the DNA repair protein poly(ADP-ribose) polymerase (PARP). This class of drugs was identified through a functional genomics approach and found to have marked preclinical in vitro and in vivo activity against Ewing sarcoma [49]. Although efficacy as monotherapy may be limited [50], the combination of a PARP inhibitor with temozolomide is now being explored in multiple trials, due to the potentiated effects of PARP inhibition following temozolomide-mediated DNA damage [51]. Stewart et al. have recently reported that further preclinical benefit may be seen by combining PARP inhibitors with both temozolomide and irinotecan [52].

Other molecular approaches include the targeting of Wee1, which helps regulate the response to DNA damage by inhibiting CDK1. Wee1 can be targeted with the small molecule MK-1775, which showed in vitro activity against a variety of sarcoma cell lines [53]. Combination with oral irinotecan is now being explored in a COG Phase I trial (ClinicalTrials.gov identifier NCT02095132), based on preclinical synergy with of this combination in neuroblastoma models [54].

It is important to note that not all irinotecan combinations may show benefit for sarcoma, even if used commonly for other tumor types. Although widely employed to treat high-grade glioma, the combination of irinotecan and the anti-VEGF antibody bevacizumab has shown no evidence to date of compelling activity in sarcoma in the limited studies to date [55, 56].

New formulations of irinotecan and SN-38

The process of pegylation joins a drug with a multimeric polyethylene glycol using a glycine linker in order to prolong exposure to the agent. This approach has been applied in an effort to prolong the exposure to irinotecan and/or SN-38. These approaches are attractive in that preclinical studies have demonstrated responses even in irinotecan-resistant xenografts [57], and the schedule of administration is less frequent and therefore more convenient for patients. In a dose-finding study of pegylated SN-38 (EZN-2208), a maximum tolerated dose of 24 mg/m^2 once every 3 weeks was identified, which was higher than the adult MTD of 16.5 mg/m^2 [58]. Some gastrointestinal toxicity was seen at lower doses, with myelosuppression being dose-limiting at the higher doses. Unfortunately, no responses were seen in the 12 sarcoma patients treated on this phase I trial.

The pegylated irinotecan compound etirinotecan (NKTR-102) has shown promising activity in phase II studies of breast and ovarian cancer using a once every 3 weeks schedule [59, 60], and is moving forward in phase III trials. With this formulation, dehydration and diarrhea were the most common grade 3–4 toxicities, occurring in just over 20 % of patients. No trials have yet been reported which partner either of these drugs with other agents, and the long-term future of these agents likely awaits a review of their benefits in larger upcoming trials.

Liposomal preparations of irinotecan have also been developed, and may preferentially accumulate in tumor cells through enhanced permeability and retention [61]. Nanoliposomal irinotecan (MM-398) also minimizes exposure of drug in the serum and so stabilizes the active lactone form of irinotecan versus the inactive carboxylate form [62]. This drug has superior activity over comparably dosed conventional irinotecan in mouse models of Ewing sarcoma [63], and is currently being evaluated in a pediatric clinical trial together with cyclophosphamide (ClinicalTrials.gov identifier NCT02013336).

Conclusions

The role of irinotecan in combination with other agents is becoming more established for the treatment of rhabdomyosarcoma, as well as for relapsed Ewing sarcoma. The d × 5 schedule may be as effective as more protracted administration, and is being used for many current and planned irinotecan trials. Oral administration is feasible for the majority of patients, may have similar activity and toxicity, and offers reduced cost and time away from the clinic. For these reasons, oral administration using a 5-day schedule is now commonly employed in the relapse setting at our institution, as well as in several ongoing clinical trials. Prophylaxis with cephalosporins is an important way to reduce severe irinotecan-associated diarrhea, and is necessary for all patients receiving oral administration of irinotecan. At present there is not a reliable way to identify patients at greatest risk of toxicity, and antibiotic prophylaxis is not routinely necessary for patients receiving intravenous irinotecan at standard doses. The single-agent activity of irinotecan is limited, although its toxicity profile allows for ready combination with a variety of other chemotherapy drugs, especially vincristine and temozolomide. Particularly exciting is the potential for combining irinotecan-based backbones with newer targeted therapies, and the opportunities for testing of the new longer-acting preparations either alone or in combination with other drugs.

Acknowledgements
This work was supported by DanceBlue, an effort of the University of Kentucky student community to support pediatric oncology care and research.

Compliance with ethical guidelines

Competing interests
The author declares no competing interests.

References
1. Furman WL, Stewart CF, Poquette CA, Pratt CB, Santana VM, Zamboni WC, et al. Direct translation of a protracted irinotecan schedule from a xenograft model to a phase I trial in children. J Clin Oncol. 1999;17:1815–24.
2. Houghton PJ, Cheshire PJ, Hallman JD 2nd, Lutz L, Friedman HS, Danks MK, et al. Efficacy of topoisomerase I inhibitors, topotecan and irinotecan, administered at low dose levels in protracted schedules to mice bearing xenografts of human tumors. Cancer Chemother Pharmacol. 1995;36:393–403.
3. Vassal G, Couanet D, Stockdale E, Geoffray A, Geoerger B, Orbach D, et al. Phase II trial of irinotecan in children with relapsed or refractory rhabdomyosarcoma: a joint study of the French Society of Pediatric Oncology and the United Kingdom Children's Cancer Study Group. J Clin Oncol. 2007;25:356–61.
4. Morland B, Platt K, Whelan JS. A phase II window study of irinotecan (CPT-11) in high risk Ewing sarcoma: a Euro-E.W.I.N.G. study. Pediatr Blood Cancer. 2014;61:442–5.

5. Bomgaars L, Kerr J, Berg S, Kuttesch J, Klenke R, Blaney SM. A phase I study of irinotecan administered on a weekly schedule in pediatric patients. Pediatr Blood Cancer. 2006;46:50–5.

6. Shitara T, Shimada A, Hanada R, Matsunaga T, Kawa K, Mugishima H, et al. Irinotecan for children with relapsed solid tumors. Pediatr Hematol Oncol. 2006;23:103–10.

7. Bomgaars LR, Bernstein M, Krailo M, Kadota R, Das S, Chen Z, et al. Phase II trial of irinotecan in children with refractory solid tumors: a Children's Oncology Group Study. J Clin Oncol. 2007;25:4622–7.

8. Cosetti M, Wexler LH, Calleja E, Trippett T, LaQuaglia M, Huvos AG, et al. Irinotecan for pediatric solid tumors: the Memorial Sloan-Kettering experience. J Pediatr Hematol Oncol. 2002;24:101–5.

9. Bisogno G, Riccardi R, Ruggiero A, Arcamone G, Prete A, Surico G, et al. Phase II study of a protracted irinotecan schedule in children with refractory or recurrent soft tissue sarcoma. Cancer. 2006;106:703–7.

10. Mascarenhas L, Lyden ER, Breitfeld PP, Walterhouse DO, Donaldson SS, Paidas CN, et al. Randomized phase II window trial of two schedules of irinotecan with vincristine in patients with first relapse or progression of rhabdomyosarcoma: a report from the Children's Oncology Group. J Clin Oncol. 2010;28:4658–63.

11. Takasuna K, Hagiwara T, Hirohashi M, Kato M, Nomura M, Nagai E, et al. Involvement of beta-glucuronidase in intestinal microflora in the intestinal toxicity of the antitumor camptothecin derivative irinotecan hydrochloride (CPT-11) in rats. Cancer Res. 1996;56:3752–7.

12. Wagner LM, Crews KR, Stewart CF, Rodriguez-Galindo C, McNall-Knapp RY, et al. Reducing irinotecan-associated diarrhea in children. Pediatr Blood Cancer. 2008;50:201–7.

13. Furman WL, Crews KR, Billups C, Wu J, Gajjar AJ, Daw NC, et al. Cefixime allows greater dose escalation of oral irinotecan: a phase I study in pediatric patients with refractory solid tumors. J Clin Oncol. 2006;24:563–70.

14. McGregor LM, Stewart CF, Crews KR, Tagen M, Wozniak A, Wu J, et al. Dose escalation of intravenous irinotecan using oral cefpodoxime: a phase I study in pediatric patients with refractory solid tumors. Pediatr Blood Cancer. 2012;58:372–9.

15. Pappo AS, Lyden E, Breitfeld P, Donaldson SS, Wiener E, Parham D, et al. Two consecutive phase II window trials of irinotecan alone or in combination with vincristine for the treatment of metastatic rhabdomyosarcoma: the Children's Oncology Group. J Clin Oncol. 2007;25:362–9.

16. O'Dwyer PJ, Catalano RB. Uridine diphosphate glucuronosyltransferase (UGT) 1A1 and irinotecan: practical pharmacogenomics arrives in cancer therapy. J Clin Oncol. 2006;24:4534–8.

17. Stewart CF, Panetta JC, O'Shaughnessy MA, Throm SL, Fraga CH, Owens T, et al. UGT1A1 promoter genotype correlates with SN-38 pharmacokinetics, but not severe toxicity in patients receiving low-dose irinotecan. J Clin Oncol. 2007;25:2594–600.

18. Wagner LM, Villablanca JG, Stewart CF, Crews KR, Groshen S, Reynolds CP, et al. Phase I trial of oral irinotecan and temozolomide for children with relapsed high-risk neuroblastoma: a new approach to neuroblastoma therapy consortium study. J Clin Oncol. 2009;27:1290–6.

19. Drengler RL, Kuhn JG, Schaaf LJ, Rodriguez GI, Villalona-Calero MA, Hammond LA, et al. Phase I and pharmacokinetic trial of oral irinotecan administered daily for 5 days every 3 weeks in patients with solid tumors. J Clin Oncol. 1999;17:685–96.

20. Wagner LM, Perentesis JP, Reid JM, Ames MM, Safgren SL, Nelson MD Jr, et al. Phase I trial of two schedules of vincristine, oral irinotecan, and temozolomide (VOIT) for children with relapsed or refractory solid tumors: a Children's Oncology Group phase I consortium study. Pediatr Blood Cancer. 2010;54:538–45.

21. Bagatell R, Norris R, Ingle AM, Ahern C, Voss S, Fox E, et al. Phase 1 trial of temsirolimus in combination with irinotecan and temozolomide in children, adolescents and young adults with relapsed or refractory solid tumors: a Children's Oncology Group Study. Pediatr Blood Cancer. 2014;61:833–9.

22. Brennan RC, Furman W, Mao S, Wu J, Turner DC, Stewart CF, et al. Phase I dose escalation and pharmacokinetic study of oral gefitinib and irinotecan in children with refractory solid tumors. Cancer Chemother Pharmacol. 2014;74:1191–8.

23. Wagner LM. Oral irinotecan for treatment of pediatric solid tumors: ready for prime time? Pediatr Blood Cancer. 2010;54:661–2.

24. Stewart CF, Leggas M, Schuetz JD, Panetta JC, Cheshire PJ, Peterson J, et al. Gefitinib enhances the antitumor activity and oral bioavailability of irinotecan in mice. Cancer Res. 2004;64:7491–9.

25. Furman WL, Navid F, Daw NC, McCarville MB, McGregor LM, Spunt SL, et al. Tyrosine kinase inhibitor enhances the bioavailability of oral irinotecan in pediatric patients with refractory solid tumors. J Clin Oncol. 2009;27:4599–604.

26. Vassal G, Terrier-Lacombe MJ, Bissery MC, Vénuat AM, Gyergyay F, Bénard J, et al. Therapeutic activity of CPT-11, a DNA-topoisomerase I inhibitor, against peripheral primitive neuroectodermal tumour and neuroblastoma xenografts. Br J Cancer. 1996;74:537–45.

27. McNall-Knapp RY, Williams CN, Reeves EN, Heideman RL, Meyer WH. Extended phase I evaluation of vincristine, irinotecan, temozolomide, and antibiotic in children with refractory solid tumors. Pediatr Blood Cancer. 2010;54:909–15.

28. Thompson J, George EO, Poquette CA, Cheshire PJ, Richmond LB, de Graaf SS, et al. Synergy of topotecan in combination with vincristine for treatment of pediatric solid tumor xenografts. Clin Cancer Res. 1999;5:3617–31.

29. Hawkins DS, Anderson JR, Mascarenhas L, McGowage GB, Rodeberg DA, Wolden SL, et al. Vincristine, dactinomycin, cyclophosphamide (VAC versus VAC/V plus irinotecan for intermediate-risk rhabdomyosarcoma: a report from the Children's Oncology Group Soft Tissue sarcoma Committee. J Clin Oncol. 2014;32:suppl abstr 10004.

30. Houghton PJ, Stewart CF, Cheshire PJ, Richmond LB, Kirstein MN, Poquette CA, et al. Antitumor activity of temozolomide combined with irinotecan is partly independent of O6-methylguanine-DNA methyltransferase and mismatch repair phenotypes in xenograft models. Clin Cancer Res. 2000;6:4110–8.

31. Patel VJ, Elion GB, Houghton PJ, Keir S, Pegg AE, Johnson SP, et al. Schedule-dependent activity of temozolomide plus CPT-11 against a human central nervous system tumor-derived xenograft. Clin Cancer Res. 2000;6:4154–7.

32. Pourquier P, Waltman JL, Urasaki Y, Loktionova NA, Pegg AE, Nitiss JL, et al. Topoisomerase I-mediated cytotoxicity of N-methyl-N'-nitro-N-nitrosoguanidine: trapping of topoisomerase I by the O6-methylguanine. Cancer Res. 2001;61:53–8.

33. Kurucu N, Sari N, Ilhan IE. Irinotecan and temozolamide treatment for relapsed Ewing sarcoma: a single-center experience and review of the literature. Pediatr Hematol Oncol. 2015;32:50–9.

34. Wagner LM, McAllister N, Goldsby RE, Rausen AR, McNall-Knapp RY, McCarville MB, et al. Temozolomide and intravenous irinotecan for treatment of advanced Ewing sarcoma. Pediatr Blood Cancer. 2007;48:132–9.

35. Casey DA, Wexler LH, Merchant MS, Chou AJ, Merola PR, Price AP, et al. Irinotecan and temozolomide for Ewing sarcoma: the Memorial Sloan-Kettering experience. Pediatr Blood Cancer. 2009;53:1029–34.

36. Raciborska A, Bilska K, Drabko K, Chaber R, Pogorzala M, Wyrobek E, et al. Vincristine, irinotecan, and temozolomide in patients with relapsed and refractory Ewing sarcoma. Pediatr Blood Cancer. 2013;60:1621–5.

37. Mixon BA, Eckrich MJ, Lowas S, Engel ME. Vincristine, irinotecan, and temozolomide for treatment of relapsed alveolar rhabdomyosarcoma. J Pediatr Hematol Oncol. 2013;35:e163–6.

38. Dharmarajan KV, Wexler LH, Wolden SL. Concurrent radiation with irinotecan and carboplatin in intermediate- and high-risk rhabdomyosarcoma: a report on toxicity and efficacy from a prospective pilot phase II study. Pediatr Blood Cancer. 2013;60:242–7.

39. McGregor LM, Spunt SL, Furman WL, Stewart CF, Schaiquevich P, Krailo MD, et al. Phase 1 study of oxaliplatin and irinotecan in pediatric patients with refractory solid tumors: a children's oncology group study. Cancer. 2009;115:1765–75.

40. Hartmann C, Weinel P, Schmid H, Grigull L, Sander A, Linderkamp C, et al. Oxaliplatin, irinotecan, and gemcitabine: a novel combination in the therapy of progressed, relapsed, or refractory tumors in children. J Pediatr Hematol Oncol. 2011;33:344–9.

41. Zak D, Styler MJ, Rosenbluth JZ, Brodsky I. Combination of gemcitabine and irinotecan for recurrent metastatic osteogenic sarcoma. Clin Adv Hematol Oncol. 2005;3:297–9.

42. Crews KR, Stewart CF, Liu T, Rodriguez-Galindo C, Santana VM, Daw NC. Effect of fractionated ifosfamide on the pharmacokinetics of irinotecan in pediatric patients with osteosarcoma. J Pediatr Hematol Oncol. 2004;26:764–7.

43. Yoon JH, Kwon MM, Park HJ, Park SY, Lim KY, Joo J, et al. A study of docetaxel and irinotecan in children and young adults with recurrent or refractory Ewing sarcoma family of tumors. BMC Cancer. 2014;14:622.

44. Geoerger B, Kieran MW, Grupp S, Perek D, Clancy J, Krygowski M, et al. Phase II trial of temsirolimus in children with high-grade glioma, neuroblastoma, and rhabdomyosarcoma. Eur J Cancer. 2012;48:253–62.

45. Mascarenhas L, Meyer WH, Lyden E, Rodeberg DA, Indelicato DJ, Linardic CM, et al. Randomized phase II trial of bevacizumab and temsirolimus in combination with vinorelbine and cyclophosphamide for first relapse/disease progression of rhabdomyosarcoma: a report from the Children's Oncology Group. J Clin Oncol. 2014;32:suppl abstr 10003.

46. Olmos D, Tan DS, Jones RL, Judson IR. Biological rationale and current clinical experience with anti-insulin-like growth factor 1 receptor monoclonal antibodies in treating sarcoma: twenty years from the bench to the bedside. Cancer J. 2010;16:183–94.

47. Malempati S, Weigel B, Ingle AM, Ahern CH, Carroll JM, Roberts CT, et al. Phase I/II trial and pharmacokinetic study of cixutumumab in pediatric patients with refractory solid tumors and Ewing sarcoma: a report from the Children's Oncology Group. J Clin Oncol. 2012;30:256–62.

48. Weigel B, Malempati S, Reid JM, Voss SD, Cho SY, Chen HX, et al. Phase 2 trial of cixutumumab in children, adolescents, and young adults with refractory solid tumors: a report from the Children's Oncology Group. Pediatr Blood Cancer. 2014;61:452–6.

49. Garnett MJ, Edelman EJ, Heidorn SJ, Greenman CD, Dastur A, Lau KW, et al. Systematic identification of genomic markers of drug sensitivity in cancer cells. Nature. 2012;483:570–5.

50. Choy E, Butrynski JE, Harmon DC, Morgan JA, George S, Wagner AJ, et al. Phase II study of olaparib in patients with refractory Ewing sarcoma following failure of standard chemotherapy. BMC Cancer. 2014;14:813.

51. Smith MA, Reynolds CP, Kang MH, Kolb EA, Gorlick R, Carol H, et al. Synergistic activity of PARP inhibition by talazoparib (BMN 673) with temozolomide in pediatric cancer models in the pediatric preclinical testing program. Clin Cancer Res. 2015;21:819–32.

52. Stewart E, Goshorn R, Bradley C, Griffiths LM, Benavente C, Twarog NR, et al. Targeting the DNA repair pathway in Ewing sarcoma. Cell Rep. 2014;9:829–41.

53. Kreahling JM, Gemmer JY, Reed D, Letson D, Bui M, Altiok S. MK1775, a selective Wee1 inhibitor, shows single-agent antitumor activity against sarcoma cells. Mol Cancer Ther. 2012;11:174–82.

54. Russell MR, Levin K, Rader J, Belcastro L, Li Y, Martinez D, et al. Combination therapy targeting the Chk1 and Wee1 kinases shows therapeutic efficacy in neuroblastoma. Cancer Res. 2013;15(73):776–84.

55. Wagner L, Turpin B, Nagarajan R, Weiss B, Cripe T, Geller J. Pilot study of vincristine, oral irinotecan, and temozolomide (VOIT regimen) combined with bevacizumab in pediatric patients with recurrent solid tumors or brain tumors. Pediatr Blood Cancer. 2013;60:1447–51.

56. Okada K, Yamasaki K, Tanaka C, Fujisaki H, Osugi Y, Hara J. Phase I study of bevacizumab plus irinotecan in pediatric patients with recurrent/refractory solid tumors. Jpn J Clin Oncol. 2013;43:1073–9.

57. Pastorino F, Loi M, Sapra P, Becherini P, Cilli M, Emionite L, et al. Tumor regression and curability of preclinical neuroblastoma models by PEGylated SN38 (EZN-2208), a novel topoisomerase I inhibitor. Clin Cancer Res. 2010;16:4809–21.

58. Norris RE, Shusterman S, Gore L, Muscal JA, Macy ME, Fox E, et al. Phase 1 evaluation of EZN-2208, a polyethylene glycol conjugate of SN38, in children adolescents and young adults with relapsed or refractory solid tumors. Pediatr Blood Cancer. 2014;61:1792–7.

59. Awada A, Garcia AA, Chan S, Jerusalem GH, Coleman RE, Huizing MT, et al. Two schedules of etirinotecan pegol (NKTR-102) in patients with previously treated metastatic breast cancer: a randomised phase 2 study. Lancet Oncol. 2013;14:1216–25.

60. Vergote IB, Garcia A, Micha J, Pippitt C, Bendell J, Spitz D, et al. Randomized multicenter phase II trial comparing two schedules of etirinotecan pegol (NKTR-102) in women with recurrent platinum-resistant/refractory epithelial ovarian cancer. J Clin Oncol. 2013;31:4060–6.

61. Kalra AV, Kim J, Klinz SG, Paz N, Cain J, Drummond DC, Nielsen UB, Fitzgerald JB. Preclinical activity of nanoliposomal irinotecan is governed by tumor deposition and intratumor prodrug conversion. Cancer Res. 2014;74:7003–13.

62. Drummond DC, Noble CO, Guo Z, Hong K, Park JW, Kirpotin DB. Development of a highly active nanoliposomal irinotecan using a novel intraliposomal stabilization strategy. Cancer Res. 2006;66:3271–7.

63. Kang MH, Wang J, Makena MR, Lee JS, Paz N, Hall CP, et al. Activity of MM-398, nanoliposomal irinotecan (nal-IRI), in Ewing's family tumor xenografts is associated with high exposure of tumor to drug and high SLFN11 expression. Clin Cancer Res. 2015;21:1139–50.

7

Two years survival of primary cardiac leiomyosarcoma managed by surgical and adjuvant therapy

K. Behi*◉, M. Ayadi, E. Mezni, K. Meddeb, A. Mokrani, Y. Yahyaoui, F. Ksontini, H. Rais, N. Chrait and A. Mezlini

Abstract

Background: Cardiac tumors are a very rare entity. Leiomyosarcoma represents less than 1% of cases.

Case presentation: a 51-year-old woman diagnosed with primary left atrium leiomyosarcoma. She was treated by optimal surgery and adjuvant chemotherapy. She is still alive after a follow-up of 24 months without evidence of local or distant recurrence.

Conclusions: Cardiac leiomyosarcoma is a rare tumor with a dismal prognosis. Surgery is the mainstay of treatment. Adjuvant treatment is still controversial.

Keywords: Leiomyosarcoma, Cardiac tumors, Survival, Chemotherapy

Background

Cardiac tumors are a very rare entity with an incidence of 0.02%. Only 25% are malignant with a prevalence ranging from 0.001% to 0.28 [1]. Primary cardiac cancers are scarcer than cardiac metastases [2]. Most frequent histologic types are Angiosarcomas followed by rhabdomyosarcomas, mesotheliomas and fibrosarcomas. Leiomyosarcoma represents less than 1% of cases [3]. In spite of improvement of multidisciplinary treatment including surgery, chemotherapy and radiotherapy, the prognosis remains (Fig. 1) poor with a median survival of 6 months [3].

This case aimed to describe the clinical, histological, therapeutic and prognostic features of this rare pathology.

Case report

We present the case of a 51-year-old woman, with past medical history of hypertension, who consulted in September 2014 for bilateral lower limb pain and lower extremity edema since 6 months. The diagnosis of hypertrophic osteoarthropathy was suspected. In this context, a CT

scan revealed a 6 cm defect, involving the right atrium and the right inferior pulmonary vein, which appears markedly enlarged. This aspect evoked a large intracavitary thrombus. A transesophageal cardiac ultrasound showed a 30 × 26 mm, with little mobility, lobed tumor, in the left atrium, connected to the atrial septum. The tumor wasn't obstructive. Cardiac chambers dimensions and pulmonary pressure were normal. There was no systolic or diastolic left ventricular dysfunction. The patient was referred to a cardiovascular surgeon with a suspected diagnosis of left atrium myxoma. Surgery was performed through median sternotomy. The patient had a cardiopulmonary bypass (CPB) with aortic and bi-caval cannulation. The left atrium was dissected, revealing a voluminous, septal based tumor involving the right inferior pulmonary vein and the posterior wall of the left atrium, suggestive of malignancy. We did a wide en bloc excision of the tumor, extended from the posterior wall of the left atrium Fig. 2 and inferior pulmonary vein to pericardial reflection. Reconstruction of the left atrium with two pericardial patches (an anterior septal and posterior parietal) was achieved according to Sutureless de lacourt-Gayettechnique. Macroscopic examination showed a friable whitish mass measuring 40 × 30 × 30 mm.

Microscopic examination revealed the presence of conjunctival tumoral proliferation made of spindle cells with

*Correspondence: kh.elbehi@gmail.com
Medical Oncology Department, Salah Azaeiz Institute, Tunis, Tunisia

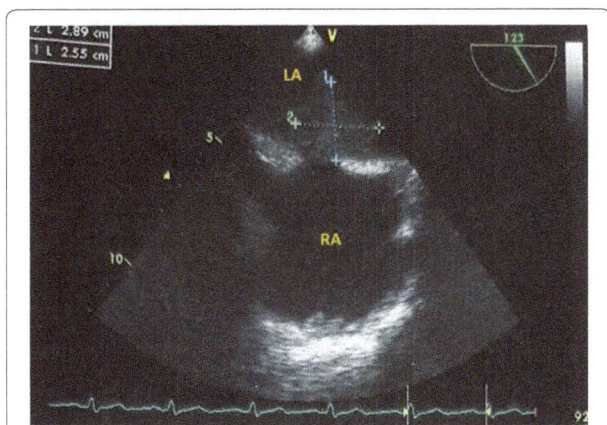

Fig. 1 Transoesophageal echocardiography showing mid esophageal 20° view. Left atrium tumor. *RA* right atrium, *LA* left atrium

a fascicular organization infiltrating myocardial fibers. A high mitotic activity was noticed. Surgical margins were clear. Immunohistochemical staining showed an intense and diffuse positivity of alpha-smooth-muscle actin and caldesmon and the negativity of PS100, desmine and myogenin. Based on these findings, diagnosis of primary cardiac leiomyosarcoma grade 3 according to FNNCLCC was confirmed.

Post-operative CT scan revealed no metastases. According to a multidisciplinary staff, an adjuvant chemotherapy consisting on six cycles of Doxorubicin and Ifosfamide was prescribed.

The patient is regularly followed. After a follow-up of 24 months, she still has no clinical or radiological evidence of recurrence.

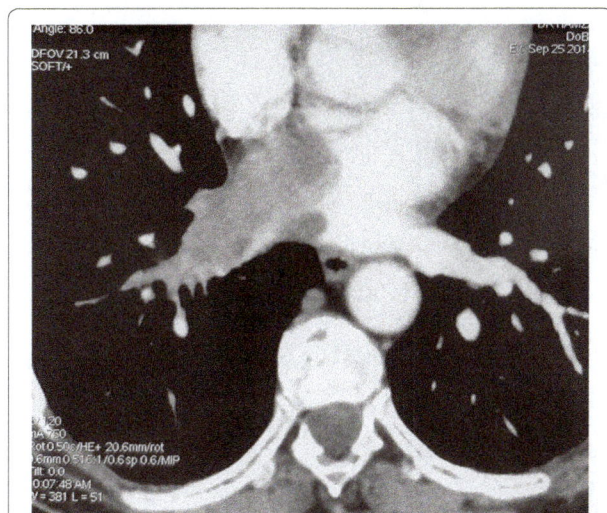

Fig. 2 Computed tomography; Transverse section: 6 cm defect involving the right atrium and the right inferior pulmonary vein, which appears markedly enlarged

Discussion

We presented a rare case of cardiac leiomyosarcoma treated by surgery followed by an adjuvant chemotherapy. The patient is still alive after a follow-up of 24 months.

Until December 2015, we found only 32 cases of primary cardiac leiomyosarcoma with available data. In most studies, it was defined as tumors originating only from cardiac chambers, excluding those located in the pericardium and great vessels [4]. Epidemiological, clinical, therapeutic features and outcomes were listed in the Table 1.

Median age at diagnosis was 48 with a female predominance [4].

This tumor has a poor prognosis due essentially to advanced stages at presentation. It usually remains asymptomatic until advanced stages. Even when it becomes symptomatic, presentation is atypical and non specific. Symptoms of obstruction especially dyspnea is found in 78.1% of cases [4]. Physical examination isn't helpful no more. In our case, the patient was asymptomatic and the diagnosis was suspected fortuitously on the findings of a CT performed for another aim.

Echocardiography, especially the trans-esophageal route, is habitually the initial imaging modality. It may show the tumor, its extent and its hemodynamic consequences (Fig. 1). CT scan and cardiac MRI provide further information about morphology, location and extent of the mass (Fig. 2). Cardiac MRI is more efficient to evaluate myocardial involvement. CT scan is useful to assess extracardiac extent and metastasis [5].

Cardiac leiomyosarcomas have a high rate of local and distant recurrence, occurring even after an optimal resection of the primary tumor.

The left atrium is the most frequent location of cardiac leiomyosarcomas (51%). That joins operative and radiological findings, in our case.

Biopsy is the gold standard for histological confirmation but this step can sometimes be overtaken and the diagnosis is then made on the examination of resected mass.

Complete surgical resection, when it's possible, is the mainstay of treatment.

Since soft tissue sarcoma is a heterogeneous group, benefits of adjuvant chemotherapy isn't clearly established. Several studies defined subgroups associated with a high risk of local and distant relapse. Risk varies depending on factors like size >5 cm, high grade, depth and chemosensitive histologies with a metastatic potential. Leiomyosarcoma belongs to the high risk group. Major drugs used are Doxorubicin, Ifosfamide and Dacarbazine [6]. It's what leaded us to propose six cycles of Doxorubicin and Ifosfamide in adjuvant setting to our patient, after a multidisciplinary team consultation.

Table 1 Epidemiological, clinical, therapeutic features and outcomes of reported cases of primary cardiac leiomyosarcomas

	Author	Age	Sex	Symptom	Site	Size (cm)	Surgery	Chemotherapy	Radiotherapy	Survival (months)
1	Kornberg [8]	21	F	N	RA	6	R2	Doxorubicin–ifosfamamide	N	3
2	Takamizawa [9]	53	M	Cough Inferior limbs oedema	RA	3	N	N	N	0.5
3	Fox [10]	61	M	Chest pain Vomiting	LV	9	R2	N	N	6
4	Ishitoya [11]	26	F	Dyspnea Inferior limbs oedema	LA	7	R0	N	N	5
5	Hattori [11]	19	M	Dyspnea Hemoptysis	LA	13	R0	N	Y	2
6	Minakata [12]	69	F	Dyspnea Cyanosis	LA	6	R0	N	N	3
7	Pins [13]	29	F	Chest pain	RV	3	R0	N	N	NA
8	Pins [13]	25	M	Syncope	RA	9	R0	Doxorubicin–ifosfamide— Actino-Doxorubicin	Y	60
9	Minardi [14]	67	M	Dyspnea Cough	LA	8 and 2	R0	N	N	7
10	Burnett [15]	60	F	Dyspnea	RV	NA	R2	N	N	0
11	Andersen [16]	86	F	Pulmonary oedema	LA	4	R0	N	N	15
12	Ogimoto [17]	73	F	Dyspnea	LA	NA	R0	N	N	3
13	Willaret [18]	70	F	Dyspnea Chest pain Palpitation	RV	4	R0	N	N	7
14	Strina [19]	33	F	Dyspnea Syncope	LA	8	R0	Doxorubicin–ifosfamide	Y	29
15	Lee [20]	45	F	Dyspnea	RV	8	R2	Doxorubicin–ifosfamide	N	NA
16	Malyshev [21]	43	F	Pulmonary oedema	LA	NA	R2	Doxorubicin–ifosfamide	N	15
17	Smith [22]	40	F	Dyspnea	LA	7	R1	N	Y	18
18	Antunes [23]	53	F	Pulmonary oedema	LA	NA	R2	Metoxantrone Dacarbazine Cyclophosphamide	N	6
19	Rastan [24]	76	F	Dyspnea	RV	6	R1	N	N	NA
20	Antunes [23]	33	F	Anorexia Tirednes, Dyspnea Chest tightness	RA	4	R0	N	N	5
21	Astarcioğlu [25]	40	F	Dyspnea	RV	9	R0	Doxorubicin	N	42
22	Glaoui [26]	47	M	Pulmonary oedema Dyspnea	RA	5	R0	Doxorubicin–ifosfamide	N	7
23	Nakanishi [27]	74	M	Dyspnea	LA	NA	R0	N	Y	8

Table 1 continued

	Author	Age	Sex	Symptom	Site	Size (cm)	Surgery	Chemotherapy	Radiotherapy	Survival (months)
24	Wilbring [28]	43	M	Paravertebral back pain Dyspnea	LA	6	R0	N	Y	9
25	Parissis [29]	36	M	Dyspnea	RA	NA	R0	Doxorubicin–Ifosfamide	N	NA
26	Mazzolla [30]	21	F	N	LA	7	R0	Doxorubicin–Ifosfamide- cis-platin	N	24
27	Esaki [31]	68	M	Dyspnea	RV	NA	R0	N	N	2
28	Guschmann [32]	61	F	Dyspnea	LA	NA	R0	Y	N	NA
29	Davis [33]	65	F	Dyspnea Chest pain	LA	6	R0	Y	N	18
30	Panday [34]	67	M	Dyspnea	RV	NA	R0	N	N	36
31	Pessotto [35]	24	M	Syncope Atrial fibrillation	LA	7	R1	Doxorubicin–Ifosfamide— Actino-Doxorubicin	Y	84
32	Lo [36]	28	F	Long term fever Body weight loss	LA	5	R0	Y	N	5

RA right atrium, *LA* left atrium, *RV* right ventricle, *LV* left ventricle, *R0* macroscopically complete resection, *R1* resection with microscopic margins, *R2* resection with macroscopic margins, *N* no, *Y*, yes, *NA*, not available

Indications of radiation therapy are mostly restrained to palliative setting. It's proposed when margins of resection are positive or for aggressive localized disease or for recurrences. Since the lack of evidence concerning the efficacy of radiotherapy in management of cardiac leiomyosarcomas and the poor tolerance, its use stills equivocal and unusual.

According to the reported cases of leiomyosarcomas with cardiac involvement, the mean survival time of patients who underwent surgery and chemotherapy was about 12 months [6]. Several factors are suspected to enworse the prognosis particularly the high grade, a high mitotic index, positive surgical margins and metastasis [7].

In the case above, our patient had a grade 3 tumor with a high mitotic activity. She underwent a carcinologic surgery and adjuvant chemotherapy. Currently, she is still alive and there is no evidence of local recurrence or metastasis, after a follow-up of 24 months.

Conclusions

Cardiac leiomyosarcoma is a rare tumor with a dismal prognosis. Wide margin resection is the mainstay of treatment. For soft tissue sarcoma, adjuvant chemotherapy is still controversial. Nevertheless, leiomyosarcoma belongs to the high risk group of soft tissue sarcoma associated with a metastatic potential. In this group, there is a trend to outcomes improvement with adjuvant chemotherapy. Drugs used in this context are Doxorubicin, Ifosfamide and Dacarbazine.

Regarding the scarcity of this disease, it's important to report all cases with a longer follow-up to refine indications and modalities of adjuvant treatment and prognostic factors.

Authors' contributions
Conception and design: FK; YY. Administrative support: AM; HR; NC. Provision of study materials or patients: AM; KM. Collection and assembly of data: EM. Data analysis and interpretation: KB; MA. Manuscript writing: All authors. All authors read and approved the final manuscript.

Acknowledgements
Not applicable.

Competing interests
The authors declare that they have no competing interests.

References
1. Smith S, Grange S, Wilson P. Leiomyosarcoma of the left atrium. A case study. Radiography. 2012;18(3):225–8.
2. Isambert N, Ray-Coquard I, Italiano A, Rios M, Kerbrat P, Gauthier M, et al. Primary cardiac sarcomas: a retrospective study of the French Sarcoma Group 1990. Eur J Cancer Oxf Engl. 2014;50(1):128–36.
3. Andersen RE, Kristensen BW, Gill S. Cardiac leiomyosarcoma, a case report. Int J Clin Exp Pathol. 2013;6(6):1197–9.
4. Wang J-G, Cui L, Jiang T, Li Y-J, Wei Z-M. Primary cardiac leiomyosarcoma: an analysis of clinical characteristics and outcome patterns. Asian Cardiovasc Thorac Ann. 2015;23(5):623–30.
5. Galeone A, Validire P, Debrosse D, Folliguet T, Laborde F. Leiomyosarcoma of the right inferior pulmonary vein: 2 years survival with multimodality therapy. Gen Thorac Cardiovasc Surg. 2013;61(9):534–7.
6. Steen S, Stephenson G. Current treatment of soft tissue sarcoma. Proc Bayl Univ Med Cent. 2008;21(4):392–6.
7. Lv Y, Pang X, Zhang Q, Jia D. Cardial leiomyosarcoma with multiple lesions involved: a case report. Int J Clin Exp Pathol. 2015;8(11):15412–6.
8. Kornberg A, Wildhirt SM, Kreuzer E, Reichart B. Asymptomatic right atrial leiomyosarcoma with tricuspid valve obstruction in a young female patient. Eur J Cardio Thorac Surg Off J Eur Assoc Cardio Thorac Surg. 1998;14:635–8.
9. Takamizawa S, Sugimoto K, Tanaka H, Sakai O, Arai T, Saitoh A. A case of primary leiomyosarcoma of the heart. Intern Med Tokyo Jpn. 1992;31:265–8.
10. Fox JP, Freitas E, McGiffin DC, Firouz-Abadi AA, West MJ. Primary leiomyosarcoma of the heart: a rare cause of obstruction of the left ventricular outflow tract. Aust N Z J Med. 1991;21:881–3.
11. Hattori Y, Iriyama T, Watanabe K, Negi K, Takeda I, Sugimura S. Rapidly growing primary cardiac leiomyosarcoma: report of a case. Surg Today. 2000;30:838–40. doi:10.1007/s005950070069.
12. Minakata K, Konishi Y, Matsumoto M, Nonaka M, Yamada N. Primary leiomyosarcoma of the left atrium. Jpn Circ J. 1999;63:414–5.
13. Pins MR, Ferrell MA, Madsen JC, Piubello Q, Dickersin GR, Fletcher CD. Epithelioid and spindle-celled leiomyosarcoma of the heart. Report of 2 cases and review of the literature. Arch Pathol Lab Med. 1999;123:782–8. doi:10.1043/0003-9985(1999)123<0782:EASCLO>2.0.CO;2.
14. Minardi G, Pulignano G, Sentinelli S, Narducci C, Giovannini M. Left atrial leiomyosarcoma: double occurrence and double recurrence—report of one case. J Am Soc Echocardiogr Off Publ Am Soc Echocardiogr. 1998;11:1171–6.
15. Burnett RA. Primary cardiac leiomyosarcoma with pulmonary metastases: a diagnostic problem. Scott Med J. 1975;20:125–8.
16. Andersen RE, Kristensen BW, Gill S. Cardiac leiomyosarcoma, a case report. Int J Clin Exp Pathol. 2013;6:1197–9.
17. Ogimoto A, Hamada M, Ohtsuka T, Hara Y, Shigematsu Y, Yokoyama A, et al. Rapid progression of primary cardiac leiomyosarcoma with obstruction of the left ventricular outflow tract and mitral stenosis. Intern Med Tokyo Jpn. 2003;42:827–30.
18. Willaert W, Claessens P, Shoja A, Heremans A, Deferm H, Roelandts J, et al. Ventricular outflow tract obstruction secondary to leiomyosarcoma of the right ventricle. Jpn Heart J. 2001;42:377–86.
19. Strina C, Zannoni M, Parolin V, Cetto GL, Zuliani S. Bone metastases from primary cardiac sarcoma: case report. Tumori. 2009;95:251–3.
20. Lee SH, Kim WH, Choi JB, Lee SR, Rhee KS, Chae JK, et al. Huge primary pleomorphic leiomyosarcoma in the right ventricle with impending obstruction of both inflow and outflow tracts. Circ J Off J Jpn Circ Soc. 2009;73:779–82.
21. Malyshev M, Safuanov A, Gladyshev I, Trushyna V, Abramovskaya L, Malyshev A. Primary left atrial leiomyosarcoma: literature review and lessons of a case. Asian Cardiovasc Thorac Ann. 2006;14:435–40. doi:10.1177/021849230601400520.
22. Smith S, Grange S, Wilson P. Leiomyosarcoma of the left atrium. A case study. Radiography. 2012;18:225–8. doi:10.1016/j.radi.2012.01.002.
23. Antunes MJ, Vanderdonck KM, Andrade CM, Rebelo LS. Primary cardiac leiomyosarcomas. Ann Thorac Surg. 1991;51:999–1001. doi:10.1016/0003-4975(91)91031-P.
24. Rastan AJ, Walther T, Mohr FW, Kostelka M. Leiomyosarcoma-an unusual cause of right ventricular outflow tract obstruction. Thorac Cardiovasc Surg. 2004;52:376–7. doi:10.1055/s-2004-821276.
25. Astarcioglu MA. Multimodality imaging of a recurrent case of right-sided cardiac leiomyosarcoma with an unusual clinical course. Turk Kardiyol Dernegi Arsivi Arch Turk Soc Cardiol. 2016. doi:10.5543/tkda.2015.09125.
26. Glaoui M, Benbrahim Z, Belbaraka R, Naciri S, Errihani H, Lescene A. An uncommon long-term survival case of primary cardiac leiomyosarcoma. World J Surg Oncol. 2014;12:338. doi:10.1186/1477-7819-12-338.

27. Nakanishi H, Furukawa K, Noguchi R, Furutachi A, Itoh M, Kamohara K, et al. Primary cardiac leiomyosarcoma originating from the left atrium. Kyobu Geka. 2012;65:1057–61.
28. Wilbring M, Kappert U, Daubner D, Matschke K, Tugtekin SM. Metastasizing primary atrial leiomyosarcoma causing a functional high-grade mitral stenosis. Heart Surg Forum. 2012;15:E108–10. doi:10.1532/HSF98.20111147.
29. Parissis H, Akbar MT, Young V. Primary leiomyosarcoma of the right atrium: a case report and literature update. J Cardiothorac Surg. 2010;5:80. doi:10.1186/1749-8090-5-80.
30. Mazzola A, Spano J-P, Valente M, Gregorini R, Villani C, Eusanio MD, et al. Leiomyosarcoma of the left atrium mimicking a left atrial myxoma. J Thorac Cardiovasc Surg. 2006;131:224–6. doi:10.1016/j.jtcvs.2005.07.061.
31. Esaki M, Kagawa K, Noda T, Nishigaki K, Gotoh K, Fujiwara H, et al. Primary cardiac leiomyosarcoma growing rapidly and causing right ventricular outflow obstruction. Intern Med Tokyo Jpn. 1998;37:370–5.
32. Guschmann M, Hofmeister J. Primary leiomyosarcoma in the left atrium—a rarity. Case report and literature review. J Pathol. 1997;18:474–9.
33. Davis GK, Jones EL, Bonser RS, Roberts DH. Coronary arteriographic and pathological findings in a case of primary leiomyosarcoma of the heart. Int J Cardiol. 1997;59:313–6. doi:10.1016/S0167-5273(97)02967-7.
34. Panday VRN, Cramer MJM, Elbers HRJ, Riviere AB, Ernst SMPG, Plokker HWT. Primary leiomyosarcoma of the heart presenting as obstruction to the pulmonary trunk. Am Heart J. 1997;133:465–6. doi:10.1016/S0002-8703(97)70191-1.
35. Pessotto R, Silvestre G, Luciani GB, Anselmi M, Pasini F, Santini F, et al. Primary cardiac leiomyosarcoma: seven-year survival with combined surgical and adjuvant therapy. Int J Cardiol. 1997;60:91–4.
36. Lo FL, Chou YH, Tiu CM, Lan GY, Hwang JH, Chern MS, et al. Primary cardiac leiomyosarcoma: imaging with 2-D echocardiography, electron beam CT and 1.5-Tesla MR. Eur J Radiol. 1998;27:72–6.

8

Clinical implications of repeated drug monitoring of imatinib in patients with metastatic gastrointestinal stromal tumour

Ivar Hompland[1,2], Øyvind Sverre Bruland[1,2], Kumari Ubhayasekhera[3], Jonas Bergquist[3] and Kjetil Boye[1,4*]

Abstract

Background: Imatinib mesylate (IM) is the preferred treatment for the majority of patients with metastatic gastrointestinal stromal tumour (GIST). Low trough IM concentration (C_{min}) values have been associated with poor clinical outcomes in GIST patients. However, there are few studies of repeated measurements of IM levels, and therapeutic drug monitoring is not yet a part of routine clinical practice. This study was conducted to reveal clinical scenarios where plasma concentration measurement of IM trough level (C_{min}) is advantageous.

Methods: Patients with advanced GIST receiving IM were included from January 2011 to April 2015. Heparin plasma was collected at each follow-up visit. Ninety-six samples from 24 patients were selected for IM concentration measurement. Associations between IM plasma concentration and clinical variables were analyzed by Students' t test, univariate and multivariate linear regression analyses.

Results: The mean IM C_{min} plasma concentrations for patients taking <400, 400 and >400 mg daily were 782, 1132 and 1665 ng/mL, respectively (p = 0.010). High IM C_{min} levels were correlated with age, low body surface area, low haemoglobin concentration, low creatinine clearance, absence of liver metastasis and no prior gastric resection in univariate analysis. In multivariate analysis age, gastric resection and liver metastasis were included in the final model. Eight patients had disease progression during the study, and mean IM levels were significantly lower at time of progression compared to the previous measurement for the same patients (770 and 1223 ng/mL, respectively; p = 0.020).

Conclusions: Our results do not support repeated monitoring of IM levels on a routine basis in all patients. However, we have revealed clinical scenarios where drug measurement could be beneficial, such as for patients who have undergone gastric resection, suspicion of non-compliance, subjectively reported side effects, in elderly patients and at the time of disease progression.

Keywords: Gastrointestinal stromal tumour, Drug monitoring, Imatinib, Plasma concentration

Background

Since the introduction of imatinib mesylate (IM) [1], the outcome of metastatic gastrointestinal stromal tumour (GIST) has improved considerably [2]. IM is an inhibitor of receptor tyrosine kinases, including the stem cell factor receptor *KIT* and the platelet-derived growth factor receptor alpha (*PDGFRA*), the main drivers of tumour development in GIST [3]. Several clinical trials have demonstrated the efficacy and safety of IM, and it has become the treatment of choice for the majority of patients with metastatic GIST [2, 4, 5]. The median duration of response to IM in metastatic GIST is 29 months [2], with approximately 20% of the responses lasting 10 years or more [6]. Still, most patients eventually progress on IM, requiring second- and third-line therapy with other tyrosine kinase inhibitors such as sunitinib and regorafinib [7].

*Correspondence: kjetil.boye@rr-research.no
[1] Department of Oncology, Norwegian Radium Hospital, Oslo University Hospital, PO Box 4953, Nydalen, 0424 Oslo, Norway
Full list of author information is available at the end of the article

In patients with chronic myeloid leukaemia (CML) and GIST, pharmacokinetic (PK) studies have shown that IM has >90% bioavailability following oral administration [8]. IM plasma concentration is influenced by various factors such age, body weight, body surface area (BSA), previous major gastric resection, white blood cell (WBC) count, haemoglobin, creatinine clearance, albumin, and alpha glycoprotein (AGP) levels [9–15]. A retrospective sub-study from the B2222 trial [4], the first trial showing safety and efficacy of IM in metastatic GIST patients, presented a significantly shorter time to progression in patients with IM trough levels (C_{min}) below 1110 ng/mL at day 29 [16]. Additionally, a retrospective study in patients with CML in chronic phase reported that C_{min} of IM could predict clinical outcome [13]. However, the optimal threshold value of IM C_{min} has yet to be determined; both in patients with GIST and CML. A prospective PK study showed a significant decrease of approximately 30% in plasma IM concentration after 90 days of treatment [17], indicating that drug monitoring should preferentially be done after 3 months. This finding was recently supported by a study in real-life practice, where C_{min} was analysed after more than 3 months of treatment, and concentrations above 760 ng/mL were associated with longer progression-free survival (PFS) [18].

Although considerable inter-patient variability in IM plasma concentrations (40–60%) has been observed in several studies [15, 16], a fixed dose of 400 mg IM is the standard of care in patients with metastatic GIST [7]. Patients that progress on 400 mg/day and patients with KIT exon 9 mutations may benefit from increasing the dose to 800 mg/day [2, 19, 20]. Treatment with 400 mg IM is generally well tolerated, but patients still experience side effects such as anaemia, periorbital oedema, muscle cramps, and diarrhoea [2, 4, 5]. Several of these can be ameliorated with supportive measures, but some patients need dose modifications [21]. Compliance, i.e. adherence to self-administered drugs, is a general challenge for patients on any long-term treatment, as also reported for patients with GIST [22]. However, the extent of non-compliance is often not known and might be a larger problem than expected. Altogether, there are several situations where IM plasma concentration measurements might have a considerable clinical impact in patients with metastatic GIST. However, at present, therapeutic drug monitoring (TDM) is not yet a part of routine clinical practice.

The aim of this study was to assess IM plasma concentration repeatedly over several years in a group of patients with metastatic GIST and thereby revealing scenarios where such measurements might have clinical implications.

Patients and methods
Patients
Patients with GIST treated with IM were included from January 2011 to April 2015. Inclusion criteria were as follows: (1) histologically confirmed GIST; (2) treatment with IM initiated >90 days prior to study entry; (3) high-risk tumour in the need of adjuvant IM, metastatic disease or inoperable primary tumour. Fifty-three patients were enrolled, of whom 19 received IM in a neoadjuvant/adjuvant setting and 34 received IM for metastatic disease or inoperable primary tumour. For the present investigation we focused on patients in advanced or metastatic setting. We further excluded eight patients who had less than three available plasma samples and two patients where drug intake was not registered. Twenty-four patients were included in the final cohort. All patients attended regular 3- to 6-month follow-up visits and were seen by the same physician (ØSB). Radiological evaluation with computed tomography of the abdomen and pelvis was performed every 3–6 months depending on the clinical scenario. Disease progression was objectively documented by an experienced radiologist. Secondary review using RECIST or CHOI criteria was not performed. Clinicopathological data were collected retrospectively by reviewing medical records. Body weight, height and biochemical parameters were measured at the time of blood sampling for PK assessment. Creatinine clearance was estimated using the Cockcroft-Gault formula: estimated creatinine clearance = (140 − age in years) × (weight in kilograms) × (0.85 if female)/(72 − serum creatinine) [23]. The study was approved by the Regional Ethics Committee (#S-06133a), and written informed consent was obtained from all patients. Patients were asked if they took the drug as prescribed, and divided into three groups based on drug compliance: Excellent compliance: Never forget to take IM; Intermediate compliance: Forget to take IM on occasions, less than once a week; Poor compliance: Not taking IM regularly with gaps for several days.

Sample collection
Three milliliter heparin plasma was collected at each follow-up visit. Within 1 h of the collection, the blood samples were centrifuged in room temperature for 15 min at 2500×g, and were stored at −20 °C until analysis. Samples were drawn in a routine clinical setting and not at the time of trough level. The time of drug intake was registered, and the validated Bayesian method developed by Gotta and colleagues [24] was used to extrapolate the measured concentrations to C_{min}.

Measurements of IM concentrations

The determination of the IM plasma concentrations followed the protocol as described in Ubhayasekhera et al. [25]. IM standard was kindly provided by Novartis (Basel, Switzerland). All chemicals including internal standard (Trazodone) and ultrapure solvents were purchased from Sigma Aldrich (Stockholm, Sweden), unless otherwise stated. The stock solutions of IM and internal standard were prepared by dissolving methanol to obtain a final concentration of 1 mg/mL. Protein precipitation was applied as a sample pretreatment. Twenty-five microliter of methanol containing 1 µg/mL internal standard and 0.5 mL of methanol were added to 100 µL of plasma, shaken in 10 min and centrifuged for 10 min at 4 °C at 14,000g. The supernatant was dried by vacuum centrifugation and the residue was reconstituted in 100 µL of 5% acetonitrile containing 0.1% formic acid. Aliquouts of 10 µL were injected into the LC–MS system. Chromatography and mass spectrometry was performed as previously described [25, 26].

Statistical analysis

All statistical analyses were performed by using SPSS 21.0 (SPSS, Chicago, IL, USA). Differences in plasma concentrations between dose groups were assessed by Kruskal–Wallis test. The IM C_{min} values were log-transformed for the subsequent analyses. To assess the characteristics of the plasma samples in a homogenous cohort, we focused on the samples being drawn in patients taking 400 mg daily (n = 69). Correlations between IM C_{min} and other variables were analysed by univariate linear regression (Pearson) and independent samples Student's t test. Variables that showed significant correlations (p < 0.05) with IM C_{min} in univariate analysis were included in a multivariate analysis using a multiple linear regression model with stepwise, backward elimination of variables. Correlations were also tested using a more stringent linear mixed models effect analysis to take into account intra-patient correlation. All tests were two-sided, and p values less than 0.05 were considered statistically significant.

Results

Patient characteristics

Ninety-six samples from 24 patients included in the study were analysed. There were 4 patients with three samples, 16 patients with four samples and 4 patients with five samples. The median duration of IM treatment prior to the first sample was 25 months (range 3–77 months). The median time from the first sample to the last sample was 32 months (range 4–48 months). All patients received IM for metastatic disease, except one patient who was medically inoperable and received IM for a large GIST in the small bowel. The median age was 69 years (range 33–88). The clinical and pathological features of all patients are listed in Table 1. Sixteen patients reported excellent compliance, seven had intermediate compliance and one patient poor compliance. No patients experienced serious life-threatening adverse events. Seven patients had dose reductions: Six patients from 400 to 200 mg due to self-reported side effects and one patient from 800 to 400 mg due to severe fluid retention and haematological toxicity.

C_{min} plasma concentrations

Plasma samples were grouped according to the IM dose at time of sampling: <400 mg group (100 mg: n = 2, 200 mg: n = 19), 400 mg (n = 69) and >400 mg (600 mg: n = 1, 700 mg: n = 1 and 800 mg: n = 4). Mean ± standard deviation values of IM C_{min} plasma concentrations were 782 ± 589, 1132 ± 712 and 1665 ± 924 ng/mL, respectively (Fig. 1a). The difference between the groups was statistically significant (p = 0.010). Intra-patient and inter-patient variability was relatively large. The mean intra-patient variability

Table 1 Baseline clinical and pathological characteristics of the 24 patients enrolled in the study

Characteristic	Number (%)
Gender	
Female	8 (33)
Male	16 (67)
Primary tumour site	
Stomach	8 (33)
Small bowel	13 (54)
Rectum	2 (8)
Unknown	1 (4)
Histological subtype	
Spindle cell	17 (71)
Epitheloid	1 (4)
Mixed	3 (13)
ND	3
Mutation analysis	
KIT exon 11	18 (75)
KIT exon 9	2 (8)
PDGFRA exon 12	1 (4)
Mutations not detected	2 (8)
ND	1
Metastatic site	
Liver	13 (54)
Intraperitoneal cavity	7 (29)
Liver + intraperitoneal cavity	3 (13)
No metastasis (inoperable primary tumour)	1 (4)

ND not determined

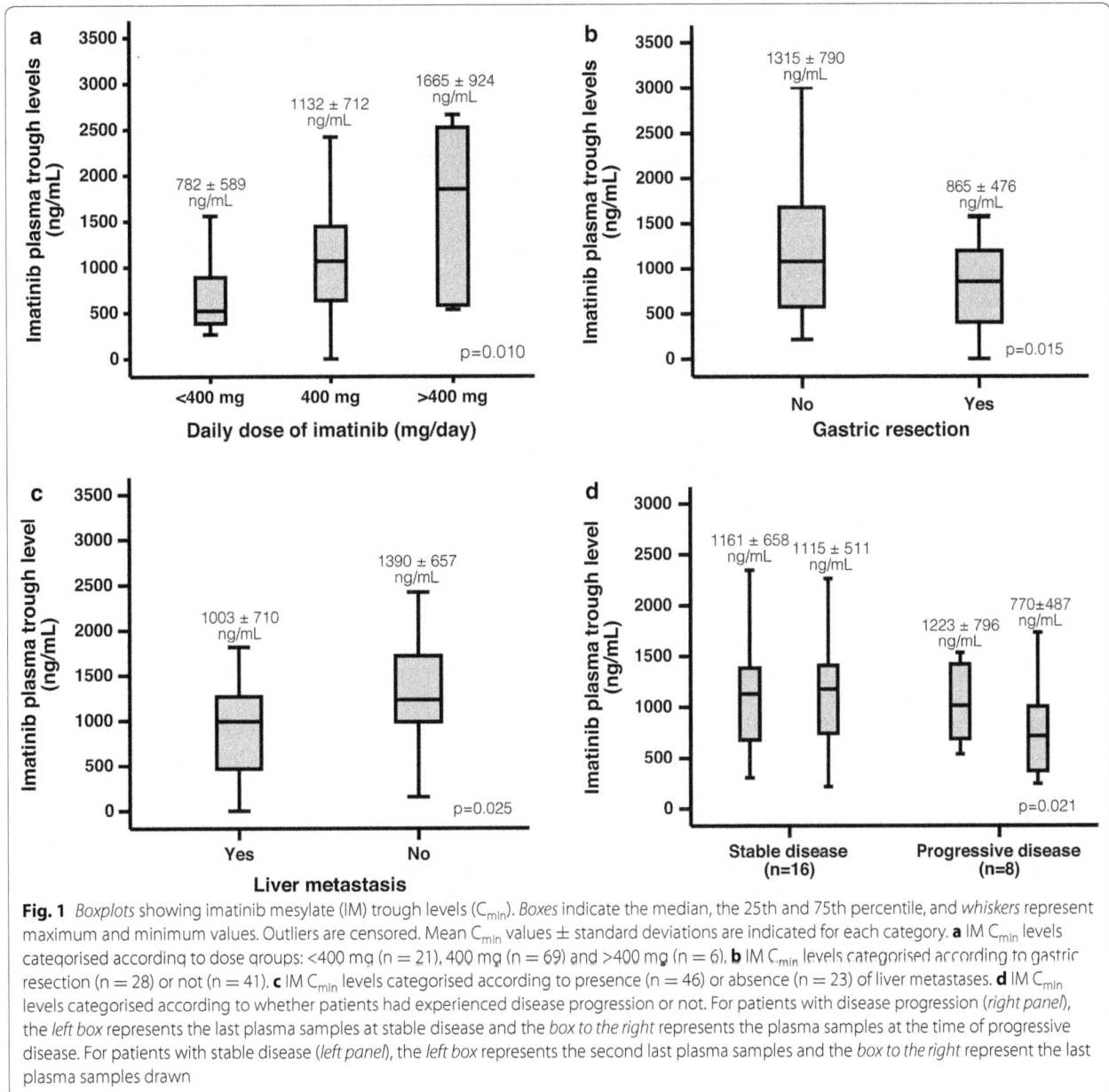

Fig. 1 *Boxplots* showing imatinib mesylate (IM) trough levels (C$_{min}$). *Boxes* indicate the median, the 25th and 75th percentile, and *whiskers* represent maximum and minimum values. Outliers are censored. Mean C$_{min}$ values ± standard deviations are indicated for each category. **a** IM C$_{min}$ levels categorised according to dose groups: <400 mg (n = 21), 400 mg (n = 69) and >400 mg (n = 6). **b** IM C$_{min}$ levels categorised according to gastric resection (n = 28) or not (n = 41). **c** IM C$_{min}$ levels categorised according to presence (n = 46) or absence (n = 23) of liver metastases. **d** IM C$_{min}$ levels categorised according to whether patients had experienced disease progression or not. For patients with disease progression (*right panel*), the *left box* represents the last plasma samples at stable disease and the *box to the right* represents the plasma samples at the time of progressive disease. For patients with stable disease (*left panel*), the *left box* represents the second last plasma samples and the *box to the right* represent the last plasma samples drawn

(coefficient of variation) in patients taking 400 mg was 36% and the highest intra-patient variability 69%, with maximum plasma concentration 1188 ng/mL and minimum of 195 ng/mL. The mean inter-patient variability in patients taking 400 mg was 68%, with the highest measured concentration of 4491 ng/mL and the lowest concentration 195 ng/mL. Among the six patients with a dose reduction to 200 mg, two had relatively high mean plasma levels of 1418 and 2242 ng/mL, whereas the other four had mean plasma concentrations of 387, 437, 565 and 521 ng/mL. Two patients started on 200 mg and had mean plasma concentrations of 1704 and 540 ng/mL.

Patient characteristics and C$_{min}$ plasma concentrations

Correlations between IM C$_{min}$ and clinical characteristics were analysed in patients receiving the standard dose 400 mg. The results presented below refer to the per-sample analysis. Linear mixed model effects analyses gave similar trends, although without reaching statistical significance. In univariate analysis, high IM C$_{min}$ was significantly correlated with age (β = 0.303, p = 0.012), BSA (β = −0.300, p = 0.010), low haemoglobin concentration (β = −0.290, p = 0.016), low creatinine clearance (β = −0.234, p = 0.050), but not with albumin (p = 0.061) or calcium level (p = 0.999), tumour diameter (p = 0.368), gender (p = 0.915), WBC (p = 0.832) or platelet count (p = 0.816).

Nine patients (38%) had undergone subtotal or total gastrectomy, and IM C_{min} was significantly lower in these patients (865 ± 476 ng/mL; n = 28) than in plasma samples from patients without gastric surgery (1315 ± 790 ng/mL; n = 41; p = 0.015) (Fig. 1b). Furthermore, IM C_{min} was significantly lower in the plasma samples from patients with liver metastases (1003 ± 710 ng/mL, n = 46) compared to patients without liver metastases (1390 ± 657 ng/mL, n = 23; p = 0.025) (Fig. 1c).

Multivariate analysis was performed including variables that were associated with IM C_{min} in univariate analysis in the 400 mg group. Gastric resection (p = 0.021), age (p = 0.049) and liver metastases (p = 0.010) were the covariates significantly associated with IM C_{min}.

Disease progression and C_{min} plasma concentrations

Eight patients had disease progression during the study. In seven of these IM C_{min} concentrations decreased at the time of progression compared to the previous measurement. The mean IM C_{min} concentration at the time of progression was 770 ± 487 ng/mL, and in the last sample from the time of stable disease from the same patients 1223 ± 796 ng/mL (p = 0.021; Student's test). In comparison, there was no statistically significant difference in IM C_{min} concentration between the two last plasma samples collected in patients with stable disease throughout the study (1161 ± 658 versus 1115 ± 511 ng/mL) (Fig. 1d).

Discussion

The role of IM C_{min} measurements in optimizing therapeutic efficacy in GIST is still investigational, despite preliminary estimates of IM blood levels that are associated with improved clinical outcomes (C_{min} > 1110 ng/mL) [16]. In this study, we assessed C_{min} in a group of patients over several years trying to determine whether there are clinical scenarios where measurements of IM C_{min} could be advantageous. To the best of our knowledge this is the first study in metastatic GIST with repeated measurements of C_{min} plasma concentrations including samples at the time of documented progression.

Low IM C_{min} was associated with major gastrectomy in both univariate and multivariate analysis, which is consistent with previous findings [14]. IM tablets dissolve more rapidly at pH 5.5 or less [8], and lack of gastric acid secretion may explain the lower concentration in such patients. Many patients with metastatic GIST have previously undergone surgery for a primary gastric GIST and one might speculate that such patients could possess an increased risk of sub-therapeutic IM plasma levels and subsequently a less favourable disease outcome. In our cohort, only eight patients had disease progression, of which three had undergone gastric resection. Thus, analysing the prognostic impact of gastric surgery

is impossible due to small patient numbers. Still, a more individualized drug dosage based on IM plasma concentrations may be beneficial in patients with prior gastric surgery.

Interestingly, in the current study patients with liver metastases had low IM C_{min} compared to patients without liver metastases. A previous study has shown that IM clearance is not affected by low volume liver disease [17], and it thus seems unlikely that the liver metastases per se affect IM metabolism in our patients. We are not aware of studies that have reported differences in IM plasma concentration in patients with or without liver metastases, and this issue could be of interest for further studies.

Older patients had higher plasma concentrations in our cohort. The well-known decline of organ functions and increased prevalence of comorbidity and concomitant medication among elderly patients may influence the pharmacokinetics and pharmacodynamics of IM. We did not prospectively register concomitant medications or co-occurring medical conditions, and are thus not able to discern the role of these factors separately. Our results could suggest that individual dosing supported by IM plasma concentration measurement could be even more useful in elderly patients, to balance side effects and antitumour efficacy more precisely.

Although there were no serious adverse events in our study, dose reduction due to subjective side effects were mandatory in seven patients. Two of these patients had relatively high C_{min} on 200 mg, suggesting that for some patients this dose is enough to ensure optimal therapeutic plasma levels of IM. The four other patients had low levels suggesting that patient-reported side effects are not necessarily associated with high plasma concentrations. Few studies have explored the relationship between IM plasma concentration and side effects. One study showed that the occurrence and number of side effects correlated with IM total and free plasma concentrations in GIST patients [27], but further studies on relations between concentration and toxicity are warranted. Unfortunately, we did not register side effects in a formal and prospective manner. However, measuring C_{min} concentrations in patients experiencing subjective side effects (e.g. muscle cramps, dizziness, fatigue etc.) that limit daily activity may help to determine whether it is safe to modify the dose of IM.

The relatively large inter- and interpatient variability in our study compared to other real-life cohorts [14, 18] could be explained by lack of compliance. Although oral cancer therapies offer patients the convenience of self-administration at home, evidence show that adherence to these therapies is far from optimal [28, 29]. The BFR14 Study evaluated the effect of IM interruption in responding patients (complete response, partial response, or stable disease) after different periods of treatment (1, 3 and 5 years), and results from the study indicated that discontinuation of IM is associated with rapid progression [30–32]. Therefore, maintaining proper adherence may be of great significance and drug monitoring could potentially improve compliance to therapy.

Interestingly, we found a decrease in C_{min} plasma concentration at the time of disease progression, which might explain loss of disease control in certain patients. Measurements of IM C_{min} in case of progressive disease could therefore be indicated if lack of patient compliance has been ascertained. A sub-therapeutic drug level at the prescribed dose could suggest that increasing the dose would be of clinical benefit, in particular in the absence of secondary KIT or PDGFRA mutations. Studies comparing 400 with 800 mg IM daily in advanced disease showed no clinical benefit of IM 800 mg daily, except for tumours with KIT exon 9 mutations [33]. Despite this, dose escalation to 800 mg can be beneficial in up to 30% of patients upon disease progression on 400 mg [2, 19, 20]. IM plasma concentration measurements have not been performed in dose escalation studies, and perhaps only patients with sub-therapeutic IM levels will benefit from this strategy, whereas the remainder should be offered second-line therapy.

Total IM plasma concentration was measured in our study. Another option is to measure free drug concentrations; i.e. the pharmacologically active fraction not bound by albumin or AGP. The area under the PK curve (AUC) for IM, which can either be measured directly or as the correction of the total drug concentration for binding to AGP, may provide a better surrogate for cellular drug exposure than total IM concentration [15, 26]. Furthermore, IM concentration measurement in the cytoplasm of the tumour cells could even more precisely predict target inhibition and clinical efficacy. A new approach to measurement of intracellular levels of IM in an in vivo setting has been developed, and there were large variation in IM concentrations between plasma, adipose tissue, and different sites within a given tumour [34]. Although only three patients were included in the latter study, this highlights the importance of further clinical investigations on measurements of intracellular IM levels in GIST tissues to understand their possible impact on patient outcome.

Among the limitations of this study are the retrospective registration of the majority of the clinical data and side effects. We neither did review of the radiology nor the pathology, but experienced sarcoma radiologists and pathologists at a major reference centre had already confirmed the diagnostic work-up at start of IM, including analyses of KIT and PDGFRA mutations that were found in all patients except three. Furthermore, patients with <3 plasma samples were excluded, and median treatment duration of IM before inclusion was 25 months. Even though patients were not excluded due to progressive disease, a bias towards patients without progression could have occurred. Moreover, the plasma samples were not drawn at trough time, but a validated method to extrapolate the samples to trough was used [25]. Even though these issues in general would be considered as shortcomings, they reflect well a routine oncology practice, and our findings could therefore easily be transferred to a routine clinical setting.

In conclusion, our results do not support repeated monitoring of IM levels on a routine basis in all patients. However, we have revealed clinical scenarios where drug measurement could be beneficial, such as for patients who have undergone gastric resection, suspicion of non-compliance, subjectively reported side effects, in elderly patients and at the time of disease progression. Whether dose escalation could be beneficial at disease progression for patients with low IM plasma concentration should be further studied.

Abbreviations

GIST: gastrointestinal stromal tumour; IM: imatinib mesylate; C_{min}: trough level; PDGFRA: platelet-derived growth factor receptor alpha; CML: chronic myeloid leukaemia; PK: pharmacokinetic; BSA: body surface area; WBC: white blood cell; AGP: alpha glycoprotein; PFS: progression-free survival; TDM: therapeutic drug monitoring.

Authors' contributions

IH, OSB and KB were responsible for the concept and design of the study. IH, OSB and KB collected and assembled the clinical data and the plasma samples. KU and JB analysed the plasma IM concentrations. IH and KB analysed the final data. All authors read and approved the final manuscript.

Author details

[1] Department of Oncology, Norwegian Radium Hospital, Oslo University Hospital, PO Box 4953, Nydalen, 0424 Oslo, Norway. [2] Institute of Clinical Medicine, University of Oslo, Oslo, Norway. [3] Department of Chemistry, Biomedical Center, Analytical Chemistry and Science for Life Laboratory, Uppsala University, Uppsala, Sweden. [4] Department of Tumor Biology, Norwegian Radium Hospital, Oslo University Hospital, Oslo, Norway.

Acknowledgements

MSc Warunika Aluthgedara is acknowledged for her kind support in the imatinib analysis and Associated Professor Manuela Zucknick for statistical advice.

Competing interests

The authors declare that they have no competing interests.

Funding

Rakel and Otto Kr Bruun's Legacy, Oslo University Hospital Foundation, the Norwegian Cancer Society (Grant 5790283) and The Swedish Research Council (Grant 621-2011-4423, 2015-4870) are acknowledged for financial support.

References

1. Joensuu H, Roberts PJ, Sarlomo-Rikala M, Andersson LC, Tervahartiala P, Tuveson D, Silberman S, Capdeville R, Dimitrijevic S, Druker B, Demetri GD. Effect of the tyrosine kinase inhibitor STI571 in a patient with a metastatic gastrointestinal stromal tumor. N Engl J Med. 2001;344:1052–6.

2. Blanke CD, Demetri GD, von Mehren M, Heinrich MC, Eisenberg B, Fletcher JA, Corless CL, Fletcher CDM, Roberts PJ, Heinz D, Wehre E, Nikolova Z, Joensuu H. Long-term results from a randomized phase II trial of standard- versus higher-dose imatinib mesylate for patients with unresectable or metastatic gastrointestinal stromal tumors expressing KIT. J Clin Oncol. 2008;26:620–5.

3. Hirota S, Isozaki K, Moriyama Y, Hashimoto K, Nishida T, Ishiguro S, Kawano K, Hanada M, Kurata A, Takeda M, Muhammad Tunio G, Matsuzawa Y, Kanakura Y, Shinomura Y, Kitamura Y. Gain-of-function mutations of c-kit in human gastrointestinal stromal tumors. Science. 1998;279:577–80.

4. Demetri G, von Mehren M, Blanke CD, Van den Abbeele AD, Eisenberg B, Roberts J, Heinrich MC, Tuveson DA, Singer S, Janicek M, Fletcher JA, Silverman SG, Silberman SL, Capdeville R, Kiese B, Peng B, Dimitrijevic S, Druker BJ, Corless C, Fletcher CD, Joensuu H. Efficacy and safety of imatinib mesylate in advanced gastrointestinal stromal tumors. N Engl J Med. 2002;347:472–80.

5. Verweij J, Casali PG, Zalcberg J, LeCesne A, Reichardt P, Blay J-Y, Issels R, van Oosterom A, Hogendoorn PC, van Glabbeke M, Bertulli R, Judson I. Progression-free survival in gastrointestinal stromal tumours with high-dose imatinib: randomised trial. Lancet. 2004;364:1127–34.

6. Demetri GD, Rankin CJ, Benjamin RS, et al. Long-term disease control of advanced gastrointestinal stromal tumors (GIST) with imatinib (IM): 10-year outcomes from SWOG phase III intergroup trial S0033. J Clin Oncol. 2014;32:5s **(suppl; abstr 10508)**.

7. The ESMO/European Sarcoma Network Working Group. Gastrointestinal stromal tumours: ESMO Clinical Practice Guidelines for diagnosis, treatment and follow-up. Ann Oncol. 2014;25(Suppl 3):iii21–6.

8. Peng B, Lloyd P, Schran H. Clinical pharmacokinetics of imatinib. Clin Pharmacokinet. 2005;44:879–94.

9. Judson I, Ma P, Peng B, Verweij J, Racine A, di Paola ED, van Glabbeke M, Dimitrijevic S, Scurr M, Dumez H, van Oosterom A. Imatinib pharmacokinetics in patients with gastrointestinal stromal tumour: a retrospective population pharmacokinetic study over time. EORTC Soft Tissue and Bone Sarcoma Group. Cancer Chemother Pharmacol. 2004;55:379–86.

10. Delbaldo C, Chatelut E, Re M, Deroussent A, Seronie-Vivien S, Jambu A, Berthaud P, Le Cesne A, Blay JY, Vassal G. Pharmacokinetic-pharmacodynamic relationships of imatinib and its main metabolite in patients with advanced gastrointestinal stromal tumors. Clin Cancer Res. 2006;12:6073–8.

11. Menon-Andersen D, Mondick JT, Jayaraman B, Thompson PA, Blaney SM, Bernstei M, Bond M, Champagne M, Fossler MJ, Barrett JS. Population pharmacokinetics of imatinib mesylate and its metabolite in children and young adults. Cancer Chemother Pharmacol. 2008;63:229–38.

12. Schmidli H, Peng B, Riviere GJ, Capdeville R, Hensley M, Gathmann I, Bolton AE, Racine-Poon A. Population pharmacokinetics of imatinib mesylate in patients with chronic-phase chronic myeloid leukaemia: results of a phase III study. Br J Clin Pharmacol. 2005;60:35–44.

13. Larson RA, Druker BJ, Guilhot F, O'Brien SG, Riviere GJ, Krahnke T, Gathmann I, Wang Y, IRIS (International Randomized Interferon vs STI571) Study Group. Imatinib pharmacokinetics and its correlation with response and safety in chronic-phase chronic myeloid leukemia: a subanalysis of the IRIS study. Blood. 2008;111:4022–8.

14. Yoo C, Ryu MH, Kang BW, Yoon SK, Ryoo BY, Chang HM, Lee JL, Beck MY, Kim TW, Kang YK. Cross-sectional study of imatinib plasma trough levels in patients with advanced gastrointestinal stromal tumors: impact of gastrointestinal resection on exposure to imatinib. J Clin Oncol. 2010;28:1554–9.

15. Widmer N, Decosterd LA, Csajka C, Leyvraz S, Duchosal MA, Rosselet A, Rochat B, Eap CB, Henry H, Biollaz J, Buclin T. Population pharmacokinetics of imatinib and the role of alpha1-acid glycoprotein. Br J Clin Pharmacol. 2006;62:97–112.

16. Demetri GD, Wang Y, Wehrle E, Racine A, Nikolova Z, Blanke CD, Joensuu H, von Mehren M. Imatinib plasma levels are correlated with clinical benefit in patients with unresectable/metastatic gastrointestinal stromal tumors. J Clin Oncol. 2009;27:3141–7.

17. Eechoute K, Fransson MN, Reyners AK, de Jong FA, Sparreboom A, van der Graaf TAW, Friberg LE, Schiavon G, Wiemer EAC, Verweij J, Loos WJ, Mathijssen RHJ, de Giorgi U. A long-term prospective population pharmacokinetic study on imatinib plasma concentrations in GIST patients. Clin Cancer Res. 2012;18:5780–7.

18. Bouchet S, Poulette S, Titier K, Moore N, Lassalle R, Abouelfath A, Italiano A, Chevreau C, Bompas E, Collard O, Duffaud F, Rios M, Cupissol D, Adenis A, Ray-Coquard I, Bouché O, Le Cesne A, Bui B, Blay JY, Molimard M. Relationship between imatinib trough concentration and outcomes in the treatment of advanced gastrointestinal stromal tumours in a real-life setting. Eur J Cancer. 2016;57:31–8.

19. Debiec-Rychter M, Sciot R, Le Cesne A, Schlemmer M, Hohenberger P, van Oosterom AT, Blay JY, Leyvraz S, Stul M, Casali PG, Zalcberg J, Verweij J, van Glabbeke M, Hagemeijer A, Judson I. KIT mutations and dose selection for imatinib in patients with advanced gastrointestinal stromal tumours. Eur J Cancer. 2006;42:1093–103.

20. Park I, Ryu MH, Sym SJ, Lee SS, Jang G, Kim TW, Chang HM, Lee JL, Lee H, Kang YK. Dose escalation of imatinib after failure of standard dose in Korean patients with metastatic or unresectable gastrointestinal stromal tumor. Jpn J Clin Oncol. 2008;39:105–10.

21. Joensuu H, Trent JC, Reichardt P. Practical management of tyrosine kinase inhibitor-associated side effects in GIST. Cancer Treat Rev. 2011;37:75–88.

22. Mazzeo F, Duck L, Joosens E, Dirix L, Focan C, Forget F, De Geest S, Muermans K, van Lierde M-A, Macdonald K, Abraham I, De Grève J. Nonadherence to imatinib treatment in patients with gastrointestinal stromal tumors: the ADAGIO study. Anticancer Res. 2011;31:1407–9.

23. Cockcroft DW, Gault MH. Prediction of creatinine clearance from serum creatinine. Nephron. 1976;16:31–41.

24. Gotta V, Widmer N, Montemurro M, Leyvraz S, Haouala A, Decosterd LA, Csajka C, Buclin T. Therapeutic drug monitoring of imatinib: Bayesian and alternative methods to predict trough levels. Clin Pharmacokinet. 2012;51:187–201.

25. Ubhayasekera SJKA, Aluthgedara W, Ek B, Bergquist J. Simultaneous quantification of imatinib and CGP74588 in human plasma by liquid chromatography-time of flight mass spectrometry (LC-TOF-MS). Anal Methods. 2016;8:3046–54.

26. Skoglund K, Richter J, Olsson-Strömberg U, Bergquist J, Aluthgedara W, Ubhayasekera SJ, Vikingsson S, Svedberg A, Söderlund S, Sandstedt A, Johnsson A, Aagesen J, Alsenhed J, Hägg S, Peterson C, Lotfi K, Gréen H. In vivo cytochrome P450 3A isoenzyme activity and pharmacokinetics of imatinib in relation to therapeutic outcome in patients with chronic myeloid leukemia. Ther Drug Monit. 2016;38(2):230–238

27. Widmer N, Decosterd LA, Leyvraz S, Duchosal MA, Rosselet A, Debiec-Rychter M, Csajka C, Biollaz J, Buclin T. Relationship of imatinib-free plasma levels and target genotype with efficacy and tolerability. Br J Cancer. 2008;98:1633–40.

28. Osterberg L, Blaschke T. Adherence to medication. N Engl J Med. 2005;353:487–97.

29. Noens L, van Lierde MA, de Bock R, Verhoef G, Zachée P, Berneman Z, Martiat P, Mineur P, van Eygen K, Macdonald K, de Geest S, Albrecht T, Abraham I. Prevalence, determinants, and outcomes of nonadherence to imatinib therapy in patients with chronic myeloid leukemia: the ADAGIO study. Blood. 2009;113:5401–11.

30. Blay J-Y, Le Cesne A, Ray-Coquard I, Bui B, Duffaud F, Delbaldo C, Adenis A, Viens P, Rios M, Bompas E, Cupissol D, Guillemet C, Kerbrat P, Fayette J, Chabaud S, Berthaud P, Pérol D. Prospective multicentric randomized phase III study of imatinib in patients with advanced gastrointestinal stromal tumors comparing interruption versus continuation of treatment beyond 1 year: the French Sarcoma Group. J Clin Oncol. 2007;25:1107–13.

31. Le Cesne A, Ray-Coquard I, Bui BN, Adenis A, Rios M, Bertucci F, Duffaud F, Chevreau C, Cupissol D, Cioffi A, Emile J-F, Chabaud S, Pérol D, Blay J-Y. Discontinuation of imatinib in patients with advanced gastrointestinal stromal tumours after 3 years of treatment: an open-label multicentre randomised phase 3 trial. Lancet Oncol. 2010;11:942–9.

Clinical implications of repeated drug monitoring of imatinib in patients with metastatic gastrointestinal...

75

32. Patrikidou A, Chabaud S, Ray-Coquard I, Bui BN, Adenis A, Rios M, Bertucci F, Duffaud F, Chevreau C, Cupissol D, Domont J, Perol D, Blay JY, le Cesne A. Influence of imatinib interruption and rechallenge on the residual disease in patients with advanced GIST: results of the BFR14 prospective French Sarcoma Group randomised, phase III trial. Ann Oncol. 2013;24:1087–93.

33. Gastrointestinal Stromal Tumor Meta-Analysis Group (MetaGIST). Comparison of two doses of imatinib for the treatment of unresectable or metastatic gastrointestinal stromal tumors: a meta-analysis of 1640 patients. J Clin Oncol. 2010;28:1247–53.

34. Berglund E, Ubhayasekera SJKA, Karlsson F, Akcakaya P, Aluthgedara W, Åhlen J, Fröbom R, Nilsson IL, Lui WO, Larsson C, Zedenius J, Bergquist J, Bränström R. Intracellular concentration of the tyrosine kinase inhibitor imatinib in gastrointestinal stromal tumor cells. Anticancer Drugs. 2014;25:415–22.

9

IDH1 or *-2* mutations do not predict outcome and do not cause loss of 5-hydroxymethylcytosine or altered histone modifications in central chondrosarcomas

Arjen H. G. Cleven[1], Johnny Suijker[1], Georgios Agrogiannis[2], Inge H. Briaire-de Bruijn[1], Norma Frizzell[3], Attje S. Hoekstra[4], Pauline M. Wijers-Koster[1], Anne-Marie Cleton-Jansen[1] and Judith V. M. G. Bovée[1]*

Abstract

Background: Mutations in *isocitrate dehydrogenase (IDH)1* or *-2* are found in ~50% of conventional central chondrosarcomas and in up to 87% of their assumed benign precursors enchondromas. The mutant enzyme acquires the activity to convert α-ketoglutarate into the oncometabolite D-2-hydroxyglutarate (D-2-HG), which competitively inhibits α-ketoglutarate dependent enzymes such as histone- and DNA demethylases.

Methods: We therefore evaluated the effect of *IDH1* or *-2* mutations on histone modifications (H3K4me3, H3K9me3 and H3K27me3), chromatin remodeler ATRX expression, DNA modifications (5-hmC and 5-mC), and TET1 subcellular localization in a genotyped cohort (*IDH*, succinate dehydrogenase (*SDH*) and fumarate hydratase (*FH*)) of enchondromas and central chondrosarcomas (n = 101) using immunohistochemistry.

Results: *IDH1* or *-2* mutations were found in 60.8% of the central cartilaginous tumours, while mutations in *FH* and *SDH* were absent. The mutation status did not correlate with outcome. Chondrosarcomas are strongly positive for the histone modifications H3K4me3, H3K9me3 and H3K27me3, which was independent of the *IDH1* or *-2* mutation status. Two out of 36 chondrosarcomas (5.6%) show complete loss of ATRX. Levels of 5-hmC and 5-mC are highly variable in central cartilaginous tumours and are not associated with mutation status. In tumours with loss of 5-hmC, expression of TET1 was more prominent in the cytoplasm than the nucleus (p = 0.0001).

Conclusions: In summary, in central chondrosarcoma *IDH1* or *-2* mutations do not affect immunohistochemical levels of 5-hmC, 5mC, trimethylation of H3K4, -K9 and K27 and outcome, as compared to wildtype.

Keywords: 5-Hydroxymethylcytosine, 5-Methylcytosine, Histone methylation, Chondrosarcoma, Isocitrate dehydrogenase, Bone tumour, Enchondroma

Background

Mutations in *isocitrate dehydrogenase (IDH)-1* or *-2* (which we commonly refer to as *IDH*) are found in gliomas (60–80% [1, 2], acute myeloid leukemia (~20%) [3], cholangiocarcinomas (7–28%) [4–6] and in benign and malignant central cartilaginous tumours [7–9]. Isocitrate dehydrogenase (IDH) is an enzyme involved in the conversion of isocitrate to α-ketoglutarate in the tricarboxylic acid (TCA) cycle (Fig. 1). Mutations are exclusively found on the arginine residues R132 of *IDH1* and in R140 and R172 of *IDH2*.

Cartilaginous neoplasias affect the bone and can be roughly divided into benign (enchondromas and osteochondromas), and malignant (chondrosarcomas of different subtypes) [10]. Enchondromas occur in the medulla of bone [10], and occasionally they can present with

*Correspondence: J.V.M.G.Bovee@lumc.nl
[1] Department of Pathology, Leiden University Medical Center, L1-Q, P.O. Box 9600, 2300 RC Leiden, The Netherlands
Full list of author information is available at the end of the article

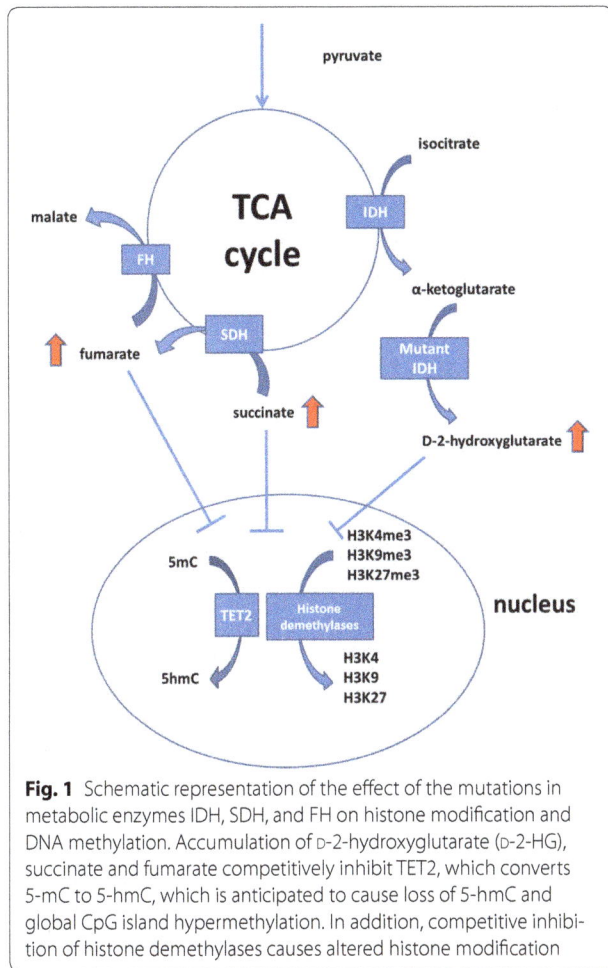

Fig. 1 Schematic representation of the effect of the mutations in metabolic enzymes IDH, SDH, and FH on histone modification and DNA methylation. Accumulation of D-2-hydroxyglutarate (D-2-HG), succinate and fumarate competitively inhibit TET2, which converts 5-mC to 5-hmC, which is anticipated to cause loss of 5-hmC and global CpG island hypermethylation. In addition, competitive inhibition of histone demethylases causes altered histone modification

multiple lesions in non-hereditary Ollier disease or Maffucci syndrome [11]. Conventional central chondrosarcoma is the most common chondrosarcoma subtype, affecting the medulla of bone, which can arise from a pre-existing benign enchondroma. Peripheral conventional chondrosarcoma affects the surface of the bone and arises from a preexisting benign osteochondroma. The best prognostic marker for chondrosarcoma so far is histological grading, since atypical cartilaginous tumour/grade I chondrosarcomas behave locally aggressive and only metastasize in exceptional cases. Grade II and III chondrosarcomas are more cellular and the chance of metastasis is increased (up to 70% of the patients for grade III) [12, 13].

Mutations in *IDH* are found in ~50% (38–86%) of conventional central chondrosarcomas, in ~54% of dedifferentiated and ~15% of periosteal chondrosarcoma, and in up to 87% of benign enchondromas [7–9], while being absent in peripheral, mesenchymal and clear cell chondrosarcoma. Patients with Ollier disease and Maffucci syndrome carry *IDH* mutations in a somatic mosaic

fashion [8, 9]. While in gliomas the *IDH* mutations are associated with a more favorable outcome [2, 14, 15], in intrahepatic cholangiocarcinoma, as well as in leukemia, its prognostic value could not unequivocally be shown [16, 17].

The mutant enzyme acquires the ability to convert α-ketoglutarate into the oncometabolite D-2-hydroxyglutarate (D-2-HG), which shows structural similarities with α-ketoglutarate. Indeed, increased levels of D-2-HG have been found in cartilage tumours with an *IDH* mutation [8]. Elevated levels of D-2-HG were shown to competitively inhibit α-ketoglutarate dependent enzymes such as histone demethylases [18] (Fig. 1), specifically affecting trimethylation of the transcriptionally permissive histone mark H3K4, and the repressive histone marks H3K9 and H3K27 [19–21]. In addition, D-2-HG inhibits the ten-eleven translocation (TET) enzymes [18] (Fig. 1). TET enzymes are involved in DNA demethylation by catalyzing the conversion of 5-methylcytosine (5-mC) into 5-hydroxymethylcytosine (5-hmC) [22, 23]. Indeed, methylation arrays confirmed global hypermethylation in *IDH1* mutant enchondromas [9], and decreased levels of 5-hmC were detected in myeloproliferative disorders harboring *TET2* mutations [24]. Furthermore, nuclear exclusion of TET1 was shown to be related to loss of 5-hmC in gliomas without *IDH* mutations [25]. Wiestler et al. described that loss of ATRX (an ATP-dependent helicase that belongs to the SWI/SNF family of chromatin remodeling proteins and facilitates access to nucleosomal DNA) was almost exclusively found in gliomas harboring *IDH* mutations [26]. Germline mutations in *ATRX* are associated with X-linked intellectual disability with alpha-thalassemia (ATRX) syndrome, and generally cause loss of protein expression [27].

Other TCA cycle enzymes involved in cancer are succinate dehydrogenase (*SDH*) in hereditary paragangliomas [28–31] and gastrointestinal stromal tumour (GIST) [32], and fumarate hydratase (*FH*) in hereditary leiomyomas and renal cell cancer (HLRCC) [33]. Mutations in either *SDH* or *FH* lead to loss of function, resulting in accumulation of succinate and fumarate, respectively. Similar to D-2-HG, elevated levels of succinate and fumarate inhibit α-ketoglutarate dependent enzymes [34–36] (Fig. 1). In *SDH* mutant paragangliomas and GIST, and in *FH* deficient smooth muscle tumours, 5-hmC was low to absent [37, 38].

In this study, our aim was to evaluate the effect of *IDH* mutations on outcome, and on histone modifications (H3K4me3, H3K9me3 and H3K27me3), DNA modifications (5-hmC and 5-mC), chromatin remodeling (ATRX), and subcellular localization of TET1 in a cohort of enchondromas and central chondrosarcomas for which we determined mutation status of *IDH*, *SDH* and *FH*.

Methods
Patient series [tissue microarray (TMA)]
The first cohort of cartilaginous tumours used for the tissue microarray (TMA) has been described previously [39] and includes nine enchondromas, 11 osteochondromas, 92 central chondrosarcomas (of which 42 atypical cartilaginous tumours/grade I; 36 grade II and 14 grade III) and 45 peripheral chondrosarcomas (of which 31 atypical cartilaginous tumours/grade I; 11 grade II and 3 grade III). Thus, this TMA contains a cohort of 101 central cartilaginous tumours. Cores from skin, colon, tonsil, prostate, breast carcinoma, spleen and liver were included for control and orientation purposes.

A second cohort of enchondromatosis related tumours was used for which details were also described previously [40]. This second TMA was exclusively used for 5mC and 5hmC immunohistochemistry as a second separate independent series, and was analyzed in the same way as the first cohort. In total, the TMA contains cores from 86 tumours, of which 65 were enchondromatosis related (51 Ollier disease, 13 Maffucci syndrome, 1 polyostotic chondrosarcoma) and 21 solitary enchondromas and chondrosarcomas. Cores from growth plate, articular cartilage, breast carcinoma, prostate, colon, skin and tonsil were included for control and orientation purposes.

Whole sections derived from normal articular cartilage (n = 3) and growth plate (n = 3) were also taken along as controls. All controls were acquired from pathological resections unrelated to cartilaginous tumours. All samples were handled in a coded manner according to the ethical guidelines as described in the Code for Proper Secondary Use of Human Tissue in The Netherlands of the Dutch Federation of Medical Scientific Societies. Follow-up data were available for all subjects (range 7–344 months, mean 150, 9 months).

Analysis of IDH, SDH and FH mutation status
Immunohistochemistry to detect the *IDH1* R132H mutation was previously reported for the first cohort and 6 out of 101 central cartilaginous tumours were shown to be positive [9]. For the 95 cases that were negative, we isolated the corresponding DNA. When available, we used frozen tissue, otherwise DNA was isolated from formalin-fixed, paraffin embedded tissue (FFPE). DNA isolation from fresh frozen material was performed using the wizard genomic DNA purification kit (Promega, Madison, WI) according to the manufacturer's instructions. DNA isolation from paraffin embedded tissue was performed as described [41]. Hydrolysis probes assay for *IDH1* R132C and R132H was performed as described previously [9]. Subsequently, PCR amplification of exon 4 of *IDH1* was performed for 76 samples that were negative in the hydrolysis probes assay. After each PCR run,

melting curves were inspected in order to check the formation of a single product. The PCR products were purified using the QIAquick PCR Purification Kit (Qiagen, Hilden, Germany) according to the manufacturer's manual and Sanger sequencing was performed, as described previously [9]. For the remaining 64 samples without an *IDH1* mutation, exon 4 of *IDH2* was amplified and sequenced for mutations. Oligonucleotide sequences for PCR are shown in Additional file 1: Table S1. Bidirectional Sanger sequencing was performed by Macrogen Europe (Amsterdam, The Netherlands). The sequence results were evaluated using Mutation Surveyor software (Soft-Genetics). To exclude that *IDH* wildtype cartilage tumours harbor mutations in *SDH* or *FH*, TMAs were stained for SDHB (Atlas antibodies, HPA002868) and S-2-succinocysteine (2-SC) [42, 43] as described [37]. Mutations in SDH subunits destabilize the complex, which leads to degradation and loss of staining for SDHB, which is therefore widely used as a marker to screen for mutations in the SDH subunits [44]. Mutations in *FH* lead to accumulation of fumarate leading to aberrant succination of proteins. Positive staining for (S)-2-succinocysteine (2SC) was shown to be a reliable marker to screen for mutations in *FH* [42, 43].

Immunohistochemistry
Immunohistochemistry was performed as described previously [37], for histone modifications (H3K4me3; Millipore, 07-473; H3K9me3, Abcam, ab8898; H3K27me3, Millipore, 07-449); a chromatin remodeler (ATRX; Sigma, HPA001906); DNA modifications (5-hmC; Active Motif, 39,769 and 5-mC; Millipore, 33D3) as well as for TET1 (Genetex, N3C1).

Evaluation and scoring of immunohistochemistry
All slides were evaluated by two observers (JVMGB, JS, AHGC, GA in variable combination) independently and discrepancies were discussed to reach consensus. Scoring for both intensity (0 = negative, 1 = weak, 2 = moderate, 3 = strong) and the percentage of positive tumour cells (0 = 0%, 1 = <25%, 2 = 25–50%, 3 = 50–75%, 4 = 75–100%) were added up to a total sum score [45]. The average was taken of the three different cores for further analysis. Since nuclear exclusion of TET1 was associated with loss of 5-hmC in *IDH* wildtype gliomas, we specifically scored the subcellular localization of TET1 (N = nuclear, C = cytoplasmic, N>C=more nuclear staining than cytoplasmic, C>N=more cytoplasmic staining than nuclear) as described [25].

Statistical analysis
Statistical significance between groups was determined using ANOVA with Tukey as posthoc analysis and Chi

square test as appropriate. Kaplan–Meier curves were plotted for the different stainings to determine the effect on overall survival and metastasis free survival, statistical significance was determined using Log Rank test. Data was analyzed using the IBM SPSS Statistics 23 software.

Results

IDH mutations in 60.8% of central cartilaginous tumours

In total, the *IDH* mutation status could be determined for 74 out of 101 central cartilaginous tumours of the first cohort. Thirty-seven tumours contained a mutation in *IDH1* at the R132 position, for which the mutational spectrum is shown in Fig. 2a. In addition, eight samples harbored an *IDH2* R172S mutation. Furthermore, 27 tumours were confirmed to lack *IDH* hotspot mutations, two of which contained an *IDH1* G105G polymorphism. These two cases were excluded from analysis since this polymorphism was recently suggested to be a possible prognostic marker in leukemia [46]. Mutation analysis failed for 27 samples due to poor quality of the DNA derived from decalcified FFPE tissue. The clinicopathological data of the genetically confirmed *IDH* mutant versus wildtype patients are shown in Table 1.

No association between *IDH* mutation and outcome

There was no significant difference in disease specific survival between *IDH* mutant and *IDH* wildtype chondrosarcomas in the first cohort (p = 0.183, Fig. 2b), independent from grade (data not shown). Also, when the different mutations were analyzed separately (R132C, R132H, R132G, R132l, R132S, R172S and wild-type) or in combination (the most common R132C and R132G

versus the others) no difference in outcome was found (Additional file 2: Figure S1, p = 0.726), although numbers are small. Likewise, metastasis free survival was not associated with *IDH* mutation status (p = 0.96, data not shown).

SDH and *FH* mutations were absent in chondrosarcoma

We excluded mutations in other metabolic enzymes in the 27 cartilaginous tumours that were wildtype for *IDH*, since all tumours were positive for SDHB immunohistochemical staining, suggesting an intact SDH complex and thereby excluding mutations in the different SDH subunits [44] (Additional file 3: Figure S2A; Additional file 4: Table S2). Furthermore, all primary tumours were

Table 1 Clinicopathological data of the *IDH* mutant versus wild-type group

	IDH wild-type (n = 29)	*IDH* mutation (n = 45)
Male	9 (31%)	19 (42%)
Median age at diagnosis	51 (21–79)	51 (22–85)
Histology		
Enchondroma	1 (15%)	6 (85%)
ACT/grade I	14 (50%)	14 (50%)
Grade II	9 (34%)	18 (66%)
Grade III	5 (42%)	7 (58%)
Metastasis	4 (45%)	5 (55%)
Median follow-up (months)	137 (7–278)	121 (11–312)

ACT atypical cartilaginous tumour

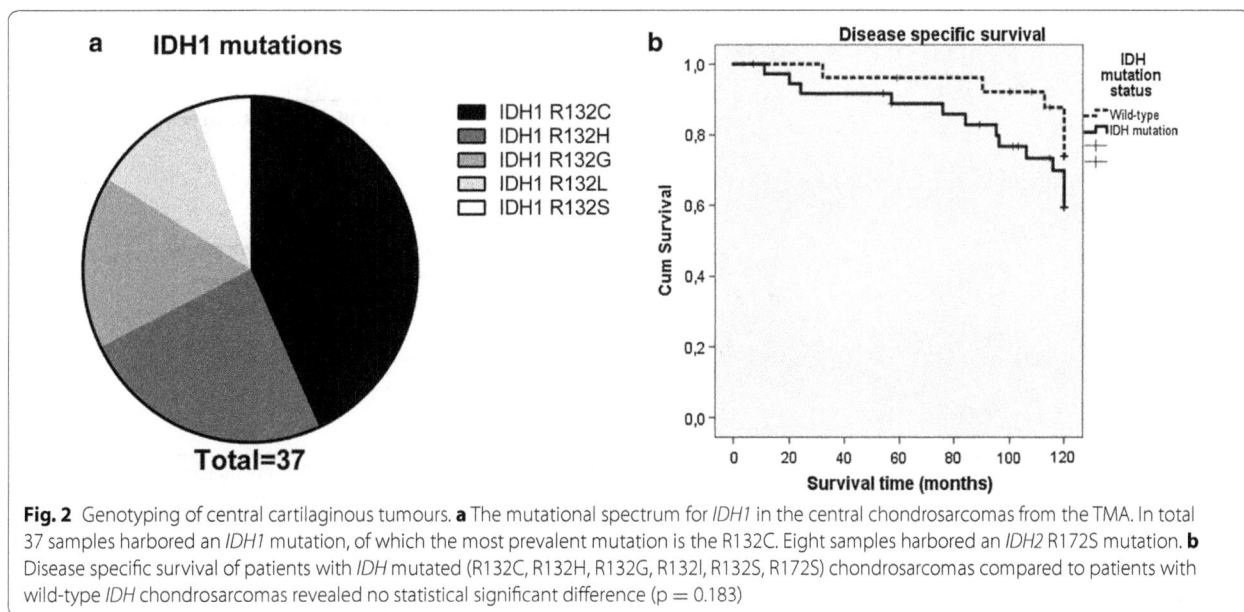

Fig. 2 Genotyping of central cartilaginous tumours. **a** The mutational spectrum for *IDH1* in the central chondrosarcomas from the TMA. In total 37 samples harbored an *IDH1* mutation, of which the most prevalent mutation is the R132C. Eight samples harbored an *IDH2* R172S mutation. **b** Disease specific survival of patients with *IDH* mutated (R132C, R132H, R132G, R132l, R132S, R172S) chondrosarcomas compared to patients with wild-type *IDH* chondrosarcomas revealed no statistical significant difference (p = 0.183)

negative for the presence of 2-SC (Additional file 3: Figure S2B; Additional file 4: Table S2), which was shown to be a robust biomarker for mutations in *FH* [42, 43].

Trimethylation of H3K4, H3K9 and H3K27 was highly abundant in chondrosarcoma

The histone modification marks H3K4me3, H3K9me3 and H3K27me3 were abundantly expressed in the vast majority of central chondrosarcomas in the first cohort (Fig. 3a, c, e). Therefore, no difference in the levels of trimethylated H3K4, H3K9 or H3K27 could be detected between *IDH* mutant and wildtype central cartilaginous tumours (Fig. 3b, d, f, p = 0.54, 0.46 and 0.78, respectively), nor between central and peripheral

chondrosarcomas (data not shown). Furthermore, studying the low grade and high grade central chondrosarcomas in separate groups revealed no significant differences, and there was no correlation with histological grade (p = 0.24, 0.51 and 0.89, respectively) (data not shown). Also, levels of trimethylation of H3K4, H3K9 and H3K27 were not associated with overall or metastasis free survival (data not shown).

Loss of ATRX in 5.6% of conventional central chondrosarcomas

Since in gliomas loss of the chromatin remodeler ATRX can be found in *IDH* mutant tumours [26], we evaluated a possible co-occurrence in chondrosarcoma. Two

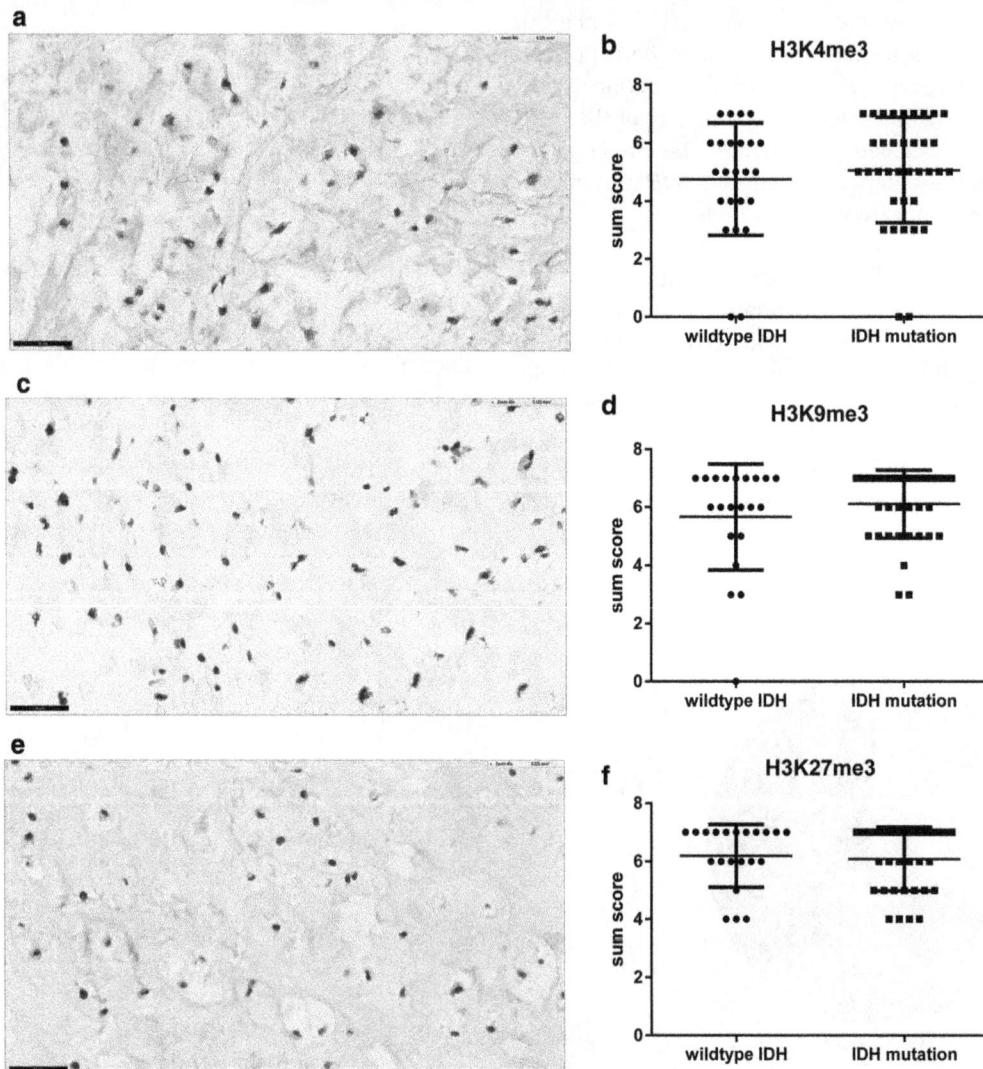

Fig. 3 No difference in trimethylation of histone marks H3K4, H3K9 and H3K27 in central chondrosarcomas. Strong nuclear positivity for H3K4me3 (**a**), H3K9me3 (**c**) and H3K27me3 (**e**) in *IDH* wildtype central chondrosarcomas as well as central chondrosarcomas harboring an *IDH* mutation. Staining was scored as the sum of the intensity and the percentage of positive tumour cells (**b, d, f**). (Scores were rounded to zero decimal places and *black bar* indicates 50 μm)

out of 36 (5.6%) conventional chondrosarcomas in the first cohort for which staining was evaluable show complete loss of ATRX (data not shown). One of these two tumours harbored an *IDH1* R132 mutation, whereas the other tumour was confirmed to be wildtype for *IDH*.

Variable levels of 5-hydroxymethylcytosine (5-hmC) and 5-methylcytosine (5-mC) in chondrosarcomas

Since D-2-HG competitively inhibits the TET enzymes [18], which catalyze the conversion of 5-mC into 5-hmC, we evaluated the distribution of 5-mC as well as 5-hmC.

Levels of 5-hmC (Fig. 4a) and 5-mC (Fig. 4c) were highly variable in chondrosarcoma. In most tumours only a fraction of the tumour cells were positive. However, no significant difference could be observed in the levels of 5-hmC (Fig. 4b) or 5-mC (Fig. 4d) between *IDH* wildtype and *IDH* mutant chondrosarcomas, considering sum score, or considering intensity and percentage of positive tumour cells separately. Interestingly, in high grade chondrosarcomas the percentage of 5-mC positive tumour cells was significantly higher as compared to low grade chondrosarcomas, which was independent of the *IDH*

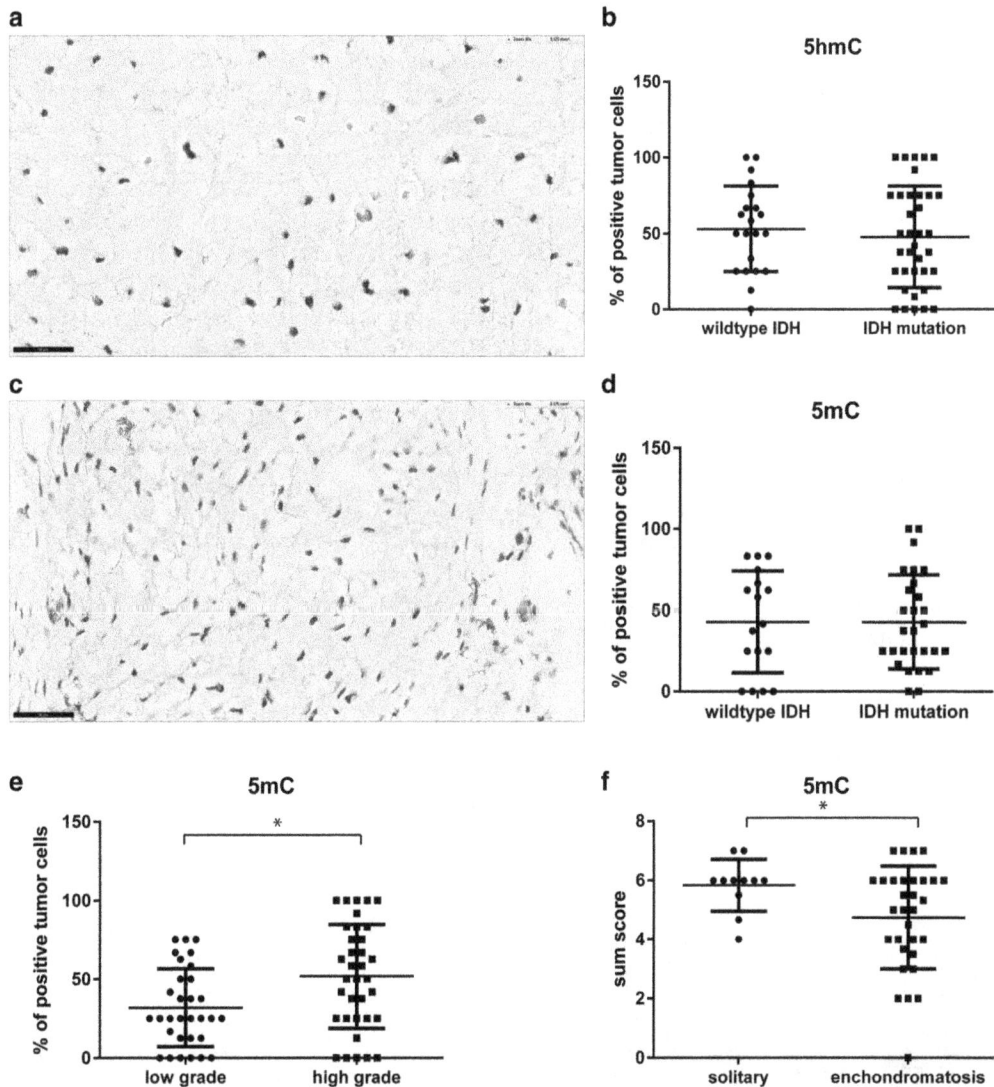

Fig. 4 Variable levels of 5-hydroxymethylcytosine (5-hmC) and 5-methylcytosine (5-mC) in chondrosarcomas. Percentage of tumour cells positive for 5hmC (**a, b**) and 5mC (**c, d**) in *IDH* mutant versus *IDH* wildtype tumours (*black bar* indicates 50 μm). The percentage of 5-mC positive tumour cells was significantly higher in high grade chondrosarcomas as compared to low grade, which was independent of the *IDH* mutation status (**e**). Solitary chondrosarcomas showed significantly higher levels of 5mC compared to enchondromatosis related chondrosarcomas, independent of the histological grade (**f**)

mutation status (p = 0.013) (Fig. 4e). This was however not reflected by a detectable decrease in 5hMC (data not shown). To increase the number of enchondromas and to compare enchondromatosis and solitary tumours, we additionally evaluated the second cohort of enchondromatosis related cartilaginous tumours for 5mC and 5hmC levels. Levels of 5mC were significantly higher in solitary tumours compared to tumours occurring in the context of enchondromatosis (p = 0.012) (Fig. 4f), which was independent of histological grade. No difference was detectable for 5hmC (data not shown).

Nuclear exclusion of TET1 is associated with loss of 5hmC in chondrosarcoma

Since we detected loss of 5-hmC in a subset of chondrosarcomas, which was not correlated with *IDH* mutation status, we evaluated whether, similar to gliomas [26], loss of 5-hmC was associated with nuclear exclusion of TET1. The majority of chondrosarcomas showed predominantly nuclear staining (N>C). No complete exclusion from the nucleus was seen in any of the chondrosarcomas (Fig. 5a). Chondrosarcomas with predominantly cytoplasmic expression of TET1 (C>N) showed significantly more often loss of 5hmC (p = 0.0001)(Fig. 5b).

Discussion

We here report the analysis of mutations in genes encoding the metabolic enzymes IDH, SDH and FH in a cohort of ~100 central cartilaginous tumours, and demonstrate that the prevalence of mutations in *IDH1* or -2 is ~60%, which is comparable to previously published data [8, 9]. As approximately 40% of the central chondrosarcomas lack detectable mutations in *IDH*, we investigated the possible involvement of two additional TCA cycle enzymes that are mutated in tumours, SDH and FH.

Mutations in components of the SDH-complex and *FH* cause upregulation of succinate and fumarate, respectively, which, similar to D-2-HG, inhibit the TET enzymes [34–36] (Fig. 1). Using immunohistochemistry as a surrogate for mutation analysis, we show that *SDH* and *FH* mutations are not involved in the subset of chondrosarcomas that are wildtype for *IDH*. Moreover, it is unlikely that mutations in *TET2* are playing a prominent role in chondrosarcoma, since Tarpey et al. demonstrated *TET2* mutations in only one out of 49 (2%) chondrosarcomas subjected to whole-exome sequencing [47].

In contrast to gliomas, we here show that in chondrosarcoma, mutations in *IDH* are not significantly correlated with outcome. Disease specific survival and metastasis free survival did not differ between wild type and *IDH* mutant tumours of 63 patients. In a previous, separate series, we also found no prognostic value of these mutations [9]. Interestingly, patients with gliomas harboring *IDH* mutations have a more favorable outcome, independent of grade, as compared to gliomas that are wildtype for *IDH* [2, 14, 15]. In intrahepatic cholangiocarcinoma, as well as in leukemia, the prognostic significance of *IDH* mutations has remained controversial. The most recent studies however fail to demonstrate prognostic significance of the *IDH* mutation in these two tumour types [16, 17], which is comparable to chondrosarcoma.

Our aim was to evaluate the effect of *IDH* mutations on histone modifications, DNA modifications, chromatin remodeling, and subcellular localization of TET1 in a cohort of central cartilaginous tumours with known *IDH* mutation status. Immunoreactivity for the histone modification marks H3K4me3, H3K9me3 and H3K27me3 was observed in the majority of chondrosarcomas, irrespective of mutation status or histological grade. In contrast, we previously showed increased H3K9me3 in *SDH*

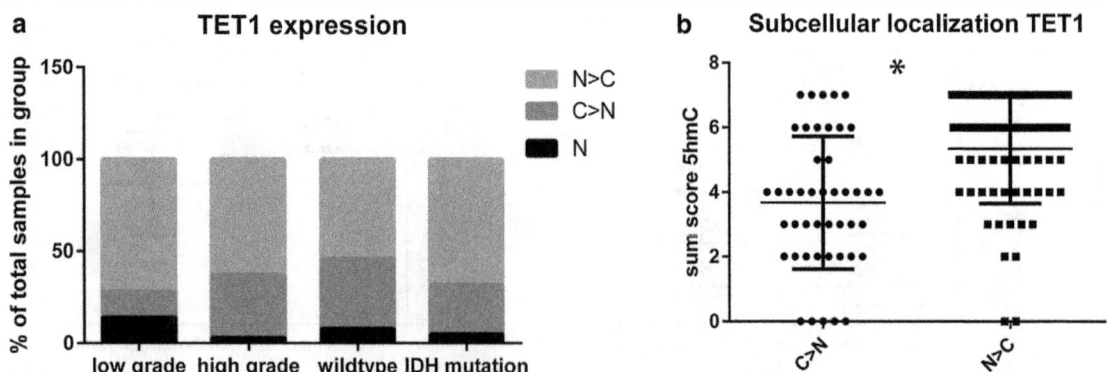

Fig. 5 Lower 5hmC levels in tumours with decreased nuclear staining for TET1. **a** There is no significant difference in subcellular localization of TET1 in *IDH* mutant versus *IDH* wildtype chondrosarcomas, and complete nuclear exclusion of TET1 was absent. **b** In tumours in which the staining was predominantly cytoplasmic, 5-hmC levels were significantly lower as compared to tumours in which staining was predominantly nuclear (scores were rounded to zero decimal places)

mutant paragangliomas and *FH* mutant smooth muscle tumours using the same immunohistochemical methods. This was supported using SDH knockdown in cell lines, which demonstrates that our approach can detect differences in the methylation of these lysine residues [37]. Lu et al. showed increased H3K9me3 levels in *IDH1* mutant gliomas as compared to the *IDH* wildtype counterparts, which were almost negative for H3K9me3 [48]. Rohle et al. reported removal of the repressive H3K9me3 and H3K27me3 marks after inhibition of mutant IDH1 using AGI-5198 in *IDH1* mutant glioma cells [49]. In contrast to these findings in other tumour types, we showed previously that inhibition of mutant IDH1 in chondrosarcoma cell lines did not alter trimethylation of H3K4, H3K9 and H3K27 [50], which is in concordance with the present immunohistochemical results.

In addition to these covalent histone modifications, ATP-dependent chromatin remodeling complexes facilitate access of nucleosomal DNA. ATRX is an example of such a chromatin remodeler. We investigated expression of ATRX, since in gliomas loss of ATRX can be found in *IDH* mutant tumours [26]. Again, results are different from glioma as we found a low prevalence of loss of ATRX (5.6%), without any correlation to *IDH* mutation status in chondrosarcoma. The observed differences between *IDH* mutated chondrosarcomas versus *IDH* mutated gliomas on DNA and histone modifications, is likely attributable to additional genetic alterations that cooperate with mutant IDH to initiate cancer, e.g. *ATRX* and *TP53* mutations in *IDH* mutant gliomas and *COL2A1*, *YEATS2*, *NRAS*, *TP53*, Rb- and Hh- signaling mutations in chondrosarcomas [47, 51–53]. D-2-HG competitively inhibits the TET enzymes [18] which is expected to result in inhibition of the conversion of 5-mC to 5-hmC [54]. Thus, loss of 5hmC expression is expected in tumours harbouring mutations in *IDH*, *FH*, *SDH*, similar to leukemias with mutations in *TET2* [54]. Indeed, we previously showed loss of 5-hmC in *SDH* mutant paragangliomas and *FH* mutant smooth muscle tumours, again verifying our methodology [37]. Also in SDH deficient GIST, 5-hmC was low to absent [38]. For *IDH* mutant gliomas, however, reports have been conflicting [55, 56] and we now show that also in chondrosarcomas a correlation between mutations in *IDH* and loss of 5-hmC is absent. Despite this, we confirmed a correlation between loss of 5-hmC and diminished nuclear staining for TET1, which was also found in *IDH* wildtype gliomas [25] and SDH deficient paragangliomas [37].

Thus, overall we did not detect any differences in trimethylation of histone marks H3K4, -K9 and K27, and in 5-mC and 5-hmC levels between *IDH* mutant and *IDH* wildtype chondrosarcomas. Recently, Thienpont and colleagues reported that tumour hypoxia causes DNA hypermethylation and loss of 5hmC by reducing TET activity [57]. Interestingly, cartilage tissue and chondrosarcomas are known to have a hypoxic microenvironment [58, 59]; [60]; [61]. They also demonstrated a large overlap between genes hypermethylated in hypoxic versus *IDH1* mutant glioblastomas [57]. Thus, as tumour hypoxia may have the same effect as an *IDH* mutation in chondrosarcoma, this may explain why we did not detect any differences using immunohistochemistry.

Moreover, we previously demonstrated that mutant IDH1 is not essential for chondrosarcoma cell proliferation and survival, as its inhibition using AGI-5198 decreased levels of D-2-HG without affecting tumourigenic properties of chondrosarcoma cell lines [50]. We also showed that trimethylation of H3K4, H3K9 and H3K27 did not change using AGI-5198 [50]. On the other hand, we and others have shown that mutant IDH1 plays a crucial role in the early development of benign enchondromas, as osteoblast differentiation was inhibited while promoting chondrogenic differentiation of mesenchymal stem cells [62, 63]. Moreover, Jin et al. have shown that during this process the repressive mark H3K9me3 and the active mark H3K4me3 were increased [63]. Thus, taken together, these data suggest that *IDH* mutations, and the resulting epigenetic changes, are only important for the initiation of enchondroma. However, once these enchondromas have matured, and after progression to chondrosarcoma, other processes are likely involved, since detectable changes in histone marks or 5-hmC are lacking and there is no correlation between *IDH* mutation and prognosis in central cartilaginous tumours.

Additional files

Additional file 1: Table S1. IDH primer sequences.

Additional file 2: Figure S1. No statistical significant difference was observed in disease specific survival between different *IDH* mutations (R132C, R132H, R132G, R132 I, R132S, R172S) compared to *IDH* wild-type chondrosarcomas (n = 63, p = 0.726).

Additional file 3: Figure S2. (A) All cartilage tumours on TMA were positive for SDHB, indicating absence of *SDH* mutations. (B) All cartilage tumours on TMA lacked detection of succinated protein using 2-SC staining, indicating absence of *FH* mutations, inset shows positive staining for 2-SC in a leiomyoma derived from a patient with a germline *FH* mutation as positive control (Scores were rounded to zero decimal places).

Additional file 4: Table S2. Mutation status for *SDH* (SDHB) and *FH* (2-SC) defined by immunohistochemistry on the TMA.

Authors' contributions
AHGC wrote the manuscript, collecting immunohistochemistry data, data analysis. JS collecting immunohistochemistry data, data analysis, reviewed the manuscript. GA collecting immunohistochemistry data, reviewed the manuscript. IHBB performed the experiments, reviewed the manuscript. NF generated and provided the 2SC antibody, reviewed the manuscript. ASH collecting immunohistochemistry data, reviewed the manuscript. PMW-K performed the experiments, reviewed the manuscript. A-MC-J supervision experiments,

reviewed the manuscript. JVMGB design of the study, scoring immunohisto-chemistry, primary supervisor of the project and writer. All authors read and approved the final manuscript.

Author details
[1] Department of Pathology, Leiden University Medical Center, L1-Q, P.O. Box 9600, 2300 RC Leiden, The Netherlands. [2] 1st Department of Pathology, Laikon General Hospital, Athens University School of Medicine, Athens, Greece. [3] Department of Pharmacology, Physiology & Neuroscience, School of Medicine, University of South Carolina, Columbia, USA. [4] Department of Human Genetics, Leiden University Medical Center, Leiden, The Netherlands.

Acknowledgements
The authors would like to thank Jolieke van Oosterwijk and Twinkal Pansuriya for construction of tissue microarrays, Yvonne de Jong for data analysis, Laura Paardekooper for technical assistance during the *IDH* mutation analysis, and Silvère M. van der Maarel for fruitful discussions.

Competing interests
The authors declare that they have no competing interests.

Funding
The study was financially supported by the Dutch Cancer Society (KWF Grant Number UL 2013-6103).

References
1. Yan H, Parsons DW, Jin G, McLendon R, Rasheed BA, Yuan W, et al. IDH1 and IDH2 mutations in gliomas. N Engl J Med. 2009;360:765–73.
2. Hartmann C, Meyer J, Balss J, Capper D, Mueller W, Christians A, et al. Type and frequency of IDH1 and IDH2 mutations are related to astrocytic and oligodendroglial differentiation and age: a study of 1010 diffuse gliomas. Acta Neuropathol. 2009;118:469–74.
3. Mardis ER, Ding L, Dooling DJ, Larson DE, McLellan MD, Chen K, et al. Recurring mutations found by sequencing an acute myeloid leukemia genome. N Engl J Med. 2009;361:1058–66.
4. Kipp BR, Voss JS, Kerr SE, Barr Fritcher EG, Graham RP, Zhang L, et al. Isocitrate dehydrogenase 1 and 2 mutations in cholangiocarcinoma. Hum Pathol. 2012;43:1552–8.
5. Borger DR, Tanabe KK, Fan KC, Lopez HU, Fantin VR, Straley KS, et al. Frequent mutation of isocitrate dehydrogenase (IDH)1 and IDH2 in cholangiocarcinoma identified through broad-based tumor genotyping. Oncologist. 2012;17:72–9.
6. Wang P, Dong Q, Zhang C, Kuan PF, Liu Y, Jeck WR, et al. Mutations in isocitrate dehydrogenase 1 and 2 occur frequently in intrahepatic cholangiocarcinomas and share hypermethylation targets with glioblastomas. Oncogene. 2013;32:3091–100.
7. Amary MF, Bacsi K, Maggiani F, Damato S, Halai D, Berisha F, et al. IDH1 and IDH2 mutations are frequent events in central chondrosarcoma and central and periosteal chondromas but not in other mesenchymal tumours. J Pathol. 2011;224:334–43.
8. Amary MF, Damato S, Halai D, Eskandarpour M, Berisha F, Bonar F, et al. Ollier disease and Maffucci syndrome are caused by somatic mosaic mutations of IDH1 and IDH2. Nat Genet. 2011;43:1262–5.
9. Pansuriya TC, van Eijk R, d'Adamo P, van Ruler MA, Kuijjer ML, Oosting J, et al. Somatic mosaic IDH1 and IDH2 mutations are associated with enchondroma and spindle cell hemangioma in Ollier disease and Maffucci syndrome. Nat Genet. 2011;43:1256–61.
10. Lucas DR, Bridge JA. Chondromas: enchondroma, periosteal chondroma. In: Fletcher CDM, Bridge JA, Hogendoorn PCW, Mertens F, editors. WHO Classification of Tumours of Soft Tissue and Bone. Lyon: International Agency for Research on Cancer (IARC); 2013. p. 252–4.
11. Pansuriya TC, Kroon HM, Bovee JVMG. Enchondromatosis: insights on the different subtypes. Int J Clin Exp Pathol. 2010;3:557–69.
12. Hogendoorn PCW, Bovée JVMG, Nielsen GP. Chondrosarcoma (grades I-III), including primary and secondary variants and periosteal chondrosarcoma. In: Fletcher CDM, Bridge JA, Hogendoorn PCW, Mertens F, editors. WHO Classification of Tumours of Soft Tissue and Bone. Lyon: IARC; 2013. p. 264–8.
13. Evans HL, Ayala AG, Romsdahl MM. Prognostic factors in chondrosarcoma of bone. A clinicopathologic analysis with emphasis on histologic grading. Cancer. 1977;40:818–31.
14. Sanson M, Marie Y, Paris S, Idbaih A, Laffaire J, Ducray F, et al. Isocitrate dehydrogenase 1 codon 132 mutation is an important prognostic biomarker in gliomas. J Clin Oncol. 2009;27:4150–4.
15. Nobusawa S, Watanabe T, Kleihues P, Ohgaki H. IDH1 mutations as molecular signature and predictive factor of secondary glioblastomas. Clin Cancer Res. 2009;15:6002–7.
16. Goyal L, Govindan A, Sheth RA, Nardi V, Blaszkowsky LS, Faris JE, et al. Prognosis and clinicopathologic features of patients with advanced stage isocitrate dehydrogenase (IDH) mutant and IDH wild-type intrahepatic cholangiocarcinoma. Oncologist. 2015;20:1019–27.
17. DiNardo CD, Ravandi F, Agresta S, Konopleva M, Takahashi K, Kadia T, et al. Characteristics, clinical outcome, and prognostic significance of IDH mutations in AML. Am J Hematol. 2015;90:732–6.
18. Xu W, Yang H, Liu Y, Yang Y, Wang P, Kim SH, et al. Oncometabolite 2-hydroxyglutarate is a competitive inhibitor of alpha-ketoglutarate-dependent dioxygenases. Cancer Cell. 2011;19:17–30.
19. Sasaki M, Knobbe CB, Munger JC, Lind EF, Brenner D, Brustle A, et al. IDH1(R132H) mutation increases murine haematopoietic progenitors and alters epigenetics. Nature. 2012;488:656–9.
20. Koch CM, Andrews RM, Flicek P, Dillon SC, Karaoz U, Clelland GK, et al. The landscape of histone modifications across 1% of the human genome in five human cell lines. Genome Res. 2007;17:691–707.
21. Barski A, Cuddapah S, Cui K, Roh TY, Schones DE, Wang Z, et al. High-resolution profiling of histone methylations in the human genome. Cell. 2007;129:823–37.
22. Tahiliani M, Koh KP, Shen Y, Pastor WA, Bandukwala H, Brudno Y, et al. Conversion of 5-methylcytosine to 5-hydroxymethylcytosine in mammalian DNA by MLL partner TET1. Science. 2009;324:930–5.
23. Ito S, Shen L, Dai Q, Wu SC, Collins LB, Swenberg JA, et al. Tet proteins can convert 5-methylcytosine to 5-formylcytosine and 5-carboxylcytosine. Science. 2011;333:1300–3.
24. Pronier E, Almire C, Mokrani H, Vasanthakumar A, Simon A, da Mor CRM, et al. Inhibition of TET2-mediated conversion of 5-methylcytosine to 5-hydroxymethylcytosine disturbs erythroid and granulomonocytic differentiation of human hematopoietic progenitors. Blood. 2011;118:2551–5.
25. Muller T, Gessi M, Waha A, Isselstein LJ, Luxen D, Freihoff D, et al. Nuclear exclusion of TET1 is associated with loss of 5-hydroxymethylcytosine in IDH1 wild-type gliomas. Am J Pathol. 2012;181:675–83.
26. Wiestler B, Capper D, Holland-Letz T, Korshunov A, von Deimling A, Pfister SM, et al. ATRX loss refines the classification of anaplastic gliomas and identifies a subgroup of IDH mutant astrocytic tumors with better prognosis. Acta Neuropathol. 2013;126:443–51.
27. Argentaro A, Yang JC, Chapman L, Kowalczyk MS, Gibbons RJ, Higgs DR, et al. Structural consequences of disease-causing mutations in the ATRX-DNMT3-DNMT3L (ADD) domain of the chromatin-associated protein ATRX. Proc Natl Acad Sci USA. 2007;104:11939–44.
28. Baysal BE, Ferrell RE, Willett-Brozick JE, Lawrence EC, Myssiorek D, Bosch A, et al. Mutations in SDHD, a mitochondrial complex II gene, in hereditary paraganglioma. Science. 2000;287:848–51.
29. Niemann S, Muller U. Mutations in SDHC cause autosomal dominant paraganglioma, type 3. Nat Genet. 2000;26:268–70.
30. Astuti D, Latif F, Dallol A, Dahia PL, Douglas F, George E, et al. Gene mutations in the succinate dehydrogenase subunit SDHB cause susceptibility to familial pheochromocytoma and to familial paraganglioma. Am J Hum Genet. 2001;69:49–54.
31. Burnichon N, Briere JJ, Libe R, Vescovo L, Riviere J, Tissier F, et al. SDHA is a tumor suppressor gene causing paraganglioma. Hum Mol Genet. 2010;19:3011–20.
32. Janeway KA, Kim SY, Lodish M, Nose V, Rustin P, Gaal J, et al. Defects in succinate dehydrogenase in gastrointestinal stromal tumors lacking KIT and PDGFRA mutations. Proc Natl Acad Sci USA. 2011;108:314–8.

33. Tomlinson IP, Alam NA, Rowan AJ, Barclay E, Jaeger EE, Kelsell D, et al. Germline mutations in FH predispose to dominantly inherited uterine fibroids, skin leiomyomata and papillary renal cell cancer. Nat Genet. 2002;30:406–10.

34. Smith EH, Janknecht R, Maher LJ III. Succinate inhibition of alpha-ketoglutarate-dependent enzymes in a yeast model of paraganglioma. Hum Mol Genet. 2007;16:3136–48.

35. Xiao M, Yang H, Xu W, Ma S, Lin H, Zhu H, et al. Inhibition of alpha-KG-dependent histone and DNA demethylases by fumarate and succinate that are accumulated in mutations of FH and SDH tumor suppressors. Genes Dev. 2012;26:1326–38.

36. Letouze E, Martinelli C, Loriot C, Burnichon N, Abermil N, Ottolenghi C, et al. SDH mutations establish a hypermethylator phenotype in paraganglioma. Cancer Cell. 2013;23:739–52.

37. Hoekstra AS, de Graaff MA, Briaire-de Bruijn IH, Ras C, Seifar RM, van Minderhout I, et al. Inactivation of SDH and FH cause loss of 5hmC and increased H3K9me3 in paraganglioma/pheochromocytoma and smooth muscle tumors. Oncotarget. 2015;6:38777–88.

38. Mason EF, Hornick JL. Succinate dehydrogenase deficiency is associated with decreased 5-hydroxymethylcytosine production in gastrointestinal stromal tumors: implications for mechanisms of tumorigenesis. Mod Pathol. 2013;26:1492–7.

39. Waaijer CJ, de Andrea CE, Hamilton A, van Oosterwijk JG, Stringer SE, Bovee JVMG. Cartilage tumour progression is characterized by an increased expression of heparan sulphate 6O-sulphation-modifying enzymes. Virchows Arch. 2012;461:475–81.

40. Pansuriya TC, Oosting J, Krenacs T, Taminiau AH, Verdegaal SH, Sangiorgi L, et al. Genome-wide analysis of Ollier disease: is it all in the genes? Orphanet J Rare Dis. 2011;6:2.

41. Gruis NA, Abeln ECA, Bardoel AFJ, Devilee P, Frants RR, Cornelisse CJ. PCR-based microsatellite polymorphisms in the detection of loss of heterozygosity in fresh and archival tumour tissue. Br J Cancer. 1993;68:308–13.

42. Bardella C, El-Bahrawy M, Frizzell N, Adam J, Ternette N, Hatipoglu E, et al. Aberrant succination of proteins in fumarate hydratase-deficient mice and HLRCC patients is a robust biomarker of mutation status. J Pathol. 2011;225:4–11.

43. Ternette N, Yang M, Laroyia M, Kitagawa M, O'Flaherty L, Wolhulter K, et al. Inhibition of mitochondrial aconitase by succination in fumarate hydratase deficiency. Cell Rep. 2013;3:689–700.

44. Kirmani S, Young WF. Hereditary Paraganglioma–Pheochromocytoma Syndromes. In: Pagon RA, Adam MP, Ardinger HH, Wallace SE, Amemiya A, Bean LJ, et al., editors. Gene reviews. Seattle: University of Washington; 2008.

45. van Oosterwijk JG, Meijer D, van Ruler MA, van den Akker BE, Oosting J, Krenacs T, et al. Screening for potential targets for therapy in mesenchymal, clear cell, and dedifferentiated chondrosarcoma reveals Bcl-2 family members and TGFbeta as potential targets. Am J Pathol. 2013;182:1347–56.

46. Wagner K, Damm F, Gohring G, Gorlich K, Heuser M, Schafer I, et al. Impact of IDH1 R132 mutations and an IDH1 single nucleotide polymorphism in cytogenetically normal acute myeloid leukemia: SNP rs11554137 is an adverse prognostic factor. J Clin Oncol. 2010;28:2356–64.

47. Tarpey PS, Behjati S, Cooke SL, Van LP, Wedge DC, Pillay N, et al. Frequent mutation of the major cartilage collagen gene COL2A1 in chondrosarcoma. Nat Genet. 2013;45:923–6.

48. Lu C, Ward PS, Kapoor GS, Rohle D, Turcan S, Abdel-Wahab O, et al. IDH mutation impairs histone demethylation and results in a block to cell differentiation. Nature. 2012;483:474–8.

49. Rohle D, Popovici-Muller J, Palaskas N, Turcan S, Grommes C, Campos C, et al. An inhibitor of mutant IDH1 delays growth and promotes differentiation of glioma cells. Science. 2013;340:626–30.

50. Suijker J, Oosting J, Koornneef A, Struys EA, Salomons GS, Schaap FG, et al. Inhibition of mutant IDH1 decreases D-2-HG levels without affecting tumorigenic properties of chondrosarcoma cell lines. Oncotarget. 2015;6:12505.

51. Clark O, Yen K, Mellinghoff IK. Molecular pathways: isocitrate dehydrogenase mutations in cancer. Clin Cancer Res. 2016;22:1837–42.

52. Totoki Y, Yoshida A, Hosoda F, Nakamura H, Hama N, Ogura K, et al. Unique mutation portraits and frequent COL2A1 gene alteration in chondrosarcoma. Genome Res. 2014;24:1411–20.

53. Zhang YX, van Oosterwijk JG, Sicinska E, Moss S, Remillard SP, Van Wezel T, et al. Functional profiling of receptor tyrosine kinases and downstream signaling in human chondrosarcomas identifies pathways for rational targeted therapy. Clin Cancer Res. 2013;19:3796–807.

54. Pronier E, Almire C, Mokrani H, Vasanthakumar A, Simon A, da Mor BD, et al. Inhibition of TET2-mediated conversion of 5-methylcytosine to 5-hydroxymethylcytosine disturbs erythroid and granulomonocytic differentiation of human hematopoietic progenitors. Blood. 2011;118(9):2551–5.

55. Zhu J, Zuo J, Xu Q, Wang X, Wang Z, Zhou D. Isocitrate dehydrogenase mutations may be a protective mechanism in glioma patients. Med Hypotheses. 2011;76:602–3.

56. Jin SG, Jiang Y, Qiu R, Rauch TA, Wang Y, Schackert G, et al. 5-Hydroxymethylcytosine is strongly depleted in human cancers but its levels do not correlate with IDH1 mutations. Cancer Res. 2011;71:7360–5.

57. Thienpont B, Steinbacher J, Zhao H, D'Anna F, Kuchnio A, Ploumakis A, et al. Tumour hypoxia causes DNA hypermethylation by reducing TET activity. Nature. 2016;537:63–8.

58. Gibson JS, Milner PI, White R, Fairfax TP, Wilkins RJ. Oxygen and reactive oxygen species in articular cartilage: modulators of ionic homeostasis. Pflugers Arch. 2008;455:563–73.

59. Kubo T, Sugita T, Shimose S, Matsuo T, Arihiro K, Ochi M. Expression of hypoxia-inducible factor-1alpha and its relationship to tumour angiogenesis and cell proliferation in cartilage tumours. J Bone Joint Surg Br. 2008;90:364–70.

60. Ayala G, Liu C, Nicosia R, Horowitz S, Lackman R. Microvasculature and VEGF expression in cartilaginous tumors. Hum Pathol. 2000;31:341–6.

61. Boeuf S, Bovee JV, Lehner B, Hogendoorn PC, Richter W. Correlation of hypoxic signalling to histological grade and outcome in cartilage tumours. Histopathology. 2010;56:641–51.

62. Suijker J, Baelde HJ, Roelofs H, Cleton-Jansen AM, Bovee JVMG. The oncometabolite D-2-hydroxyglutarate induced by mutant IDH1 or -2 blocks osteoblast differentiation in vitro and in vivo. Oncotarget. 2015;20:14832–42.

63. Jin Y, Elalaf H, Watanabe M, Tamaki S, Hineno S, Matsunaga K, et al. Mutant IDH1 dysregulates the differentiation of mesenchymal stem cells in association with gene-specific histone modifications to cartilage- and bone-related genes. PLoS ONE. 2015;10:e0131998.

10

Dendritic and mast cell involvement in the inflammatory response to primary malignant bone tumours

Y. Inagaki[1,2], E. Hookway[1], K. A. Williams[1], A. B. Hassan[1], U. Oppermann[1], Y. Tanaka[2], E. Soilleux[1] and N. A. Athanasou[1*]

Abstract

Background: A chronic inflammatory cell infiltrate is commonly seen in response to primary malignant tumours of bone. This is known to contain tumour-associated macrophages (TAMs) and lymphocytes; dendritic cells (DCs) and mast cells (MCs) have also been identified but whether these and other inflammatory cells are seen commonly in specific types of bone sarcoma is uncertain.

Methods: In this study we determined the nature of the inflammatory cell infiltrate in 56 primary bone sarcomas. Immunohistochemistry using monoclonal antibodies was employed to assess semiquantitatively CD45+ leukocyte infiltration and the extent of the DC, MC, TAM and T and B lymphocyte infiltrate.

Results: The extent of the inflammatory infiltrate in individual sarcomas was very variable. A moderate or heavy leukocyte infiltrate was more commonly seen in conventional high-grade osteosarcoma, undifferentiated pleomorphic sarcoma and giant cell tumour of bone (GCTB) than in Ewing sarcoma, chordoma and chondrosarcoma. CD14+/CD68+ TAMs and CD3+ T lymphocytes were the major components of the inflammatory cell response but (DC-SIGN/CD11c+) DCs were also commonly noted when there was a significant TAM and T lymphocyte infiltrate. MCs were identified mainly at the periphery of sarcomas, including the osteolytic tumour-bone interface.

Discussion: Our findings indicate that, although variable, some malignant bone tumours (e.g. osteosarcoma, GCTB) are more commonly associated with a pronounced inflammatory cell infiltrate than others (e.g. chondrosarcoma. Ewing sarcoma); the infiltrate is composed mainly of TAMs but includes a significant DC, T lymphocyte and MC infiltrate.

Conclusion: Tumours that contain a heavy inflammatory cell response, which includes DCs, TAMs and T lymphocytes, may be more amenable to immunomodulatory therapy. MCs are present mainly at the tumour edge and are likely to contribute to osteolysis and tumour invasion.

Keywords: Immunity, Bone sarcomas, Dendritic cells, Mast cells, Macrophages, Lymphocytes

Background

Host defence against primary bone sarcomas is evidenced by the presence of a chronic inflammatory cell infiltrate both within the tumour and in the 'pseudocapsule'

around the tumour [1, 2]. The inflammatory cell response to malignant tumours, including sarcomas, is composed mainly of tumour-associated macrophages (TAMs) and lymphocytes, but is known to include dendritic cells (DCs) and mast cells (MCs) [2–5]. Tumour cells and stromal cells in the tumour microenvironment are known to release chemokines, cytokines and growth factors which attract inflammatory cells; these cells in turn release numerous humoral factors that are implicated in

*Correspondence: nick.athanasou@ndorms.ox.ac.uk
[1] Nuffield Department of Orthopaedics, Rheumatology
and Musculoskeletal and Sciences, University of Oxford, Nuffield
Orthopaedic Centre, Oxford OX3 7HE, UK
Full list of author information is available at the end of the article

promoting tumour growth, angiogenesis and modulation of the immune response [5, 6].

The cellular components of the peri-tumoural inflammatory infiltrate reflect the nature of the innate and adaptive host immune response to a particular tumour. Specific inflammatory cell components have been shown to produce both positive and negative effects on tumour growth and spread. In some cancers, a high TAM infiltrate has been shown to correlate with poor prognosis, leading to the suggestion that these cells could represent a potential therapeutic target for cancer immunotherapy [7–9]. In contrast, lymphocytic infiltration, predominantly of T lymphocytes, correlates with improved survival in several cancers [10–12]. The role of other myeloid cells known to be present in cancer-related inflammation, such as DCs and MCs, is less well-defined. Some but by no means all studies have shown that DC infiltration of carcinomas is associated with increased survival and reduced incidence of metastasis; accordingly, immunotherapeutic strategies to treat solid tumours have been developed that exploit the specific role of DCs to coordinate the innate and adaptive immune response [13, 14]. MCs have been shown to play a role in regulating the adaptive immune response and in mediating vascular and stromal changes in tumour tissues [4, 15, 16]. MCs have also been shown to influence the extent of the DC, TAM and lymphocyte infiltrate through the release of mediators which enhance migration and proliferation of these cells [17–20].

Although immunotherapies targeting TAMs, lymphocytes and DCs have been investigated in some bone and soft tissue sarcomas [21–24], there has been little analysis of the number of these inflammatory cells in specific primary malignant bone tumours. In this study our aim has been to examine the nature and extent of myeloid and lymphoid inflammatory cells found in different types of primary malignant bone tumour. In this way we have sought to determine not only whether TAMs, lymphocytes, DCs and MCs are likely to play a role in influencing tumour growth and spread but also whether these cells are present in sufficient numbers to provide a target for immunotherapy in specific sarcomas.

Methods

Cases examined and specimen processing

Samples of 56 primary malignant bone tumours were obtained from archival surgical material at the Department of Histopathology, Nuffield Orthopaedic Centre, Oxford, UK. Samples of primary aggressive or malignant bone tumours included 14 cases of conventional osteosarcoma, 8 cases of Grade I chondrosarcoma, 4 cases of Grade II/III chondrosarcoma, 2 cases of dedifferentiated chondrosarcoma, 11 cases of giant cell tumour of bone

(GCTB), 12 cases of Ewing sarcoma, 2 cases of chordoma and 3 cases of undifferentiated pleomorphic sarcoma of bone. None of the patients had received immunomodulatory neo-adjuvant therapies.

Several osteolytic benign bone tumours were also assessed for MC infiltration. These included 4 cases of fibrous dysplasia, 4 cases of non-ossifying fibroma, 2 cases of osteoblastoma, 2 cases of aneurysmal bone cyst and 2 cases of chondroblastoma.

Control tissues included samples of normal bone obtained from amputation specimens and, for mast cell staining, samples of bone obtained from two cases of systemic mastocytosis. All samples were fixed in 10 % neutral buffered formalin and decalcified in 5 % nitric acid prior to processing and embedding in paraffin wax. Serial sections of 5 μm were cut and mounted on charged microscope slides (Surgipath, UK) for immunohistochemical staining.

Immunohistochemistry

Monoclonal antibodies employed in this study and their specificity are shown in Table 1. Sections were incubated at 37 °C for at least 24 h to improve tissue adhesion before immunohistochemistry. Tissue sections were dewaxed in xylene and rehydrated by successive immersion in graded alcohol and water. Endogenous peroxidase was blocked by treating the sections with 0.2 % hydrogen peroxide (BDH, UK) in 80 % alcohol for 30 min. Antigen retrieval was required for all antibodies. This involved microwave heat treatment in 500 ml 10 mM Tris/1 M EDTA (BDH, UK) buffer, pH 8.5.

Immunohistochemistry was performed using an indirect immunoperoxidase technique with 3,3-diaminobenzidine chromogen (ChemMate Envision, Dako, UK). Sections were incubated with primary antibodies for 30 min at room temperature followed by 30 min incubation with labelled polymer and 10 min in 3,3-diaminobenzidene. The sections were then counterstained using Mayer's haematoxylin (RA Lamb, UK) for 3 min and blued in 2 % hydrogen sodium carbonate (BDH, UK).

Histological analysis

Areas of tumour containing the maximum inflammatory response were scored, as previously described, by a modified semi quantitative technique as sparse (<2 %), moderate (2–10 %) or dense (>10 %) after counting 500 cells in five high-powered (×400) fields and determining the number of cells expressing CD45 (leukocyte common antigen) [25, 26]. Areas of tumour necrosis were not included in this assessment. In parallel sections stained with immunophenotypic markers, identifying B and T lymphocytes, TAMs, MCs and DCs (Table 1), the number of these infiltrating cells was scored relative to the

Table 1 Monoclonal antibodies used in this study

Antigen	Antibody (clone)	Specificity	Source	Dilution	Pre-treatment
CD3	(F7.2.38)	T cells	Dako	1:25	MW 20 min
CD11c	(5D11)	DCs, histiocytes	Novocastra	1:100	MW 20 min
CD14	(7)	Macrophages, monocytes	Novocastra	1:50	MW 20 min
CD20	(L26)	B cells	Dako	1:100	—
CD45	(PD7/26;2B11)	Leucocyte common antigen	Dako	1:100	MW 10 min
CD68	(KP1)	Macrophages, monocytes, neutrophils, NK cells	Dako	1:1000	MW 10 min
DC-SIGN	(120,507)	Immature DCs	R&D Systems	1:500	MW 10 min
S100	(polyclonal)	DCs, histiocytes, chondrocytes	Dako	1:1000	—
Mast cell tryptase	AA1	Mast cells	Dako	1:100	MW 10 min

MW microwave, – no pre-treatment required

number of CD45+ cells as: +low (<5 % positive cells); ++moderate (6–25 % positive cells); +++heavy (>25 % positive cells).

Results

Results of the immunohistochemical findings are summarised in Table 2.

The extent of the CD45+ inflammatory cell infiltrate in the malignant bone tumours analysed was highly variable, not only between different types of bone sarcoma but also between sarcomas of a single type. The inflammatory infiltrate was not uniformly distributed throughout these tumours; all GCTBs contained a dense CD45+ inflammatory infiltrate while osteosarcoma and undifferentiated pleomorphic sarcomas often contained areas with a moderate CD45+ infiltrate (Fig. 1). In contrast, chondrosarcomas, chordomas and Ewing sarcomas contained a sparse inflammatory cell infiltrate. In all bone sarcomas, CD68+ TAMs comprised the largest sub-population of inflammatory cells in the tumour followed by CD3+ T cells and DCs. CD20+ B cells were absent or very rarely identified in the bone sarcomas analysed.

Where there was a high number of CD68+ TAMs and CD3+ T lymphocytes in bone sarcomas, DC-SIGN-expressing DCs were noted; some of these cells stained for CD11c and S100 but they did not stain for CD1a. The most common pattern seen in conventional osteosarcoma, undifferentiated pleomorphic sarcoma and GCTB

was that of a moderate or heavy (++/+++) TAM infiltrate, with a low/moderate (+/++) CD3+ T cell and DC infiltrate (Fig. 2). DCs were absent or present in low numbers (+) in chondrosarcoma, chordoma and most but not all Ewing sarcomas. All Grade 1 chondrosarcomas contained a sparse inflammatory cell infiltrate (Fig. 3a). A few (+) TAMs were noted in areas of matrix degeneration or mineralisation but there were few or no T cells or DCs identified in the tumour stroma. Grade II and III chondrosarcomas also contained few or no inflammatory cells, although some TAMs, T cells and DCs were seen in areas of matrix degeneration in fibrous tissue separating lobules of tumour cartilage. DCs were not present in the low-grade cartilaginous component but were seen in the spindle cell component of dedifferentiated chondrosarcoma (Fig. 3c). These tumours also contained numerous TAMs and T cells.

MCs were not present or very few in number in the main tumour mass of most bone sarcomas. However, MCs (+/++) were commonly found at the periphery of invasive bone tumours in the fibrous pseudocapsule at the soft tissue margin and at the host bone-tumour interface where there was osteolysis (Fig. 4). The finding of an MC association with tumour osteolysis in sarcomas prompted us to examine MC infiltration in lytic benign bone tumours. We found that MCs were commonly sited at the host bone-tumour interface in all cases of chondroblastoma (Fig. 4d), osteoblastoma, aneurysmal bone cyst,

Table 2 Tumour-infiltrating leucocyte antigen expression

	CD45	CD68	CD14	CD3	CD20	DC-SIGN	Mast cell[a] tryptase
Giant cell tumour of bone	Dense	+++	++	+	–	+	+/++
Osteosarcoma; Undifferentiated pleomorphic sarcoma dedifferentiated chondrosarcoma	Moderate	++	+/++	+	–	+	+/++
Ewing sarcoma Chondrosarcoma Chordoma	Sparse	+/++	+/++	–/+	–	–/+	+/++

Inter/intra-tumour variability of leucocyte antigen expression noted. For details, see "Results" section

[a] Mast cells (+/++) were identified at the periphery of all osteolytic bone tumours

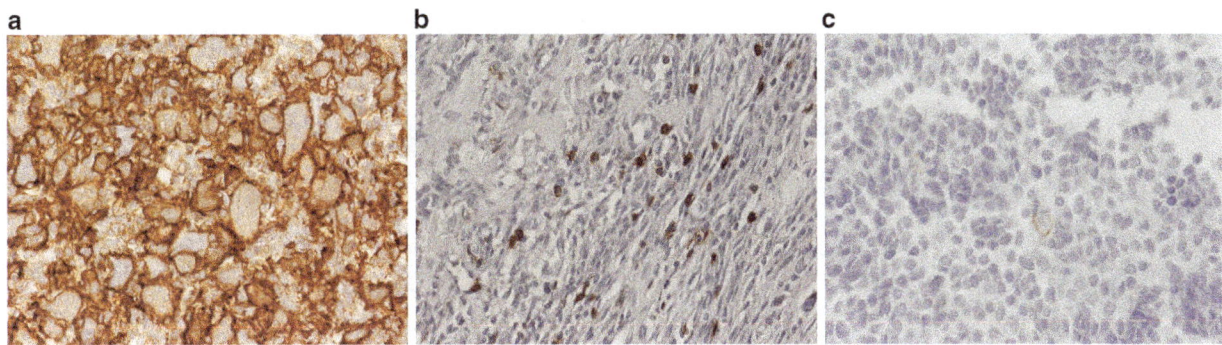

Fig. 1 Immunohistochemistry for the leucocyte marker CD45 showing that the inflammatory cell infiltrate is: **a** heavy in GCTB. **b** Moderate in osteosarcoma. **c** Sparse in Ewing sarcoma

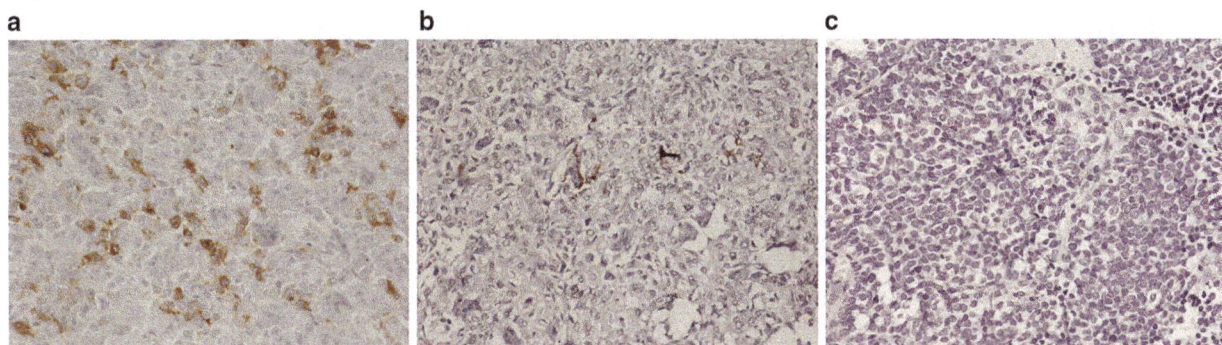

Fig. 2 Immunohistochemistry for the DC marker for DC-SIGN showing: **a** moderate (++) expression in GCTB. **b** Low (+) expression in osteosarcoma. **c** Absence of expression in Ewing sarcoma

Fig. 3 Immunohistochemistry for the macrophage marker CD68 in chondrosarcoma showing: **a** absence of TAMs in low-grade chondrosarcoma. **b** Scattered (+) TAMs in areas of matrix mineralisation within the tumour. **c** Absence of TAMs in the low-grade cartilaginous component (*left*) but scattered (+) TAMs in the high-grade sarcomatous component (*right*) of a dedifferentiated chondrosarcoma

non-ossifying fibroma and fibrous dysplasia. A few (+) MCs were also noted in fibrotic areas of undifferentiated pleomorphic sarcomas and osteosarcomas of bone. MCs (++) were also commonly seen in the fibrous component of benign bone lesions such as non-ossifying fibroma and fibrous dysplasia.

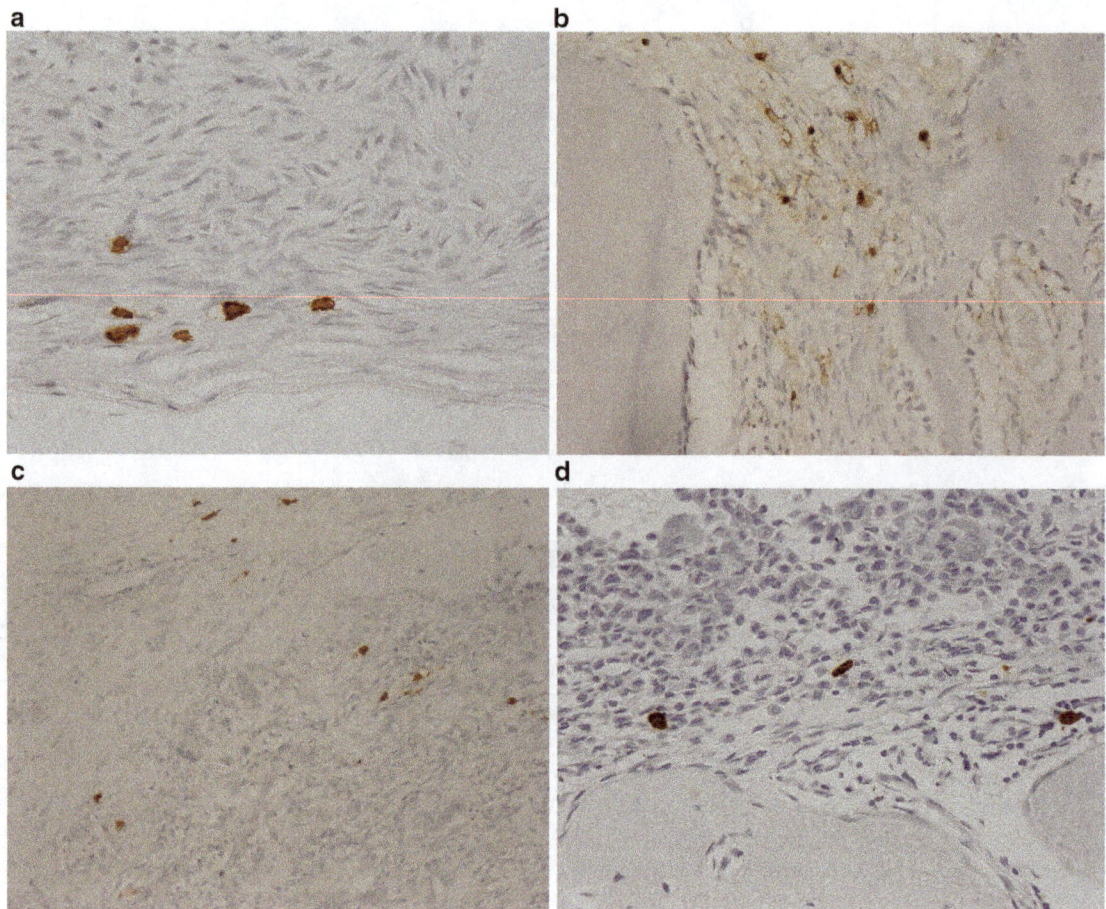

Fig. 4 Immunohistochemistry for mast cell tryptase showing MCs in: **a** the pseudocapsule and **b** tumour-bone interface of an osteosarcoma. **c** The soft tissue margin of an aggressive GCTB. **d** The osteolytic margin of a chondroblastoma

Discussion

This study has shown that myeloid and lymphoid cells, which play a role in innate and adaptive immunity are present in the inflammatory response to primary aggressive/malignant bone tumours. A significant inflammatory cell infiltrate was commonly seen in osteosarcoma, undifferentiated pleomorphic sarcoma, GCTB and dedifferentiated chondrosarcomas. Inflammation was less pronounced in Ewing sarcoma, chordoma and chondrosarcoma. TAMs formed the major component of the inflammatory cell infiltrate in all bone tumours; there was also a variable population of CD3+ T cells and DCs. In general, the extent of DC infiltration corresponded to that of TAMs and T cells. MCs were found mainly at the osteolytic bone-tumour interface in bone sarcomas as well as other benign primary bone tumours.

As in carcinomas and soft tissue sarcomas, the major subpopulation of leukocytes noted in bone sarcomas was that of TAMs [5, 26]. TAMs have been shown to promote tumour progression in several carcinomas by suppressing the immune response, increasing expression of matrix metalloproteinases and promoting tumour angiogenesis [5, 7–9]. The role of TAMs in bone sarcomas has not been extensively investigated. TAMs have been associated with reduced metastasis and improved survival in high-grade osteosarcoma [30]. In contrast, TAM infiltration has been associated with a poor prognosis in Ewing sarcoma [31]. Osteoclasts, which carry out the bone resorption associated with growth of a bone tumour are derived from TAMs by a RANKL-dependent mechanism [32, 33], and it would be expected that a heavy TAM infiltrate would promote tumour growth and spread. Ewing sarcoma and osteosarcoma tumour cells have been shown to express RANKL and to support macrophage-osteoclast differentiation [33–36]. Although we found that the majority of Ewing sarcomas in our study induced a relatively low inflammatory cell response, we noted that most of the cells in the infiltrate were TAMs. Paradoxically, it has been shown in some reports that there is an inverse relationship between the number of osteoclasts and the extent of pulmonary metastasis [37, 38]. Further studies are required to establish the role of TAMs in high-grade bone sarcomas as these cells constitute the major subpopulation of inflammatory cells in these tumours.

DCs and CD3+ T lymphocytes were noted in all types of bone sarcoma and in general their number corresponded with the extent of TAM infiltration. DCs are efficient antigen-presenting cells that have the ability to prime naïve T cells and initiate a specific immune response [37, 38]. DCs exist in two functionally and phenotypically distinct stages, immature and mature. Immature DCs have high endocytic activity, specialise in antigen capture and processing and reside in peripheral tissues. Upon exposure to pathogen-derived products or innate pro-inflammatory signals, DCs lose their phagocytic activity and migrate to draining lymph nodes where they become mature DCs. Mature DCs have high antigen-presenting capability and interact with antigen-specific T cells to initiate a specific immune response. In tumours there is a disturbance of DC differentiation, survival and function [13, 14, 38]. A C-type lectin, a DC-specific ICAM-grabbing non-integrin (DC-SIGN), has been identified and shown to mediate strong adhesion between DCs and intracellular adhesion molecule 3 (ICAM-3) on resting T cells [39, 40]. We noted that CD3+ T lymphocytes were more commonly found in osteosarcomas than Ewing sarcomas although considerable variation was observed regarding the density and distribution of these cells, some of which have been shown to be cytotoxic against osteosarcoma tumour cells and to promote adaptive antitumor immunity in Ewing sarcoma [41, 42]. Tumour-derived factors such as vascular endothelial growth factor can induce immature DCs from the bone marrow to migrate to osteosarcomas [43, 44]. Although showing some variability, fewer DCs were seen in Ewing sarcomas where the TAM and T-lymphocyte response was also reduced. The suppression of DC antigen and function can induce immune tolerance to tumour antigens in sarcomas [39]; specifically, the alteration of carbohydrates on the cell surface is thought to influence the interaction between C-type lectins on DCs and tumour cells, thus interfering with antigen presentation [45]. DC-SIGN is a useful immunohistochemical marker of immature and mature DCs and may be useful in assessing the efficacy of DC-based immunotherapy against sarcomas [46, 47]. Antibodies targeting DC-SIGN have been used to induce a T cell response, and vaccines comprising autologous antigen-loaded DCs have been shown to prime tumour immunity [48, 49].

MCs are found throughout the body and are usually located in connective tissues, particularly around blood and lymphatic vessels as well as peripheral nerves; they are present in low numbers in normal human bone marrow [50]. MCs are mobilised to infiltrate tumours by means of stem cell factor (SCF) [16, 18]. Production of SCF and the receptor for SCF (c-kit) have been identified in several bone sarcomas, including Ewing sarcoma and osteosarcoma [51–53]. Mechanisms whereby MCs may influence tumour progression include stimulation of the release of growth factors essential for tumour growth and suppression of the host immune response to tumour cells [16, 18]. MC-derived humoral factors are known to influence the migration and function of TAMs, T-lymphocytes and DCs [18–20]. We noted that MCs were found mainly at the tumour-bone interface where there was tumour-associated osteolysis. MCs have been identified at the periphery of tumours in aggressive breast cancer and malignant melanoma [16]. MCs are known to promote osteoclastic bone resorption and to play a role in inflammatory osteolysis, renal osteodystrophy and other bone conditions where there is increased remodelling activity [50, 54]. Mediators produced by MCs which promote osteoclastic resorption include the prostaglandins E2 and D2, and cytokines such as tumour necrosis factor alpha (TNFα) [16, 19]. The latter has been shown to simulate osteoclast formation by a RANKL-independent mechanism [55], it has been shown that TAM-osteoclast differentiation in Ewing sarcoma can be induced by TNFα [33]. This may play a role in promoting tumour metastases in Ewing sarcoma which is modulated by stem cell factor and its receptor c-kit [56].

Conclusions

Our findings show that the inflammatory response to primary malignant bone tumours is variable and to some extent depends on tumour type. TAMs and T-lymphocytes are the major inflammatory cell types seen in bone sarcomas but there is also a significant DC component within some tumours. MCs are likely to contribute to tumour osteolysis as they are almost exclusively found at the tumour-bone interface. Using specific myeloid and lymphoid inflammatory cell subpopulations as targets for immunomodulatory therapy has been proposed for bone sarcomas but the efficacy of such treatment is likely to depend of the presence of a significant inflammatory response in the tumour; our findings show that this can be highly variable, and it may thus be useful to assess the extent and nature of the inflammatory cell response in a bone sarcoma before instituting this type of therapy.

Abbreviations

TAMs: tumour-associated macrophages; DCs: dendritic cells; MCs: mast cells; GCTB: giant cell tumour of bone; DC-SIGN: DC-specific ICAM-grabbing non-integrin; SCF: stem cell factor; TNFα: tumour necrosis factor alpha.

Authors' contributions
KAW/YI/ES—supplied reagents and carried out methods and analysed results.
NAA/EH/ABH/UO/YT—contributed to analysing the results and writing the manuscript. All authors read and approved the final manuscript.

Author details
[1] Nuffield Department of Orthopaedics, Rheumatology and Musculoskeletal and Sciences, University of Oxford, Nuffield Orthopaedic Centre, Oxford OX3 7HE, UK. [2] Department of Orthopaedic Surgery, Nara Medical University, Kashihara, Japan.

Acknowledgements
None applicable.

Competing interests
The authors declare that they have no competing interests.

Funding
This was solely supported by the funding from the European Union through EuroBoNet and EuroSarc consortiums as well as by funding from the Oxford NIHR BRU, The Rosetrees Trust, Sarcoma (UK) and the Bone Cancer Research Trust. The funding bodies had no role in the design of the study, the collection of data, interpretation of data, writing of the manuscript of decision to publish.

References
1. Enneking WF. Musculoskeletal tumor surgery. New York: Churchill Living-stone; 1983. p. 3–27.
2. Miura Y, Suda A, Watanabe Y, Yamakawa M, Imai Y. Inflammatory cells in the pseudocapsule of osteosarcoma. A clinicopathologic analysis. Clin Orthop Relat Res. 1994;300:225–32.
3. Theoleyre S, Mori K, Cherrier B, Rassuti Nm Louin F, Redini F, Heymann D. Phenotypic and functional analysis of lymphocytes infiltrating osteolytic tumors: use as a possible therapeutic approach of osteosarcoma. BMC Cancer. 2005;5:123.
4. Murdoch C, Muthana M, Coffelt SB, Lewis CE. The role of myeloid cells in the promotion of tumour angiogenesis. Nat Rev Cancer. 2008;8:618–31.
5. Mantovani A, Allavena P, Sica A, Balliwill F. Cancer-related inflammation. Nature. 2008;454:436–44.
6. Del Prete A, Allavena P, Santoro G, Fumarolo R, Corsi MM, Mantovani A. Molecular pathways in cancer-related inflammation. Biochem Med (Zagreb). 2011;21:264–75.
7. Siveen KS, Kuttan G. Role of macrophages in tumour progression. Immunol Lett. 2009;123:97–102.
8. Allavena P, Mantovani A. Immunology in the clinic review series; focus on cancer: tumour-associated macrophages: undisputed stars of the inflammatory tumour microenvironment. Clin Exp Immunol. 2012;167:195–205.
9. Cook J, Hagemann T. Tumour-associated macrophages and cancer. Curr Opin Pharmacol. 2013;13:595–601.
10. Pages F, Berger A, Camus M, Sanchev-Cabo F, Costes A, Molidor R, Mlecnik B, Kirilovsky A, Nilsson M, Damotte D, Meatchi T, Bruneval P, Cugnenc PH, Trajanoski Z, Fridman WH, Galon J. Effector memory T cells, early metastasis, and survival in colorectal cancer. N Engl J Med. 2005;353:2654–66.
11. Zhang L, Conejo-Garcia JR, Katsaros D, Gimotty PA, Massobria M, Regani G, Makrigiannakis A, Gray H, Schlienger K, Liebman MN, Rubin SC, Coukos G. Intratumoral T cells, recurrence, and survival in epithelial ovarian cancer. N Engl J Med. 2003;348:203–13.
12. Nishikawa H, Sakaguchi S. Regulatory T cells in tumor immunity. Int J Cancer. 2010;127:759–67.
13. Demaria S, Pikarsky E, Karin M, Coussens LM, Chen YC, EL-Omar EM, Trinchieri G, Dubinett SM, Mao JT, Szabo E, Krieg A, Weiner GJ, Fox BA, Coukos G, Wang E, Abraham RT, Carbone M, Lotze MT. Cancer and inflammation: promise for biologic therapy. J Immunother. 2010;33:335–51.
14. Karthaus N, Torensma R, Tel J. Deciphering the message broadcast by tumor-infiltrating dendritic cells. Am J Pathol. 2012;181:733–42.
15. Stockmann C, Schadendorf D, Klose R, Helifrich I. The impact of the immune system on tumor: angiogenesis and vascular remodeling. Front Oncol. 2014;4:69.
16. Maltby S, Khazaie K, McNagny KM. Mast cells in tumour growth: angiogenesis, tissue remodelling and immune-modulation. Biochem Biophys Acta. 2009;1796:19–26.
17. Sayed BA, Brown MA. Mast cells are modulators of T-cell responses. Immuno Rev. 2007;217:53–64.
18. Wasiuk A, de Vries VC, Hartmann K, Roers A, Noelle RJ. Mast cells as regulators of adaptive immunity to tumours. Clin Exp Immunol. 2009;155:140–6.
19. Suto H, Nakae S, Kakurai M, Sedgewick JD, Tsai M, Galli SJ. Mast cell-associated TNF promotes dendritic cell migration. J Immunol. 2006;176:4102–12.
20. Nakae S, Suto H, Iikura M, Kakurai M, Sedgwick JD, Tsai M, Galli SJ. Mast cells enhance T cell activation: importance of mast cell costimulatory molecules and secreted TNF. J Immunol. 2006;176:2238–48.
21. D'Angelo SP, Tap WD, Schwartz GK, Carajal RD. Sarcoma immunotherapy: past approaches and future directions. Sarcoma. 2014;2014:391967.
22. Kansara M, Teng MW, Smyth MJ, Thomas DM. Transitional biology of osteosarcoma. Nat Rev Cancer. 2014;14:722–35.
23. Robert SS, Chou AJ, Cheung NK. Immunotherapy of childhood sarcomas. Front Oncol. 2015;5:181.
24. Burgess M, Tawbi H. Immunonotherapeutic approaches to sarcoma. Curr Treat Options Oncol. 2015;16:26.
25. Lee CH, Espinosa I, Vrijaldenhoven S, Subramanian S, Montgomery KD, Zhu S, Marinelli RJ, Peterse JL, Poulin N, Neilson TO, West RB, Gilks CB, Van den Rijn M. Prognostic significance of macrophage infiltration in leiomyosarcomas. Clin Cancer Res. 2008;14:1423–30.
26. Yang TT, Sabokbar A, Gibbons CL, Athanasou NA. Human mesenchymal tumour-assocated macrophages diffentiate into osteoclastic bone-resorbing cells. J Bone Joint Surg Br. 2002;84:452–6.
27. Buddingh EP, Kuijjer ML, Duim RA, Bürger H, Agelopoulos K, Myklebost O, Serra M, Mertens F, Hogendoorn PC, Lankester AC, Cleton-Jansen AM. Tumor-infiltrating macrophages are associated with metastasis suppression in high-grade osteosarcoma: a rationale for treatment with macrophage activating agents. Clin Cancer Res. 2011;17(8):2110–9.
28. Fujiwara T, Fukushi J, Yamamoto S, Matsumoto Y, Setsu N, Oda Y, Yamada H, Okada S, Watari K, Ono M, Kuwano M, Kamura S, Iida K, Okada Y, Koga M, Iwamoto Y. Macrophage infiltration predicts a poor prognosis for human ewing sarcoma. Am J Pathol. 2011;179(3):1157–70.
29. Lau YS, Danks L, Sun SG, Fox S, Sabokbar A, Harris A, Athanasou NA. RANKL-dependent and RANKL-independent mechanisms of macrophage-osteoclast differentiation in breast cancer. Breast Cancer Res Treat. 2007;105(1):7–16
30. Lau YS, Adamopoulos IE, Sabokbar A, Giele H, Gibbons CL, Athanasou NA. Cellular and humoral mechanisms of osteoclast formation in Ewing's sarcoma. Br J Cancer. 2007;4:1716–22.
31. Kinpara K, Mogi M, Kuzushima M, Togari A. Osteoclast differentiation factor in human osteosarcoma cell line. J Immunoassay. 2000;21:327–40.
32. Miyamoto N, Higuchi Y, Mori K, Ito M, Tsurudome M, Nishio M, Yamada H, Sudo A, Kato K, Uchida A, Ito Y. Human osteosarcoma-derived cell lines produce soluble factors(s) that induces differentiation of blood monocytes to osteoclast-like cells. Int Immunopharmacol. 2002;2:25–38.
33. Sun SG, Lau YS, Itonaga I, Sabokbar A, Athanasou NA. Bone stromal cells in pagetic one and Paget's sarcoma express RANKL and support human osteoclast formation. J Pathol. 2006;209:114–20.
34. Taylor R, Knowles HJ, Athanasou NA. Ewing sarcoma cells express RANKL and support osteoclastogenesis. J Pathol. 2011;225:195–202.
35. Endo-Munoz L, Evdokiou A, Saunders NA. The role of osteoclasts and tumour associated macrophages in osteosarcoma metastasis. Biochem Biophys Acta. 2012;1862:434–42.
36. Endo-Munoz L, Cummin A, Rickwood D, Wilson D, Cueva C, Ng C, Strutton G, Cassady AI, Evdokiou A, Sommerville S, Dickinson I, Guminiski A, Saunders NA. Loss of osteoclasts contributes to the development of osteosarcoma pulmonary metastases. Cancer Res. 2010;70:7063–72.

37. Geissmann F, Manz MG, Jung S, Sieweke MH, Merad M, Ley K. Development of monocytes, macrophages and dendritic cells. Science. 2010;327:656–61.

38. Fricke I, Gabrilovich DI. Dendritic cells and the tumour microenvironment: a dangerous liaisom. Immunol Invest. 2006;35:459–83.

39. Geijtenbeek TBH, Torensma R, van Vlier SJ, van Duijnhoven GCF, Adema SJ, van Kooyk Y, Figdor CG. Identification of DC-SIGN, a novel dendritic cell-specific ICAM-3 receptor that supports primary immune responses. Cell. 2000;100:575–85.

40. Zhou T, Chen Y, Hao L, Zhang Y. DC-SIGN and Immunoregulation. Cell Mol Immunol. 2006;3:279–83.

41. Berghuis D, Santos SJ, Baelde HJ, Taminiau AH, Egeler RM, Schilham MW, Hogendoorn PC, Lankester AC. Pro-inflammatory chemokine-chemokine receptor interactions within the Ewing sarcoma microenvironment determine CD8. J Pathol. 2011;223:347–57.

42. Huang G, Yu L, Cooper LJ, Hollomon M, Huls H, Kleinerman ES. Genetically modified T cells targeting interleukin-11 receptor of α-chain kill human osteosarcoma cells and induce the regression of established osteosarcoma lung metastases. Cancer Res. 2012;72:271–81.

43. Yu XW, Wu TY, Yi X, Ren WP, Zhou ZB, Sun YQ, Zhang CQ. Prognostic significance of VEGF expression in osteosarcoma; a meta-analysis. Tumour Biol. 2014;35:155–60.

44. Zhuang Y, Wei M. Impact of vascular endothelial growth factor expression on overall survival in patients with osteosarcoma: a meta-analysis. Tumour Biol. 2014;35:1745–9.

45. Aarnoudse CA, Garcia Vallejo JJ, Saeland E, van Kooyk Y. Recognition of tumour glycans by antigen-presenting cells. Curr Opin Immunol. 2006;18:105–11.

46. Soilleux EJ, Morris LS, Leslie G, Chehimi J, Luo Q, Levroney E, Trowsdale J, Montaner LJ, Doms RW, Weissman D, Coleman N, Lee B. Constitutive and induced expression of DC-SIGN on dendritic cell and macrophage subpopulations in situ and in vitro. J Leucoc Biol. 2002;71:445–57.

47. Soilleux EJ, Rous B, Love K, Vowler S, Morris LS, Fisher C, Coleman N. Myxofibrosarcomas contain large numbers of infiltrating immature dendritic cells. Am J Clin Pathol. 2003;119:540–5.

48. Engleman EG, Fong L. Induction of immunity to tumor-associated antigens following dendritic cell vaccination of cancer patients. Clin Immunol. 2003;106:10–5.

49. Kim R, Emi M, Tanabe K. Functional roles of immature dendritic cells in impaired immunity of solid tumour and their targeted strategies for provoking tumour immunity. Clin Exp Immunol. 2006;146:189–96.

50. Ellis HA, Peart KM. Iliac bone marrow mast cells in relation to the renal osteodystrophy of patients treated by haemodialysis. J Clin Pathol. 1976;29:502–16.

51. Smithey BE, Pappo AS, Hill DA. C-kit expression in paediatric solid tumours: a comparative immunohistochemical study. Am J Surg Pathol. 2001;26:486–92.

52. Hitora T, Yamamoto T, Akisue T, Marui T, Nakatani T, Kawamoto T, Nagira K, Yoshiya S, Kurosaka M. Establishment and characterisation of a KIT-positive and stem cell factor-producing cell line, KTHOS, derived from human osteosarcoma. Pathol Int. 2005;55:41–7.

53. Bozzi F, Tamborini E, Negri T, Pastore E, Ferrari A, Luksch R, Cassanova M, Pierotti MA, Bellani FF, Pilotti S. Evidence of activation of KIT, PDGFRalpha and PDGFRbeta receptors in the Ewing sarcoma family of tumours. Cancer. 2007;109:1638–45.

54. Chiappetta N, Gruber B. The role of mast cells in osteoporosis. Semin Arthritis Rheum. 2006;36:32–6.

55. Kudo O, Fujikawa Y, Itonaga I, Sabokbar A, Torisu T, Athanasou NA. Proinflammatory cytokine (TNFalpha/IL-alpha) induction of human osteoclast formation. J Pathol. 2002;198:220–7.

56. Landuzzi L, De Giovanni C, Nicoletti G, Rossi I, Ricci C, Astolfi A, Scopece L, Scotlandi K, Serra M, Bagnara GP, Nanni P, Lollini PL. The metastatic ability of Ewing's sarcoma cells is modulated by stem cell factor and by its receptor c-kit. Am J Pathol. 2000;157:2123–31.

11

Older soft tissue sarcoma patients experience increased rates of venous thromboembolic events

Sumitra Shantakumar[1]*, Alexandra Connelly-Frost[2], Monica G Kobayashi[3], Robert Allis[3] and Li Li[4]

Abstract

Background: Venous thromboembolic co-morbidities can have a significant impact on treatment response, treatment options, quality of life, and ultimately, survival from cancer. There is a dearth of published information on venous thromboembolic co-morbidity among older soft tissue sarcoma patients.

Methods: SEER-Medicare linked data (1993–2005) was utilized for this retrospective cohort analysis (n = 3,480 soft tissue sarcoma patients). Non-cancer patients were frequency-matched by age to cancer patients at a ratio of 1:1; coverage and follow-up requirements were the same as for soft tissue sarcoma cases. Venous thromboembolic events were divided into three groups of interest: deep vein thrombosis, pulmonary embolism, and other thromboembolic events. Relative incidence rates of venous thromboembolic events in soft tissue sarcoma patients with a recent history of cardiovascular event or venous thromboembolic event (12 months before diagnosis) versus soft tissue sarcoma patients without such a recent history were calculated using the Cox proportional hazard models. The Cox proportional hazard model was used to build predictive models to identify important risk factors for each venous thromboembolic event of interest among soft tissue sarcoma patients. Relative incidence rate of VTEs in cancer patients (12 months after diagnosis) versus non-cancer cases (12 months after index date) was calculated using multi-variable Cox proportional hazard models.

Results: We observed that among older soft tissue sarcoma patients, 10.6% experienced a deep vein thrombosis, 3.0% experienced a pulmonary embolism, and 3.1% experienced other thromboembolic events in the 12 months after sarcoma diagnosis. On average, 60% of venous thromboembolic events occurred in the first 90 days after sarcoma diagnosis. The highest rates of deep vein thrombosis and pulmonary embolism after sarcoma diagnosis were seen in patients with sarcoma not otherwise specified (deep vein thrombosis: 204/1,000 p-y and pulmonary embolism: 50/1,000 p-y). Recent history of a venous thromboembolic event was the strongest predictor of a subsequent venous thromboembolic event after soft tissue sarcoma diagnosis.

Conclusion: Venous thromboembolic events are common and serious co-morbidities that should be closely monitored in older soft tissue sarcoma patients.

Keywords: Soft tissue sarcoma, Venous thromboembolic events, Deep vein thrombosis, Pulmonary embolism, Co-morbidity, Elderly

*Correspondence: sumitra.y.shantakumar@gsk.com
[1] Worldwide Epidemiology, Research and Development, GlaxoSmithKline, 150 Beach Road, #26-00 Gateway West, Singapore 189720, Singapore
Full list of author information is available at the end of the article

Background

Venous thromboembolic co-morbidities among cancer patients can have a significant impact on quality of life, treatment options, treatment response, and ultimately, survival from cancer [1–3]. A small body of evidence is developing for brain, breast, lung, ovarian, and pancreatic cancers, suggesting that the incidence of venous thromboembolic events (VTEs) VTEs varies substantially by cancer subtype [2, 4–13]. Estimates for the occurrence of VTEs in these cancers range from as low as 0.4% up to 26.0%, depending on the cancer type, study population, and the length of follow-up [12]. Because the risk of VTEs differs by the histological type of each cancer, it is important to carefully characterize this co-morbidity by cancer subtype.

There is a dearth of information on the extent of venous thromboembolic co-morbidity among older soft tissue sarcoma (STS) patients in the literature. VTE incidence among STS patients has rarely been addressed, timing of VTEs has not been investigated, co-factors have not been considered, soft tissue and bone sarcomas are usually combined, and older populations have not been studied. It is important to understand the scope of VTEs, before and after diagnosis, in order to offer STS patients optimal care and improved quality of life.

The main goals of this study were (1) to estimate the incidence of VTEs before STS diagnosis and during 90-day time periods after STS diagnosis and (2) to produce adjusted relative risk estimates of VTEs for STS patients with and without a cardiovascular disease or VTE history and (3) to compare risk of VTEs for STS patients versus age-matched non-cancer individuals.

Methods

Study population

SEER-Medicare data is a linkage of US cancer registry data with Medicare claims data. This database combines two large, population-based, geographically diverse US data sources, providing detailed information about older persons ($\geq$65 years) with and without cancer. Data from 1993 to 2005 were utilized for this retrospective cohort analysis. Patients 65 years of age and over who were diagnosed with STS and had at least 24 months of continuous non-HMO Medicare coverage (Parts A and B) before diagnosis and 1–12 months of follow-up information after diagnosis were included in the cancer cohort. Duration of patient follow-up after diagnosis (maximum 12 months) was the number of months until the patient died or lost Medicare coverage. If neither of these events occurred before the end of the planned follow-up time after diagnosis, the patient was followed for the full 12 months. Non-cancer patients were frequency-matched by age to cancer patients at a ratio of

1:1; and coverage and follow-up requirements were the same as for STS cases. VTEs of interest were deep vein thrombosis (DVT), pulmonary embolism (PE), and other thromboembolic events (OTE). Thromboembolic events included in the OTE category were as follows: central retinal vein occlusion, venous tributary (branch) occlusion, nonpyogenic thrombosis of intracranial venous sinus, phlebitis/thrombophlebitis of superficial veins of lower and upper extremities, phlebitis/thrombophlebitis of other sites, gout with other specified manifestations, Budd–Chiari syndrome, venous embolism/thrombosis of renal vein, and portal vein thrombosis. ICD-9 diagnosis codes were used to identify VTEs and ICD-O-3 codes were used to identify STS patients (overall and by subtype). Types and definitions of STS by ICD-O-3 histology codes are as follows: GIST (8935, 8936), leiomyosarcoma (8890–91, 8894–97), malignant fibrous histiocytoma (8830), liposarcoma (8850–8855, 8858), dermatofibrosarcoma (8832, 8833), rhabdomyosarcoma (8900–8902, 8910, 8912, 8920), angiosarcoma (9120, 9130, 9133, 9170), nerve sheath tumor (9540, 9560–62), fibrosarcoma (8810, 8811, 8814, 8815), sarcoma NOS (not otherwise specified) (8800–8805), Ewing Sarcoma/primitive neuroectodermal tumor (9260, 9364, 9365, 9473), extraskeletal osteosarcoma (9180, 9181), extraskeletal chondrosarcoma (9220, 9231, 9240), synovial sarcoma (9040–9043), clear cell sarcoma (9044), myxosarcoma (8840), malignant hemangiopericytoma (9150), malignant giant cell tumor (9251, 9252), malignant granular cell tumor (9580), alveolar soft part sarcoma (9581), and desmoplastic small round cell tumor (8806). Bone and joint sites were excluded for all above mentioned diagnoses as were non-malignant tumor types. DVT was captured using ICD-9 codes of 451.1 (451.11, 451.19) 451.2, 451.81, 451.83, 451.84, 453.1, 453.2, 453.4 (453.40, 453.41, 453.42) 453.8, and 453.9; PE was captured using ICD-9 codes of 415.1 and 415.19; and OTEs were captured using ICD-9 codes of 362.35, 362.36, 437.6, 451.0, 451.82, 451.89, 451.9, 453.0, 453.3, and 452.

Statistical analysis

STS patients

Incidence rates of each VTE (a) in the 12 months before diagnosis and (b) in the 12 months after diagnosis were described by age, race, sex, stage at diagnosis, and year of diagnosis. The numerator is the number of events that occurred over the respective 12-month period and the denominator was the person-years at risk. Events in the 12 months after diagnosis were further described as the proportion of cases with a first event in discrete time intervals of follow-up time (0–90 days, 91–180 days, 181–270 days, and 271–365 days). The numerator of each incidence proportion is the number of persons with their first event of interest during that time period only, while the denominator represents the persons who were alive and free of events at the beginning of the period.

Relative incidence rates of VTEs in STS patients with a recent history of cardiovascular event (CV) or VTE event (12 months before diagnosis) versus STS patients without such a recent history were calculated using the Cox proportional hazard models. Using a commonly used definition present in the literature, history of CV event was defined as any of the following events in the 12 months before STS diagnosis: myocardial infarction, ischemic stroke, congestive heart failure, angina, or TIA in the prior 12 months. The first VTE outcome was counted for each patient from time of diagnosis up to 12 months after diagnosis. Potential confounders, identified through ICD-9 diagnosis and procedure codes, were as follows: age at diagnosis, race, sex, diabetes, hypercholesterolemia, atherosclerosis, varicose veins, recent high-risk surgical procedure, central venous catheter, kidney disease, stage at diagnosis, surgery of primary tumor, chemotherapy, history of cancer. Results are presented by major STS subtypes [angiosarcoma, fibrosarcoma, GIST, leiomyosarcoma, liposarcoma, malignant fibrous histiosarcoma (MFH), nerve sheath tumor, and sarcoma NOS] where cell sizes permit.

The Cox proportional hazard model was used to build predictive models to identify important risk factors for each VTE of interest among STS patients. Potential risk factors included in the initial (full) model were as follows: age at diagnosis, race, sex, diabetes, hypercholesterolemia, atherosclerosis, varicose veins, recent high-risk surgical procedure, central venous catheter, kidney disease, stage at diagnosis, chemotherapy, hormone therapy, surgery of primary tumor, history of cancer, and recent history of VTE of interest. After stepwise backwards elimination, risk factors with a multivariable p value <0.1 were retained in the final multivariable predictive model.

STS vs. non-cancer patients

A matched-cohort design was utilized to evaluate the relative incidence rate of VTEs in STS patients (12 months before diagnosis) versus non-cancer cases (12 months before index date). Multivariable logistic regression modeling was performed. Potential confounders assessed were as follows: race, sex, diabetes, hypercholesterolemia, atherosclerosis, varicose veins, recent high-risk surgical procedure, central venous catheter, kidney disease, recent history of cardiovascular or VTEs. All models were adjusted for age to account for the age-matched design.

Relative incidence rate of VTEs in cancer patients (12 months after diagnosis) versus non-cancer cases (12 months after index date) was calculated using multivariable Cox proportional hazard models. Matching was

accounted for by including the matching variable (age) in the STRATA statement. Potential confounders assessed were the same as in aforementioned logistic regression models. Where possible, results are presented by major STS subtypes [angiosarcoma, fibrosarcoma, GIST, leiomyosarcoma, liposarcoma, malignant fibrous histiosarcoma (MFH), nerve sheath tumor, sarcoma NOS]. Sas 9.1 was used to perform all analyses.

Results

The study population for the first series of analyses consisted of 3,480 STS patients 65 years of age and older (median age = 77). Eighty-five percent of the population was white, 9% of the population was black, and 6% was another race. Forty-seven percent of STS patients were male. The distribution of cases by stage was as follows: 43% localized, 23% regional, 21% distant, and 14% unstaged. The most common STS subtypes in our data were sarcoma NOS (40.9%), GIST (24.3%), leiomyosarcoma (7.6%), MFH (6.4%), and angiosarcoma (5.3%) (Table 1). The two most common primary sites were connective or subcutaneous tissue (35.0%) and the digestive system (31.8%) (Table 1). The non-cancer comparison cohort (n = 3,480) was similar in its distribution of age, race, and sex (Table 1).

STS patients

Among STS patients, DVTs occurred at the highest rate (149/1,000 person-years) of all VTEs after diagnosis (Table 2). The unadjusted incidence rate of VTEs was 1.7–4.1 times higher during the 12-month period after STS diagnosis than the 12-month period prior to cancer diagnosis (Table 2). Regardless of VTE type, over half of VTEs occurred in the first 90 days after STS diagnosis: DVT: 62% (228/367), PE: 67% (70/105), and OTE: 51% (55/108). This pattern did not vary by STS subtype (data not shown).

When STS cases were stratified further by subtype, the highest rates of DVT and PE were seen in sarcoma NOS patients (DVT: 204/1,000 p-y and PE: 50/1,000 p-y). Rates of OTEs ranged from 18/1,000 to 50/1,000; however, estimates for most subtypes were based on very small numbers (Table 3). Unadjusted analyses revealed that STS patients with a recent history of a VTE had substantially higher rates of that specific VTE after STS diagnosis than those without history of that VTE (Table 3). STS patients with a recent history of a CVD event had slightly higher rates of VTEs after STS diagnosis than those without history of a CVD event. Patients of advanced or regional STS stage had higher rates of VTEs after diagnosis compared to patients with localized disease. Patients who were treated with chemotherapy were also more likely compared to patients without chemotherapy to

Table 1 SEER-Medicare study population (1993–2005): soft tissue sarcoma patients (n = 3,480) and non-cancer controls (n = 3,480)

	Cancer		Non-cancer	
	n	%	N	%
Age in years				
65–69	475	13.7	549	15.8
70–74	825	23.7	836	24.0
75–79	880	25.3	853	24.5
80–84	744	21.4	715	20.6
85+	556	16.0	527	15.1
Race				
Black	300	8.6	301	8.7
White	2,967	85.3	2,945	84.6
Other/unknown race	213	6.1	234	6.7
Sex				
Female	1,843	53.0	1,972	56.7
Male	1,637	47.0	1,508	43.3
STS subtype				
Sarcoma NOS	1,422	40.9	na	na
GIST	845	24.3	na	na
Leiomyosarcoma	264	7.6	na	na
Maligant fibrous histiocytoma	224	6.4	na	na
Angiosarcoma	184	5.3	na	na
Liposaroma	136	3.9	na	na
Nerve sheath tumor	118	3.4	na	na
Fibrosarcoma	64	1.8	na	na
Synovial Sarcoma	49	1.4	na	na
Osteosarcoma	44	1.3	na	na
Rhabdomyosarcoma	25	0.7	na	na
Chondrosarcoma	25	0.7	na	na
Dermatofibrosaroma	22	0.6	na	na
Ewing sarcoma	19	0.5	na	na
Maligant hemangiopericytoma	15	0.4	na	na
Clear cell sarcoma	<11	0.3	na	na
Myxosarcoma	<11	0.2	na	na
Alveolar soft part	<11	0.1	na	na
Maligant granular cell tumor	<11	0.1	na	na
Maligant giant cell tumor	<11	0.0	na	na
Primary site				
Connective/subcutaneous tissue	1,217	35.0	na	na
Digestive system	1,107	31.8	na	na
Respiratory system	279	8.0	na	na
Breast	178	7.7	na	na
Other non-epithelial skin	167	5.1	na	na
Female genital system	160	4.8	na	na
Urinary system	105	4.6	na	na
Other and unknown	267	3.0	na	na
Stage				
Unstaged	482	13.9	na	na
Localized	1,482	42.6	na	na

Table 1 continued

	Cancer		Non-cancer	
	n	%	N	%
Regional	800	23.0	na	na
Distant	716	20.5	na	na

Per SEER Medicare data use agreement, cell sizes <11 cannot be displayed.
na not applicable.

experience a VTE after STS diagnosis. Patients who were treated with surgery of their primary tumor were half as likely as patients without surgery to experience a VTE after STS diagnosis.

Multivariable modeling was conducted to more closely evaluate the association between VTE history and incidence of VTEs after sarcoma diagnosis by STS subtype. Overall, history of a VTE in the 12 months before sarcoma diagnosis substantially increased the risk of a subsequent VTE in the 12 months after STS diagnosis (HR range = 6.4–49.3) (Table 4). Although all age-adjusted associations were strong, the most marked associations were seen in patients with leiomyosarcoma (HR = 49.3, 95% CI = 22.2–109.0), GIST (HR = 20.9, 95% CI = 13.6–32.2), and liposarcoma (HR = 19.1, 95% CI = 4.2–87.4) (Table 4).

Predictors of each VTE subtype after sarcoma diagnosis were evaluated among the combined group of STS patients. There were only two statistically significant predictors of increased risk of PE after STS diagnosis: atherosclerosis and recent history of PE. There were four predictors of increased risk of OTE after STS diagnosis: atherosclerosis, hormone therapy, recent history of OTE and varicose veins. There were multiple predictors of both increased risk and decreased risk of DVT among the combined group of STS patients. Predictors of increased risk of DVT included kidney disease, radiation treatment, regional or distant stage and varicose veins; predictors of decreased risk of DVT included surgery of primary, high risk surgery, and central venous catheter. By far, the strongest predictor of all VTE events after STS diagnosis was a history of that same event in the 12 months before diagnosis (DVT: HR = 7.6, 95% CI = 5.7–10.1; PE: HR = 17.6, 95% CI = 9.4–33.0; OTE: HR = 16.6, 95% CI = 10.8–25.4) (data not shown). Presence of atherosclerosis was also an important predictor for all VTE events, associated with a 1.8–2.5 times greater risk of VTE (DVT: HR = 1.8, 95% CI = 1.4–2.3; PE: HR = 2.0, 95% CI = 1.3–3.1; OTE: HR = 2.5, 95% CI = 1.7–3.8) (data not shown).

STS patients compared to an age-matched, non-cancer population

Angiosarcoma and sarcoma NOS patients were more likely to have experienced a VTE in the recent past

Table 2 Unadjusted incidence rates of venous thromboembolic events, before and after STS diagnosis

n = 3,480 STS[a] patients	Incidence 12 months before STS diagnosis	Incidence 12 months after STS diagnosis
DVT[a]		
n/person-years[b]	137/3,418	367/2,468
Rate/1,000[c]	40.1 (33.7–164.7)	148.7 (133.9–164.7)
Rate ratio (after vs. before)[d]	*–*	*3.7 (3.0–4.5)*
PE[a]		
n/person-years[b]	34/3,463	105/2,589
Rate/1,000[c]	9.8 (6.8–49.1)	40.6 (33.2–49.1)
Rate ratio (after vs. before)[d]	*–*	*4.1 (2.8–6.1)*
OTE[a]		
n/person-years[b]	82/3,438	106/2,590
Rate/1,000[c]	23.9 (19.0–49.5)	40.9 (33.5–49.5)
Rate ratio (after vs. before)[d]	*–*	*1.7 (1.3–2.3)*

Rate ratios are highlighted in italics.

[a] *VTE* venous thromboembolic events, *STS* soft tissue sarcoma, *DVT* deep vein thrombosis, *PE* pulmonary embolism, *OTE* other thromboembolic event. OTE category includes the following diagnoses: central retinal vein occlusion, venous tributary (branch) occlusion, nonpyogenic thrombosis of intracranial venous sinus, phlebitis/thrombophlebitis of superficial vessels of lower extremities, phlebitis/thrombophlebitis of superficial veins of upper extremities, phlebitis/thrombophlebitis of other sites, gout with other specified manifestations, Budd–Chiari syndrome, and venous embolism/thrombosis of renal vein.

[b] *n* number of VTE events, *p-y* person-years.

[c] Rates are per 1,000 person-years and are unadjusted. Age adjustment is unnecessary as these rates are intentionally representative of the older subpopulation (ages 65+) of STS patients. Only first VTE counted in rate estimates.

[d] Rate ratios are unadjusted.

(i.e. 12 month prior to STS diagnosis/index date) than non-cancer individuals (Table 5). A strong association between STS and VTE after diagnosis (or index date for non-cancer patients) was observed in most STS subtypes. The strongest comparisons of VTE after diagnosis for cancer versus non-cancer patients were among angiosarcoma (HR = 9.1, 95% CI = 2.1–39.5), leiomyosarcoma (HR = 5.5, 95% CI = 2.1–15.0) and sarcoma NOS patients (HR = 5.2, 95% CI = 3.8–6.9) (Table 5).

Discussion

We studied the incidence of venous thromboembolic events before and after soft tissue sarcoma diagnosis. There are only four published studies, to our knowledge, that have investigated VTEs in adult STS patients. Two of these are large studies of thromboembolic events among cancer patients that include sarcomas as a cancer site [6, 7]. Khorana et al. [6] reported results from a retrospective cohort study (n = 1,597 sarcoma patients) including patients receiving chemotherapy at any one of 115

University HealthSystem Consortium locations between the years of 1995 and 2002. During their first hospitalization for neutropenia, 4.8% of sarcoma patients had a VTE. Khorana et al. [7] conducted a retrospective cohort study (n = 21,989 sarcoma cases) of the same health consortium and found that 2.9% of sarcoma patients experienced a VTE during one hospitalization following cancer diagnosis. Results from these two large studies are difficult to compare to our incidence proportions for several reasons: in these studies, bone sarcomas were included in their sarcoma category, median age of the sarcoma group was not stated, and incidence proportions were based on a VTE diagnosis during a single hospitalization. Our analysis evaluated incidence proportions and incidence rates (Table 2) over the full 12-month period (or death) after diagnosis.

Two studies reported incidence of venous thromboembolic events (VTEs) among soft tissue sarcoma patients, specifically [14, 15]. Mitchell et al. [15] conducted a retrospective cohort study of VTE events among trunk/extremity soft tissue or bone sarcoma patients presenting to their unit between 1998 and 2003. Among STS patients (n = 158), 5.0% experienced a DVT and 1.3% experienced a PE after diagnosis. Damron et al. [14] conducted a retrospective cohort study of patients receiving surgery for bone and soft tissue sarcoma of the head, neck, upper extremity and lower extremity. There were 120 STS cases included and 4.2% of those cases experienced one or more VTE following surgery (2.5% DVT and 2.5% PE). Incidence proportions from these two studies were lower than what we found in our study (10.6% DVT and 3.0% PE). Both of these studies, however, were very small and had much younger patient populations than ours.

Our study found that STS patients undergoing chemotherapy were roughly 50% more likely (DVT: RR = 1.7, PE: RR = 1.5, OTE: RR = 1.4) to experience a DVT, PE or OTE after diagnosis, although only about 10% of our STS patients received chemotherapy treatment (Table 3). Damron et al. [14] reported a similar result; STS patients undergoing chemotherapy treatment were at an increased risk of VTE compared to those not receiving chemotherapy (p = 0.04).

An important component of our analysis was the evaluation of VTE history as a risk factor for future VTE events. Our results suggest that VTE history is the most important factor to consider in evaluating risk of future VTE in STS patients. There are no other studies in the current literature that quantify the association between VTE history and future events among STS patients; however, this result is consistent with broader studies of VTE among cancer patients [16, 17].

The major risk factors for VTEs among cancer patients reported in the literature are increased age, female sex, African American race, renal disease, infection,

Table 3 Unadjusted incidence rates of venous thromboembolic events after cancer diagnosis among older STS patients

	DVT[a]		PE[a]		OTE[a]	
	N/P-Y[b]	Rate/1,000[c] (95% CI)	N/P-Y[b]	Rate/1,000[c] (95% CI)	N/P-Y[b]	Rate/1,000[c] (95% CI)
By major STS subtype						
Angiosarcoma (n = 184)	14/147	95.4 (52.1, 160.0)	<11	26.5 (7.2, 68.0)	<11	39.8 (14.6, 86.6)
Fibrosarcoma (n = 64)	<11	72.1 (19.6, 184.5)	0	0	<11	17.6 (0.4, 97.8)
GIST (n = 845)	94/683	137.6 (111.2, 168.4)	33/721	45.7 (31.5, 64.2)	23/730	31.5 (20.0, 47.3)
Leiomyosarcoma (n = 264)	19/210	90.6 (54.5, 141.4)	<11	28.0 (10.3, 60.8)	<11	32.6 (13.1, 67.1)
Liposarcoma (n = 224)	13/118	110.1 (58.6, 188.2)	<11	24.5 (5.1, 71.7)	<11	24.5 (5.0, 71.5)
MFH (n = 184)	20/178	112.2 (68.5, 173.3)	<11	21.9 (6.0, 55.9)	<11	27.3 (8.9, 63.6)
Nerve sheath tumor (n = 118)	15/93	160.8 (90.0, 265.3)	<11	40.7 (11.1, 104.2)	<11	49.8 (16.2, 116.3)
Sarcoma, NOS (n = 1,422)	166/812	204.4 (174.5, 237.9)	41/862	47.5 (34.1, 64.5)	41/858	47.8 (34.3, 64.8)
By history of VTE[e]						
Yes	61/51	1199.2 (917.3–1540.5)	11/14	785.5 (392.3–1406.0)	30/50	599.2 (404.3–855.4)
No	306/2,417	126.6 (112.8–141.6)	94/2,575	27.6 (24.3–31.1)	76/2,540	29.9 (23.6–37.5)
Rate ratio (yes vs. no)[d]	–	*9.5 (7.2–12.5)*	–	*21.5 (11.5–40.2)*	–	*20.0 (13.1–30.6)*
By history of CVD event[f]						
Yes	120/579	207.3 (171.9–247.9)	29/623	46.6 (31.2–66.9)	39/619	63.1 (44.8–86.2)
No	247/1,889	130.8 (115.0–148.1)	76/1,966	38.7 (30.5–48.4)	67/1,971	34.0 (26.3–43.2)
Rate ratio (yes vs. no)[d]	–	*1.6 (1.3–2.0)*	–	*1.2 (0.8–1.8)*	–	*1.9 (1.3–2.8)*
By disease stage						
Localized	133/1,236	107.6 (90.1–127.5)	38/1,290	29.5 (20.9–40.4)	34/1,295	26.3 (18.2–36.7)
Regional	93/586	158.7 (128.1–194.4)	26/614	42.3 (27.7–62.1)	34/610	55.7 (38.6–77.9)
Distant	86/380	238.9 (191.1–295.0)	25/385	65.0 (42.1–95.9)	19/387	49.1 (29.6–76.7)
Rate ratio (regional and distant. vs. local)[d]	–	*1.5 (1.1–1.9)*	–	*1.4 (0.9–2.4)*	–	*2.1 (1.3–3.4)*
By chemotherapy						
Yes	74/324	227.9 (178.9–286.1)	20/348	57.5 (35.1–88.7)	19/346	54.9 (33.0–85.7)
No	293/2,413	136.7 (121.5–153.3)	85/2,241	37.9 (30.3–46.9)	87/2,244	38.8 (31.1–47.8)
Rate ratio (yes vs. no)[d]	–	*1.7 (1.3–2.2)*	–	*1.5 (0.9–2.5)*	–	*1.4 (0.9–2.3)*
By surgery of primary tumor						
Yes	247/1,976	125.0 (109.9–141.6)	72/2,065	34.9 (27.3–43.9)	76/2,064	36.8 (29.0–46.1)
No	115/467	246.4 (203.5–295.8)	32/498	64.2 (43.9–90.7)	29/501	57.9 (38.8–83.1)
Rate ratio (yes vs. no)[d]	–	*0.5 (0.4–0.6)*	–	*0.5 (0.4–0.8)*	–	*0.6 (0.4–1.0)*
By Primary site						
Connective/subcutaneous	136/830	163.9 (137.5–193.8)	33/877	37.6 (25.9–52.8)	37/875	42.3 (29.8–58.3)
Digestive system	120/832	144.2 (119.5–172.4)	38/879	43.2 (30.6–59.4)	29/885	32.8 (22.0–47.1)
Other/unknown[g]	111/805	137.8 (113.3–165.9)	34/833	40.8 (28.3–57.0)	40/830	48.2 (34.4–65.7)

Per SEER-Medicare data use agreement, cell sizes <11 cannot be displayed, nor can estimates that could be used to derive the undisplayed numbers <11. Rate ratios are highlighted in italics.

[a] *DVT* deep vein thrombosis, *PE* pulmonary embolism, *OTE* other thromboembolic event. OTE category includes the following diagnoses: central retinal vein occlusion, venous tributary (branch) occlusion, nonpyogenic thrombosis of intracranial venous sinus, phlebitis/thrombophlebitis of superficial vessels of lower extremities, phlebitis/thrombophlebitis of superficial veins of upper extremities, phlebitis/thrombophlebitis of other sites, gout with other specified manifestations, Budd–Chiari syndrome, and venous embolism/thrombosis of renal vein.

[b] *N* number of VTE events, *P-Y* person-years.

[c] Rates are per 1,000 person-years and are unadjusted. Age adjustment is unnecessary as these rates are intentionally representative of the older subpopulation (≥65 years) of STS patients. Only first VTE counted in rate estimates.

[d] Rate ratios are unadjusted.

[e] History of VTE of interest in the 12 months before STS diagnosis.

[f] History of CVD is defined as a history of any of the following events in the 12 months before STS diagnosis: myocardial infarction, ischemic stroke, onset congestive heart failure, angina, or TIA.

[g] Other/unknown category includes primary sites of the breast, female genital system, other non-epithelial, respiratory system, urinary system, other sites and unknown sites.

Table 4 Relative risk of VTE after STS diagnosis, recent versus no recent VTE history

STS subtype[a]	Hazard ratio	95% confidence interval
Angiosarcoma	6.4	$(1.9–21.8)^+$
GIST	20.9	$(13.6–32.2)^+$
Leiomyosarcoma	49.3	$(22.2–109.0)^+$
Liposarcoma	19.1	$(4.2–87.4)^+$
MFH[b]	11.9	$(3.6–39.4)^+$
NST[c]	15.8	$(5.8–42.7)^+$
Sarcoma NOS[d]	15.4	$(10.9–21.8)^+$

All models adjusted for age. Recent VTE history = history of VTE in the 12 months before STS diagnosis. *VTE* venous thromboembolic event, including deep vein thrombosis, pulmonary embolism, and other thromboembolic events. The other thromboembolic event category includes the following diagnoses: central retinal vein occlusion, venous tributary (branch) occlusion, nonpyogenic thrombosis of intracranial venous sinus, phlebitis/thrombophlebitis of superficial vessels of lower extremities, phlebitis/thrombophlebitis of superficial veins of upper extremities, phlebitis/thrombophlebitis of other sites, gout with other specified manifestations, Budd–Chiari syndrome, and venous embolism/thrombosis of renal vein.

[a] Hazard ratios for STS subtypes other than those listed were not estimable due to small numbers.

[b] Maligant fibrous histiocytoma.

[c] Nerve sheath tumor.

[d] Sarcoma not otherwise specified.

[+] Statistically significant.

Table 5 Relative risk of VTEs before and after STS diagnosis/index date: STS versus non-cancer cohort

STS subtype[a]	Before odds ratio (95% CI)	After hazard ratio (95% CI)
Angiosarcoma	$4.0 (1.4, 11.1)^+$	$9.1 (2.1, 39.5)^+$
Fibrosarcoma	0.5 (0.1, 2.0)	1.0 (0.1, 16.0)
GIST	1.0 (0.7, 1.4)	$4.0 (2.8, 5.7)^+$
Leiomyosarcoma	1.5 (0.6, 3.5)	$5.5 (2.1, 15.0)^+$
Liposarcoma	Not estimable	2.5 (0.9, 7.6)
MFH[b]	1.4 (0.6, 3.3)	$19.7 (3.7, 106.0)^+$
NST[c]	2.1 (0.8, 5.4)	$4.4 (1.1, 17.5)^+$
Sarcoma NOS[d]	$1.9 (1.4, 2.6)^+$	$5.2 (3.8, 6.9)^+$

All models adjusted for age at index/diagnosis date. Estimates represent the relative risk of VTE event in the 12 months before or after diagnosis/index date. *STS patients* 3,840; non-cancer patients = 3,480. *VTE* Venous Thromboembolic Event (including deep vein thrombosis, pulmonary embolism, and other thromboembolic events). OTE category includes the following diagnoses: central retinal vein occlusion, venous tributary (branch) occlusion, nonpyogenic thrombosis of intracranial venous sinus, phlebitis/thrombophlebitis of superficial vessels of lower extremities, phlebitis/thrombophlebitis of superficial veins of upper extremities, phlebitis/thrombophlebitis of other sites, gout with other specified manifestations, Budd-Chiari syndrome, and venous embolism/thrombosis of renal vein.

[a] Hazard ratios for STS subtypes other than those listed were not estimable due to small numbers.

[b] Maligant fibrous histiocytoma.

[c] Nerve sheath tumor.

[d] Sarcoma not otherwise specified.

[+] Statistically significant.

pulmonary disease, obesity, arterial thromboembolism, inherited prothrombotic mutations, prior history of VTE, performance status, advanced stage cancer, major surgery, hospitalization, chemotherapy, hormone therapy, anti-angiogenic agents, erythropoiesis-stimulating agents, transfusions, and central venous catheters [7, 12, 18]. In our predictive models, many of these risk factors proved to be predictors of VTEs in the 12 months after STS diagnosis.

A few interesting differences are worth discussion. Atherosclerosis was a strong predictor for DVT, PE and OTE events in our data. This condition is not generally mentioned as a risk factor for VTE among cancer patients; however, cardiovascular literature has suggested a link between these two conditions [19–22]. We also observed that central venous catheterization, high-risk surgery, and surgery of primary were associated with a decreased risk of DVT after STS diagnosis. Decreased risk in this subgroup of patients is likely due to the close monitoring and prophylactic treatment for venous thromboses in surgical and catheterization situations.

Finally, our analysis compared the risk of VTE events in STS versus non-cancer patients both before and after STS diagnosis. Our study found that patients with angiosarcoma and sarcoma NOS were more likely to have experienced a VTE in the recent past (i.e. 12 month before STS diagnosis) than non-cancer individuals. These results support the theory that VTE could be a risk marker for an ensuing STS diagnosis or, perhaps, a misdiagnosis. Several authors of case studies suggested that STSs may present as or be mistaken for a VTE, underlining the importance of investigating potential tumors when diagnosing VTE. In particular, STSs of the lower extremities have been misdiagnosed as DVTs [23–26] and pulmonary sarcomas/leiomyosarcomas have been misdiagnosed as pulmonary embolisms [27–40].

There are several strengths of note for this study. To our knowledge, this is the first study to examine VTEs among older STS patients. In this analysis we were able to focus on STS patients in particular, rather than the broader category of sarcoma which includes bone sarcomas. The STS patient cohort was large (n = 3,840) allowing us to provide data by STS subtype. The wealth of the data in the SEER-Medicare database allowed us to quantify the occurrence of TE events before STS diagnosis and during various time periods after STS diagnosis, and to make comparisons between STS patients and age-matched non-cancer individuals. Furthermore, we were able to adjust for and/or stratify by important covariates in our analysis. No previous studies performed multivariate analyses on STS patients nor did they investigate the timing of VTE events among STS patients.

As in any study, limitations were present. Many effect estimates are imprecise, present with wide confidence intervals, and should be interpreted cautiously with the direction of the effect emphasized over the magnitude. The STS classification of MFH was changed in 2002 because the large majority of tumors formerly classified as MFH can be more meaningfully classified as other tumor types. However, due to the timeframe of SEER-Medicare data collection, the old categorization had to be used for this study. The results based on this older cohort (i.e., 65 years or older) are generalizable only to those of the same age group. Also, information on some behavioral risk factors such as smoking, sedentary lifestyle, immobility, and CVD family history was unavailable. Finally, we had no access to information about potential predictive biomarkers such as elevated platelet or leukocyte counts, tissue factor, soluble p-Selectin, D-dimer, factor V Leiden, and prothrombin 20210A mutations [12, 41, 42].

Conclusion

This is the first study to perform an in depth analysis of VTEs among older STS patients. Our results indicate that STS patients are at increased risk of VTEs after cancer diagnosis and that patients with a history of VTE are much more likely to have a subsequent VTE in the 12 months after their sarcoma diagnosis. VTEs are common and serious co-morbidities that should be closely monitored in older STS patients, particularly during the first 3 months after diagnosis and among those with a recent history of a VTE.

Authors' contributions

SS participated in study conception and design, data analysis, data interpretation and manuscript drafting. ACF participated in study design, data analysis, data interpretation and manuscript drafting. MK participated in study design, data analysis and manuscript drafting. RA participated in data analysis and data interpretation. LL participated in data analysis and data interpretation. All authors read and approved the final manuscript.

Author details

[1] Worldwide Epidemiology, Research and Development, GlaxoSmithKline, 150 Beach Road, #26-00 Gateway West, Singapore 189720, Singapore. [2] Frost Consulting, Epidemiologic Research and Grant Writing, Charlotte, NC, USA. [3] Worldwide Epidemiology, Research and Development, GlaxoSmithKline, Research Triangle Park, NC, USA. [4] Center for Observational Data Analytics, Amgen, Thousand Oaks, CA, USA.

Acknowledgements

This study used the linked SEER-Medicare database. The interpretation and reporting of these data are the sole responsibility of the authors. The authors acknowledge the efforts of the Applied Research Program, NCI; the Office of Research, Development and Information, CMS; Information Management Services (IMS), Inc.; and the Surveillance, Epidemiology, and End Results (SEER) Program tumor registries in the creation of the SEER-Medicare database. We would like to thank Sue Hall, Jerzy Tyczynski, and Annette Beiderbeck for their contributions to the original objectives and variable definitions for this project. We are also grateful to Jeanenne Nelson for reviewing results throughout the analysis process.

Competing interests

The authors declare that they have no competing interests.

References

1. Sorensen HT, Mellemkjaer L, Olsen JH, Baron JA (2000) Prognosis of cancers associated with venous thromboembolism. N Engl J Med 343:1846–1850
2. Chew HK, Wun T, Harvey D, Zhou H, White RH (2006) Incidence of venous thromboembolism and its effect on survival among patients with common cancers. Arch Intern Med 166:458–464
3. Khorana AA, Francis CW, Culakova E, Kuderer NM, Lyman GH (2007) Thromboembolism is a leading cause of death in cancer patients receiving outpatient chemotherapy. J Thromb Haemost 5:632–634
4. Agnelli G, Bolis G, Capussotti L, Scarpa RM, Tonelli F, Bonizzoni E et al (2006) A clinical outcome-based prospective study on venous thromboembolism after cancer surgery: the @RISTOS project. Ann Surg 243:89–95
5. Blom JW, Vanderschoot JP, Oostindier MJ, Osanto S, van der Meer FJ, Rosendaal FR (2006) Incidence of venous thrombosis in a large cohort of 66,329 cancer patients: results of a record linkage study. J Thromb Haemost 4:529–535
6. Khorana AA, Francis CW, Culakova E, Fisher RI, Kuderer NM, Lyman GH (2006) Thromboembolism in hospitalized neutropenic cancer patients. J Clin Oncol 24:484–490
7. Khorana AA, Francis CW, Culakova E, Kuderer NM, Lyman GH (2007) Frequency, risk factors, and trends for venous thromboembolism among hospitalized cancer patients. Cancer 110:2339–2346
8. Khorana AA, Kuderer NM, Culakova E, Lyman GH, Francis CW (2008) Development and validation of a predictive model for chemotherapy-associated thrombosis. Blood 111:4902–4907
9. Levitan N, Dowlati A, Remick SC, Tahsildar HI, Sivinski LD, Beyth R et al (1999) Rates of initial and recurrent thromboembolic disease among patients with malignancy versus those without malignancy. Risk analysis using Medicare claims data. Medicine (Baltimore) 78:285–291
10. Sallah S, Wan JY, Nguyen NP (2002) Venous thrombosis in patients with solid tumors: determination of frequency and characteristics. Thromb Haemost 87:575–579
11. Stein PD, Beemath A, Meyers FA, Skaf E, Sanchez J, Olson RE (2006) Incidence of venous thromboembolism in patients hospitalized with cancer. Am J Med 119:60–68
12. Khorana AA, Connolly GC (2009) Assessing risk of venous thromboembolism in the cancer patient. J Clin Oncol 27(29):4839–4847
13. Wun T, White RH (2009) Venous thromboembolism (VTE) in patients with cancer: epidemiology and risk factors. Cancer Invest 27(Suppl 1):63–74
14. Damron TA, Wardak Z, Glodny B, Grant W (2010) Risk of venous thromboembolism in bone and soft-tissue sarcoma patients undergoing surgical intervention: a report from prior to the initiation of SCIP measures. J Surg Oncol 103(7):643–647
15. Mitchell SY, Lingard EA, Kesteven P, McCaskie AW, Gerrand CH (2007) Venous thromboembolism in patients with primary bone or soft-tissue sarcomas. J Bone Joint Surg Am 89:2433–2439
16. Lee AY, Levine MN (2003) Venous thromboembolism and cancer: risks and outcomes. Circulation 107:I17–I21
17. Anderson FA Jr, Spencer FA (2003) Risk factors for venous thromboembolism. Circulation 107:I9–16
18. Sousou T, Khorana A (2009) Identifying cancer patients at risk for venous thromboembolism. Hamostaseologie 29:121–124
19. Agnelli G, Becattini C (2006) Venous thromboembolism and atherosclerosis: common denominators or different diseases? J Thromb Haemost 4:1886–1890
20. Prandoni P, Bilora F, Marchiori A, Bernardi E, Petrobelli F, Lensing AW et al (2003) An association between atherosclerosis and venous thrombosis. N Engl J Med 348:1435–1441

21. Prandoni P (2007) Venous thromboembolism and atherosclerosis: is there a link? J Thromb Haemost 5(Suppl 1):270–275

22. van der Hagen PB, Folsom AR, Jenny NS, Heckbert SR, O'Meara ES, Reich LM et al (2006) Subclinical atherosclerosis and the risk of future venous thrombosis in the Cardiovascular Health Study. J Thromb Haemost 4:1903–1908

23. Benns M, Dalsing M, Sawchuck A, Wurtz LD (2006) Soft tissue sarcomas may present with deep vein thrombosis. J Vasc Surg 43:788–793

24. Emori M, Naka N, Hamada K, Tomita Y, Takami H, Araki N (2010) Soft-tissue sarcomas in the inguinal region may present as deep vein thrombosis. Ann Vasc Surg 24:951

25. Arumilli BR, Babu VL, Paul AS (2008) Painful swollen leg–think beyond deep vein thrombosis or Baker's cyst. World J Surg Oncol 6:6

26. Singh NK, Kolluri R (2009) Liposarcoma of thigh presenting as deep venous thrombosis. Phlebology 24:139–141

27. Kruger I, Borowski A, Horst M, de Vivie ER, Theissen P, Gross-Fengels W (1990) Symptoms, diagnosis, and therapy of primary sarcomas of the pulmonary artery. Thorac Cardiovasc Surg 38:91–95

28. Chang SK, Wang TL, Teh M (1996) Extraskeletal Ewing's sarcoma presenting with pulmonary embolism. Australas Radiol 40:175–178

29. Cox JE, Chiles C, Aquino SL, Savage P, Oaks T (1997) Pulmonary artery sarcomas: a review of clinical and radiologic features. J Comput Assist Tomogr 21:750–755

30. Richards AM, Tiernan EP, Cole RP, Hobby JE (1997) Are soft-tissue sarcomas of the thigh particularly prone to thromboembolic phenomena? Plast Reconstr Surg 100:1074–1075

31. Kanjanauthai S, Kanluen T, Ray C (2008) Pulmonary artery sarcoma masquerading as saddle pulmonary embolism. Heart Lung Circ 17:417–419

32. Sandhu A, Yates TJ, Kuriakose P (2008) Pulmonary artery sarcoma mimicking a pulmonary embolism. Indian J Cancer 45:27–29

33. Minakata K, Konishi Y, Matsumoto M, Aota M, Nonaka M, Yamada N (2000) Primary leiomyosarcoma of the pulmonary artery mimicking massive pulmonary thromboembolism. Jpn Circ J 64:783–784

34. Hoffmeier A, Semik M, Fallenberg EM, Scheld HH (2001) Leiomyosarcoma of the pulmonary artery—a diagnostic chameleon. Eur J Cardiothorac Surg 20:1049–1051

35. Hollenbeck ST, Grobmyer SR, Kent KC, Brennan MF (2003) Surgical treatment and outcomes of patients with primary inferior vena cava leiomyosarcoma. J Am Coll Surg 197:575–579

36. Hilliard NJ, Heslin MJ, Castro CY (2005) Leiomyosarcoma of the inferior vena cava: three case reports and review of the literature. Ann Diagn Pathol 9:259–266

37. Dew J, Hansen K, Hammon J, McCoy T, Levine EA, Shen P (2005) Leiomyosarcoma of the inferior vena cava: surgical management and clinical results. Am Surg 71:497–501

38. Shindo S, Katsu M, Kaga S, Inoue H, Ogata K, Matsumoto M (2009) Leiomyosarcoma of a femoral vein misdiagnosed as deep vein thrombosis. J Vasc Interv Radiol 20:689–691

39. Parissis H, Akbar MT, Young V (2010) Primary leiomyosarcoma of the right atrium: a case report and literature update. J Cardiothorac Surg 5:80

40. Neragi-Miandoab S, Kim J, Vlahakes GJ (2007) Malignant tumours of the heart: a review of tumour type, diagnosis and therapy. Clin Oncol (R Coll Radiol) 19:748–756

41. Blom JW, Doggen CJ, Osanto S, Rosendaal FR (2005) Malignancies, prothrombotic mutations, and the risk of venous thrombosis. JAMA 293:715–722

42. Kessler CM (2009) The link between cancer and venous thromboembolism: a review. Am J Clin Oncol 32:S3–S7

12

Overexpressed PRAME is a potential immunotherapy target in sarcoma subtypes

Jason Roszik[1,2]*⬥, Wei-Lien Wang[3], John A. Livingston[4], Christina L. Roland[5], Vinod Ravi[4], Cassian Yee[1], Patrick Hwu[1,4], Andrew Futreal[2], Alexander J. Lazar[3], Shreyaskumar R. Patel[4] and Anthony P. Conley[4]

Abstract

Background: PRAME (preferentially expressed antigen in melanoma), a member of the cancer-testis antigen family, has been shown to have increased expression in solid tumors, including sarcoma, and PRAME-specific therapies are currently in development for other cancers such as melanoma.

Methods: To map the landscape of PRAME expression in sarcoma, we used publicly available data from The Cancer Genome Atlas (TCGA) and the Cancer Cell Line Encyclopedia (CCLE) projects and determined which sarcoma subtypes and subsets are associated with increased PRAME expression. We also analyzed how PRAME expression correlates with survival and expression of markers related to antigen presentation and T cell function. Furthermore, tumor and normal tissue expression comparisons were performed using data from the genotype-tissue expression (GTEx) project.

Results: We found that uterine carcinosarcoma highly overexpresses the PRAME antigen, and synovial sarcomas and multifocal leiomyosarcomas also show high expressions suggesting that PRAME may be an effective target of immunotherapies of these tumors. However, we also discovered that PRAME expression negatively correlates with genes involved in antigen presentation, and in synovial sarcoma MHC class I antigen presentation deficiencies are also present, potentially limiting the efficacy of immunotherapies of this malignancy.

Conclusions: We determined that uterine carcinosarcoma, synovial sarcoma, and leiomyosarcoma patients would potentially benefit from PRAME-specific immunotherapies. Tumor escape through loss of antigen presentation needs to be further studied.

Keywords: PRAME, Cancer testis antigen, Immunotherapy, Sarcoma, Sarcoma subtypes

Background

Preferentially expressed antigen in melanoma (PRAME) was first discovered in melanomas and it was associated with cytotoxic T cell activation [1]. Shortly after its discovery, it was also shown to be expressed in acute leukemia cells [2]. The function of PRAME appears to be extensive though it was first identified as a repressor of the retinoic acid receptor pathway [3]. PRAME also inhibits myeloid differentiation in a retinoic acid-dependent and independent manner as well [4]. PRAME,

like other cancer-testis antigens, has been shown be minimally expressed in adult human organs except for gonadal tissues and various human cancers including sarcomas.

Cancer-testis antigens such as MAGE-A and NY-ESO-1 have been widely explored, and these tumor-associated antigens have served as the therapeutic target of various vaccine strategies and adoptive cellular therapies. Objective tumor regressions of cutaneous metastases of melanoma patients have been documented with a MAGE-3.A1 peptide [5]. Similarly, patients with synovial sarcoma treated with genetically engineered autologous T cells with NY-ESO-1 recognition experienced RECIST partial responses as noted in 11 of 18 cases (61%) [6].

*Correspondence: jroszik@mdanderson.org
[1] Department of Melanoma Medical Oncology, The University of Texas MD Anderson Cancer Center, 1515 Holcombe Blvd., Houston, TX 77030, USA
Full list of author information is available at the end of the article

Various subtypes of sarcomas have demonstrated expression of cancer-testis antigens including synovial sarcomas, myxoid liposarcomas, chondrosarcomas, and osteosarcomas. Co-expression of PRAME and NY-ESO-1 has been shown to correlate with high-grade histologic features and a worse overall survival in patients with myxoid liposarcomas [7] and synovial sarcomas [8]. High protein expression levels of PRAME have been shown to correlate with a worse overall survival in osteosarcoma, and the expression of PRAME was more common in metastases compared to primary tumors [9]. In chondrosarcoma, a disease with low expression of PRAME at baseline, induction of PRAME with 5-aza-2-deoxycitabine rendered chondrosarcoma cells targetable by PRAME-specific CD8+ T cells [10].

The goal of this study is to evaluate the expression of PRAME across multiple sarcoma subtypes and normal tissues using three large public datasets. We report statistically significant associations to guide PRAME-specific therapies of sarcoma. To our knowledge this is the first comprehensive analysis of PRAME in multiple sarcoma subtypes and clinical subsets. In addition, we evaluated associations of T cell and antigen expression markers with PRAME expression to show how these may affect immunotherapies targeting this antigen.

Methods

Data sources

RNA expression and clinical data from the TCGA were downloaded from public repositories (https://tcga-data.nci.nih.gov). In the sarcoma TCGA, the following histologies were represented: leiomyosarcoma (LMS) (n = 106 samples), undifferentiated pleomorphic sarcoma/myxofibrosarcoma (UPS/MFS) (n = 76), dedifferentiated liposarcoma (DDLPS) (n = 58), synovial sarcoma (n = 10), and malignant peripheral nerve sheath tumors (MPNST) (n = 10). Data from carcinosarcoma cases (n = 57) were downloaded similarly from the uterine carcinosarcoma (UCS) TCGA project. Normal tissue expressions were obtained from the Genotype-Tissue Expression (GTEx, https://www.gtexportal.org/home/) project [11]. Homogeneous normal tissues were collapsed into a smaller number of groups the reduce figure complexity. Expression data of PRAME in cancer cell lines (n = 46) were downloaded from the website of the Cancer Cell Line Encyclopedia (CCLE) [12].

Analysis of expression and clinical data

Clinical and mRNA expression data were merged into an input table using the TCGA sample identifiers. We included only those cases where both clinical and expression data were available. When comparing expressions from RNA sequencing from the TCGA and GTEx

databases, we used the transcripts per million (TPM) unit, which was found to be most suitable unit for comparing RNA sequencing data [13]. For the analysis of PRAME expression in multifocal tumors, we used the *tumor_multifocal* TCGA clinical variable. Figures were created using the Tableau Desktop software. Kaplan–Meier analyses were performed using the 'survival' package of the R programming language. CCLE expression analyses were performed using microarray and also RNA-sequencing data. The TPM unit was used for RNA-seq, and in the case of microarray we used RMA-normalized data, which is calculated using a quantile normalization approach.

Statistical analyses

For comparisons of two groups we performed two-tailed Student's t-tests. When comparing multiple groups, we used Kruskal–Wallis rank sum tests followed by a post-hoc Kruskal-Nemenyi test when $p < 0.05$. All differences were considered significant when $p < 0.05$, and a trend towards significance was noted when $0.05 \leq p < 0.1$.

Results

PRAME is expressed in sarcoma and shows high overexpression in uterine carcinosarcoma

To determine the relevance of PRAME as a target in sarcoma, we compared all normal (GTEx, n = 30 tissue types, n = 8153 samples) and tumor tissue (TCGA, n = 33 cancers) expressions (Fig. 1). Expression of PRAME in the uterine carcinosarcoma TCGA (n = 57) was significantly higher ($p < 0.001$) compared to the sarcoma TCGA as a whole, and only skin cutaneous melanoma showed a higher PRAME expression among all normal and tumor tissue types. Furthermore, PRAME expression was significantly higher ($p < 0.001$) in uterine carcinosarcoma than in normal uterus (n = 83).

PRAME is expressed in sarcoma cell lines

In the CCLE cell line data (n = 46 with microarray, n = 40 with RNA-sequencing data) we found that sarcoma subtypes show diverse PRAME expressions (Fig. 2), however, in the microarray data, all four chondrosarcoma lines had lower expressions than other bone sarcoma cell lines such as Ewing's sarcoma ($p < 0.01$) and osteosarcoma ($p < 0.1$). Analysis of the RNA-sequencing data confirmed chondrosarcoma—Ewing's sarcoma difference ($p < 0.05$), and we also observed a trend for overexpression in rhabdomyosarcoma compared to chondrosarcoma ($p < 0.1$). Notably, with the exception of chondrosarcoma, PRAME over-expressing cell line(s) were found in all CCLE sarcoma types.

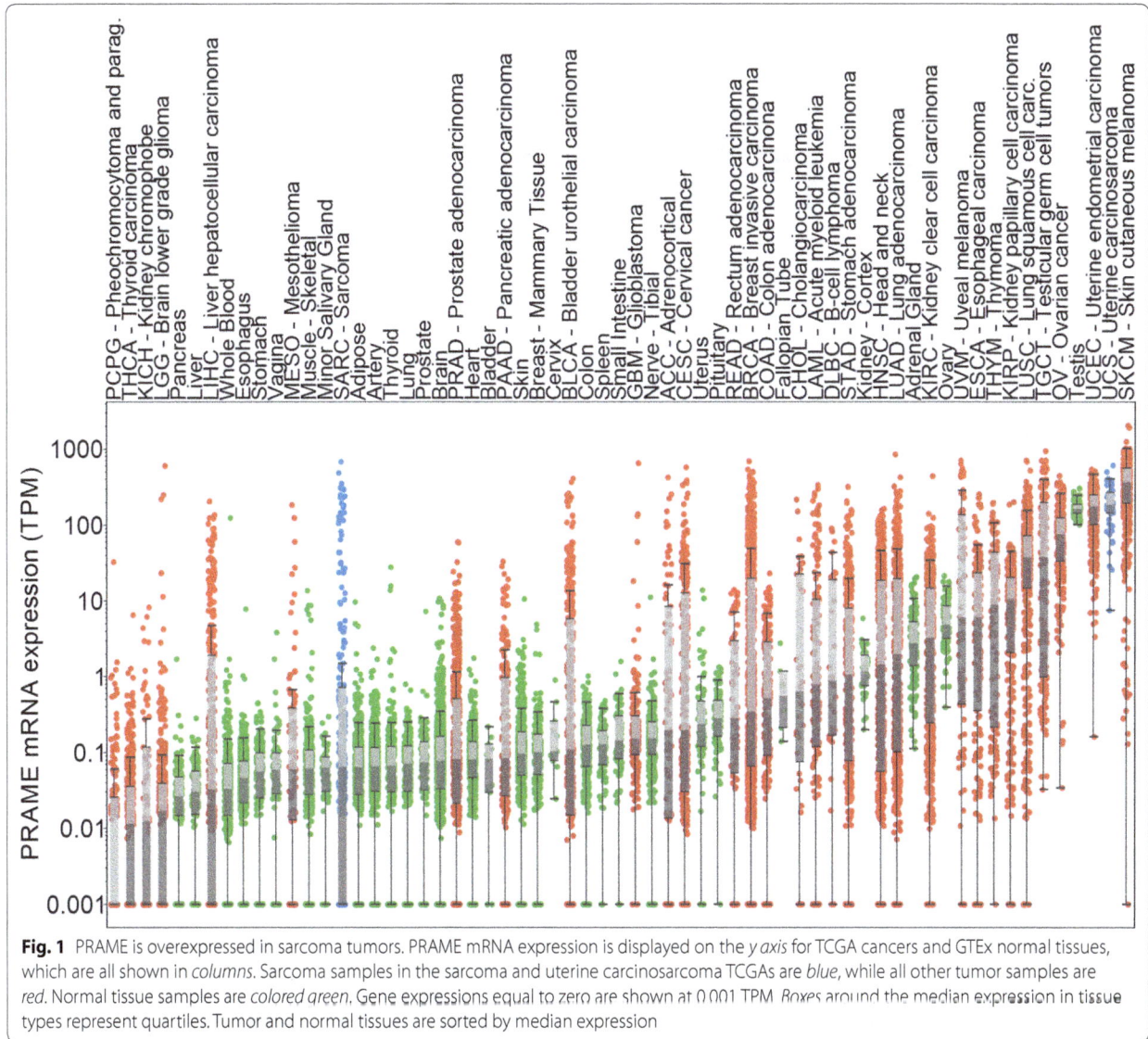

Fig. 1 PRAME is overexpressed in sarcoma tumors. PRAME mRNA expression is displayed on the *y axis* for TCGA cancers and GTEx normal tissues, which are all shown in *columns*. Sarcoma samples in the sarcoma and uterine carcinosarcoma TCGAs are *blue*, while all other tumor samples are *red*. Normal tissue samples are *colored green*. Gene expressions equal to zero are shown at 0.001 TPM. Boxes around the median expression in tissue types represent quartiles. Tumor and normal tissues are sorted by median expression

PRAME is overexpressed in synovial sarcoma and in multifocal leiomyosarcoma

Analyzing the expression of PRAME in sarcoma subtypes, we found that PRAME was highly expressed in all synovial sarcomas (Fig. 3a). The PRAME expression in these samples was significantly higher (p < 0.001) than in LMS, UPS/MFS, and DDLPS, while LMS expression was significantly lower (p < 0.05) than UPS/MFS, DDLPS, and MPNST PRAME expression (Fig. 3a). Importantly, a few of the LMS, UPS/MFS, DDLPS, and MPNST tumors also showed high PRAME expressions, suggesting that in addition to synovial sarcomas, these subtypes may also be considered for immunotherapies targeting PRAME. Although PRAME median expression was low in LMS, it showed a significantly higher (p < 0.05) expression

in multifocal LMS compared to non-multifocal LMS (Fig. 3b), therefore PRAME may be a relevant target in multifocal LMS cases.

PRAME expression negatively correlates with genes involved in antigen presentation

We have determined that PRAME expression was not associated with overall survival in dedifferentiated liposarcoma (Fig. 4a), leiomyosarcoma (Fig. 4b), and UPS/MFS (Fig. 4c), subtypes where a sufficient number of samples were available for Kaplan–Meier analyses.

We also determined whether antigen presentation and other immune-related genes (B2M, CD3E, CD4, CD8A, GZMA, GZMB, HLA-A, HLA-B, HLA-C, IFNG, LCK, PRF1, LMP7, LMP2, TAP1, and TAP2) are associated

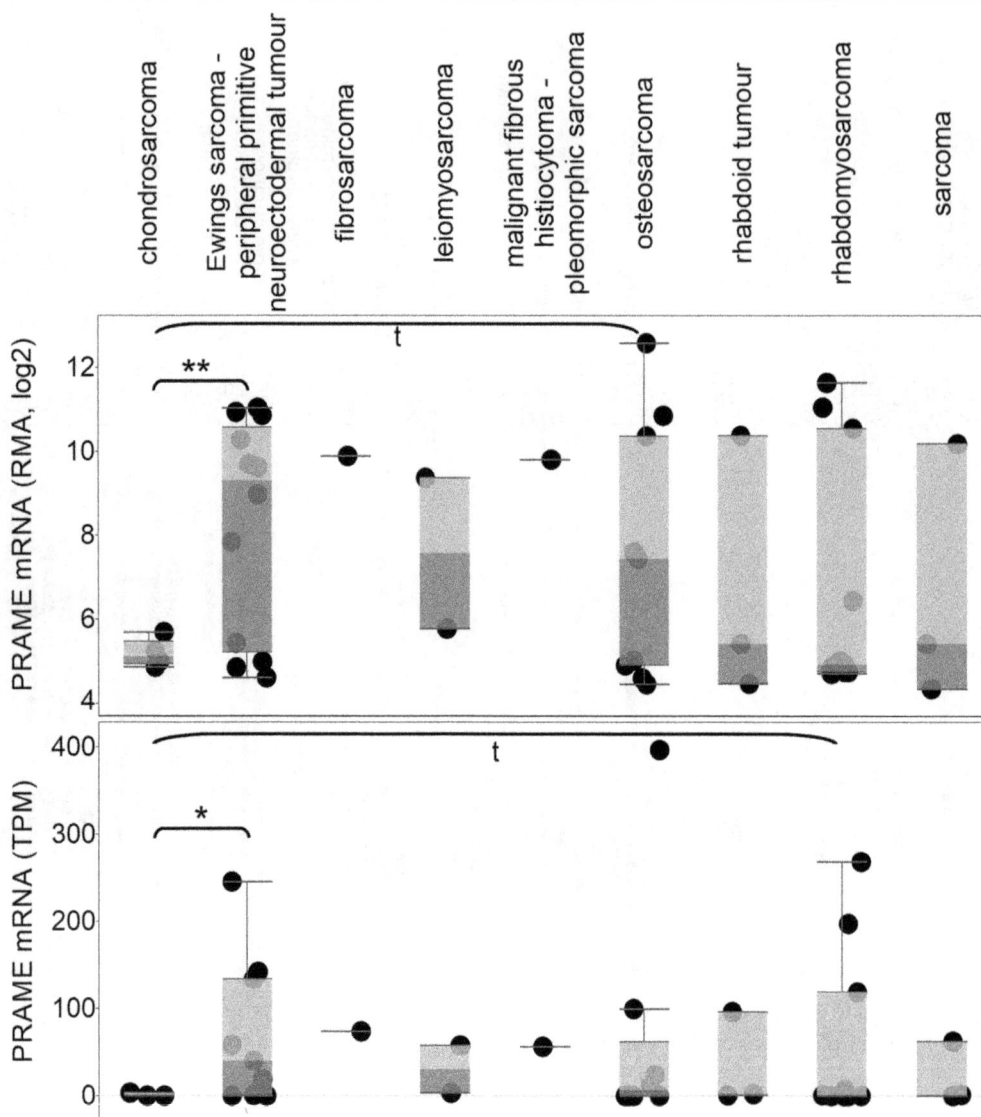

Fig. 2 PRAME is expressed in sarcoma cell lines. Cancer Cell Line Encyclopedia sarcoma cell lines are shown in *columns*, each *dot* representing a cell line. PRAME expression is shown on the *y axis*. **p < 0.01, *p < 0.05, while t denotes a trend with 0.05 ≤ p < 0.1

with PRAME and found that expression of multiple genes involved in antigen presentation (HLA-B, HLA-C, B2M, LMP2, LMP7, TAP2) negatively correlate with PRAME expression in dedifferentiated liposarcoma and leiomyosarcoma (Fig. 4d). PD-L1 and PRAME expression also negatively correlated in dedifferentiated liposarcoma. The other three subtypes did not show significant (p < 0.05) correlations. Furthermore, we found that synovial sarcoma, which overexpresses PRAME, showed a significantly lower B2M and CD8A expressions compared to other subtypes (Fig. 4e). Interestingly, CTAG1B (NY-ESO-1) expression was significantly higher in synovial sarcoma than in the other sarcoma types (Fig. 4e).

Furthermore, PD-1 expression was significantly higher (p < 0.05) in synovial sarcoma and UPS/MFS compared to leiomyosarcoma. Interestingly, PD-L1 was expressed in most subtypes except synovial sarcoma, where the expression level was significantly lower than in leiomyosarcoma (p < 0.001), UPS/MFS (p < 0.001), dedifferentiated liposarcoma (p < 0.05), and MPNST (p < 0.05).

Discussion

Sarcomas represent a rare collection of neoplasms of mesenchymal origin that make up less than 1% of all cancer cases diagnosed each year in the United States [14]. While surgery can be curative for low-grade/low-stage

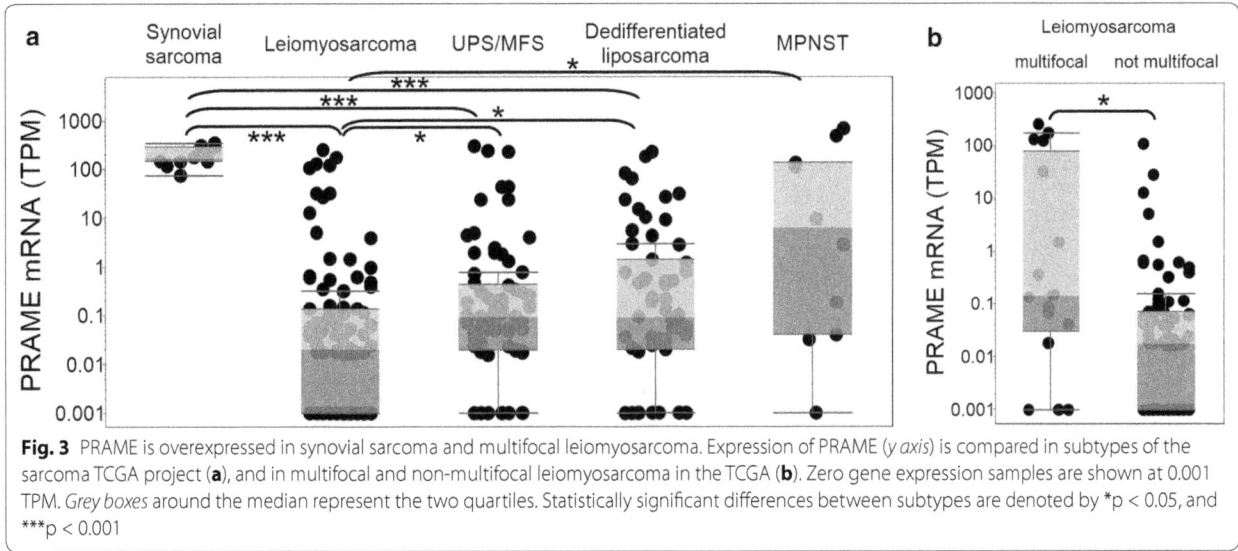

Fig. 3 PRAME is overexpressed in synovial sarcoma and multifocal leiomyosarcoma. Expression of PRAME (*y axis*) is compared in subtypes of the sarcoma TCGA project (**a**), and in multifocal and non-multifocal leiomyosarcoma in the TCGA (**b**). Zero gene expression samples are shown at 0.001 TPM. *Grey boxes* around the median represent the two quartiles. Statistically significant differences between subtypes are denoted by *p < 0.05, and ***p < 0.001

disease, unresectable/metastatic disease is treated with systemic therapies. These therapies for soft tissue sarcomas have improved in slow incremental steps over the last 40 years with limited success [15]. Treatment of sarcoma is also difficult because more than one hundred subtypes have been identified. The success of immunotherapies in certain tumors provide a new avenue for investigation for the treatment of sarcoma. In fact, a recent phase II study (SARC028) of pembrolizumab for advanced/metastatic sarcomas demonstrated a response rate of 17% [16]. In the current study, we show that PRAME could be an effective immunotherapy target in specific sarcoma subtypes. Furthermore, we show that PD-1 and PD-L1 are also expressed in a heterogeneous manner, supporting further evaluation of anti-PD-1 and anti-PD-L1 therapies in sarcomas.

We determined that uterine carcinosarcoma, a disease that lacks standard therapies, highly overexpresses the PRAME antigen. Other cancer testis antigens have been identified as potential immunotherapy targets for this malignancy, including MAGE-A4 and NY-ESO-1 [17]. We propose that PRAME might also be an effective and broadly expressed target. Although the other sarcoma tumors included in the sarcoma TCGA showed a lower expression, a subset of samples was clearly characterized by PRAME overexpression. Multiple CCLE cell lines that were derived from sarcoma tumors retained PRAME expression, with the exception of chondrosarcoma, which was not included in the sarcoma TCGA.

Our analysis of PRAME expression associations with subtypes and clinical variables revealed that PRAME is overexpressed in synovial sarcoma and in multifocal leiomyosarcoma. Notably, all other sarcoma subtypes showed a highly heterogeneous PRAME expression, from zero to very high expression. This is in line with heterogeneity of sarcomas, which represents a major challenge. Cancer testis antigens, focusing primarily on NY-ESO-1, are currently being tested in clinical trials and show promise as targets of adoptive immunotherapies and cancer vaccines to treat sarcoma [18]. PRAME co-overexpression with NY-ESO-1 in synovial sarcoma suggests that this antigen may also be targeted efficiently by these immunotherapy approaches.

The negative correlation that we identified between PRAME and expression of antigen presentation-related genes also supports that tumor-associated antigens derived from the PRAME protein can be recognized by the immune system, and tumors lose expression of genes involved in antigen presentation to avoid an effective immune response. Indeed, in the PRAME-overexpressing synovial sarcoma, beta2-microglobulin (B2M) loss appears to be a mechanism by which the tumor avoids immune recognition, evidenced by low expression of the CD8A cytotoxic T cell marker. However, we also found non-zero interferon gamma (IFNG) expression in half of the synovial sarcoma samples that we analyzed, therefore we hypothesize that there are functional and active T cells in those tumors that may be exploited to develop effective immunotherapies. Furthermore, MHC class I recovery approaches [19] might also be needed to ensure the success of T cell-based immunotherapy of sarcoma.

Conclusions

Our analysis of sarcoma subtypes shows that uterine carcinosarcoma, synovial sarcoma, and multifocal leiomyosarcoma samples overexpress this antigen and patients with these malignancies would potentially benefit from

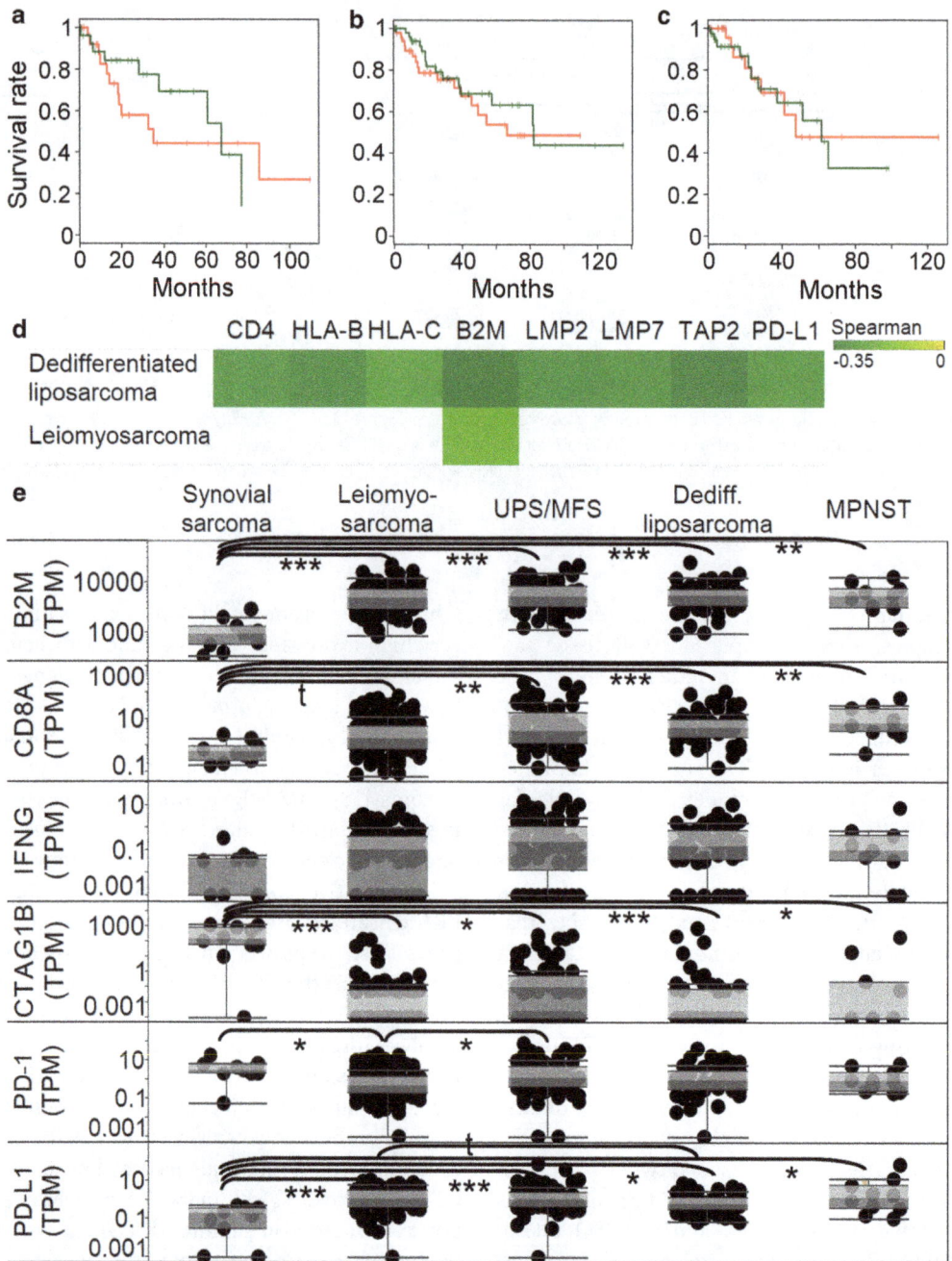

Fig. 4 Survival and immune correlations of PRAME. Kaplan–Meier plots comparing low (*green*, below median expression samples) and high (*red*, above median expression) in dedifferentiated liposarcoma (**a**), leiomyosarcoma (**b**), and UPS/MFS (**c**) show no statistically significant associations. Spearman's rank correlation coefficients of PRAME and antigen presentation and immune related genes are displayed in *panel* **d** (only p < 0.05 correlations are shown). Expression of B2M, CD8A, IFNG, CTAG1B (NY-ESO-1), PD-1, and PD-L1 are compared in sarcoma subtypes (**e**), where t: p < 0.1, *p < 0.05, **p < 0.01, and ***p < 0.001

PRAME-specific immunotherapies. We also found a negative correlation between PRAME and expression of genes involved in antigen presentation, which may provide a way for tumors to avoid immune recognition.

Abbreviations

LMS: leiomyosarcoma; UPS/MFS: undifferentiated pleomorphic sarcoma/myxofibrosarcoma; DDLPS: dedifferentiated liposarcoma; MPNST: malignant peripheral nerve sheath tumors; TCGA: The Cancer Genome Atlas; GTEx: genotype-tissue expression project; TPM: transcripts per million.

Authors' contributions
JR and APC conceived the study. JR, APC, WLW, JAL, CLR, VR, CY, PH, AF, AJL, SRP, and APC contributed to analysis of data and interpretation of results. JR and APC drafted the manuscript. All authors read and approved the final manuscript.

Author details
[1] Department of Melanoma Medical Oncology, The University of Texas MD Anderson Cancer Center, 1515 Holcombe Blvd., Houston, TX 77030, USA. [2] Department of Genomic Medicine, The University of Texas MD Anderson Cancer Center, 1515 Holcombe Blvd., Houston, TX 77030, USA. [3] Department of Pathology, The University of Texas MD Anderson Cancer Center, 1515 Holcombe Blvd., Houston, TX 77030, USA. [4] Department of Sarcoma Medical Oncology, The University of Texas MD Anderson Cancer Center, 1515 Holcombe Blvd., Houston, TX 77030, USA. [5] Department of Surgical Oncology, The University of Texas MD Anderson Cancer Center, 1515 Holcombe Blvd, Houston, TX 77030, USA.

Acknowledgements
We thank the generous philanthropic contributions to The University of Texas MD Anderson Moon Shots Program.

Competing interests
The authors declare that they have no competing interests.

Funding
The University of Texas MD Anderson Moon Shots Program.

References
1. Ikeda H, Lethe B, Lehmann F, van Baren N, Baurain JF, de Smet C, et al. Characterization of an antigen that is recognized on a melanoma showing partial HLA loss by CTL expressing an NK inhibitory receptor. Immunity. 1997;6(2):199–208.
2. van Baren N, Chambost H, Ferrant A, Michaux L, Ikeda H, Millard I, et al. PRAME, a gene encoding an antigen recognized on a human melanoma by cytolytic T cells, is expressed in acute leukaemia cells. Br J Haematol. 1998;102(5):1376–9.
3. Epping MT, Wang L, Edel MJ, Carlee L, Hernandez M, Bernards R. The human tumor antigen PRAME is a dominant repressor of retinoic acid receptor signaling. Cell. 2005;122(6):835–47.
4. Oehler VG, Guthrie KA, Cummings CL, Sabo K, Wood BL, Gooley T, et al. The preferentially expressed antigen in melanoma (PRAME) inhibits myeloid differentiation in normal hematopoietic and leukemic progenitor cells. Blood. 2009;114(15):3299–308.
5. Marchand M, van Baren N, Weynants P, Brichard V, Dreno B, Tessier MH, et al. Tumor regressions observed in patients with metastatic melanoma treated with an antigenic peptide encoded by gene MAGE-3 and presented by HLA-A1. Int J Cancer. 1999;80(2):219–30.
6. Robbins PF, Kassim SH, Tran TL, Crystal JS, Morgan RA, Feldman SA, et al. A pilot trial using lymphocytes genetically engineered with an NY-ESO-1-reactive T-cell receptor: long-term follow-up and correlates with response. Clin Cancer Res. 2015;21(5):1019–27.
7. Iura K, Kohashi K, Hotokebuchi Y, Ishii T, Maekawa A, Yamada Y, et al. Cancer-testis antigens PRAME and NY-ESO-1 correlate with tumour grade and poor prognosis in myxoid liposarcoma. J Pathol Clin Res. 2015;1(3):144–59.
8. Iura K, Maekawa A, Kohashi K, Ishii T, Bekki H, Otsuka H, et al. Cancer-testis antigen expression in synovial sarcoma: NY-ESO-1, PRAME, MAGEA4, and MAGEA1. Hum Pathol. 2017;61:130–9.
9. Tan P, Zou C, Yong B, Han J, Zhang L, Su Q, et al. Expression and prognostic relevance of PRAME in primary osteosarcoma. Biochem Biophys Res Commun. 2012;419(4):801–8.
10. Pollack SM, Li Y, Blaisdell MJ, Farrar EA, Chou J, Hoch BL, et al. NYESO-1/LAGE-1 s and PRAME are targets for antigen specific T cells in chondrosarcoma following treatment with 5-Aza-2-deoxycitabine. PLoS ONE. 2012;7(2):e32165.
11. Consortium GT. The genotype-tissue expression (GTEx) project. Nat Genet. 2013;45(6):580–5.
12. Barretina J, Caponigro G, Stransky N, Venkatesan K, Margolin AA, Kim S, et al. The Cancer Cell Line Encyclopedia enables predictive modelling of anticancer drug sensitivity. Nature. 2012;483(7391):603–7.
13. Wagner GP, Kin K, Lynch VJ. Measurement of mRNA abundance using RNA-seq data: RPKM measure is inconsistent among samples. Theory Biosci. 2012;131(4):281–5.
14. Siegel RL, Miller KD, Jemal A. Cancer statistics, 2016. CA Cancer J Clin. 2016;66(1):7–30.
15. Ratan R, Patel SR. Chemotherapy for soft tissue sarcoma. Cancer. 2016;122(19):2952–60.
16. Tawbi HA, Burgess MA, Crowley J, Van Tine BA, Hu J, Schuetze S, et al. Safety and efficacy of PD-1 blockade using pembrolizumab in patients with advanced soft tissue (STS) and bone sarcomas (BS): results of SARC028—a multicenter phase II study. J Clin Oncol 2016; 34(suppl; abstr 11006).
17. Resnick MB, Sabo E, Kondratev S, Kerner H, Spagnoli GC, Yakirevich E. Cancer-testis antigen expression in uterine malignancies with an emphasis on carcinosarcomas and papillary serous carcinomas. Int J Cancer. 2002;101(2):190–5.
18. Mitsis D, Francescutti V, Skitzki J. Current immunotherapies for sarcoma: clinical trials and rationale. Sarcoma. 2016;2016:9757219.
19. Garrido F, Aptsiauri N, Doorduijn EM, Garcia Lora AM, van Hall T. The urgent need to recover MHC class I in cancers for effective immunotherapy. Curr Opin Immunol. 2016;39:44–51.

13

High nuclear expression of proteasome activator complex subunit 1 predicts poor survival in soft tissue leiomyosarcomas

Sha Lou[1], Arjen H. G. Cleven[2], Benjamin Balluff[3], Marieke de Graaff[2], Marie Kostine[2], Inge Briaire-de Bruijn[2], Liam A. McDonnell[1,2,4] and Judith V. M. G. Bovée[2]*

Abstract

Background: Previous studies on high grade sarcomas using mass spectrometry imaging showed proteasome activator complex subunit 1 (PSME1) to be associated with poor survival in soft tissue sarcoma patients. PSME1 is involved in immunoproteasome assembly for generating tumor antigens presented by MHC class I molecules. In this study, we aimed to validate PSME1 as a prognostic biomarker in an independent and larger series of soft tissue sarcomas by immunohistochemistry.

Methods: Tissue microarrays containing leiomyosarcomas (n = 34), myxofibrosarcomas (n = 14), undifferentiated pleomorphic sarcomas (n = 15), undifferentiated spindle cell sarcomas (n = 4), pleomorphic liposarcomas (n = 4), pleomorphic rhabdomyosarcomas (n = 2), and uterine leiomyomas (n = 7) were analyzed for protein expression of PSME1 using immunohistochemistry. Survival times were compared between high and low expression groups using Kaplan–Meier analysis. Cox regression models as multivariate analysis were performed to evaluate whether the associations were independent of other important clinical covariates.

Results: PSME1 expression was variable among soft tissue sarcomas. In leiomyosarcomas, high expression was associated with overall poor survival (p = 0.034), decreased metastasis-free survival (p = 0.002) and lower event-free survival (p = 0.007). Using multivariate analysis, the association between PSME1 expression and metastasis-free survival was still significant (p = 0.025) and independent of the histological grade.

Conclusions: High expression of PSME1 is associated with poor metastasis-free survival in soft tissue leiomyosarcoma patients, and might be used as an independent prognostic biomarker.

Keywords: Proteasome activator complex subunit 1, Prognostic biomarker, Sarcoma, Leiomyosarcoma, Soft tissue sarcoma, Immunohistochemistry

Background

Soft tissue sarcomas are a heterogeneous group of rare malignancies often having poor outcome [1]. Soft tissue sarcomas constitute less than 1 % of all cancers [1] while there are more than 50 histological subtypes with sometimes overlapping histological features [2]. Distinction is essential as subtypes differ in biological behaviour and sensitivity to chemotherapy, and as such an adequate histological diagnosis, is crucial for clinical decision making [3]. Fifty-six percent of soft tissue sarcomas present as localized disease at the time of diagnosis, and surgery is the mainstay of treatment, sometimes combined with radiotherapy or chemotherapy [4].

From the molecular point of view, soft tissue sarcomas can be distinguished into two categories. The first class includes sarcomas with a simple genome, in which recurrent translocations, amplifications or specific mutations can be found. The second class includes sarcomas with a complex genome, characterized by a multitude

*Correspondence: J.V.M.G.Bovee@lumc.nl
[2] Department of Pathology, Leiden University Medical Center, Leiden, The Netherlands
Full list of author information is available at the end of the article

of chromosomal alterations and genomic instability, often reflected by pleomorphic histological features [3]. This group includes high grade leiomyosarcoma, myxofibrosarcoma, undifferentiated pleomorphic sarcoma, undifferentiated spindle cell sarcoma, pleomorphic liposarcoma, and pleomorphic rhabdomyosarcoma.

Leiomyosarcomas constitute 5–10 % of all soft tissue sarcomas, displaying smooth-muscle differentiation [1]. Studies showed for leiomyosarcoma that the metastasis-free 5-year survival rate is about 60 % [5]. Histological grade is the most important prognostic factor for most soft tissue sarcomas. By using FNCLCC grading system, which is the most widely used 3-grade system, soft tissue sarcomas are divided into low, intermediate and high grade based on the sum score of three histologic parameters including tumor differentiation, mitotic count and tumor necrosis. About 65 % of leiomyosarcomas are reported to have high-grade areas [6]. High grade leiomyosarcomas often have poor patient outcome [4]. Until now, the genetics and pathology of leiomyosarcomas are not completely understood and as they have a complex genome, no molecular diagnostic tests or specific therapeutic targets are available. Hence, there is a strong need for new molecular markers that can aid in the stratification of leiomyosarcomas patients with respect to their disease outcome.

In a previous study, we used imaging mass spectrometry to compare these soft tissue sarcomas with a complex genome. A panel of protein signatures that could distinguish between different subtypes, or were associated to patient survival were discovered [7]. Among them, proteasome activator complex subunit 1 (PSME1) was found indicative of poor survival in soft tissue sarcomas. PSME1 (also known as REGalpha and PA28A), is a multicatalytic proteinase complex, implicated in immunoproteasome assembly and required for efficient antigen processing [8]. Intriguingly, PSME1 was also found to associate with diagnosis or prognosis in other tumor types, e.g. prostate cancer [9], breast cancer [10] and ovarian cancer [11, 12].

In this study, we used tissue microarrays of soft tissue sarcomas with complex genomes, to evaluate whether PSME1 expression can predict clinical outcome in soft tissue sarcomas, especially leiomyosarcomas.

Methods

Tissue microarrays

Tissue microarrays were previously constructed from paraffin embedded formalin fixed tissues using a semi-automated TMA apparatus (TMA Master; 3D Histech, Budapest, Hungary) [13]. Clinicopathological details were described previously [14]. In brief, analysed samples include 34 leiomyosarcomas, 14 myxofibrosarcomas, 15 undifferentiated pleomorphic sarcomas, four

undifferentiated spindle cell sarcomas, four pleomorphic liposarcomas, two pleomorphic rhabdomyosarcomas, and seven uterine leiomyomas. Clinicopathological data for the leiomyosarcomas, as described previously [14], are summarized in Additional file 1: Table S1. All tumor samples are present at least in triplicates with a diameter of 1.5 mm (a surface area of around 1.767 mm^2). Cores from colon, liver, placenta, prostate, skin, and tonsil were included for control and orientation purposes. Four micrometre thick sections were transferred by using a tape-transfer system to coated glass slides for analysis.

The histological diagnosis of all samples was confirmed by reviewing the hematoxylin and eosin—stained slides by expert pathologist (J. V. M. G. B.). Malignant tumors were graded according to the FNCLCC (French Fédération Nationale des Centres de Lutte Contre le Cancer) grading system [1]. All samples were handled according to the Dutch code of proper secondary use of human material as accorded by the Dutch society of pathology (Federa). The samples were handled in a coded manner. All study methods were approved by the LUMC ethical board (B16.025).

PSME1 immunohistochemistry

Four micrometre thick sections were dried overnight at 37 °C. Immunohistochemistry was performed using anti-PSME1 antibody (clone [EPR10968(B)], abcam, Cambridge, UK) according to protocols described previously [15]. Briefly, slides underwent deparaffinization, blocking of endogenous peroxidase, antigen retrieval (10 min microwave in citrate, pH 6.0), pre-incubation, and addition of the primary antibody in a dilution of 1:1500 overnight. Next, slides were incubated with Poly-HRP-GAM/R/R [Immunologic BV, Duiven, The Netherlands (DPVO110HRP)], visualized with DAB+Substrate Chromogen System (DAKO, Heverlee, Belgium) and counterstained with hematoxylin. Colon tissue was used as a positive control. As a negative control slides were incubated with PBS/1 % BSA instead of the primary antibody.

Scoring of immunohistochemistry

Slides were scored independently by two observers (J.V.M.G.B and A.H.G.C) as described previously [16]. In brief, staining intensity (0, absent; 1, weak; 2, moderate; 3, strong) and percentage of positive tumor cells (0, 0 %; 1, 1–24 %; 2, 25–49 %; 3, 50–74 %; 4, 75–100 %) were assessed. Afterwards, scores of staining intensity and percentage of positive tumor cells were added to obtain the sum score; for later statistical analysis, the average sum score was calculated over all cores belonging to the same tumor. Proteasomes are present both in the nucleus as well as in the cytoplasm of eukaryotic cells, although their relative abundance within these compartments can be highly variable [8, 17–20]. We therefore evaluated cytoplasmic and nuclear staining separately. Cores in which tissue was lost or with not enough tumor area were excluded from the analysis. Cores with differences on sum score from two observers more than two were re-evaluated to reach consensus.

Statistical analysis

Only primary tumour samples were used in statistical analysis. First, the distribution of sum score data was evaluated by Shapiro–Wilk normality test. As this test showed that the score data was not normally distributed, nonparametric Spearman correlation coefficient was used as a measure of the statistical dependence between the histological grades and PSME1 expression. Further statistical two-group comparisons between controls (uterine leiomyoma) and the different histological grades of soft tissue sarcomas were calculated by Dunn's multiple-comparison test. Spearman correlation was performed in R environment (R Foundation for statistical Computing, Vienna, Austria), scatter plots and Dunn's test results were generated in GraphPad Prism version 6.00 for Windows (GraphPad Software, La Jolla, California, USA, http://www.graphpad.com). All two-sided p values equal or lower than 0.05 were considered statistically significant.

For survival analysis, patients were dichotomized into two groups. We dichotomized leiomyosarcoma patients into high and low expression groups according to the sum scores of immunohistochemistry, for which we chose the cut-off at the 3rd quartile—Experience shows that molecular subgroups are usually found in 10–25 % of the patients (e.g. HER2 overexpression [21], KRAS mutation [22]). Differences in overall survival, metastasis-free survival and event-free survival between these groups were investigated using Kaplan–Meier curves and the log-rank test. Independent variables predicting survival were evaluated in a multivariable model using Cox Regression analyses. Survival analysis was performed in R environment (R Foundation for statistical Computing, Vienna, Austria) using *Survival* package and all two-sided p values lower or equal than 0.05 were considered statistically significant.

Results
Variable nuclear and cytoplasmic expression of PSME1 in soft tissue sarcomas

In soft tissue sarcomas, PSME1 protein expression was found in the majority of the cases, both in the nucleus as well as in the cytoplasm. In contrast, expression in benign leiomyoma was low or absent (Fig. 1a, b). Representative images of immunohistochemistry are shown in Fig. 2.

Increased expression of PSME1 with increasing histological grade in leiomyosarcomas

The leiomyosarcoma subgroup was large enough to analyse a possible correlation with histological grade. Indeed, while expression was low to absent in uterine leiomyoma, expression gradually increased with increasing histological grade in both nucleus ($p_{overall} = 0.000357$) and cytoplasm ($p_{overall} = 0.00045$) in leiomyosarcomas (Fig. 1c, d). Further statistical two groups comparisons between control and any histological grade by Dunn's multiple comparisons test showed that both nuclear and cytoplasmic staining significantly differed in uterine leiomyomas versus leiomyosarcomas grade 2 ($p \leq 0.05$) and uterine leiomyomas versus leiomyosarcomas grade 3 ($p \leq 0.01$).

High nuclear expression of PSME1 predicts poor outcome in leiomyosarcoma patients

To investigate a possible correlation of PSME1 expression with clinical outcome, leiomyosarcoma patients were dichotomized into high and low PSME1 expression groups according to the sum scores of immunohistochemistry. High PSME1 expression was associated with poor overall survival ($p = 0.034$), decreased metastasis-free survival ($p = 0.002$) and lower event-free survival ($p = 0.007$) (Fig. 3).

High nuclear expression of PSME1 as an independent prognostic factor in leiomyosarcoma patients

Using multivariable Cox Regression analyses including clinically relevant co-factors such as histological grade, age and gender, we showed that high nuclear expression of PSME1 was independently associated with metastasis-free survival ($p = 0.03$) (Table 1). The independent predictive power of nuclear PSME1 expression for overall and event-free survival was at the border of significance ($p = 0.07$) (Table 1).

Discussion

Using imaging mass spectrometry we previously identified PSME1 as a prognostic biomarker indicating poor survival in soft tissue sarcoma patients [7]. Imaging mass spectrometry is a sensitive discovery tool (zepto-molar sensitivity [23]) enabling the detection of hundreds of molecules directly from tissue [24, 25]. To further explore the prognostic value of PSME1 we analysed PSME1 expression in a larger, independent set of soft tissue sarcomas using immunohistochemistry on tissue microarrays. PSME1 (or PA28A) encodes a subunit of the proteasome system, which is a major source for generation of tumor antigens presented by MHC class I molecules [26, 27]. Escape of immune response is one of the hallmarks of cancer [28]. In addition, elevated proteasome activity in tumor cells has been described to

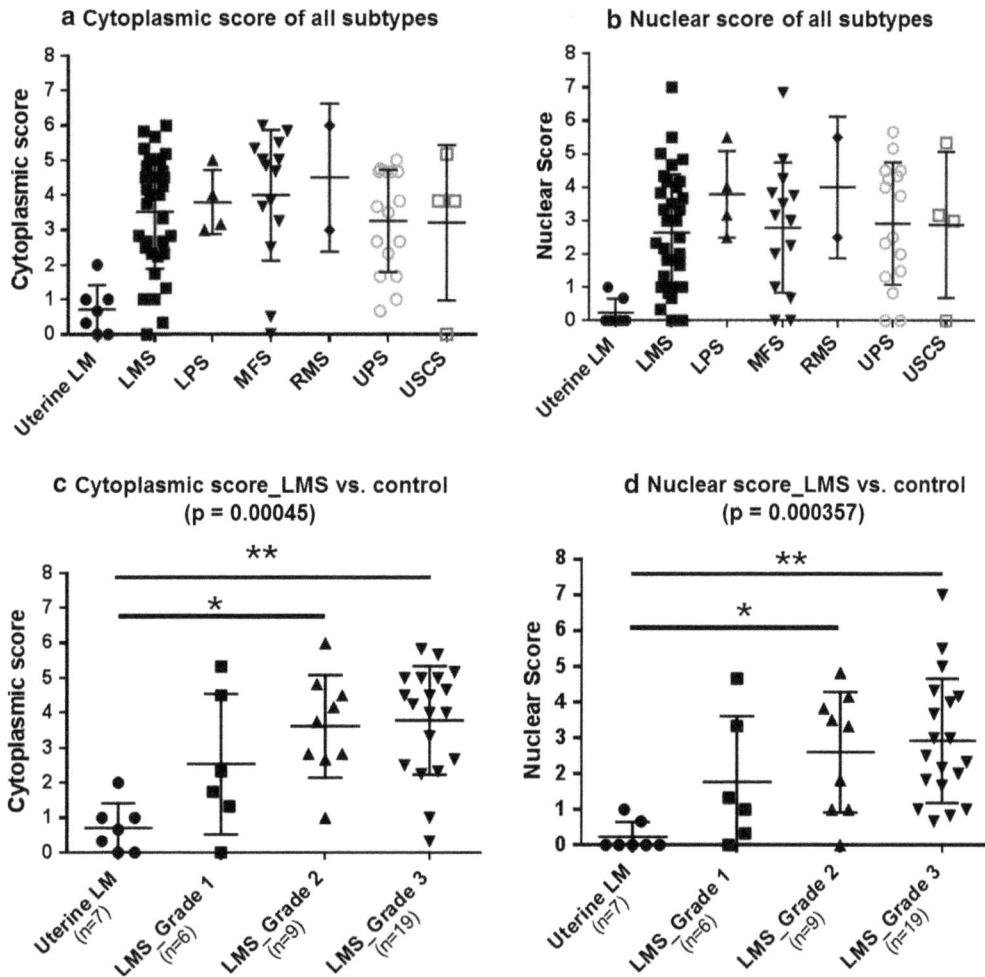

Fig. 1 Summary of PSME1 immunohistochemistry results. Variable expression of PSME1 both in the cytoplasm (**a**) as well as in the nucleus (**b**) in soft tissue sarcomas, while expression in uterine leiomyoma (LM; control) is low. *LMS* leiomyosarcomas, *LPS* pleomorphic liposarcomas, *MFS* myxofi-brosarcomas, *RMS* pleomorphic rhabdomyosarcomas, *UPS* undifferentiated pleomorphic sarcomas, and *USCS* undifferentiated spindle cell sarcomas. In leiomyosarcomas, both cytoplasmic (**c**) and nuclear (**d**) expression increased with increasing histological grade (p = 0.00045 and p = 0.000357). In addition, both cytoplasmic and nuclear expression of PSME1 was significantly higher in intermediate and high grade leiomyosarcomas as compared to uterine leiomyomas (p ≤ 0.05/p ≤ 0.01). All score data for each group were presented in mean ± SD

influence transcription factors involved in cell survival or apoptosis [29, 30]. Novel strategies using the proteasome have been proposed for cancer treatment for example by alternating the $NAD^+/NADH$ ratio to change kinetics of proteasomal degradation [30] or inhibiting proteasome to induce apoptosis [31–34].

PSME1 is expressed in many different cell types, especially antigen presenting cells, and its expression can be controlled by interferon gamma. Both chemotherapy and TNF-alpha may induce a local inflammatory reaction within the tumor microenvironment and therefore may influence expression of PSME1. It is of interest that all sarcoma subtypes included in our study expressed PSME1 to a variable extent, while neoadjuvant

chemotherapy or treatment with interferon gamma is not standard practice in our hospital. As far as clinical data were available, only four patients received preoperative chemotherapy or TNF-alpha, and expression levels were not significantly different. In the control group, consisting of uterine leiomyomas, expression was low to absent, both in the nucleus as well as in the cytoplasm.

High PSME1 expression was also described in other tumors. For example, increased PSME1 expression was also found in primary and metastatic human prostate cancer and was suggested as a potential target for therapeutic intervention [9]. PSME1 was previously also detected using imaging mass spectrometry in other tumors: Dekker et al. detected PSME1 as a marker of

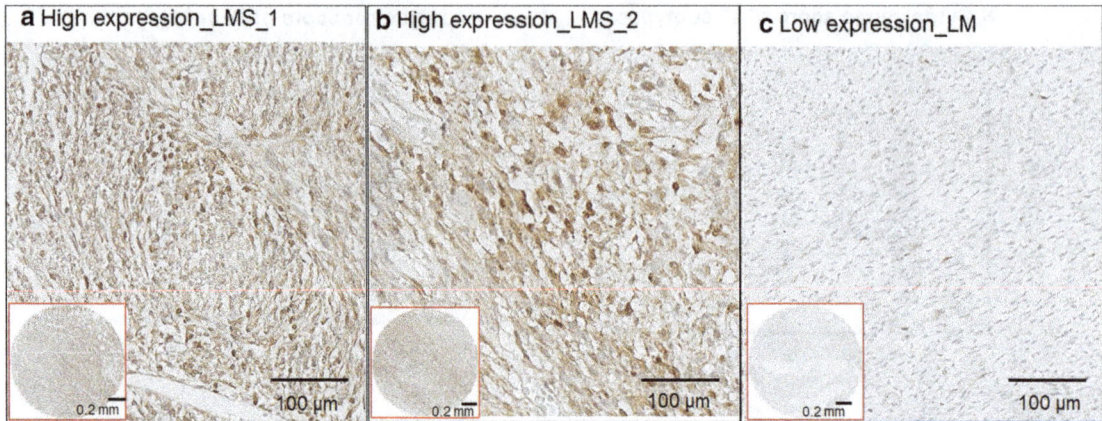

Fig. 2 Representative images of immunohistochemistry of PSME1. **a** and **b** are two leiomyosarcoma (LMS) samples with high expression of PSME1. **c** A uterine leiomyoma (LM) control sample with low expression of PSME1. Images in *red squares* are the overviews of expression the tissue microarray cores for respective samples

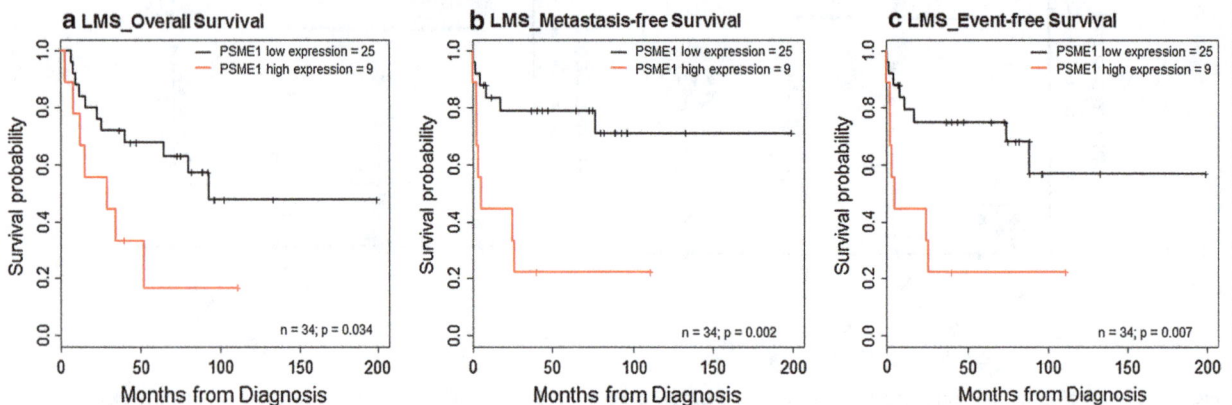

Fig. 3 Kaplan–Meier survival plots of PSME1. Kaplan–Meier plots comparing the different survival data of leiomyosarcoma patients with respect to a high and low nuclear expression of PSME1 (cut-off: 3rd quartile). High nuclear expression of PSME1 in leiomyosarcoma was significantly associated with decreased overall survival, metastasis-free survival and event-free survival (log-rank test; $p \leq 0.05$)

stromal activation in breast cancer [10]. Previous studies also showed that PSME1 could be a molecular signature to discriminate between benign and malignant ovarian tumors [11, 35], and an early diagnosis and tumor-relapse biomarker [12]. Zhang et al. detected PSME1 as a tumor marker in human oesophageal squamous cell carcinoma [36]. The proteasome can be present in the cytoplasm as well as in the nucleus of all eukaryotic cells, although their distribution and function can be variable [17]. We here show that in soft tissue sarcomas with a complex genome, PSME1 is expressed both in the cytoplasm and in the nucleus. Proteasome-dependent protein degradation is important in the cytoplasm for MHC class 1 antigen presentation [8]. In the nucleus, PSME1 plays an important role in maintaining the nuclear

function including gene expression and cell proliferation [19, 37].

To further evaluate its clinical relevance, we analysed the largest subgroup, comprising 34 leiomyosarcomas of different histological grade, in more detail. Both nuclear as well as cytoplasmic expression of PSME1 significantly increased with increasing histological grade. Moreover, high nuclear expression of PSME1 was significantly associated to poor outcome (overall survival, metastasis-free survival and event-free survival) in leiomyosarcoma patients, although the patient cohort is rather small (n = 34). In multivariate analysis only the association with decreased metastasis-free survival was independent of histological grade, while an independent association to poor overall survival and decreased

Table 1 Results of multivariable analysis of factors influencing survival

Clinical association	Variable	Hazards ratio	95 % Confidence interval	p value
Metastasis-free survival				
	PSME1 high nuclear expression	3.685	1.177–11.541	0.025*
	Histological grade	1.831	0.710–4.723	0.211
	Age	0.974	0.932–1.017	0.225
	Gender (M)	0.377	0.070–2.039	0.257
Event-free survival				
	PSME1 high nuclear expression	2.667	0.919–7.743	0.071
	Histological grade	2.216	0.882–5.569	0.090
	Age	0.975	0.937–1.015	0.215
	Gender (M)	0.339	0.068–1.695	0.188
Overall survival				
	PSME1 high nuclear expression	2.612	0.916–7.448	0.072
	Histological grade	2.552	0.953–6.837	0.062
	Age	1.005	0.972–1.039	0.758
	Gender (M)	2.071	0.660–6.502	0.212

* p value reaches statistically significant level ($p \leq 0.05$)

event-free survival was at the border of significance. Although PMSE1 expression is a promising biomarker, our results need to be validated in an independent cohort of leiomyosarcomas.

In summary, we found elevated expression of the proteasome subunit PSME1 in leiomyosarcomas compared to control tissues, and an association of the expression with increasing histological grade in leiomyosarcoma. Moreover, high nuclear PSME1 expression was found to be an independent predictor of metastasis-free survival in leiomyosarcoma patients. Our results suggest that the expression of proteasome subunits such as PSME1 could be taken into account for leiomyosarcoma patients when considering immunotherapeutic strategies in these tumors [38].

Conclusions

We show variable expression of PSME1 in different soft tissue sarcoma subtypes with complex genomes. Our results showed that high nuclear expression of proteasome activator complex subunit 1 is an independent poor prognostic factor in leiomyosarcomas, which suggests that the proteasome could be exploited as a possible novel target for the treatment of leiomyosarcomas.

Abbreviations

PSME1: proteasome activator complex subunit one; LMS: leiomyosarcomas; MFS: myxofibrosarcomas; UPS: undifferentiated pleomorphic sarcomas; Uterine LM: uterine leiomyomas; LPS: pleomorphic liposarcomas; RMS: pleomorphic rhabdomyosarcomas; USCS: undifferentiated spindle cell sarcomas.

Authors' contributions

SL: data analysis and interpretation, writing of manuscript. AHGC: immunohistochemistry scoring, data interpretation. BB: statistical analysis. MG: tissue microarrays' construction. MK: data collection and analysis. IBB: experimental work. LAM: design and supervision of the study. JVMGB: immunohistochemistry scoring, design and supervision of the study, writing of manuscript. All authors read and approved the final manuscript.

Author details

[1] Center for Proteomics and Metabolomics, Leiden University Medical Center, Albinusdreef 2, Postzone L1-Q, Postbus 9600, 2300 RC Leiden, The Netherlands. [2] Department of Pathology, Leiden University Medical Center, Leiden, The Netherlands. [3] Maastricht MultiModal Molecular Imaging Institute (M4I), Maastricht University, Maastricht, The Netherlands. [4] Fondazione Pisana per la Scienza ONLUS, Pisa, Italy.

Acknowledgements

The authors would like to thank B.E.W.M. van den Akker for technical assistance.

Competing interests

The authors declare that they have no competing interests.

Funding

The authors would like to acknowledge financial support from COMMIT, Cyttron II and the ZonMW Zenith project Imaging Mass Spectrometry-Based Molecular Histology: Differentiation and Characterization of Clinically Challenging Soft Tissue Sarcomas (No. 93512002). BB is funded by the Marie Curie Action of the European Union (SITH FP7-PEOPLE-2012-IEF No. 331866).

References

1. Fletcher CDM, Bridge JA, Hogendoorn PCW, Mertens F. WHO classification of tumors of soft tissue and bone. 4th ed. Lyon: WHO Press; 2013. p. 14–8.
2. Taylor B, Barretina J, Maki R, Antonescu C, Singer S, Ladanyi M. Advances in sarcoma genomics and new therapeutic targets. Nat Rev Cancer. 2011;11:541–57.
3. Jain S, Xu R, Prieto VG, Lee P. Molecular classification of soft tissue sarcomas and its clinical applications. Int J Clin Exp Pathol. 2010;3:416–28.

References

1. Fletcher CDM, Bridge JA, Hogendoorn PCW, Mertens F. WHO classification of tumors of soft tissue and bone. 4th ed. Lyon: WHO Press; 2013. p. 14–8.
2. Taylor B, Barretina J, Maki R, Antonescu C, Singer S, Ladanyi M. Advances in sarcoma genomics and new therapeutic targets. Nat Rev Cancer. 2011;11:541–57.
3. Jain S, Xu R, Prieto VG, Lee P. Molecular classification of soft tissue sarcomas and its clinical applications. Int J Clin Exp Pathol. 2010;3:416–28.
4. Arifi S, Belbaraka R, Rahhali R, Ismaili N. Treatment of adult soft tissue sarcomas: an overview. Rare Cancers Ther. 2015;3:69–87.
5. Coindre JM, Terrier P, Guillou L, Le Doussal V, Collin F, Ranchère D, et al. Predictive value of grade for metastasis development in the main histologic types of adult soft tissue sarcomas: a study of 1240 patients from the French Federation of Cancer Centers Sarcoma Group. Cancer. 2001;91:1914–26.
6. Pisters PW, Leung DH, Woodruff J, Shi W, Brennan MF. Analysis of prognostic factors in 1041 patients with localized soft tissue sarcomas of the extremities. J Clin Oncol. 1996;14:1679–89.
7. Lou S, Balluff B, de Graaff MA, Cleven AH, Briaire-de Bruijn IH, Bovée JV, et al. High grade sarcoma diagnosis and prognosis: biomarker discovery by mass spectrometry imaging. Proteomics. 2016;16:1802–13.
8. Vigneron N, van den Eynde BJ. Proteasome subtypes and regulators in the processing of antigenic peptides presented by class I molecules of the major histocompatibility complex. Biomolecules. 2014;4:994–1025.
9. Sanchez-Martin D, Martinez-Torrecuadrada J, Teesalu T, Sugahara KN, Alvarez-Cienfuegos A, Ximenez-Embun P, et al. Proteasome activator complex PA28 identified as an accessible target in prostate cancer by in vivo selection of human antibodies. Proc Natl Acad Sci USA. 2013;110:13791–6.
10. Dekker TJ, Balluff BD, Jones EA, Schone CD, Schmitt M, Aubele M, et al. Multicenter matrix-assisted laser desorption/ionization mass spectrometry imaging (MALDI MSI) identifies proteomic differences in breast-cancer-associated stroma. J Proteome Res. 2014;13:4730–8.
11. Lemaire R, Menguellet SA, Stauber J, Marchaudon V, Lucot JP, Collinet P, et al. Specific MALDI imaging and profiling for biomarker hunting and validation: fragment of the 11S proteasome activator complex, Reg alpha fragment, is a new potential ovary cancer biomarker. J Proteome Res. 2007;6:4127–34.
12. Longuespee R, Boyon C, Castellier C, Jacquet A, Desmons A, Kerdraon O, et al. The C-terminal fragment of the immunoproteasome PA28S (Reg alpha) as an early diagnosis and tumor-relapse biomarker: evidence from mass spectrometry profiling. Histochem Cell Biol. 2012;138:141–54.
13. de Graaff MA, Cleton-Jansen AM, Szuhai K, Bovée JV. Mediator complex subunit 12 exon 2 mutation analysis in different subtypes of smooth muscle tumors confirms genetic heterogeneity. Hum Pathol. 2013;44:1597–604.
14. de Graaff MA, de Rooij MA, van den Akker BE, Gelderblom H, Chibon F, Coindre JM, et al. Inhibition of Bcl-2 family members sensitises soft tissue leiomyosarcomas to chemotherapy. Br J Cancer. 2016;24:1219–26.
15. Baranski Z, Booij TH, Cleton-Jansen AM, Price LS, van de Water B, Bovée JV, et al. Aven-mediated checkpoint kinase control regulates proliferation and resistance to chemotherapy in conventional osteosarcoma. J Pathol. 2015;236:348–59.
16. Hoekstra AS, de Graaff MA, Briaire-de Bruijn IH, Ras C, Seifar RM, van Minderhout I, et al. Inactivation of SDH and FH cause loss of 5hmC and increased H3K9me3 in paraganglioma/pheochromocytoma and smooth muscle tumors. Oncotarget. 2015;6:38777–88.
17. Wójcik C, DeMartino GN. Intracellular localization of proteasomes. Int J Biochem Cell Biol. 2003;35:579–89.
18. Groettrup M, Soza A, Eggers M, Kuehn L, Dick TP, Schild H, et al. A role for the proteasome regulator PA28alpha In antigen presentation. Nature. 1996;381:166–8.
19. von Mikecz A. The nuclear ubiquitin-proteasome system. J Cell Sci. 2006;119:1977–84.
20. Muratani M, Tansey WP. How the ubiquitin-proteasome system controls transcription. Nat Rev Mol Cell Biol. 2003;4:192–201.
21. Hetzel DJ, Wilson TO, Keeney GL, Roche PC, Cha SS, Podratz KC. HER-2/neu expression: a major prognostic factor in endometrial cancer. Gynecol Oncol. 1992;47:179–85.
22. Ohtaki Y, Shimizu K, Kakegawa S, Nagashima T, Nakano T, Atsumi J, et al. Postrecurrence survival of surgically resected pulmonary adenocarcinoma patients according to EGFR and KRAS mutation status. Mol Clin Oncol. 2014;2:187–96.
23. Jungmann J, Heeren R. Emerging technologies in mass spectrometry imaging. J Proteom. 2012;75:5077–92.
24. McDonnell LA, Heeren RM. Imaging mass spectrometry. Mass Spectrom Rev. 2007;26:606–43.
25. McDonnell LA, Corthals GL, Willems SM, van Remoortere A, van Zeijl RJ, Deelder AM. Peptide and protein imaging mass spectrometry in cancer research. J Proteom. 2010;73:1921–44.
26. Sijts A, Sun Y, Janek K, Kral S, Paschen A, Schadendorf D, et al. The role of the proteasome activator PA28 in MHC class I antigen processing. Mol Immunol. 2002;39:165–9.
27. Hochstrasser M. Ubiquitin-dependent protein degradation. Annu Rev Genet. 1996;30:405–39.
28. Hanahan D, Weinberg RA. Hallmarks of cancer: the next generation. Cell. 2011;144:646–74.
29. Zhu Q, Wani G, Yao J, Patnaik S, Wang QE, El-Mahdy MA, et al. The ubiquitin–proteasome system regulates p53-mediated transcription at p21waf1 promoter. Oncogene. 2007;26:4199–208.
30. Tsvetkov P, Reuven N, Shaul Y. Ubiquitin-independent p53 proteasomal degradation. Cell Death Differ. 2010;17:103–8.
31. Almond JB, Cohen GM. The proteasome: a novel target for cancer chemotherapy. Leukemia. 2002;16:433–43.
32. Montagut C, Rovira A, Albanell J. The proteasome: a novel target for anticancer therapy. Clin Transl Oncol. 2006;8:313–7.
33. Voorhees PM, Orlowski RZ. The proteasome and proteasome inhibitors in cancer therapy. Annu Rev Pharmacol Toxicol. 2006;46:189–213.
34. Orlowski R, Dees EC. The role of the ubiquitination-proteasome pathway in breast cancer: applying drugs that affect the ubiquitin-proteasome pathway to the therapy of breast cancer. Breast Cancer Res. 2003;5:1–7.
35. El Ayed M, Bonnel D, Longuespée R, Castelier C, Franck J, Vergara D, et al. MALDI imaging mass spectrometry in ovarian cancer for tracking, identifying, and validating biomarkers. Med Sci Monit. 2010;16(8):BR233–45.
36. Zhang J, Wang K, Zhang J, Liu SS, Dai L, Zhang JY. Using proteomic approach to identify tumor-associated proteins as biomarkers in human esophageal squamous cell carcinoma. J Proteome Res. 2011;10:2863–72.
37. von Mikecz A, Chen M, Rockel T, Scharf A. The nuclear ubiquitin-proteasome system: visualization of proteasomes, protein aggregates, and proteolysis in the cell nucleus. Methods Mol Biol. 2008;463:191–202.
38. Lim J, Poulin NM, Nielsen TO. New strategies in sarcoma: linking genomic and immunotherapy approaches to molecular subtype. Clin Cancer Res. 2015;21:4753–9.

14

High-grade focal areas in low-grade central osteosarcoma: high-grade or still low-grade osteosarcoma?

Alberto Righi[1*], Anna Paioli[2], Angelo Paolo Dei Tos[1,4], Marco Gambarotti[1], Emanuela Palmerini[2], Manuela Cesari[2], Emanuela Marchesi[2], Davide Maria Donati[3], Piero Picci[1] and Stefano Ferrari[2]

Abstract

Background: High-grade foci (grade 3 according to Broder's grading system) are sometimes detected in low-grade (grade 1 and 2) central osteosarcoma. The aim of this study was to retrospectively evaluate the clinical outcome in patients upgraded to high grade (grade 3) after a first diagnosis of low-grade osteosarcoma, following the detection of high-grade areas (grade 3) in the resected specimen.

Methods: Of the 132 patients with a diagnosis of low-grade central osteosarcoma at surgical biopsy at our Institute, 33 patients were considered eligible for the study.

Results: Median age was 37 (range 13–58 years). Location was in an extremity in 29 patients (88 %). Post-operative chemotherapy was given in 22 (67 %) patients. Follow-up data were available for all patients, with a median observation time of 115 months (range 4–322 months). After histological revision, areas of high-grade (grade 3) osteosarcoma accounting for less than 50 % of the tumor were found in 20 (61 %) patients, whereas the majority of the tumor was composed of a high-grade (grade 3) component in 13 (39 %) patients. In the 20 cases of low-grade osteosarcoma with high-grade foci (grade 3) in less than 50 % of the tumor, 9 patients did not receive adjuvant chemotherapy; only one of them died, of unrelated causes. In the adjuvant chemotherapy group (11 out of 20 patients), one patient developed multiple lung metastases and died of disease 39 months after the first diagnosis. In the other 13 cases of low-grade osteosarcoma with high-grade foci (grade 3) in more than 50 % of the tumor, 12 patients received adjuvant chemotherapy: 2 had recurrence, 4 developed multiple lung metastases and 3 died of disease. The only patient who did not receive chemotherapy is alive without disease 232 months after complete surgical remission.

Conclusion: Our data indicate that patients with a diagnosis of low-grade osteosarcoma where the high-grade (grade 3) component is lower than 50 % of the resected specimen, may not require chemotherapy, achieving high survival rates by means of complete surgical resection only.

Keywords: Low-grade osteosarcoma, Central, High-grade, Chemotherapy, Prognosis

Background

The grading of malignant bone tumors has traditionally been based on a combination of histologic diagnosis and Broder's grading system, which assesses cellularity and degree of anaplasia [1]. The 7th edition of the AJCC Cancer Staging Manual recommends a 4 grade system, with grades 1 and 2 being considered "low-grade" and grades 3 and 4 "high-grade". The World Health Organization endorses the use of a two-tier system designating an osteosarcoma as low-grade (grades 1 and 2 in a four-tier system) or high-grade (grades 3 and 4 in a four-tier system) [2].

Histologic grading of osteosarcoma has an important impact on clinical outcome: the risk of distant metastases is low in grade 1–2 (low-grade) and high in cases of

*Correspondence: alberto.righi@ior.it
[1] Department of Pathology, Rizzoli Institute, Via di Barbiano 1/10, 40136 Bologna, Italy
Full list of author information is available at the end of the article

grade 3–4 (high-grade) osteosarcoma, making chemotherapy mandatory in patients with a diagnosis of grade 3–4 (high-grade) osteosarcoma [3, 4].

Low-grade central osteosarcoma is an uncommon variant, accounting for approximately 1–2 % of all osteosarcomas composed of low-grade, mostly fibroblastic, osteogenic proliferation featuring mild cytological atypia [5, 6]. The low-grade central osteosarcoma series published in the literature report an incidence of areas of high-grade osteosarcoma ranging between 10 and 36 % of cases [3–5, 7–12]. Some authors regard the high-grade component of low-grade central osteosarcoma as a separate entity from conventional high-grade osteosarcoma, and consider it a form of morphologic progression (dedifferentiation) of a low-grade osteosarcoma [7–9, 11, 12]. While this distinction is controversial and not uniformly accepted, it appears that low-grade tumors with focal high-grade progression actually behave differently than their conventional high-grade counterparts [7–9, 11]. Unfortunately there are no established criteria (such as the percentage of the overall tumor with a high-grade component) to categorize these tumors as typical high-grade (grade 3–4) osteosarcoma [3–5]. In principle, the presence of any high-grade area in a low-grade lesion makes the tumor high-grade, thereby prompting systemic adjuvant treatment [13–15]. Nevertheless, there is little data in support of such therapeutic approach, and it is not well established whether low-grade (grade 1–2) central osteosarcoma with areas of high-grade (grade 3) osteosarcoma actually differs from high-grade (grade 3–4) osteosarcoma, with regard to rates of local recurrence, metastasis, and survival.

The aim of this study was to retrospectively evaluate the clinical outcome in patients who, after a first diagnosis of low-grade central osteosarcoma based on surgical biopsy, were upgraded to high-grade (grade 3) osteosarcoma following evaluation of the surgical specimen at resection.

Methods

The medical records were retrieved of a consecutive series of patients diagnosed and treated for low-grade osteosarcoma (grade 1–2 according to Broder's grading system) at the Rizzoli Institute, Bologna, Italy, between January 1981 and June 2014 (Fig. 1a, b). The resected specimens and radiological imaging were reviewed. No patients received preoperative chemotherapy. A statement on consent to use the data for scientific purposes was obtained from all patients. Inclusion criteria were: (a) availability of the histologic slides of both the biopsy and surgical specimens, in which systematic mapping of the entire tumor featured a low-grade osteosarcoma

according to the protocol for the examination of bone tumor specimens [16]. Three pathologists (A.R., M.G., A.D.T.) independently reviewed the slides stained with hematoxylin and eosin, evaluating diagnosis, subtype, and grade. On the basis of the predominant morphology of the neoplastic cells and quality of the intercellular matrix, osteosarcomas were classified in surgical specimens by the following subtypes: osteoblastic, chondroblastic and fibroblastic. Tumours were graded according to the 4-tiered Broder's grading system by assessing cellularity and degree of atypia [1]. Where high-grade (grade 3) areas were detected (defined as the presence of increased cellularity, absence of the typical architectural pattern of growth of low-grade osteosarcoma and higher nuclear atypia), tumor maps were examined and the percentage of high-grade (grade 3) areas scored (Fig. 2a–c).

After definitive surgical treatment, the use of postoperative chemotherapy was mainly based on clinical experience, as no specific guidelines were available. For patients younger than 40 years, the chemotherapy regimen was based on the protocol adopted at the time for non metastatic osteosarcoma. The remaining patients received a chemotherapy regimen without methotrexate and usually including doxorubicin, cisplatin and ifosfamide. All patients, regardless of the use of adjuvant chemotherapy, were followed up every 2–3 months in the first 2–3 years and then every 4–6 months. Survival analysis was performed according to Kaplan–Meier. All analyses were performed using Stata/SE statistical software (version 10.0; StataCorp LT, College Station, TX, USA).

Results

Of the 132 patients with a diagnosis of low-grade (grade 1 and 2) osteosarcoma at surgical biopsy, 33 patients were considered eligible for the study. The clinical and pathological features are summarized in Table 1. The median age was 37 years (range 13–58 years) with a slight prevalence of females. Most of the tumours were located in the extremities. The majority of the patients (26 cases, 79 %) had a diagnosis of fibroblastic osteosarcoma (of these, 4 cases had the fibrous dysplasia-like variant), followed by osteoblastic osteosarcoma (5 cases, 15 %) and chondroblastic osteosarcoma (2 cases, 6 %). All patients were surgically treated with wide surgical margins. Twenty-two (67 %) patients received adjuvant chemotherapy.

Follow-up data were available for all patients with a median observation time of 115 months (range 4–322 months). Twenty (61 %) patients showed areas of high-grade (grade 3) osteosarcoma accounting for less than 50 % of the tumor, whereas 13 (39 %) patients showed a high-grade (grade 3) component in the majority of the tumor (Table 1).

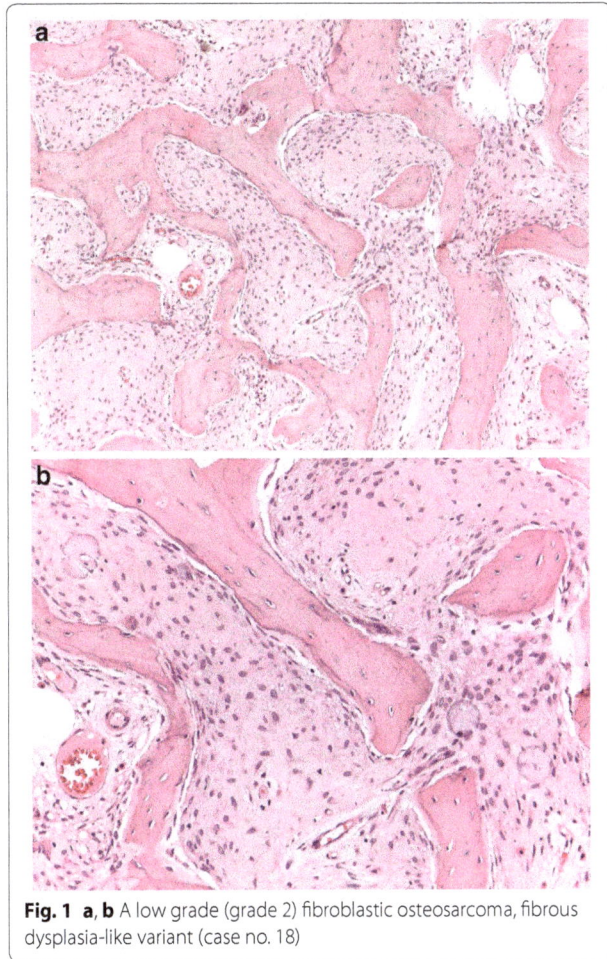

Fig. 1 a, b A low grade (grade 2) fibroblastic osteosarcoma, fibrous dysplasia-like variant (case no. 18)

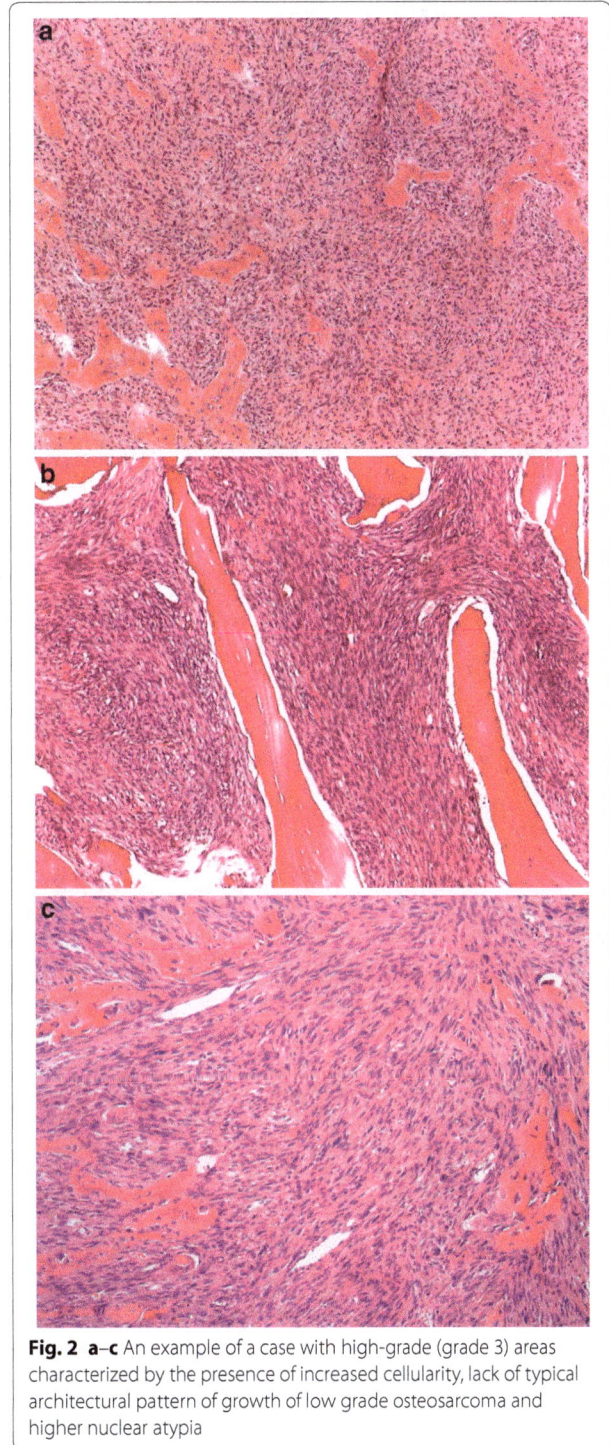

Fig. 2 a–c An example of a case with high-grade (grade 3) areas characterized by the presence of increased cellularity, lack of typical architectural pattern of growth of low grade osteosarcoma and higher nuclear atypia

Low-grade osteosarcoma with high-grade foci (grade 3 in less than 50 % of the tumor: 20 patients)

None of the patients belonging to this group showed metastatic lesions at the staging workup. Adjuvant chemotherapy was not given to 9 (45 %) patients. One patient (case 8) showed a local recurrence in the soft tissue 53 months after surgical resection. Recurrence was surgically removed and morphologically it was associated with progression to a higher grade (grade 4, fibroblastic and osteoblastic osteosarcoma). Therefore the patient received adjuvant chemotherapy and at the last follow-up (232 months after the surgical bone resection) is alive without disease. Another patient (case 18) developed a single bone metastasis in the thoracic vertebra, which was surgically removed. Morphologically the vertebral lesion showed the same features as the primitive osteosarcoma (grade 2 fibroblastic osteosarcoma, fibrous dysplasia-like variant). The patient started adjuvant chemotherapy and at the last follow-up (57 months after the surgical bone resection) is alive without disease. Another patient of this group (case 12) died of unrelated causes. The remaining patients are disease-free at last follow-up. Adjuvant chemotherapy was given to 11 (55 %) patients. One patient (case 2) developed multiple lung metastases 13 months after surgery. Histologically, the lung metastases were diagnosed as grade 4 osteoblastic

Table 1 The clinical and pathological features of 33 cases of low-grade central osteosarcoma with areas of high-grade (grade 3)

Case	Age/sex	Site	% high-grade (grade 3) areas	Histotype	Adjuvant chemotherapy	Local recurrence (months after surgery)	Metastases (months after surgery)	Follow-up (months after surgery)
1	56/F	Distal femur	2	Osteoblastic	No			NED (55)
2	39/M	Proximal humerus	4	Fibroblastic (fibrous dysplasia-like)	Yes		Lung (13)	DOD (39)
3	19/M	Distal femur	4	Osteoblastic	No			NED (157)
4	34/F	Proximal humerus	4	Fibroblastic	No			NED (120)
5	35/F	Distal femur	4	Fibroblastic	Yes			NED (225)
6	44/M	Proximal humerus	4	Fibroblastic	Yes			NED (56)
7	23/M	Distal femur	4	Fibroblastic	Yes			NED (69)
8	25/F	Distal femur	4	Fibroblastic	No	Yes (53)		NED (284)
9	13/F	Clavicle	9	Fibroblastic (fibrous dysplasia-like)	Yes			NED (103)
10	22/F	Proximal femur	9	Fibroblastic	Yes			NED (132)
11	32/F	Proximal humerus	9	Fibroblastic	No			NED (109)
12	58/F	Proximal femur	11	Fibroblastic	No			DOC (136)
13	27/M	Proximal tibia	16	Fibroblastic	No			NED (231)
14	45/M	Distal tibia	16	Fibroblastic	Yes			NED (45)
15	24/F	Distal femur	16	Osteoblastic	Yes			NED (45)
16	41/M	Proximal tibia	16	Osteoblastic	No			NED (89)
17	55/F	Pelvis	31	Osteoblastic	Yes			NED (33)
18	28/M	Proximal humerus	31	Fibroblastic (fibrous dysplasia-like)	No		Bone thoracic vertebra (51)	NED (57)
19	50/M	Distal femur	35	Fibroblastic	No			NED (262)
20	21/M	Distal femur	40	Fibroblastic	Yes			NED (151)
21	42/M	Proximal femur	51	Fibroblastic	Yes	Yes (21)	Lung (46; 65)	DOD (108)
22	38/F	proximal humerus	51	Fibroblastic (fibrous dysplasia-like)	Yes			NED (134)
23	59/M	Proximal humerus	51	Fibroblastic	Yes		Lung (37; 85)	NED (137)
24	35/F	Distal ulna	51	Fibroblastic	Yes			NED (4)
25	25/M	Lumbar vertebra	51	Fibroblastic	Yes			NED (10)
26	24/M	Proximal humerus	51	Osteoblastic	Yes			NED (65)
27	40/M	Proximal tibia	81	Fibroblastic	Yes		Lung (10)	DOD (32)
28	53/F	Proximal tibia	81	Fibroblastic	Yes	Yes (2)		DOD (5)
29	46/F	Distal femur	81	Fibroblastic	Yes		Lung (14;38;50)	NED (132)
30	49/F	Distal femur	81	Chondroblastic	Yes			NED (164)
31	42/F	Pelvis	81	Fibroblastic	Yes			NED (27)
32	20/F	Proximal femur	81	Chondroblastic	No			NED (250)
33	48/F	Distal femur	81	Fibroblastic	Yes			NED (322)

osteosarcoma. After surgical resection of the lung metastases the patient underwent second line chemotherapy and died of disease 39 months after the first diagnosis.

Overall 18 (90 %) of the 20 patients with an area of high-grade (grade 3) osteosarcoma accounting for less than 50 % of the tumor were alive without disease, none of the patients who did not receive adjuvant chemotherapy died of disease. The median observation time was 109 months (from 29 to 284 months). The probability of evidence-free survival and overall survival at 5 years was 88 % (95 % CI 72–100 %) and 95 % (95 % CI 84–100 %), respectively.

High-grade focal areas in low-grade central osteosarcoma: high-grade or still low-grade...

121

Low-grade osteosarcoma with high-grade foci (grade 3) in more than 50 % of the tumor (13 patients)

Twelve patients received adjuvant chemotherapy. Of these, two patients had recurrent disease in the soft tissues (cases 21, 28) after 2 and 21 months of follow-up, respectively, and one of them (case 28) died of disease 5 months after the surgical resection. Four patients developed lung metastases (cases 21, 23, 27, 29) after a mean follow-up of 27 months (range 10–46 months). Three of these 4 patients (cases 21, 23, 29) developed other multiple lung metastases following the first lung metastasectomies. Both the two recurrences and lung metastases were histologically associated with progression to a higher grade (grade 4) osteosarcoma.

Two of 4 patients with lung metastases (cases 21, 27) died of disease after 108 and 32 months, respectively. The patient (case 32) who did not receive chemotherapy is alive without disease 232 months after complete surgical remission.

Overall 10 (77 %) of the 13 patients with areas of high-grade (grade 3) osteosarcoma accounting for more than 50 % of the tumor were alive without disease, 5 (38.5 %) patients experienced recurrent disease, with distant metastases in 4 and local recurrence in only one patient. The median observation time was 120 months (from 4 to 322 months). The probability of evidence-free survival and overall survival at 5 years was 68 % (95 % CI 42–94 %) and 83 % (95 % CI 61–100 %), respectively.

Discussion

The grading of osteosarcoma is based on morphologic observation of a set of parameters that have proved relatively reproducible [1, 2, 4]. Some discrepancies are unavoidable when comparing biopsy material with the corresponding surgical specimen, in which variable amounts of higher grade malignancy can be seen. It is our experience that areas of high-grade (grade 3) osteosarcoma can be found in patients with a bioptic diagnosis of low-grade (grade 1–2) osteosarcoma, even when the biopsy was obtained from the site showing the greatest aggressiveness on imaging studies [6–8, 17, 18].

Interestingly, the group of patients forming the study population exhibit clinical features that differ from those observed in patients with conventional high-grade osteosarcoma. The age of our patients was higher than the age reported for classic osteosarcoma, with most of the patients being adults [1, 2, 4]. Another observed difference was the histologic subtype. It is well known that osteoblastic osteosarcoma is the most frequent subtype [1, 2, 4], whereas most low-grade osteosarcomas with high-grade areas were fibroblastic osteosarcoma.

High-grade dedifferentiation or progression to a higher grade in low-grade central osteosarcoma represents an exceedingly rare event, which can be seen in the primary tumor, but more commonly in recurrences [7–12, 19]. Our series reports a 25 % rate of progression to high-grade (grade 3) osteosarcoma (33/132 cases), which to some extent overlaps with the range of 10–36 % of cases reported in the literature [3–5, 7–12]. Previous reports have documented the association between inadequate surgical resection, local recurrence, and morphologic progression to higher grade, which was associated with a poor prognosis [7, 8, 19]. While surgery alone is deemed adequate for low-grade central osteosarcoma, even in the absence of published guidelines, the addition of chemotherapy is being suggested as an option for those patients featuring areas of histologic progression (also defined by some authors as dedifferentiation) [7–15, 19].

This study shows that the presence of areas of high-grade (grade 3) progression in patients with low-grade osteosarcoma does not by itself imply biological systemic aggressiveness. Furthermore we have shown a correlation between the percentage of high-grade (grade 3) areas and risk of metastatic spread. In our retrospective analysis, those patients with low-grade osteosarcoma with a high-grade (grade 3) component of less than 50 % of the tumor did in fact have a very high probability of survival regardless of the use of adjuvant chemotherapy. By contrast, the clinical behaviour of tumors featuring a high-grade (grade 3) osteosarcoma component greater than 50 % overlaps with that reported for conventional high-grade osteosarcoma [1, 2, 4, 17, 18].

In surgical pathology it is broadly accepted that the grade of any tumor is based on the highest grade observed in the surgical specimen [20]. Our study seems to suggest that this general rule cannot be applied systematically to all osteosarcomas.

The standard treatment of high-grade (grade 3–4) osteosarcoma is surgical removal of the tumor and adjuvant (or neo-adjuvant) chemotherapy [3, 13–15]. A pathology report describing areas of high-grade (grade 3–4) osteosarcoma would currently represent the rationale for the use of chemotherapy [3, 13–15].

Conclusion

Our data indicate that not all patients with a diagnosis of osteosarcoma featuring a high-grade (grade 3) component would benefit from systemic treatment. In particular, in patients with small foci with high-grade (grade 3) progression or in whom the high-grade (grade 3) component is less than 50 % of the resected specimen at tumour map examination, high survival rates can only be achieved by means of complete surgical resection.

Authors' contributions

AR, MG, ADT and PP reviewed the histological slides of all cases. EM, EP, MC, AP participated in the design of the study and performed the statistical analysis. ADT, DD, SF conceived the study, participated in its design and coordination, and helped to draft the manuscript. All authors read and approved the final manuscript.

Author details

[1] Department of Pathology, Rizzoli Institute, Via di Barbiano 1/10, 40136 Bologna, Italy. [2] Department of Oncology, Rizzoli Institute, Bologna, Italy. [3] Department of Orthopaedic Oncology, Rizzoli Institute, Bologna, Italy. [4] Department of Pathology, Treviso Regional Hospital, Treviso, Italy.

Competing interests

The authors declare that they have no competing interests.

References

1. Unni KK. Osteosarcoma of bone. New York: Churchill Livingstone; 1988.
2. Grimer RJ, Hogendoorn PCW, Vanel D. Tumours of bone: introduction. In: Fletcher CDM, Bridge JA, Hogendoorn PCW, Mertens F, editors. World Health organization classification of tumours. Pathology and genetics of tumours of soft tissue and bone. 4th ed. Lyon: IARC Press; 2013. p. 244–7.
3. Bielack S, Carrle D, Casali PG, ESMO Guidelines Working Group. Osteosarcoma: ESMO clinical recommendations for diagnosis, treatment and follow-up. Ann Oncol. 2009;20:137–9.
4. Klein MJ, Siegal GP. Osteosarcoma: anatomic and histologic variants. Am J Clin Pathol. 2006;125(4):555–81.
5. Inwards C, Squire J. Low-grade central osteosarcoma. In: Fletcher CDM, Bridge JA, Hogendoorn PCW, Mertens F, editors. World Health Organization Classification of Tumours. Pathology and genetics of tumours of soft tissue and bone. 4th ed. Lyon: IARC Press; 2013. p. 281.
6. Bertoni F, Bacchini P, Fabbri N, Mercuri M, Picci P, Ruggieri T, Campanacci M. Low grade intraosseous-type osteosarcoma, histologically resembling parosteal osteosarcoma, fibrous dysplasia, and desmoplastic fibroma. Cancer. 1993;71:338–45.
7. Kurt AM, Unni KK, McLeod RA, Pritchard DJ. Low-grade intraosseous osteosarcoma. Cancer. 1990;65(6):1418–28.
8. Schwab JH, Antonescu CR, Athanasian EA, Boland PJ, Healey JH, Morris CD. A comparison of intramedullary and juxtacortical low-grade osteogenic sarcoma. Clin Orthop Relat Res. 2008;466(6):1318–22.
9. Wenger DE, Sundaram M, Unni KK, Janney CG, Merkel K. Microscopic correlation of radiographically disparate appearing well differentiated osteosarcoma. Skeletal Radiol. 2002;31(8):488–92.
10. Ogose A, Hotta T, Emura I, Imaizumi S, Takeda M, Yamamura S. Repeated dedifferentiation of low-grade intraosseous osteosarcoma. Hum Pathol. 2000;31:615–8.
11. Yoshida A, Ushiku T, Motoi T, Beppu Y, Fukayama M, Tsuda H, Shibata T. MDM2 and CDK4 immunohistochemical coexpression in high-grade osteosarcoma: correlation with a dedifferentiated subtype. Am J Surg Pathol. 2012;36:423–31.
12. Antonescu CR, Huvos AG. Low-grade osteogenic sarcoma arising in medullary and surface osseous locations. Am J Clin Pathol. 2000;114:S90–103.
13. Luetke A, Meyers PA, Lewis I, Juergens H. Osteosarcoma treatment—where do we stand? A state of the art review. Cancer Treat Rev. 2014;40:523–32.
14. Manoso MW, Healey JH, Boland PJ, Athanasian EA, Maki RG, Huvos AG, Morris CD. De novo osteogenic sarcoma in patients older than forty: benefit of multimodality therapy. Clin Orthop Relat Res. 2005;438:110–5.
15. Meyers PA, Heller G, Healey J, Huvos A, Lane J, Marcove R, Applewhite A, Vlamis V, Rosen G. Chemotherapy for nonmetastatic osteogenic sarcoma: the Memorial Sloan-Kettering experience. J Clin Oncol. 1992;10:5–15.
16. Rubin BP, Antonescu CR, Gannon FH, Hunt JL, Inwards CY, Klein MJ, Kneisl JS, Montag AG, Peabody TD, Reith JD, Rosenberg AE, Krausz T, Members

of the Cancer Committee, College of American Pathologists. Protocol for the examination of specimens from patients with tumors of bone. Arch Pathol Lab Med. 2010;134:e1–7.
17. Kenan S, Ginat DT, Steiner GC. Dedifferentiated high-grade osteosarcoma originating from low-grade central osteosarcoma of the fibula. Skeletal Radiol. 2007;36(4):347–51.
18. Iemoto Y, Ushigome S, Fukunaga M, Nikaido T, Asanuma K. Case report 679. Central low-grade osteosarcoma with foci of dedifferentiation. Skeletal Radiol. 1991;20(5):379–82.
19. Choong PF, Pritchard DJ, Rock MG, Sim FH, McLeod RA, Unni KK. Low grade central osteogenic sarcoma. A long-term follow-up of 20 patients. Clin Orthop Relat Res. 1996;322:198–206.
20. Rosai J, Ackerman LV. Surgical pathology. 10th ed. USA: Mosby Elsevier; 2011.

15

Central venous access related adverse events after trabectedin infusions in soft tissue sarcoma patients; experience and management in a nationwide multi-center study

Michiel C. Verboom[1*], Jan Ouwerkerk[1], Neeltje Steeghs[2], Jacob Lutjeboer[3], J. Martijn Kerst[2],
Winette T. A. van der Graaf[4,5], Anna K. L. Reyners[6], Stefan Sleijfer[7] and Hans Gelderblom[1]

Abstract

Background: Trabectedin has shown efficacy against soft tissue sarcomas (STS) and has manageable toxicity. Trabectedin is administered through central venous access devices (VAD), such as subcutaneous ports with tunneled catheters, Hickman catheters and PICC lines. Venous access related adverse events are common, but have not yet been reported in detail.

Methods: A retrospective analysis of patient files of STS patients receiving trabectedin monotherapy between 1999 and 2014 was performed in all five STS referral centers in the Netherlands. This survey focused on adverse events related to the VAD and the actions taken in response to these events.

Results: In the 127 patients included in this analysis, 102 venous access ports (VAP), 15 Hickman catheters and 10 PICC lines were used as primary means of central venous access. The most frequently reported adverse events at the VAD site were erythema (30.7%), pain (28.3%), inflammation (11.8%) and thrombosis (11.0%). Actions taken towards these adverse events include oral antibiotics (17.3%), VAD replacement (15.0%) or a wait-and-see policy (13.4%). In total, 45 patients (35.4%) with a subcutaneous port developed a varying degree of inflammation along the trajectory of the tunneled catheter. In all but three patients, this was a sterile inflammation, which was considered a unique phenomenon for trabectedin. Microscopic leakage of trabectedin along the venous access device and catheter was considered the most plausible cause for this adverse event. Placing the catheter deeper under the skin resolved the issue almost completely.

Conclusion: Trabectedin infusion commonly leads to central venous access related adverse events. Sterile inflammation along the catheter trajectory is one of the most common adverse events and can be prevented by placing the catheter deeper under the skin.

Keywords: Trabectedin, Central venous catheters, Adverse events, Soft tissue sarcoma

Background

Cytostatic drugs infused directly into peripheral veins can have very damaging effects on these blood vessels. To ensure safe and durable administration of such agents,

several methods have been developed in the past, like the arteriovenous shunt, which is no longer used for the infusion of chemotherapy [1]. In 1982, a central venous access device was introduced, that used a subcutaneous reservoir and a tunneled catheter to provide access to the superior vena cava [2]. This type of central venous catheters (CVC) allows for easy access to a patient's circulation, incur minimal restriction in normal activities and usually at a low risk of complications [3]. Next to VAPs,

*Correspondence: m.c.verboom@lumc.nl
[1] Department of Medical Oncology, Leiden University Medical Center, Postbus 9600, 2300 RC Leiden, The Netherlands
Full list of author information is available at the end of the article

other methods have also been introduced, such as the Hickman catheter and peripherally inserted CVC (PICC) lines [4, 5]. However, all devices constitute some risk of venous access related adverse events (VARAE).

As anticancer drug, trabectedin stands out as a drug with a unique mechanism of action, having effect both at the level of tumor DNA and on the tumor microenvironment [6]. It is one of the few drugs active in STS [7]. The drug has a manageable toxicity profile, but life-threatening toxicity due to uncommon adverse events has been reported [8]. Thus far several papers have mentioned VARAE, including reports on trabectedin extravasation and associated thrombi on the line tip, but no papers focusing on VARAE in detail have been published [9–12]. This article aims to systematically study VARAE observed in 127 consecutive sarcoma patients treated with trabectedin and to evaluate the measures taken to handle these problems.

Methods

A retrospective analysis of VARAE in all patients treated with trabectedin was performed in all five participating Dutch sarcoma referral centers: the Leiden University Medical Center (LUMC), the Netherlands Cancer Institute Antoni van Leeuwenhoek (NKI-AvL), the Erasmus MC Cancer Institute (EMC), the Radboud University Medical Center (RUMC) and the University Medical Center Groningen (UMCG). Patients were eligible when treated with trabectedin monotherapy for advanced STS. Data on patient characteristics were reported as well as the type of venous access device, its placement, adverse events related to its usage and the interventions to counter these events. Adverse events related to the VAD placement were ignored, as these have no direct relation with trabectedin infusions. Hence, all events described occurred after at least one cycle of trabectedin had been given.

To test for a difference in the number of cycles per VAD, a Kruskal–Wallis non-parametric test was used. To assess differences between VARAE per VAD cross tables and the Chi square were computed. All statistical analyses were performed using SPSS version 20.

Results

Patients

In total, 127 advanced STS patients were treated with single agent trabectedin between November 1999 and November 2014. Almost all patients were treated as part of an observational phase IV study or of the TRUSTS trial [13, 14]. Due to the inclusion criteria of these studies, trabectedin was given either as first line (15.0%), second line (59.1%), third line (16.5%), fourth line (7.1%) or as a further line of treatment (2.4%). The trabectedin treatment

regimen was given at a dosage of 1.5 mg/m^2 as 24 h infusion every three weeks in 89.8% of patients, the remaining patients received a lower dose (1.1–1.3 mg/m^2) and/or a 3 h infusion. The most prevalent types of STS histology were leiomyosarcoma (40.9%), liposarcoma (26.0%) and synovial sarcoma (12.6%), as shown in Table 1.

VADs inserted

The VAP was used in 102 (80.3%) patients, of which 87 were identified as a Smith Medical Port-a-Cath®. Hickman catheters and PICC lines were inserted in 15 (11.8%) and 10 (7.9%) of patients, respectively. A total of 540 cycles of trabectedin were given with a median number of 4 cycles for the entire patient group. The number of cycles given did not differ significantly per VAD (data not shown).

Each hospital had a clear preference for a particular type of VAD that was initially inserted; in the LUMC VAPs (100% of patients), in the NKI-AvL VAPs (95%), in the EMC the Hickman catheter (100%), in the RUMC a PICC line (66.7%) and in the UMCG VAPs (100%). VADs were inserted by a dedicated team of health care workers

Table 1 Patient characteristics

	N (%)
Sex	
Female	66 (52.0)
Male	61 (48.0)
Age	
Median (years)	54.3
Range (years)	25.6–79.5
WHO performance score	
0	52 (40.9)
1	66 (52.0)
2	9 (7.1)
Histology	
Leiomyosarcoma	52 (40.9)
Liposarcoma	33 (26.0)
Synovial sarcoma	16 (12.6)
Various others	26 (20.5)
Best response	
Partial response	8 (6.3)
Stable disease	64 (50.4)
Progressive disease	45 (35.4)
Not evaluable	10 (7.9)
Hospital	
LUMC	48 (37.8)
NKI-AvL	40 (31.5)
EMC	15 (11.8)
RUMC	12 (9.4)
UMCG	12 (9.4)

to ensure low incidence of complications related to the VAD placement.

Of all patients, only three patients with a Hickman catheter requested their VAD to be replaced by another type of VAD. Two of these patients preferred a VAP, but did not have a VARAE at the time of replacement. In another patient, the catheter was chronically obstructed due to a thrombus at the catheter tip, which required catheter flushing by a radiologist, despite adequate antithrombotic treatment.

Sterile inflammation along the catheter trajectory

Out of the 127 patients, 45 patients (35.4%) with a VAP developed a varying degree of inflammation along the catheter trajectory, which could include erythema, pain or swelling, as shown in Fig. 1. In between cycles these symptoms waned, but a few days after the following infusion a flare up was often noted. Fever was neither reported by patients, nor observed during physical examination at admission or at the outpatient clinic. The skin surrounding the port's reservoir was not affected and the VAD could be used for infusions normally. Bacterial cultures could not identify an etiological micro-organism for these symptoms in all, but three patients.

In the first instances these symptoms were deemed a result of cellulitis and oral antibiotics were prescribed (flucloxacillin 500 mg four times daily). However, the symptoms abated only mildly and the erythema remained unchanged for weeks and existed even after the discontinuation of trabectedin therapy. Extra intravenous infusion of normal saline fluids during trabectedin infusion appeared to ease the symptoms, especially the pain.

In a single patient with port VAD, the inflammation became rampant and in the course of several weeks it led to severe skin erosion along the catheter trajectory, as shown in Fig. 2. At progression of the inflammatory

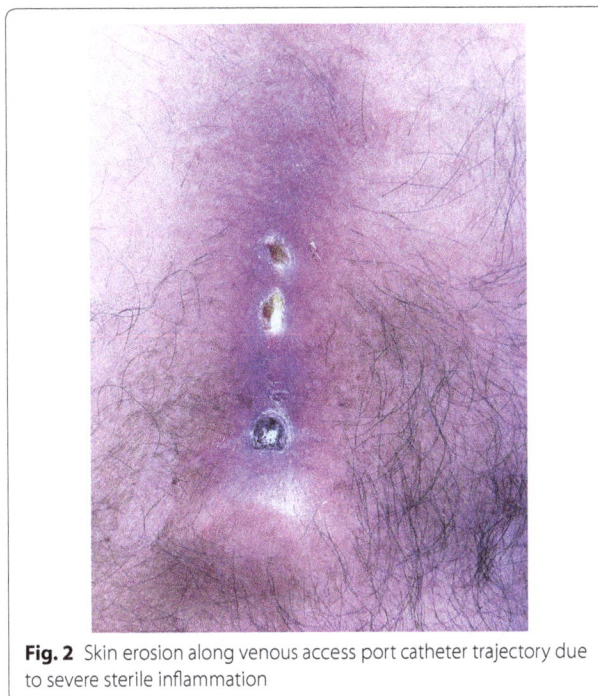

Fig. 2 Skin erosion along venous access port catheter trajectory due to severe sterile inflammation

aspect of the skin, the patient was treated with oral antibiotics. Due to the skin destruction, a local secondary cellulitis developed. Despite this, the patient did not feel ill. As the patient did not show symptoms of acute infection, it was decided to continue trabectedin treatment. After trabectedin was stopped due to progressive disease, the VAP remained in place and was used for dacarbazine cycles without VARAE.

Remarkably, this complication appeared only in patients from one hospital and only after receiving several trabectedin cycles, and did not occur with any other type of cytostatic agent. As the same brand and type of VAD was used in another hospital without this complication, the dedicated teams compared their respective methods of VAD insertion. The only apparent difference found, was in the depth of the subcutaneous insertion for tunneling the catheter. Catheter insertion can be performed more or less deeper under the skin and the latter method was associated with the sterile inflammation along the catheter trajectory. Upon changing the local protocol to deepen the tunneling of the catheter, no further events of sterile inflammation of the catheter trajectory were observed.

Adverse events related to VAD

All types of VADs used had VARAE, as shown in Table 2. For the whole patient cohort, the most common adverse events were erythema (30.7%) and pain (28.3%) at the VAD site or along the catheter trajectory. In 11.8% of

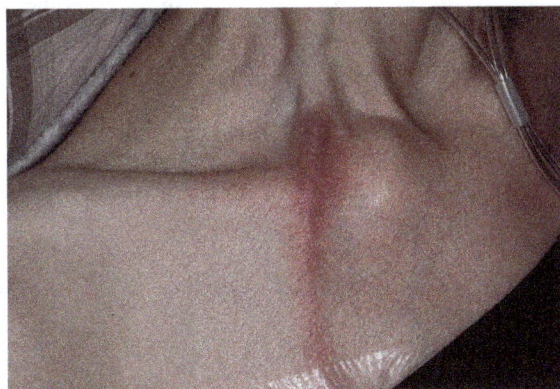

Fig. 1 Typical sterile inflammation along the venous access port catheter trajectory

Table 2 Adverse events at VAD site/trajectory per venous access device

N (%)	Inflammation	Erythema	Pain	Infection	Thrombosis	Impairment	Erosion	Extravasation	All AE[a]
Venous access port (102)	35 (34.3)	30 (29.4)	28 (27.5)	9 (8.8)	11 (10.8)	5 (4.9)	1 (1.0)	0 (0.0)	44 (43.1)
Hickman line (15)	5 (33.3)	4 (26.7)	4 (26.7)	3 (20.0)	1 (6.7)	3 (20.0)	0 (0.0)	1 (6.7)	7 (46.7)
PICC line (10)	5 (50.0)	5 (50.0)	4 (40.0)	3 (30.0)	2 (20.0)	1 (10.0)	0 (0.0)	0 (0.0)	5 (50.0)
Total	45 (35.4)	39 (30.7)	36 (28.3)	15 (11.8)	14 (11.0)	9 (7.1)	1 (0.8)	1 (0.8)	56 (44.1)

[a] Summary of all types of adverse events per venous access device

patients these symptoms were diagnosed as an inflammation and/or infection, where inflammation consisted of swelling, painfulness and erythema. Blood cultures did not grow pathogenic micro-organisms. In some of these patients the 'infection' diagnosis could retrospectively be reclassified as the previously described sterile inflammation with near certainty. Several patients (11.0%) had a thrombus at the catheter tip at one or several instances. Often, these thrombi could be flushed with urokinase solution before proceeding to administer the trabectedin infusion without further complications. However, catheter thrombosis could also lead to VAD impairment. Remarkably, all of these patients were treated in the same hospital, which was also the hospital were VAPs were inserted with tunneled catheters deep in the epidermis. Thrombosis at the catheter tip and the sterile inflammation were not significantly associated (data not shown). The skin erosion and extravasation of trabectedin were seldom seen. Dislocation or pinch-off was not seen in any patient. Due to the small number of patients with a Hickman catheter or PICC line, no statistical differences in the incidence of VARAE could be detected. Only a single patient (0.8%), who had a Hickman catheter, had an extravasation.

Interventions for VARAE

Oral antibiotics were given in 17.3% of patients, most often flucloxacillin, as shown in Table 3. Some patients received a prescription for oral antibiotics to be taken in case VAD related symptoms worsened. Although this was not sufficient to stop the erythema along the catheter trajectory, it may have helped against a secondary infection. In 5 patients (3.9%) VAD an infection necessitated IV antibiotics (2 patients with a VAP, 3 patients with

a PICC line). Due to the severity of symptoms or VAD impairment VAD replacement was needed in 15.0% of patients. Patients with a VAP usually had the same type of VAP inserted at the contralateral side, patients with a Hickman catheter or PICC line most often received a VAP. As the problem of the sterile inflammation and other VARAE were better understood and recognized, in due course a wait-and-see policy was applied in a considerable number of patients (13.4%). Despite frequent complaints of pain at the VAD site, analgesics were only needed in a minority of these patients.

Discussion

Trabectedin is one of the proven active drugs in the treatment of soft tissue sarcoma and is given through a central venous catheter to avoid peripheral vein damage. As treatment continues until progressive disease or unacceptable toxicity, is it important to evaluate catheter related complications. The sterile inflammation along the catheter trajectory found in this study was an unexpected VARAE and was initially poorly understood. Erythema or pain is usually taken as a sign of skin infection and treated as such. However, there were no other signs of infection such as positive cultures, and the severity of the skin complications appeared to be related to the administration of trabectedin. In addition, the erythema was most prominent along the catheter trajectory, which made a porous catheter likely to be the cause. A direct effect of trabectedin on the tissue surrounding the catheter could cause the inflammation, but this catheter porosity implies that only a small quantity of trabectedin permeates. This small quantity leads to fewer symptoms compared to a full trabectedin extravasation, as has been reported in literature [11].

Table 3 Interventions for VAD related adverse events per venous access device

N (%)	Antibiotics (oral)	VAD replaced	Wait-and-see	Analgesics	Urokinase (IV)	Antibiotics (IV)
Venous access port (102)	19 (18.6)	10 (9.8)	13 (12.7)	8 (7.8)	8 (7.8)	2 (2.0)
Hickman line (15)	1 (6.7)	6 (40.0)	3 (20.0)	2 (13.3)	1 (6.7)	0 (0.0)
PICC line (10)	2 (20.0)	3 (30.0)	1 (10.0)	0 (0.0)	0 (0.0)	3 (30.0)
Total	22 (17.3)	19 (15.0)	17 (13.4)	10 (7.9%)	9 (7.1)	5 (3.9)

To investigate the hypothesis of catheter porosity, the manufacturer of trabectedin, PharmaMar, offered to test a used catheter. A VAP was available that was previously used in a patient who had received several cycles of trabectedin with symptoms of sterile inflammation alongside the catheter trajectory and from whom the VAP was removed because of disease progression. The objective of the test was to determine if trabectedin permeates from the internal surface to the outside of the catheter during a 24 h infusion. High-performance liquid chromatography with diode array detection (HPLC–DAD) and multi-syringe flow injection system (MS-FIA) methods were used for detection of trabectedin in the dextrose 5% solution the VAP was submerged in. Neither test could detect trabectedin in samples taken from the dextrose 5% solution, which ruled out gross catheter porosity (PharmaMar communication). In our view, however, this could not rule out sub lower-limit of quantification leakage.

Non-infectious inflammation of the VAD site of various severity was also reported by Hoicyk et al. in addition of thrombi at the catheter tip. It was hypothesized that increased resistance due to small thrombi may be associated with drug backspill [12]. In the current study, neither an association of sterile inflammation and thrombosis was found, nor was reduced flow through the catheter observed. Catheter thrombosis occurred in several patients, which was treated by flushing the catheter with an urokinase solution. Thrombosis prophylaxis was not initiated at the start of trabectedin therapy in any of the participating centres.

In the patient cohort only a small number of patients had PICC lines. A larger retrospective series of STS and ovarian cancer patients was reported by Martella and colleagues. Out of 45 patients with a PICC line receiving trabectedin a device dislocation was reported in two patients and an infection in another two. PICC line malfunction or VARAE requiring VAD removal did not occur [10]. This implies that PICC lines may have lower incidence of associated toxicity than our current cohort suggests. However, the number of VARAE in patients using a PORT was also lower. Due to the retrospective nature of this patient series, relative underreporting compared to our study may have occurred, as almost all patient in this cohort where treated as part of a clinical trial.

The usage of a disposable elastomeric pump to administer a 24-h trabectedin infusion has been described [9]. Patients could choose for a regular VAP or a Baxter LV10 Pump which allowed patients to spend the night at home. Out of 28 patients 21 chose the ambulatory pump. This method was considered feasible and safe. However, most patients will receive trabectedin trough conventional VAPs reported on in this paper, and no data is available comparing these different techniques.

Compared to published safety data, the rate of observed trabectedin extravasation of 0.8% in our series was similar to 0.5% reported in large pooled analysis of 1132 patients who received single agent trabectedin [8].

Conclusions

Despite the use of central venous access devices, trabectedin can cause local sterile inflammation along the catheter trajectory, in particular in venous access ports. Positioning the port's catheter deeper in the subcutis appears to be the most efficient way to prevent this complication.

Abbreviations
STS: soft tissue sarcomas; VAD: venous access devices (any type); PICC line: peripherally inserted CVC line; CVC: central venous catheter; VAP: venous access ports (such as a Port-a-Cath); VARAE: venous access related adverse events.

Authors' contributions
HG designed the study, MV collected, analysed the data and drafted the first manuscript, all authors participated in patient care and manuscript writing. All authors read and approved the final manuscript.

Author details
[1] Department of Medical Oncology, Leiden University Medical Center, Postbus 9600, 2300 RC Leiden, The Netherlands. [2] Department of Medical Oncology, Antoni van Leeuwenhoek-Netherlands Cancer Institute, Postbus 90203, 1006 BE Amsterdam, The Netherlands. [3] Department of Radiology, Interventional Radiology Section, Leiden University Medical Center, Postbus 9600, 2300 RC Leiden, The Netherlands. [4] Department of Medical Oncology, Radboud University Medical Center, Postbus 9101, 6500 HB Nijmegen, The Netherlands. [5] The Institute of Cancer Research and the Royal Marsden NHS Foundation Trust, 123 Old Brompton Road, London SW7 3RP, UK. [6] Department of Medical Oncology, University of Groningen, University Medical Center Groningen, Postbus 30.001, 9700 RB Groningen, The Netherlands. [7] Department of Medical Oncology, Erasmus MC Cancer Institute, Postbus 2040, 3000 CA Rotterdam, The Netherlands.

Acknowledgements
Not applicable.

Competing interests
HG: PharmaMar provided a research grant to the Leiden University Medical Center to perform a health outcomes study, which was also supported by a ZonMW grant. This study is a sub-study of the health outcomes study. MV: PharmaMar provided a research grant to perform this study, as sub-study of a health outcomes study. None for the other authors.

References
1. Lemmers NW, Gels ME, Sleijfer DT, Plukker JT, van der Graaf WT, de Langen ZJ, et al. Complications of venous access ports in 132 patients with disseminated testicular cancer treated with polychemotherapy. J Clin Oncol. 1996;14:2916–22.
2. Niederhuber JE, Ensminger W, Gyves JW, Liepman M, Doan K, Cozzi E. Totally implanted venous and arterial access system to replace external catheters in cancer treatment. Surgery. 1982;92:706–12.
3. Di Carlo I, Pulvirenti E, Mannino M, Toro A. Increased use of percutaneous technique for totally implantable venous access devices. Is it real progress? A 27-year comprehensive review on early complications. Ann Surg Oncol. 2010;17:1649–56.
4. Hickman RO, Buckner CD, Clift RA, Sanders JE, Stewart P, Thomas ED. A modified right atrial catheter for access to the venous system in marrow transplant recipients. Surg Gynecol Obstet. 1979;148:871–5.
5. Hoshal VL Jr. Total intravenous nutrition with peripherally inserted silicone elastomer central venous catheters. Arch Surg. 1975;110:644–6.

6. D'Incalci M, Badri N, Galmarini CM, Allavena P. Trabectedin, a drug acting on both cancer cells and the tumour microenvironment. Br J Cancer. 2014;111:646–50.

7. Le Cesne A, Cresta S, Maki RG, Blay JY, Verweij J, Poveda A, et al. A retrospective analysis of antitumour activity with trabectedin in translocation-related sarcomas. Eur J Cancer. 2012;48:3036–44.

8. Le Cesne A, Yovine A, Blay JY, Delaloge S, Maki RG, Misset JL, et al. A retrospective pooled analysis of trabectedin safety in 1132 patients with solid tumors treated in phase II clinical trials. Invest New Drugs. 2012;30:1193–202.

9. Schoffski P, Cerbone L, Wolter P, De Wever I, Samson I, Dumez H, et al. Administration of 24-h intravenous infusions of trabectedin in ambulatory patients with mesenchymal tumors via disposable elastomeric pumps: an effective and patient-friendly palliative treatment option. Onkologie. 2012;35:14–7.

10. Martella F, Salutari V, Marchetti C, Pisano C, Di NM, Pietta F, et al. A retrospective analysis of trabectedin infusion by peripherally inserted central venous catheters: a multicentric Italian experience. Anticancer Drugs. 2015;26:990–4.

11. Theman TA, Hartzell TL, Sinha I, Polson K, Morgan J, Demetri GD, et al. Recognition of a new chemotherapeutic vesicant: trabectedin (ecteinascidin-743) extravasation with skin and soft tissue damage. J Clin Oncol. 2009;27:e198–200.

12. Hoiczyk M, Grabellus F, Podleska L, Ahrens M, Schwindenhammer B, Taeger G, et al. Trabectedin in metastatic soft tissue sarcomas: role of pretreatment and age. Int J Oncol. 2013;43:23–8.

13. Bui-Nguyen B, Butrynski JE, Penel N, Blay JY, Isambert N, Milhem M, et al. A phase IIb multicentre study comparing the efficacy of trabectedin to doxorubicin in patients with advanced or metastatic untreated soft tissue sarcoma: the TRUSTS trial. Eur J Cancer. 2015;51:1312–20.

14. Verboom M, Kerst M, Van der Graaf W, Sleijfer S, Reyners A, Steeghs N et al. Trabectedin in patients with advanced soft tissue sarcoma (STS): results from a prospective, observational phase IV study in the Netherlands. 20th CTOS Meeting 2014, abstract Poster 90.

16

Targeted antiangiogenic agents in combination with cytotoxic chemotherapy in preclinical and clinical studies in sarcoma

Kieuhoa T. Vo[1*], Katherine K. Matthay[1] and Steven G. DuBois[2]

Abstract

Sarcomas are a heterogeneous group of mesenchymal malignancies. In recent years, studies have demonstrated that inhibition of angiogenic pathways or disruption of established vasculature can attenuate the growth of sarcomas. However, when used as monotherapy in the clinical setting, these targeted antiangiogenic agents have only provided modest survival benefits in some sarcoma subtypes, and have not been efficacious in others. Preclinical and early clinical data suggest that the addition of conventional chemotherapy to antiangiogenic agents may lead to more effective therapies for patients with these tumors. In the current review, the authors summarize the available evidence and possible mechanisms supporting this approach.

Keywords: Sarcoma, Antiangiogenesis, Combination drug therapy, Combination chemotherapy

Background

Sarcomas are a heterogeneous group of malignancies, including soft tissue sarcomas (STS) and tumors of bone and cartilage. Conventional chemotherapy regimens for advanced or metastatic sarcomas have low survival rates, substantial toxicity, and frequent emergence of resistance, making alternative novel treatment approaches a priority.

Sarcomas express proangiogenic factors that may represent therapeutic targets, with vascular endothelial growth factor (VEGF) being the best characterized. In animal models of human sarcomas, inhibitors of angiogenesis have shown promising antitumor activity [1–3]. Antiangiogenic therapies have a number of potential advantages compared to chemotherapy including overcoming chemoresistance [4, 5], more favorable toxicity profile, and broad spectrum of activity. Since 2004, over ten drugs that target VEGF or its receptors have been approved as cancer therapeutics, with many more in clinical trials [6]. These agents have shown single-agent activity in sarcoma. Most notably, pazopanib has been approved by the US Food and Drug Administration and the European Medicines Agency for advanced STS. As monotherapy, these agents have only provided survival benefits on the order of weeks to months in some sarcoma subtypes, and have not been efficacious in others [7]. Therefore, combining antiangiogenic agents (AA) with other systemic agents active in sarcoma may lead to more effective therapies for patients with these tumors.

This review summarizes evidence supporting the use of targeted AA in combination with cytotoxic chemotherapy in sarcomas. We performed an extensive review of the available medical literature using the US National Library of Medicine's PubMed search function to find relevant primary articles based on key search terms including "angiogenesis", "antiangiogenic", "antiangiogenesis", and "antivascular". These search terms were searched with "chemotherapy" and "sarcoma", "bone tumor", or "soft tissue cancer". The "Related Articles" function of PubMed and reference lists from relevant articles were used to identify additional articles. Additionally, in order to identify recent trials not yet published, we also performed a search of abstracts presented at the American Society of Clinical Oncology (ASCO) annual meetings from 2013 to 2015.

*Correspondence: kieuhoa.vo@ucsf.edu
[1] Department of Pediatrics, UCSF School of Medicine, San Francisco School of Medicine, UCSF Benioff Children's Hospital, University of California, 550 16th Street, 4th Floor, Box 0434, San Francisco, CA 94158, USA
Full list of author information is available at the end of the article

In the current review, we provide the results of this search beginning with the preclinical data supporting AA in combination with chemotherapy in this diverse group of diseases. The review concludes with an assessment of the completed and ongoing clinical studies that have treated patients with sarcoma using this therapeutic strategy.

Preclinical efficacy of targeted AA in combination with chemotherapy

Angiogenesis is tightly regulated at the molecular level. Dysregulation of angiogenesis occurs in various pathologies and is one of the hallmarks of cancer. Concentrated efforts in this area of research are leading to the discovery of a growing number of pro- and anti-angiogenic molecules, many of which are already in clinical trials. The complex interactions among these molecules and how they affect vascular structure and function in different environments are now beginning to be elucidated [6, 8–10]. This integrated understanding is leading to the development of a number of therapeutic approaches to treat cancer, including the use of AA in combination with chemotherapy.

Biological mechanisms supporting combination approaches in solid tumor malignancies other than sarcoma

With the discovery of VEGF as a major driver of tumor angiogenesis, efforts have focused on novel therapeutics aimed at inhibiting VEGF activity. Unfortunately, clinical trials of anti-VEGF monotherapy in patients with solid tumors have resulted in only modest responses. Intriguingly, the combination of anti-VEGF therapy with conventional chemotherapy has improved survival in cancer patients compared with chemotherapy alone [6].

The proposed mechanisms of benefit from combined AA and chemotherapy include: (1) normalization of the tumor vasculature by altering vascular permeability and increasing drug accessibility (Fig. 1a); (2) synergistic effects leading to enhanced direct cytotoxicity of cancer cells and/or endothelial cells (Fig. 1b); and/or (3) decreased chemoresistance (Fig. 1c).

A paradoxical hypothesis that may explain the antitumor effect of this combination approach relies on the theory of transient "normalization" of the abnormal tumor vasculature, which results in improved blood perfusion and enhanced chemotherapy accessibility and antitumor activity (Fig. 1a) [6]. Several preclinical studies using direct and indirect AA support the normalization hypothesis [11–13]. Blockade of VEGF signaling results in transient pruning and active remodeling of the immature and leaky blood vessels of tumors in animal models so that it more closely resembled the normal vasculature. Functional improvements accompany these

morphological changes, including decreased interstitial fluid pressure (IFP), decreased tumor hypoxia, and improved penetration of macromolecules from these vessels into tumors [11–13].

Based on this hypothesis, Liu and colleagues examined the vascular density and structural changes of tumors obtained from lung cancer xenograft mice treated with bevacizumab combined with gemcitabine and cisplatin [14]. They demonstrated significant reduction in VEGF levels and microvessel density (MVD) and increased number of normal vessels as analyzed by electron microscopy in mice treated with combination therapy compared to those mice treated with chemotherapy alone [14]. The tumor volume of mice in the combined treatment group was significantly lower compared to the bevacizumab monotherapy and chemotherapy groups, which also correlated with significant survival advantage [14].

Improved chemotherapy delivery secondary to tumor vessel normalization was demonstrated in a study of bevacizumab and topotecan in neuroblastoma xenograft models. After a single bevacizumab dose, there were decreases in tumor MVD, tumor vessel permeability, and tumor IFP compared to controls [15]. Intratumoral perfusion, as assessed by contrast-enhanced ultrasonography, was also improved [15]. Moreover, intratumoral drug delivery accompanied these changes: penetration of topotecan was improved when given 1–3 days after bevacizumab, compared to concomitant administration or 7 days apart, and resulted in greater tumor growth inhibition than with monotherapy or concomitant administration of the two drugs [15]. Similarly, the increase in antitumor activity of chemotherapy during the transient vascular normalization period produced by bevacizumab has also been confirmed in animal models of colorectal cancer (irinotecan) [16] and melanoma (melphalan) [17].

In vivo [(15)O]H2O positron emission tomography (PET) imaging in a mouse model of lung cancer showed that treatment with the VEGFR/platelet-derived growth factor receptor (PDGFR) inhibitor PTK787 created a 7-day window of improved tumor blood flow when tumor vessels are transiently normalized [18]. An improvement in pericyte coverage and reduced leakiness from tumor vessels in xenografts accompanied this normalization phase [18]. Initiation of newer targeted agents during this window of vessel normalization also resulted in increased drug delivery and apoptotic efficacy of erlotinib, an epidermal growth factor receptor (EGFR) inhibitor [18]. Together, these findings offer strong supportive evidence that strategic administration of AA can promote transient vessel normalization that improves drug delivery and efficacy in a range of solid tumors.

In contrast, a study by Van der Veldt et al. in non-small cell lung cancer (NSCLC) showed that pretreatment

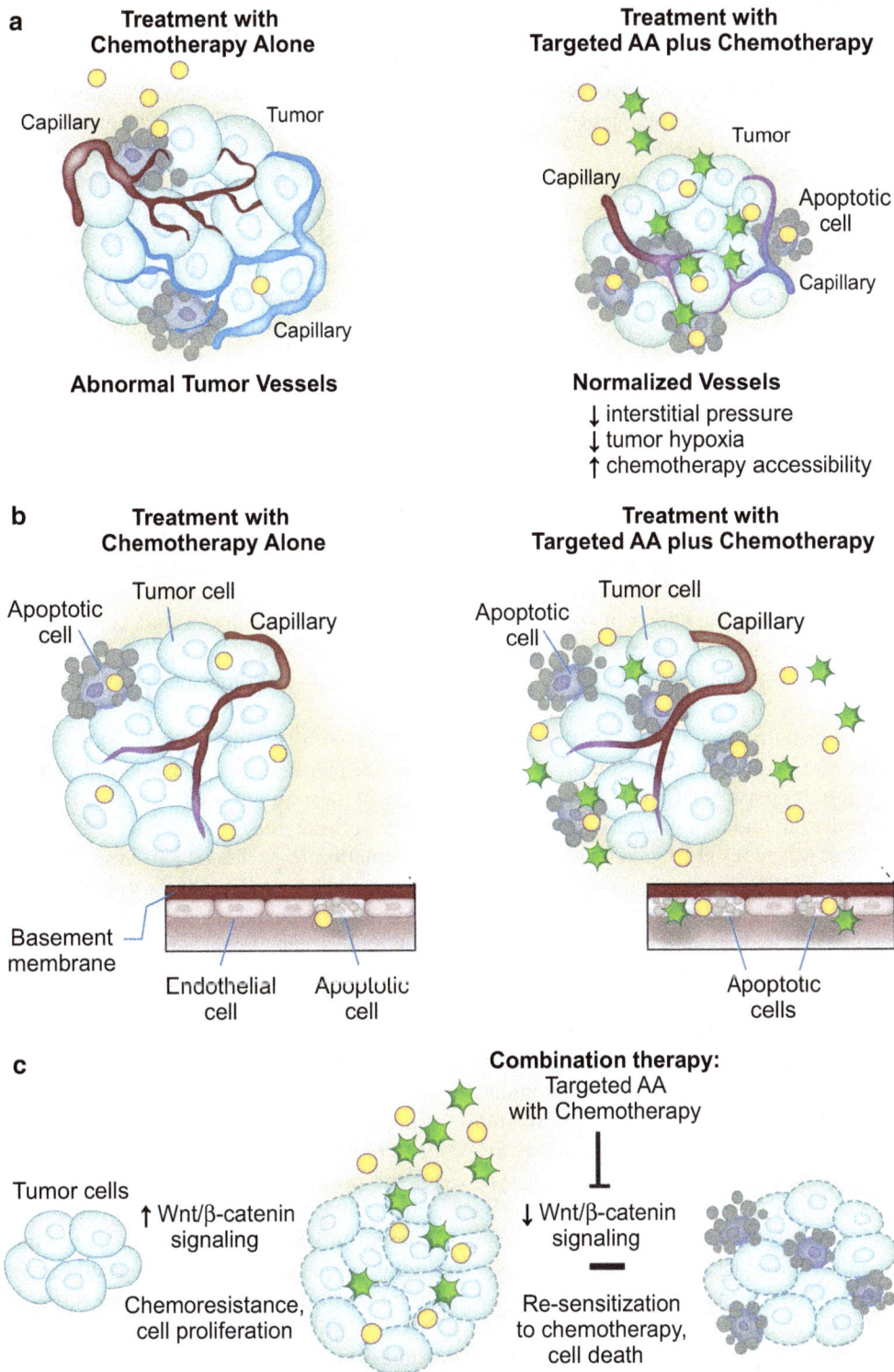

Fig. 1 Proposed biological mechanisms supporting combination antiangiogenesis approaches in sarcoma. **a** Transient "normalization" of the abnormal tumor vasculature by AA results in improved blood perfusion and enhanced chemotherapy accessibility and antitumor activity. **b** The synergistic interaction of combination therapy leads to enhanced direct cytotoxicity of tumor cells and/or endothelial cells. **c** Combination therapy leads to up- or down-regulation signaling pathways involved in chemoresistance. For example, down-regulation of the Wnt/β-catenin pathway by the combination of masitinib and gemcitabine contribute to the re-sensitization of gemcitabine-resistant pancreatic tumor cells leading to apoptotic death [27]. *AA* antiangiogenic agents

with bevacizumab reduced both perfusion and net influx rate of radiolabeled docetaxel as measured by PET with effects persisting after 4 days [19]. This study highlighted the importance of drug scheduling and advocated further studies to optimize scheduling of antiangiogenic drugs combined with cytotoxic chemotherapy.

Other preclinical studies reporting the impact of AA upon delivery of cytotoxic therapies include sunitinib, an inhibitor of VEGFR and PDGFR, combined with temozolomide in orthotopic glioma models [20, 21]. Sunitinib significantly increased temozolomide tumor distribution [21]. A "vascular normalization index" incorporating MVD and protein expression of α-SMA and collagen IV was proposed as an indication of the number of tumor vessels with relatively good quality, and significantly correlated with the unbound temozolomide AUC in tumor interstitial fluid [21].

Interestingly, when used as monotherapy, several preclinical studies have shown that the normalization of blood vessels by AA may result in paradoxical increased invasion of local vessels by the tumor and resulting metastases. A recent study of the effects of combination therapy in breast cancer model suggest that the addition of chemotherapy to AA can help prevent local invasion of vessels promoted by the AA and result in lower metastatic rate. Antiangiogenic therapy with DC101 (VEGFR2 inhibitor), while blunting tumor volume growth, was found to increase local invasion in multiple primary tumor models, including a patient-derived xenograft [22]. This effect was blocked by concurrent chemotherapy with paclitaxel [22]. Similarly, the combination of paclitaxel with DC101 caused a marked reduction of micro- or macrometastatic disease in contrast to DC101 monotherapy, which was associated with small increases in metastatic disease.

Synergistic effects of combination therapy of AA with chemotherapy have been seen in several preclinical models of solid cancers (Fig. 1b). For example, in vitro studies of bladder cancer demonstrated the efficacy of pazopanib with docetaxel, even in docetaxel-resistant bladder cancer cell lines [23]. While the mechanism(s) of these synergistic effects have not been fully elucidated, and may be dependent on the specific combination regimen used and tissue type treated, we have highlighted several examples of mechanisms related to enhanced direct cytotoxicity of cancer cells and/or endothelial cells.

Sorafenib increased apoptosis in melanoma-derived cell lines treated with melphalan or temozolomide [24]. The molecular mechanisms underlying sorafenib enhancement were investigated by analyzing the changes in signaling events in melanoma cell lines in response to sorafenib treatment alone. Response to sorafenib correlated with extracellular signal-regulated kinase (ERK) down-regulation and loss of Mcl-1 expression [24]. These results suggest that sorafenib enhanced sensitivity to chemotherapy by altering signaling in the mitogen-activated protein kinase (MAPK) and the mitochondrial apoptotic pathways. These in vitro findings highlight the potential for AA to have effects independent of classical antiangiogenic mechanisms.

The timing and sequence of AA with chemotherapy can also be critical in determination of synergy or antagonism. Troiani et al. demonstrated the sequence-dependent interactions of ZD6474 (VEGR, EGFR, and RET inhibitor) with oxaliplatin in colon cancer cell lines in vitro using three combination schedules [25]. Treatment with oxaliplatin followed by ZD6474 was highly synergistic, whereas the reverse sequence or concurrent exposure was clearly antagonistic [25]. Oxaliplatin induced a G2-M arrest, which was antagonized if the cells were previously or concurrently treated with ZD6474. ZD6474 enhanced oxaliplatin-induced apoptosis, but only when added after oxaliplatin [25].

Alternatively, Naumova and colleagues demonstrated that paclitaxel and SU6668, a VEGFR2/PDGFR inhibitor, synergistically inhibited the proliferation and increased apoptosis of endothelial cells [26]. These findings, together with the in vivo inhibition of angiogenesis in Matrigel plugs and the reduction of MVD of paclitaxel-resistant ovarian carcinoma xenograft models, support the hypothesis that the enhanced effect exerted by the combination of paclitaxel and SU6668 on tumor growth is mediated by an effect on the vasculature [26].

Another mechanism of combination therapy involves overcoming chemoresistance (Fig. 1c). Acquired drug resistance is a major problem in the treatment of cancer. Boehm et al. reported that chronic, intermittent therapy of three different mouse tumors with endostatin, an angiogenic inhibitor, did not show any evidence of acquired drug resistance [5]. In contrast, standard chemotherapy, using maximum doses of cyclophosphamide, resulted in drug resistance in lung carcinoma xenografts [5]. These results provided initial evidence that a specific angiogenic inhibitor does not induce drug resistance in three different tumor xenografts. Perhaps the most significant finding of this study was that repeated cycles of endostatin therapy induced tumor dormancy that persisted after therapy. While the mechanism(s) is not yet clear, recent studies may help to elucidate these findings.

For example, a series of in vitro and in vivo studies using preclinical models of human pancreatic cancer characterized the synergistic effects of combination therapy with gemcitabine with masitinib, a selective inhibitor of PDGFR [27]. The masitinib and gemcitabine combination synergistically inhibited proliferation of gemcitabine-refractory cell lines [27]. Analysis of gene expression profiling of gemcitabine-resistant pancreatic cells revealed differences in gene expression unique to the masitinib plus gemcitabine combination. The most significantly altered pathway involved genes associated with Wnt/β-catenin signaling [27]. This pathway is involved in pancreatic development and re-activation has been implicated in pancreatic carcinoma, suggesting a mechanism of augmented cell death with combination therapy in gemcitabine-resistant cells as compared to gemcitabine monotherapy [27].

Preclinical studies of combination approaches in sarcoma

Targeted AA and cytotoxic chemotherapy have been combined in several laboratory models of sarcoma, mainly STS, as summarized in Table 1. Most notably, studies have shown that VEGFR2 blockade by DC101 combined with chemotherapy inhibits tumor growth, metastases, and angiogenesis in STS xenografts [28, 29]. Combined DC101 and continuous low-dose doxorubicin resulted in more effective growth inhibition of STS xenografts compared to either agent alone [28]. DC101 plus doxorubicin also enhanced the inhibition of tumor angiogenesis and endothelial cell activity, as demonstrated by significantly reduced MVD and inhibition of neovascularization [28]. Additionally, this combination regimen directly exerted enhanced inhibitory effects on endothelial cell migration, proliferation, and

tube-like formation in vitro. Furthermore, the combination enhanced apoptosis of endothelial cells [28].

To elucidate the role of recombinant human $VEGF_{165}$ in STS growth, metastasis, and chemoresistance, Zhang and colleagues generated stably $VEGF_{165}$-transfected STS cell lines to study the effect of VEGF overexpression in vitro and in vivo. $VEGF_{165}$-transfected xenografts formed highly vascular tumors with shorter latency, accelerated growth, enhanced chemoresistance, and increased incidence of pulmonary metastases [29]. Combined therapy with DC101 and low-dose doxorubicin in vivo suppressed the growth of $VEGF_{165}$-overexpressing xenografts, inhibited angiogenesis, increased the vessel maturation index, and suppressed tumor cell proliferation compared to monotherapy-treated mice. The addition of DC101 induced endothelial cell sensitivity to doxorubicin and suppressed the activity of matrix metalloproteinases secreted by endothelial cells [29]. These results suggested that the antitumor effects of combined therapy with DC101 and doxorubicin were secondary to tumor-associated endothelial cell growth modulation and chemosensitization [29].

Likewise, the enhanced antitumor effects of combination therapy using low-dose topotecan and pazopanib in mouse models of osteosarcoma and rhabdomyosarcoma are thought to be related to augmented antiangiogenesis [30]. The metronomic administration of pazopanib and topotecan in vitro showed reduction in circulating

Table 1 Preclinical studies of combination approaches in sarcoma

Drug combination	Sarcoma tumor models	Results compared to models treated with chemotherapy alone	Reference
Pazopanib + topotecan	OS KHOS and RMS RH30 cell lines and xenografts	↑ Antitumor and antiangiogenic effects, ↑ Survival, ↓ Circulating endothelial cells and/or endothelial progenitor cells, ↓ MVD	[30]
VDA (OXi4503/CA1P) + doxorubicin	EWS xenografts	↑ Antitumor effects ↑ Necrosis ↓ Perfused vasculature	[59]
Bevacizumab + topotecan	ASPS xenografts	↑ Antitumor effects compared to bevacizumab monotherapy, but not topotecan alone	[60]
Vandetanib + doxorubicin	Multiple STS cell lines and xenografts	↑ Antitumor and antiangiogenic effects ↓ Local growth leiomyosarcoma ↓ Lung metastases in fibrosarcoma	[31]
DC101 + doxorubicin	Multiple STS cell lines and xenografts transfected with $VEGF_{165}$	↑ Antitumor and antiangiogenic effects ↓ Tumor growth and pulmonary metastases ↓ MVD ↑ Percentage of mature vessels ↓ Matrix metalloproteinases secreted by endothelial cells	[29]
DC101 + doxorubicin	Leiomyosarcoma SKLMS-1 and RMS RD cell lines and xenografts	↑ Antitumor and antiangiogenic effects ↓ MVD and neovascularization ↑ Apoptosis of endothelial cells ↓ Endothelial cell migration, proliferation, tube-like formation	[28]
TNP-470 + etoposide	Angiosarcoma ISOS-1 cell line and xenograft	↑ Antitumor effects ↑ Growth inhibition	[61]

ASPS alveolar soft part sarcoma, *ES* Ewing sarcoma, *MVD* microvessel density, *OS* osteosarcoma, *RMS* rhabdomyosarcoma, *STS* soft tissue sarcoma, *VDA* vascular-disrupting agent, *VEGF(R)* vascular endothelial growth factor (receptor)

endothelial cells, circulating endothelial progenitor cells, and tumor MVD which correlated with antitumor activity and enhancement in survival compared with monotherapy agents in all preclinical models [30].

Concomitant use of a dual VEGFR2/EGFR inhibitor (vandetanib) with doxorubicin resulted in additional cytotoxicity and endothelial cell growth inhibition with lowered doxorubicin doses compared to vandetanib monotherapy in leiomyosarcoma, fibrosarcoma, and uterine sarcoma models [31]. In addition, vandetanib in combination with low-dose doxorubicin resulted in significant inhibition of human fibrosarcoma xenograft lung metastases compared to control and doxorubicin-only groups [31]. Collectively, these studies suggest that AA plus chemotherapy regimens may also help to reduce the dose and therefore cumulative toxicities of cytotoxic chemotherapy.

Clinical efficacy of targeted AA in combination with chemotherapy
Clinical studies of combination approaches in solid tumors
Outside the field of sarcoma, AA have been combined with chemotherapy with varying outcomes. A retrospective study of patients with advanced solid malignancies treated on phase 1 protocols between 2004 and 2013 showed that chemotherapy concomitant with VEGF(R) inhibitors was associated with significantly higher odds ratio for clinical benefit compared with chemotherapy without VEGF(R) inhibitors [32].

For example, in lung, breast, and colorectal carcinoma, AA have shown increased activity when combined with standard chemotherapy, as highlighted below. In advanced non-small cell lung cancer, a randomized phase 2 trial showed a trend towards increased response rate and time to progression when bevacizumab was combined with paclitaxel and carboplatin [33]. Several large randomized trials in patients with metastatic breast cancer showed significantly higher response rates and increased progression-free survival (PFS) when treated with bevacizumab combined with chemotherapy compared to those treated with chemotherapy alone [34–38].

Perhaps the disease in which bevacizumab has had the greatest impact in combination with chemotherapy is metastatic colorectal cancer. After a randomized phase 2 study showed encouraging results when bevacizumab was combined with fluorouracil and leucovorin [39], a randomized phase 3 trial of irinotecan, fluorouracil, and leucovorin with bevacizumab or placebo showed that bevacizumab increased response rate, time to progression, and overall survival [40]. Given these findings, bevacizumab is now included in the first-line management of patients with metastatic colorectal cancer. These clinical findings provided proof of principle of additive activity

when AA are added to chemotherapy in patients with cancer and support clinical investigation in sarcoma.

Clinical studies of combination approaches in sarcoma
Targeted AA and chemotherapy have been combined in numerous early phase clinical trials in children and adults with advanced solid tumors. Phase 1 studies that included patients with sarcoma are summarized in Table 2. The backbone chemotherapy regimens used in these trials included taxane- and platinum-based therapies, camptothecins, and gemcitabine. Although not powered to evaluate the antitumor activity of AA combined with chemotherapy, the results of these phase 1 studies suggest that these regimens are generally well tolerated with promising clinical activity in sarcomas. In a phase 1b study of the combination of bevacizumab added to gemcitabine and docetaxel in patients with advanced STS, the overall response rate observed was 31 %, with 5 complete and 6 partial responses, and 18 patients with stable disease lasting for a median of 6 months [41]. Several pediatric phase 1 clinical trials have demonstrated the safety of combining AA, specifically bevacizumab, with cytotoxic chemotherapy in patients with advanced solid tumors, with tumor responses in patients with Ewing sarcoma [42]. In addition to those listed in Table 2, combination antiangiogenic approaches combining AA and conventional chemotherapy, such as ifosfamide and doxorubicin, studied in other malignancies, may warrant further study in sarcoma [43, 44].

There have been four reported phase 2 studies evaluating the combination of AA with chemotherapy in sarcoma. The combination of bevacizumab with doxorubicin was evaluated in 17 patients with metastatic STS [45]. While two partial responses (12 %) were observed, this response rate was not greater than that observed for single-agent doxorubicin [45]. However, 11 patients (65 %) had stable disease lasting four cycles or longer, suggesting that further consideration of this treatment regimen may be warranted in STS [45]. In general, the toxicity of bevacizumab and doxorubicin was similar to that reported for single-agent doxorubicin with one notable exception: the reported 35 % rate of grade 2 or higher cardiotoxicity with this combination regimen was greater than expected (compared to historical controls) [45]. Despite close monitoring and standard use of dexrazoxane, the observed cardiac toxicity warrants a change in the dose and/or schedule in future studies of this combination.

The Children's Oncology Group (COG) evaluated bevacizumab or temsirolimus in combination with vinorelbine (V) and cyclophosphamide (C) in a randomized phase 2 study in patients with advanced rhabdomyosarcoma. Both treatment regimens were well tolerated and

Table 2 Completed phase 1 (or pilot) trials of combination approaches that enrolled patients with sarcoma

Drug combination	Sarcoma tumor type (number enrolled)	Responses[a]	Reference
Trials with bevacizumab			
Bevacizumab + pegylated SN-38 (EZN-2208)	STS (5)	SD (2)	[62]
Bevacizumab + bendamustine	Angiosarcoma (1)	None	[63]
Bevacizumab + irinotecan	RMS (1)	None	[64]
Bevacizumab + vincristine/irinotecan/temozolomide	STS (3); OS (2); ES (1)	SD (2)	[65]
Bevacizumab + vincristine/irinotecan/temozolomide	ES (2); RMS (1); Clear cell sarcoma (1)	CR (1); PR (1)	[42]
Bevacizumab + sorafenib + cyclophosphamide	OS (2); RMS (2); Other STS (4)	PR (1); SD (3)	[66]
Bevacizumab + gemcitabine/doxetaxel	STS (36)	CR (5); PR (6); SD (18)	[41]
Bevacizumab + ifosphamide/etoposide/carboplatin	STS (7); OS (3); Chondrosarcoma (2); Undifferentiated (1)	PR (4); SD (5)	[67]
Trials with VEGFR and PDGFR inhibitors			
Pazopanib + cisplatin	Sarcoma (5)	CR (1); SD (2)	[68]
Pazopanib + topotecan	STS (6); OS (2)	Unknown	[69]
Pazopanib + ifosfamide	Sarcoma (19)	PR (3)	[70]
Pazopanib + paclitaxel/carboplatin	OS (1); Giant cell tumor (1); Other sarcoma (1)	None	[71]
PDGFR inhibitor (CP-868,596) + docetaxel ± axitinib	ES (3); Other sarcoma (5)	SD (3)	[72]
Semaxanib + cisplatin/irinotecan	GIST (2); STS (1)	None	[73]
Sorafenib + irinotecan	OS (4); Synovial sarcoma (1); DSRCT (1); MPNST (1)	Unknown	[74]
Sunitinib + pemetrexed/carboplatin	Synovial sarcoma (1)	None	[75]
Sunitinib + gemcitabine	OS (1); STS (1)	SD (1)	[76]
Sunitinib + ifosfamide	ES (2); STS (6); Other sarcoma (7)	PR (2); SD (3)	[77]
Sunitinib + irinotecan	OS (1); STS (1)	None	[78]
Sunitinib + docetaxel	OS and STS (unknown)	None	[79]
Trials with other antiangiogenic agents			
Ombrabulin (AVE8062) + docetaxel	Muscle/bone tumors (5)	None	[80]
Thrombospondin-1 mimetic (ABT-510) + gemcitabine/cisplatin	Sarcoma (1)	None	[81]
Thrombospondin-1 mimetic (ABT-510) + 5-FU/leucovorin	Synovial sarcoma (1)	None	[82]
TNP-470 + paclitaxel/carboplatin	Sarcoma (2)	None	[83]

[a] Only includes SD, PR, and CR responses among patients with sarcoma. *CR* complete response; *DRSCT* desmoplastic small round cell tumor; *ES* Ewing sarcoma; *GIST* gastrointestinal stromal tumor; *MPNST* malignant peripheral nerve sheath tumor; *OS* osteosarcoma; *PDGFR* platelet-derived growth factor receptor; *PR* partial response; *RMS* rhabdomyosarcoma; *STS* soft tissue sarcoma; *SD* stable disease; *VEGF(R)* vascular endothelial growth factor (receptor)

without unexpected toxicities. In a preliminary report, patients randomized to VC plus temsirolimus had a superior event-free survival compared to VC plus bevacizumab (65 vs. 50 %, respectively) [46]. As a VC alone arm was not included in the trial, it is not known if bevacizumab improved outcomes compared to the VC backbone.

Ray-Coquard and colleagues examined the addition of bevacizumab added to paclitaxel in a randomized phase 2 study of patients with angiosarcoma. While the combination antiangiogenic regimen was shown to be active in patients with angiosarcoma, the PFS and overall survival was similar in both arms [47]. Nevertheless, there was increased toxicity in the bevacizumab arm, which included one fatal drug-related toxicity (intestinal obstruction) [47]. The lack of benefit from bevacizumab may be due in part to key mutations in angiosarcoma

that may activate the proangiogenic pathway independently of the classic ligand-receptor activation shown in recent studies. These findings suggest that the extracellular blockade of VEGF by a monoclonal antibody, such as bevacizumab, would not interfere with angiosarcoma proliferation [47]. Given these findings, the authors did not recommend the addition of bevacizumab to paclitaxel for the treatment of advanced angiosarcoma.

Recently, the Spanish Group for Research on Sarcomas presented their findings of a phase 2 study of sorafenib and ifosfamide in 35 patients with advanced STS [48]. This combination antiangiogenic regimen had acceptable toxicity in patients previously treated with anthracyclines. The study met its primary endpoint requiring at least 19/35 patients to be free of progression at 3 months. The combination was shown to be active in patients with advanced STS. Six (17 %) patients had partial responses to this regimen. The 3-month PFS was found to be 66 % (23/35) in patients treated with sorafenib plus ifosfamide, which may exceed the 3-month PFS in patients treated with ifosfamide alone, thus warranting further investigation [48].

Additional clinical trials evaluating combination therapy with targeted AA and cytotoxic chemotherapy in patients with sarcoma are ongoing (Table 3). With early promising results, the latest phase 2 trials have been largely directed towards pediatric sarcoma. These include bevacizumab, cyclophosphamide, and topotecan in patients with relapsed/refractory Ewing sarcoma (NCT01492673); and maintenance bevacizumab therapy in high-risk Ewing sarcoma and desmoplastic small round cell tumor (NCT01946529). Furthermore, the COG is actively enrolling patients on a randomized phase 2/3 trial of preoperative chemoradiation or preoperative radiation plus or minus pazopanib in STS histologies other than rhabdomyosarcoma (NCT02180867).

In adults, phase 2 studies are evaluating pazopanib and topotecan in patients with high-risk sarcomas (NCT02357810); pazopanib plus gemcitabine in advanced STS (NCT02203760, NCT01593748 and NCT01532687); pazopanib and paclitaxel in advanced angiosarcoma (NCT02212015); sorafenib, epirubicin, ifosfamide, and radiotherapy followed by surgery in high-risk STS (NCT02050919). Lastly, there is one open randomized phase 3 trial evaluating bevacizumab versus placebo combined with docetaxel and gemicitabine in the treatment of advanced uterine leiomyosarcoma (NCT01012297).

Outside of the context of formal clinical trials, several retrospective case studies/series have also highlighted the potential efficacy of these combination regimens. A child with transformed malignant angiosarcoma was successfully treated with bevacizumab, gemcitabine, and docetaxel, which resulted in temporary tumor regression with progression free survival of 12 months [49]. Dramatic improvement was also seen in another patient with inoperable face and neck angiosarcoma who was treated with bevacizumab and paclitaxel [50]. In three pediatric patients with Ewing sarcoma or undifferentiated sarcoma who were treated with bevacizumab, gemcitabine, and docetaxel, two patients had a partial response and the third patient had stable disease for >6 months [51]. Lastly, in a retrospective analysis of 14 patients with hemangiopericytomas and malignant solitary fibrous tumors who were treated with bevacizmuab and temozolomide, 11 patients (79 %) achieved a partial response, with a median time to response of 2.5 months [52].

Extensively reviewed elsewhere [53, 54], metronomic chemotherapy is an alternative antiangiogenic strategy, involving the application of daily, low-dose chemotherapy. With this low-dose approach, apoptosis is induced in the less frequently dividing endothelial cells rather than in the tumor cells [53]. This approach has been used in sarcoma with promising results [55–58]. In a feasibility study of metronomic cyclophosphamide plus prednisolone in 26 elderly patients with inoperable or metastatic STS, the response rate was 27 % and the disease control rate (responses and stable disease >12 weeks) was 69 % [56]. Currently, there are three open phase 1 studies examining the combination of bevacizumab or pazopanib added to metronomic chemotherapy that may include eligible sarcoma patients (Table 3).

Conclusions

Advances in the biology of sarcomas have established the critical role of tumor angiogenesis and multiple signaling pathways involved in tumor development, growth, and therapy resistance. Numerous preclinical studies have demonstrated that targeting proangiogenic mechanisms

Table 3 Ongoing phase 1 (or pilot) clinical trials of combination approaches in sarcoma

Targeted antiangiogenic agent	Chemotherapy regimen	Tumor type	NCT
Bevacizumab	Doxorubicin/temsirolimus	Advanced solid tumors, including sarcoma	00761644
Bevacizumab	Doxorubicin	Advanced Kaposi sarcoma	00923936
Bevacizumab	Gemcitabine/docetaxel/valproic acid	Advanced sarcoma	01106872
Bevacizumab	Gemcitabine/paclitaxel	Advanced solid tumors, including sarcoma	01113476
Bevacizumab	Irinotecan/temozolomide + standard alkylator-based chemotherapy	Newly diagnosed DSRCT	01189643
Bevacizumab	Metronomic doxorubicin + radiation	Resectable STS	01746238
Bevacizumab	Metronomic cyclophosphamide/valproic acid/temsirolimus	Advanced solid tumors, including sarcoma	02446431
Pazopanib	Gemcitabine	Advanced leiomyosarcoma	01442662
Pazopanib	Docetaxel/gemcitabine	Operable STS	01719302
Pazopanib	Metronomic topotecan	Advanced solid tumors, including sarcoma	02303028

DSRCT desmoplastic small round cell tumor; *NCT* ClinicalTrials.gov Identifier/Number; *STS* soft tissue sarcoma

in combination with cytotoxic chemotherapy may provide a valid approach to overcoming chemoresistance and inhibiting growth of these tumors. Early clinical data are still inconclusive, but some reports suggest that the use of these AA in combination with chemotherapy may be beneficial in the treatment of patients with advanced sarcoma.

Similar to various targeted therapeutic approaches that looked straightforward initially, antiangiogenesis has turned out to be more complex and nuanced than originally thought. Although VEGF seems to have a critical role in angiogenesis, our knowledge of the other molecular determinants of angiogenesis is still in its infancy. In fact, many of these pro- and antiangiogenic molecules are context- and dose-dependent. Additional studies are needed to understand these mechanisms and expand these findings to determine how to optimize these strategies for use in the management of patients with sarcoma. Ultimately, randomized studies are needed to demonstrate the benefit of angiogenesis inhibitors combined with chemotherapy.

Abbreviations

AA: antiangiogenic agents; COG: Children's Oncology Group; EGFR: epidermal growth factor receptor; ERK: extracellular signal-regulated kinase; IFP: interstitial fluid pressure; MAPK: mitogen-activated protein kinase; MVD: microvessel density; NSCLC: non-small cell lung cancer; PET: positron emission tomography; PDGFR: platelet-derived growth factor receptor; PFS: progression-free survival; STS: soft tissue sarcoma; VEGF(R): vascular endothelial growth factor (receptor).

Authors' contributions

Conception and design: all authors; collection and assembly of data: all authors; data analysis and interpretation: all authors; manuscript writing: all authors; final approval of manuscript: all authors; accountability for all aspects of the work: all authors. All authors read and approved the final manuscript.

Author details

[1] Department of Pediatrics, UCSF School of Medicine, San Francisco School of Medicine, UCSF Benioff Children's Hospital, University of California, 550 16th Street, 4th Floor, Box 0434, San Francisco, CA 94158, USA. [2] Dana-Farber/Boston Children's Cancer and Blood Disorders Center, 450 Brookline Avenue, Dana 3, Boston, MA 02215, USA.

Acknowledgements

The authors acknowledge the assistance of Diana Lim with graphic design.

Competing interests

The authors declare that they have no competing interests.

Funding

This work was supported in part by the Alex's Lemonade Stand Foundation (KTV, KKM, SGD), the Campini Foundation (KTV, KKM, SGD), and the Mildred V. Strouss Chair (KKM). The contents are solely the responsibility of the authors and do not necessarily represent the official views of the funding agencies.

References

1. Ganjoo K, Jacobs C. Antiangiogenesis agents in the treatment of soft tissue sarcomas. Cancer. 2010;116(5):1177–83.

2. DuBois S, Demetri G. Markers of angiogenesis and clinical features in patients with sarcoma. Cancer. 2007;109(5):813–9.

3. DuBois SG, Marina N, Glade-Bender J. Angiogenesis and vascular targeting in Ewing sarcoma: a review of preclinical and clinical data. Cancer. 2010;116(3):749–57.

4. Kerbel RS. Inhibition of tumor angiogenesis as a strategy to circumvent acquired resistance to anti-cancer therapeutic agents. BioEssays. 1991;13(1):31–6.

5. Boehm T, Folkman J, Browder T, O'Reilly MS. Antiangiogenic therapy of experimental cancer does not induce acquired drug resistance. Nature. 1997;390(6658):404–7.

6. Jain RK. Antiangiogenesis strategies revisited: from starving tumors to alleviating hypoxia. Cancer Cell. 2014;26(5):605–22.

7. Sleijfer S, Ray-Coquard I, Papai Z, Le Cesne A, Scurr M, Schoffski P, Collin F, Pandite L, Marreaud S, De Brauwer A, et al. Pazopanib, a multikinase angiogenesis inhibitor, in patients with relapsed or refractory advanced soft tissue sarcoma: a phase II study from the European organisation for research and treatment of cancer-soft tissue and bone sarcoma group (EORTC study 62043). J Clin Oncol. 2009;27(19):3126–32.

8. Carmeliet P, Jain RK. Angiogenesis in cancer and other diseases. Nature. 2000;407(6801):249–57.

9. Liekens S, De Clercq E, Neyts J. Angiogenesis: regulators and clinical applications. Biochem Pharmacol. 2001;61(3):253–70.

10. Goel S, Duda DG, Xu L, Munn LL, Boucher Y, Fukumura D, Jain RK. Normalization of the vasculature for treatment of cancer and other diseases. Physiol Rev. 2011;91(3):1071–121.

11. Tong RT, Boucher Y, Kozin SV, Winkler F, Hicklin DJ, Jain RK. Vascular normalization by vascular endothelial growth factor receptor 2 blockade induces a pressure gradient across the vasculature and improves drug penetration in tumors. Cancer Res. 2004;64(11):3731–6.

12. Winkler F, Kozin SV, Tong RT, Chae SS, Booth MF, Garkavtsev I, Xu L, Hicklin DJ, Fukumura D, di Tomaso E, et al. Kinetics of vascular normalization by VEGFR2 blockade governs brain tumor response to radiation: role of oxygenation, angiopoietin-1, and matrix metalloproteinases. Cancer Cell. 2004;6(6):553–63.

13. Yuan F, Chen Y, Dellian M, Safabakhsh N, Ferrara N, Jain RK. Time-dependent vascular regression and permeability changes in established human tumor xenografts induced by an anti-vascular endothelial growth factor/vascular permeability factor antibody. Proc Natl Acad Sci USA. 1996;93(25):14765–70.

14. Liu Y, Xia X, Zhou M, Liu X. Avastin(R) in combination with gemcitabine and cisplatin significantly inhibits tumor angiogenesis and increases the survival rate of human A549 tumor-bearing mice. Exp Ther Med. 2015;9(6):2180–4.

15. Dickson PV, Hamner JB, Sims TL, Fraga CH, Ng CY, Rajasekeran S, Hagedorn NL, McCarville MB, Stewart CF, Davidoff AM. Bevacizumab-induced transient remodeling of the vasculature in neuroblastoma xenografts results in improved delivery and efficacy of systemically administered chemotherapy. Clin Cancer Res. 2007;13(13):3942–50.

16. Vangestel C, Van de Wiele C, Van Damme N, Staelens S, Pauwels P, Reutelingsperger CP, Peeters M. (99)mTc-(CO)(3) His-annexin A5 microSPECT demonstrates increased cell death by irinotecan during the vascular normalization window caused by bevacizumab. J Nucl Med. 2011;52(11):1786–94.

17. Turley RS, Fontanella AN, Padussis JC, Toshimitsu H, Tokuhisa Y, Cho EH, Hanna G, Beasley GM, Augustine CK, Dewhirst MW, et al. Bevacizumab-induced alterations in vascular permeability and drug delivery: a novel approach to augment regional chemotherapy for in-transit melanoma. Clin Cancer Res. 2012;18(12):3328–39.

18. Chatterjee S, Wieczorek C, Schottle J, Siobal M, Hinze Y, Franz T, Florin A, Adamczak J, Heukamp LC, Neumaier B, et al. Transient antiangiogenic treatment improves delivery of cytotoxic compounds and therapeutic outcome in lung cancer. Cancer Res. 2014;74(10):2816–24.

19. Van der Veldt AA, Lubberink M, Bahce I, Walraven M, de Boer MP, Greuter HN, Hendrikse NH, Eriksson J, Windhorst AD, Postmus PE, et al. Rapid decrease in delivery of chemotherapy to tumors after anti-VEGF therapy: implications for scheduling of anti-angiogenic drugs. Cancer Cell. 2012;21(1):82–91.

20. Zhou Q, Gallo JM. Differential effect of sunitinib on the distribution of temozolomide in an orthotopic glioma model. Neuro Oncol. 2009;11(3):301–10.

21. Zhou Q, Guo P, Gallo JM. Impact of angiogenesis inhibition by sunitinib on tumor distribution of temozolomide. Clin Cancer Res. 2008;14(5):1540–9.

22. Paez-Ribes M, Man S, Xu P, Kerbel RS. Potential proinvasive or metastatic effects of preclinical antiangiogenic therapy are prevented by concurrent chemotherapy. Clin Cancer Res. 2015;21(24):5488–98.

23. Li Y, Yang X, Su LJ, Flaig TW. Pazopanib synergizes with docetaxel in the treatment of bladder cancer cells. Urology. 2011;78(1):233.

24. Augustine CK, Toshimitsu H, Jung SH, Zipfel PA, Yoo JS, Yoshimoto Y, Selim MA, Burchette J, Beasley GM, McMahon N, et al. Sorafenib, a multikinase inhibitor, enhances the response of melanoma to regional chemotherapy. Mol Cancer Ther. 2010;9(7):2090–101.

25. Troiani T, Lockerbie O, Morrow M, Ciardiello F, Eckhardt SG. Sequence-dependent inhibition of human colon cancer cell growth and of pro-survival pathways by oxaliplatin in combination with ZD6474 (Zactima), an inhibitor of VEGFR and EGFR tyrosine kinases. Mol Cancer Ther. 2006;5(7):1883–94.

26. Naumova E, Ubezio P, Garofalo A, Borsotti P, Cassis L, Riccardi E, Scanziani E, Eccles SA, Bani MR, Giavazzi R. The vascular targeting property of paclitaxel is enhanced by SU6668, a receptor tyrosine kinase inhibitor, causing apoptosis of endothelial cells and inhibition of angiogenesis. Clin Cancer Res. 2006;12(6):1839–49.

27. Humbert M, Casteran N, Letard S, Hanssens K, Iovanna J, Finetti P, Bertucci F, Bader T, Mansfield CD, Moussy A, et al. Masitinib combined with standard gemcitabine chemotherapy: in vitro and in vivo studies in human pancreatic tumour cell lines and ectopic mouse model. PLoS One. 2010;5(3):e9430.

28. Zhang L, Yu D, Hicklin DJ, Hannay JA, Ellis LM, Pollock RE. Combined anti-fetal liver kinase 1 monoclonal antibody and continuous low-dose doxorubicin inhibits angiogenesis and growth of human soft tissue sarcoma xenografts by induction of endothelial cell apoptosis. Cancer Res. 2002;62(7):2034–42.

29. Zhang L, Hannay JA, Liu J, Das P, Zhan M, Nguyen T, Hicklin DJ, Yu D, Pollock RE, Lev D. Vascular endothelial growth factor overexpression by soft tissue sarcoma cells: implications for tumor growth, metastasis, and chemoresistance. Cancer Res. 2006;66(17):8770–8.

30. Kumar S, Mokhtari RB, Sheikh R, Wu B, Zhang L, Xu P, Man S, Oliveira ID, Yeger H, Kerbel RS, et al. Metronomic oral topotecan with pazopanib is an active antiangiogenic regimen in mouse models of aggressive pediatric solid tumor. Clin Cancer Res. 2011;17(17):5656–67.

31. Ren W, Korchin B, Lahat G, Wei C, Bolshakov S, Nguyen T, Merritt W, Dicker A, Lazar A, Sood A, et al. Combined vascular endothelial growth factor receptor/epidermal growth factor receptor blockade with chemotherapy for treatment of local, uterine, and metastatic soft tissue sarcoma. Clin Cancer Res. 2008;14(17):5466–75.

32. Tang C, Hess K, Jardim DL, Gagliato Dde M, Tsimberidou AM, Falchook G, Fu S, Janku F, Naing A, Piha-Paul S, et al. Synergy between VEGF/VEGFR inhibitors and chemotherapy agents in the phase I clinic. Cancer Res. 2014;20(23):5956–63.

33. Johnson DH, Fehrenbacher L, Novotny WF, Herbst RS, Nemunaitis JJ, Jablons DM, Langer CJ, DeVore RF 3rd, Gaudreault J, Damico LA, et al. Randomized phase II trial comparing bevacizumab plus carboplatin and paclitaxel with carboplatin and paclitaxel alone in previously untreated locally advanced or metastatic non-small-cell lung cancer. J Clin Oncol. 2004;22(11):2184–91.

34. Miller KD, Chap LI, Holmes FA, Cobleigh MA, Marcom PK, Fehrenbacher L, Dickler M, Overmoyer BA, Reimann JD, Sing AP, et al. Randomized phase III trial of capecitabine compared with bevacizumab plus capecitabine in patients with previously treated metastatic breast cancer. J Clin Oncol. 2005;23(4):792–9.

35. Miller K, Wang M, Gralow J, Dickler M, Cobleigh M, Perez EA, Shenkier T, Cella D, Davidson NE. Paclitaxel plus bevacizumab versus paclitaxel alone for metastatic breast cancer. N Engl J Med. 2007;357(26):2666–76.

36. Pivot X, Schneeweiss A, Verma S, Thomssen C, Passos-Coelho JL, Benedetti G, Ciruelos E, von Moos R, Chang HT, Duenne AA, et al. Efficacy and safety of bevacizumab in combination with docetaxel for the first-line treatment of elderly patients with locally recurrent or metastatic breast cancer: results from AVADO. Eur J Cancer. 2011;47(16):2387–95.

37. Robert NJ, Dieras V, Glaspy J, Brufsky AM, Bondarenko I, Lipatov ON, Perez EA, Yardley DA, Chan SY, Zhou X, et al. RIBBON-1: randomized, double-blind, placebo-controlled, phase III trial of chemotherapy with or without bevacizumab for first-line treatment of human epidermal growth factor receptor 2-negative, locally recurrent or metastatic breast cancer. J Clin Oncol. 2011;29(10):1252–60.

38. Pignata S, Lorusso D, Scambia G, Sambataro D, Tamberi S, Cinieri S, Mosconi AM, Orditura M, Brandes AA, Arcangeli V, et al. Pazopanib plus weekly paclitaxel versus weekly paclitaxel alone for platinum-resistant or platinum-refractory advanced ovarian cancer (MITO 11): a randomised, open-label, phase 2 trial. Lancet Oncol. 2015;16(5):561–8.

39. Kabbinavar F, Hurwitz HI, Fehrenbacher L, Meropol NJ, Novotny WF, Lieberman G, Griffing S, Bergsland E. Phase II, randomized trial comparing bevacizumab plus fluorouracil (FU)/leucovorin (LV) with FU/LV alone in patients with metastatic colorectal cancer. J Clin Oncol. 2003;21(1):60–5.

40. Hurwitz H, Fehrenbacher L, Novotny W, Cartwright T, Hainsworth J, Heim W, Berlin J, Baron A, Griffing S, Holmgren E, et al. Bevacizumab plus irinotecan, fluorouracil, and leucovorin for metastatic colorectal cancer. N Engl J Med. 2004;350(23):2335–42.

41. Verschraegen CF, Arias-Pulido H, Lee SJ, Movva S, Cerilli LA, Eberhardt S, Schmit B, Quinn R, Muller CY, Rabinowitz I, et al. Phase IB study of the combination of docetaxel, gemcitabine, and bevacizumab in patients with advanced or recurrent soft tissue sarcoma: the Axtell regimen. Ann Oncol. 2012;23(3):785–90.

42. Wagner L, Turpin B, Nagarajan R, Weiss B, Cripe T, Geller J. Pilot study of vincristine, oral irinotecan, and temozolomide (VOIT regimen) combined with bevacizumab in pediatric patients with recurrent solid tumors or brain tumors. Pediatr Blood Cancer. 2013;60(9):1447–51.

43. Hainsworth JD, Firdaus ID, Earwood CB, Chua CC. Pazopanib and liposomal doxorubicin in the treatment of patients with relapsed/refractory epithelial ovarian cancer: a phase Ib study of the Sarah Cannon Research Institute. Cancer Invest. 2015;33(3):47–52.

44. Vergote I, Schilder RJ, Pippitt CH Jr, Wong S, Gordon AN, Scudder S, Kridelka F, Dirix L, Leach JW, Ananda S, et al. A phase 1b study of trebananib in combination with pegylated liposomal doxorubicin or topotecan in women with recurrent platinum-resistant or partially platinum-sensitive ovarian cancer. Gynecol Oncol. 2014;135(1):25–33.

45. D'Adamo DR, Anderson SE, Albritton K, Yamada J, Riedel E, Scheu K, Schwartz GK, Chen H, Maki RG. Phase II study of doxorubicin and bevacizumab for patients with metastatic soft-tissue sarcomas. J Clin Oncol. 2005;23(28):7135–42.

46. Mascarenhas L, Meyers WH, Lyden E, Rodeberg DA. Randomized phase II trial of bevacizumab and temsirolimus in combination with vinorelbine (V) and cyclophosphamide (C) for first relapse/disease progression of rhabdomyosarcoma (RMS): a report from the Children's Oncology Group (COG). J Clin Oncol. 2014;32:5s **(suppl; abstract 10003)**.

47. Ray-Coquard IL, Domont J, Tresch-Bruneel E, Bompas E, Cassier PA, Mir O, Piperno-Neumann S, Italiano A, Chevreau C, Cupissol D, et al. Paclitaxel given once per week with or without bevacizumab in patients with advanced angiosarcoma: a randomized phase ii trial. J Clin Oncol. 2015;33(25):2797–802.

48. Del Muro XG, Maurel J, Trufero JM, Lavernia J, Lopez-Pousa A, De Las Penas R, Cubedo R, Fra J, Casado A, De Juan A et al. Phase II trial of ifosfamide in combination with sorafenib in patients with advanced soft tissue sarcoma: A Spanish Group for Research on Sarcomas (GEIS) study. J Clin Oncol. 2013; 31. **(suppl; abstr 10523)**.

49. Jeng MR, Fuh B, Blatt J, Gupta A, Merrow AC, Hammill A, Adams D. Malignant transformation of infantile hemangioma to angiosarcoma: response to chemotherapy with bevacizumab. Pediatr Blood Cancer. 2014;61(11):2115–7.

50. Fuller CK, Charlson JA, Dankle SK, Russell TJ. Dramatic improvement of inoperable angiosarcoma with combination paclitaxel and bevacizumab chemotherapy. J Am Acad Dermatol. 2010;63(4):e83–4.

51. Hingorani P, Eshun F, White-Collins A, Watanabe M. Gemcitabine, docetaxel, and bevacizumab in relapsed and refractory pediatric sarcomas. J Pediatr Hematol Oncol. 2012;34(7):524–7.

52. Park MS, Patel SR, Ludwig JA, Trent JC, Conrad CA, Lazar AJ, Wang WL, Boonsirikamchai P, Choi H, Wang X, et al. Activity of temozolomide and bevacizumab in the treatment of locally advanced, recurrent, and metastatic hemangiopericytoma and malignant solitary fibrous tumor. Cancer. 2011;117(21):4939–47.

53. Kerbel RS, Kamen BA. The anti-angiogenic basis of metronomic chemotherapy. Nat Rev Cancer. 2004;4(6):423–36.

54. Penel N, Adenis A, Bocci G. Cyclophosphamide-based metronomic chemotherapy: after 10 years of experience, where do we stand and where are we going? Crit Rev Oncol Hematol. 2012;82(1):40–50.

55. Felgenhauer JL, Nieder ML, Krailo MD, Bernstein ML, Henry DW, Malkin D, Baruchel S, Chuba PJ, Sailer SL, Brown K, et al. A pilot study of low-dose anti-angiogenic chemotherapy in combination with standard multiagent chemotherapy for patients with newly diagnosed metastatic Ewing sarcoma family of tumors: a Children's Oncology Group (COG) Phase II study NCT00061893. Pediatr Blood Cancer. 2013;60(3):409–14.

56. Mir O, Domont J, Cioffi A, Bonvalot S, Boulet B, Le Pechoux C, Terrier P, Spielmann M, Le Cesne A. Feasibility of metronomic oral cyclophosphamide plus prednisolone in elderly patients with inoperable or metastatic soft tissue sarcoma. Eur J Cancer. 2011;47(4):515–9.

57. Italiano A, Toulmonde M, Lortal B, Stoeckle E, Garbay D, Kantor G, Kind M, Coindre JM, Bui B. "Metronomic" chemotherapy in advanced soft tissue sarcomas. Cancer Chemother Pharmacol. 2010;66(1):197–202.

58. Briasoulis E, Pappas P, Puozzo C, Tolis C, Fountzilas G, Dafni U, Marselos M, Pavlidis N. Dose-ranging study of metronomic oral vinorelbine in patients with advanced refractory cancer. Clin Cancer Res. 2009;15(20):6454–61.

59. Dalal S, Burchill SA. Preclinical evaluation of vascular-disrupting agents in Ewing's sarcoma family of tumours. Eur J Cancer. 2009;45(4):713–22.

60. Vistica DT, Hollingshead M, Borgel SD, Kenney S, Stockwin LH, Raffeld M, Schrump DS, Burkett S, Stone G, Butcher DO, et al. Therapeutic vulnerability of an in vivo model of alveolar soft part sarcoma (ASPS) to antiangiogenic therapy. J Pediatr Hematol Oncol. 2009;31(8):561–70.

61. Ma G, Masuzawa M, Hamada Y, Haraguchi F, Tamauchi H, Sakurai Y, Fujimura T, Katsuoka K. Treatment of murine angiosarcoma with etoposide, TNP-470 and prednisolone. J Dermatol Sci. 2000;24(2):126–33.

62. Jeong W, Park SR, Rapisarda A, Fer N, Kinders RJ, Chen A, Melillo G, Turkbey B, Steinberg SM, Choyke P, et al. Weekly EZN-2208 (PEGylated SN-38) in combination with bevacizumab in patients with refractory solid tumors. Invest New Drugs. 2014;32(2):340–6.

63. Tsimberidou AM, Adamopoulos AM, Ye Y, Piha-Paul S, Janku F, Fu S, Hong D, Falchook GS, Naing A, Wheler J, et al. Phase I clinical trial of bendamustine and bevacizumab for patients with advanced cancer. J Natl Compr Canc Netw. 2014;12(2):194–203.

64. Okada K, Yamasaki K, Tanaka C, Fujisaki H, Osugi Y, Hara J. Phase I study of bevacizumab plus irinotecan in pediatric patients with recurrent/refractory solid tumors. Jpn J Clin Oncol. 2013;43(11):1073–9.

65. Venkatramani R, Malogolowkin M, Davidson TB, May W, Sposto R, Mascarenhas L. A phase I study of vincristine, irinotecan, temozolomide and bevacizumab (vitb) in pediatric patients with relapsed solid tumors. PLoS One. 2013;8(7):e68416.

66. Navid F, Baker SD, McCarville MB, Stewart CF, Billups CA, Wu J, Davidoff AM, Spunt SL, Furman WL, McGregor LM, et al. Phase I and clinical pharmacology study of bevacizumab, sorafenib, and low-dose cyclophosphamide in children and young adults with refractory/recurrent solid tumors. Clin Cancer Res. 2013;19(1):236–46.

67. Jordan K, Wolf HH, Voigt W, Kegel T, Mueller LP, Behlendorf T, Sippel C, Arnold D, Schmoll HJ. Bevacizumab in combination with sequential high-dose chemotherapy in solid cancer, a feasibility study. Bone Marrow Transpl. 2010;45(12):1704–9.

68. Dieras V, Bachelot T, Campone M, Isambert N, Joly F, LeTourneau C, Cassier PA, Bompas E, Fumoleau P, Noal S, et al. Pazopanib (P) and cisplatin (CDDP) in patients with advanced solid tumors: a UNICANCER phase I study. J Clin Oncol. 2014;32:2583.

69. Kerklaan BM, Lolkema MP, Devriese LA, Voest EE, Nol-Boekel A, Mergui-Roelvink M, Mykulowycz K, Stoebenau JE, Fang L, Legenne P, et al. Phase I study of safety, tolerability, and pharmacokinetics of pazopanib in combination with oral topotecan in patients with advanced solid tumors. J Clin Oncol. 2013;31:2536.

70. Hamberg P, Boers-Sonderen MJ, van der Graaf WT, de Bruijn P, Suttle AB, Eskens FA, Verweij J, van Herpen CM, Sleijfer S. Pazopanib exposure decreases as a result of an ifosfamide-dependent drug-drug interaction: results of a phase I study. Br J Cancer. 2014;110(4):888–93.

71. Burris HA 3rd, Dowlati A, Moss RA, Infante JR, Jones SF, Spigel DR, Levinson KT, Lindquist D, Gainer SD, Dar MM, et al. Phase I study of pazopanib in combination with paclitaxel and carboplatin given every 21 days in patients with advanced solid tumors. Mol Cancer Ther. 2012;11(8):1820–8.

72. Michael M, Vlahovic G, Khamly K, Pierce KJ, Guo F, Olszanski AJ. Phase Ib study of CP-868,596, a PDGFR inhibitor, combined with docetaxel with or without axitinib, a VEGFR inhibitor. Br J Cancer. 2010;103(10):1554–61.

73. Martin LK, Bekaii-Saab T, Serna D, Monk P, Clinton SK, Grever MR, Kraut EH. A phase I dose escalation and pharmacodynamic study of SU5416

74. (semaxanib) combined with weekly cisplatin and irinotecan in patients with advanced solid tumors. Onkologie. 2013;36(11):657–60.

74. Meany HJ, Dome J, Hinds PS, Bagatell R, Shusterman S, Widemann BC, Stern E, London WB, Kim A, Fox E, et al. Phase 1 study of sorafenib and irinotecan in pediatric patients with relapsed or refractory solid tumors. J Clin Oncol. 2014;32:10052.

75. Blais N, Camidge DR, Jonker DJ, Soulieres D, Laurie SA, Diab SG, Ruiz-Garcia A, Thall A, Zhang K, Chao RC, et al. Sunitinib combined with pemetrexed and carboplatin in patients with advanced solid malignancies–results of a phase I dose-escalation study. Invest New Drugs. 2013;31(6):1487–98.

76. Brell JM, Krishnamurthi SS, Rath L, Bokar JA, Savvides P, Gibbons J, Cooney MM, Meropol NJ, Ivy P, Dowlati A. Phase I trial of sunitinib and gemcitabine in patients with advanced solid tumors. Cancer Chemother Pharmacol. 2012;70(4):547–53.

77. Hamberg P, Steeghs N, Loos WJ, van de Biessen D, den Hollander M, Tascilar M, Verweij J, Gelderblom H, Sleijfer S. Decreased exposure to sunitinib due to concomitant administration of ifosfamide: results of a phase I and pharmacokinetic study on the combination of sunitinib and ifosfamide in patients with advanced solid malignancies. Br J Cancer. 2010;102(12):1699–706.

78. Boven E, Massard C, Armand JP, Tillier C, Hartog V, Brega NM, Countouriotis AM, Ruiz-Garcia A, Soria JC. A phase I, dose-finding study of sunitinib in combination with irinotecan in patients with advanced solid tumours. Br J Cancer. 2010;103(7):993–1000.

79. Robert F, Sandler A, Schiller JH, Liu G, Harper K, Verkh L, Huang X, Ilagan J, Tye L, Chao R, et al. Sunitinib in combination with docetaxel in patients with advanced solid tumors: a phase I dose-escalation study. Cancer Chemother Pharmacol. 2010;66(4):669–80.

80. Eskens FA, Tresca P, Tosi D, Van Doorn L, Fontaine H, Van der Gaast A, Veyrat-Follet C, Oprea C, Hospitel M, Dieras V. A phase I pharmacokinetic study of the vascular disrupting agent ombrabulin (AVE8062) and docetaxel in advanced solid tumours. Br J Cancer. 2014;110(9):2170–7.

81. Gietema JA, Hoekstra R, de Vos FY, Uges DR, van der Gaast A, Groen HJ, Loos WJ, Knight RA, Carr RA, Humerickhouse RA, et al. A phase I study assessing the safety and pharmacokinetics of the thrombospondin-1-mimetic angiogenesis inhibitor ABT-510 with gemcitabine and cisplatin in patients with solid tumors. Ann Oncol. 2006;17(8):1320–7.

82. Hoekstra R, de Vos FY, Eskens FA, de Vries EG, Uges DR, Knight R, Carr RA, Humerickhouse R, Verweij J, Gietema JA. Phase I study of the thrombospondin-1-mimetic angiogenesis inhibitor ABT-510 with 5-fluorouracil and leucovorin: a safe combination. Eur J Cancer. 2006;42(4):467–72.

83. Tran HT, Blumenschein GR Jr, Lu C, Meyers CA, Papadimitrakopoulou V, Fossella FV, Zinner R, Madden T, Smythe LG, Puduvalli VK, et al. Clinical and pharmacokinetic study of TNP-470, an angiogenesis inhibitor, in combination with paclitaxel and carboplatin in patients with solid tumors. Cancer Chemother Pharmacol. 2004;54(4):308–14.

17

Radiation induced angiosarcoma of the breast: outcomes from a retrospective case series

R. B. Cohen-Hallaleh, H. G. Smith, R. C. Smith, G. F. Stamp, O. Al-Muderis, K. Thway, A. Miah, K. Khabra, I. Judson, R. Jones, C. Benson and A. J. Hayes*

Abstract

Background: Radiation induced angiosarcoma (RIAS) of the breast is a rare and aggressive complication of radiotherapy. Due to the rarity of this disease, much of the evidence for its management is based on case reports or small retrospective series. We sought to describe the management and outcomes of RIAS in a large single-institution series.

Methods: All patients diagnosed with RIAS between January 2000 and January 2014 were identified from an institutional database.

Results: A total of 49 patients were identified. Median age at diagnosis was 72 years (range 51–93). Median time from completion of radiotherapy to diagnosis of RIAS was 7.5 years. Median tumour size at presentation was 5.0 cm (1.5–19.0). The majority of patients presented with localised disease (47, 95.9%). Of these, 35 (74.5%) were suitable for surgery and underwent surgery with curative intent. Twelve patients presented with localised irresectable disease. Of these, 7 received systemic chemotherapy, with a sufficient response to facilitate surgery in 3 patients. Following potentially curative surgery, 2-year local recurrence-free was 55.2%. Survival was significantly prolonged in patients presenting with resectable disease (2-year overall survival 71.1% vs 33.3%, $p < 0.001$). Tumour size >5 cm was prognostic of distant metastases-free survival and overall survival.

Conclusion: RIAS are rare, aggressive soft-tissue lesions with limited treatment options and high-rates of both local and systemic relapse.

Keywords: Radiation, Angiosarcoma, Breast

Background

Radiation-induced angiosarcoma of the breast (RIAS) is a rare and late complication of radiotherapy for breast cancer. In those patients undergoing breast conserving surgery with adjuvant radiotherapy, the estimated incidence of RIAS is 0.05–0.3% [1–4]. Although still rare, the incidence of RIAS appears to be increasing, perhaps reflecting the long latency period for the development of these tumours following the widespread adoption of adjuvant radiotherapy for breast cancer. In a large population-based cohort study, a history of prior radiotherapy as a treatment for breast cancer was associated with 26-fold increase in the risk of developing angiosarcoma when compared with non-irradiated controls [5]. The prognosis for patients with RIAS remains poor, with 5-year overall survival rates ranging from 27 to 48% [2]. Surgery, in the form of wide excision or mastectomy, is the mainstay of management in localised disease. Some studies have reported an association between R0 margins and improved survival, although this was not demonstrated to be independent of other biological factors such as tumour size [6, 7]. Although there is some evidence that neoadjuvant chemotherapy may improve outcomes in angiosarcoma, the rarity of this condition limits such evidence to case reports or small retrospective series [8–12]. The purpose of this study was to describe the

*Correspondence: Andrew.Hayes@rmh.nhs.uk
The Sarcoma Unit, The Royal Marsden Hospital NHS Foundation Trust, London, UK

management and outcomes of patients presenting with RIAS of the breast within a large single-institution case series.

Methods

All patients treated with a diagnosis of RIAS at The Royal Marsden Hospital between January 2000 and January 2014 were identified from a prospectively maintained database. Ethical approval was obtained from an institutional review board. RIAS was defined as a histologically proven diagnosis of angiosarcoma occurring in a patient with a history of irradiation of the surgical field following breast-conserving surgery for breast cancer.

Operative strategy

Patients either underwent their initial surgical management at The Royal Marsden Hospital or were referred following an initial resection elsewhere. All patients undergoing surgery at The Royal Marsden Hospital were discussed at a sarcoma multidisciplinary meeting pre-operatively. Patients were classified as having resectable disease if pre-operative assessment indicated that a 2 cm or greater negative margin could be achieved by surgery with or without plastic surgical reconstruction in the form of a single pedicled or free myocutaneous flap. If the desired negative margins would require more extensive reconstruction, such as with extensive resurfacing by large skin grafting, the patient was classified as having irresectable disease. Rapidly progressive disease, where disease volume increased over a time span of 2–3 weeks from being suitable for mastectomy alone or in combination with a pedicled flap to requiring more extensive reconstruction, was also judged irresectable in oncological terms. Pre-operative 4-quadrant punch biopsies were performed to confirm that the planned surgical margins were not involved by microscopically occult disease. Macroscopically complete resection was judged by the operating surgeon. Histologically, the resection was classified as R0 (microscopically negative) if the negative margins were >1 mm circumferentially or R1 (microscopically positive) if tumour extended to or within 1 mm of the resection margin.

Statistical analyses

The latency period to the development of RIAS was defined as the time from the date of completion of radiotherapy to the date of a histological diagnosis of RIAS. Local recurrence-free survival (LRFS) was defined as the time from histological diagnosis to the development of a local recurrence or last follow-up. Distant metastases-free survival (DMFS) was defined as the time from histological diagnosis to the development of distant metastases or last follow-up. Overall survival (OS)

was defined as the time from histological diagnosis to the date of death or last follow-up. Survival curves were constructed using the Kaplan–Meier method and compared with the log-rank test. A univariate Cox regression analysis was used to investigate the following potential prognostic variables of LRFS, DMFS and OS: age; margin status; tumour size; treatment (surgery versus surgery and adjuvant chemotherapy). Potentially confounding factors ($p < 0.1$) were then combined in a multivariate analysis with forward stepwise combination methods. The results of these analyses are presented as hazard ratios (HR) with 95% confidence intervals (CI).

Results

A total of 49 patients with a confirmed diagnosis of RIAS were identified during the study period. Patient demographics, primary breast cancer characteristics and treatment for primary breast cancer are outlined in Table 1. All patients were female, with a median age at diagnosis of RIAS of 72 years (range 51–93 years). The median time from completion of radiation therapy to the diagnosis of RIAS was 7.5 (range 1–26) years, with a median maximal tumour dimension of 5.0 cm (range 1.5–19.0 cm). None of the patients in this study had active breast cancer at the time of RIAS diagnosis, nor did any develop recurrent breast cancer during follow-up.

The majority of patients presented with localised disease (47 patients, 95.9%). Of these, 35 patients had

Table 1 Primary breast cancer characteristics and treatment in patients who developed RIAS

	N = 49 (%)
Median age at RIAS diagnosis (range)	72 (51–93)
Primary breast cancer histology	
Infiltrating ductal carcinoma	25 (51.0)
Infiltrating lobular carcinoma	3 (6.1)
Ductal carcinoma in situ	1 (2.0)
Unspecified	20 (40.8)
Surgery for primary breast cancer	
Wide local excision (WLE)	18 (36.7)
WLE and axillary lymph node dissection	29 (59.2)
Mastectomy	1 (2.0)
Mastectomy and LD flap reconstruction	1 (2.0)
Adjuvant therapies	
Chemotherapy	10 (20.4)
Endocrine therapy	36 (73.5)
Trastuzumab	3 (6.1)
Radiation dose (Gy) (range)	
Primary median	50 (40–54)
Boost median	12.5 (10–16)

LD latissimus dorsi

resectable disease at presentation and underwent surgery with curative intent (74.5%). 25 patients (74.3%) underwent their initial operation at The Royal Marsden Hospital with 10 patients (25.7%) initially treated elsewhere. Of the 10 patients undergoing initial surgery elsewhere, 8 had a simple mastectomy, with 2 undergoing mastectomy with immediate plastic reconstruction with a pedicled flap (20.0%). Of the 25 patients undergoing initial surgery at The Royal Marsden Hospital, 9 had a simple mastectomy, with 16 undergoing a mastectomy with immediate plastic reconstruction (64.0%). A microscopically complete R0 resection was performed in 32 patients (91.4%). No further therapy was given to the majority of these patients, with 2 patients receiving adjuvant chemotherapy following surgery. The decision to give adjuvant chemotherapy was made based on the extent of disease, with 1 patient requiring both a pedicled flap and skin grafting to achieve macroscopic clearance and the other having a positive deep margin on the chest wall. Interestingly, neither of these patients developed local recurrence, though both subsequently relapsed systemically.

The remaining 12 patients with localised disease at presentation were considered to have irresectable disease (25.5%). Of these, 4 patients declined or were unfit for further intervention and received best supportive care (33.3%). Debulking surgery was performed in 1 patient for symptomatic palliation. This patient presented with large volume, fungating disease and a mastectomy was performed with no prospect of achieving clearance of all macroscopic skin changes. The remaining 7 patients were treated with systemic therapy, with 2 patients treated with doxorubicin and 5 patients receiving weekly paclitaxel. A sufficient response, downsizing the tumour to allow a potentially curative resection to be performed, was achieved in 3 patients. Local disease control was achieved in 2 of these patients, although both subsequently developed distant metastases.

Two patients presented with metastatic RIAS. The first patient presented with hepatic metastases and died following spontaneous haemorrhage from these lesions 5 months after diagnosis. The second patient with metastatic hilar and axillary lymphadenopathy responded well to paclitaxel chemotherapy and was disease free after 20 months follow-up.

Outcomes

Of the 35 patients undergoing surgery for locally resectable disease, 18 developed a local recurrence (51.4%), 8 of whom presented with a synchronous systemic relapse (22.9%). 2-year LRFS was with 51.2% (95% CI 33.2–67.2). Of these 18 patients, 17 had microscopically negative margins following their initial surgery (94.4%). Resection margins in those patients who went on to develop local recurrence were significantly closer than those who did not (median clearance 1.0 cm vs 2.5 cm, p = 0.003, unpaired t test). All but 1 patient who developed local recurrence had less than 2 cm clearance. No difference in the proportion of patients developing local recurrence was noted in those undergoing reconstructive surgery and those closed primarily (44.4% vs 55.6%, p = 0.505, Fisher's exact test). A further 7 patients developed isolated distant metastases, giving a systemic failure rate of 42.9%. 2-year DMFS was 67.3% (95% CI 48.6–80.5). At the time of writing, 20 patients had died (57.1%) with a 2-year OS of 71.1% (95% CI 52.9–83.3).

Of the 12 patients with irresectable localised disease, 4 developed distant metastases (33.3%), with a 2-year DMFS of 57.3% (95% CI 21.6–81.7). At the time of writing, 11 of these patients had died (91.7%) with a 2-year OS of 33.3% (95% CI 10.3–58.8). Overall survival of patients with irresectable localised disease was significantly shorter than those with resectable disease (median OS 18 months vs 37 months, p < 0.001, log-rank test) (Fig. 1).

Univariate analyses were performed to identify prognostic factors of oncological outcomes in patients with resectable localised disease at presentation. The results are summarised in Tables 2 and 3. Tumour size and margin status were prognostic of DMFS on univariate analysis. However, with multivariate analysis, only tumour size remained prognostic of DMFS. Tumour size was also prognostic for OS, with no prognostic factors for LRFS identified.

Discussion

The widespread adoption of breast-conserving surgery and adjuvant radiotherapy in the management of primary breast cancer has been accompanied by a steady

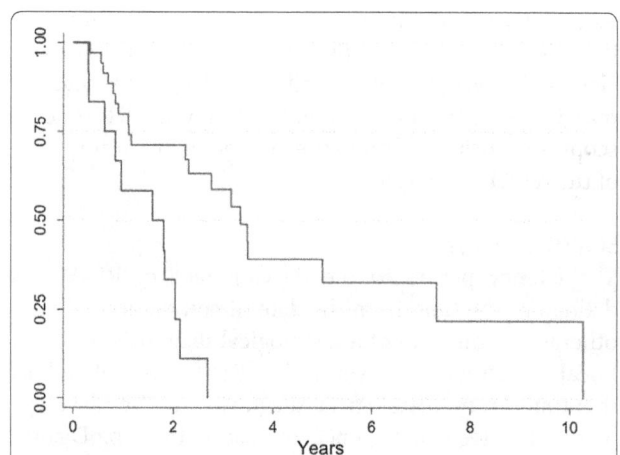

Fig. 1 Overall survival from diagnosis of RIAS in patients with localised resectable (*blue*) and localised irrespectable (*red*) disease (p < 0.001, log-rank test)

Table 2 Univariate and multivariate Cox regressional analyses for prognostic factors of distant metastases-free survival in patients with localised resectable RIAS

Variable	Univariate		Multivariate	
	HR (95% CI)	p value	HR (95% CI)	p value
Age (years)				
<70	Reference	–	*	*
≥70	1.06 (0.98–1.15)	0.146	*	*
Positive margins				
No	Reference	–	*	*
Yes	4.20 (1.12–15.67)	0.033	*	*
Tumour size (cm)				
<5	Reference	–	Reference	–
≥5	5.70 (1.18–27.50)	0.030	5.70 (1.18–27.50)	0.030
Treatment				
Surgery	Reference	–	*	*
Surgery + chemotherapy	2.08 (0.46–9.51)	0.344	*	*

*Not included in model generated by forward stepwise combination

Table 3 Univariate Cox regressional analyses for prognostic factors of overall survival in patients with localised resectable RIAS

Variable	HR (95% CI)	p value
Age (years)		
<70	Reference	–
≥70	1.94 (0.77–4.91)	0.161
Positive margins		
No	Reference	–
Yes	1.17 (0.27–5.10)	0.837
Tumour size (cm)		
<5	Reference	–
≥5	5.18 (1.41–19.0)	0.013
Treatment		
Surgery	Reference	–
Surgery + chemotherapy	1.53 (0.35–6.72)	0.575

increase in the incidence of RIAS of the breast. RIAS is typically a late complication of adjuvant radiotherapy, with a median latency of 7.5 years in our institutional series, although there is considerable variation in the time to presentation, ranging from 1 to 26 years. These findings are consistent with those previously reported in the literature and due to the substantial variability in the latency of this disease, a high index of suspicion is warranted for any patient undergoing adjuvant radiotherapy in this context [1, 3, 13].

Surgery, in the form of mastectomy with or without plastic reconstruction, is the modality of choice in patients presenting with localised disease and achieved microscopically complete (R0) resection margins in more than 90% of patients in the current series. Despite this, the majority of patients developed local recurrence with a 2-year recurrence free survival of 55%. RIAS typically present as multifocal lesions and the propensity for this pathology to form microsatellite deposits may contribute to the difficulty in obtaining local control [3, 6, 14, 15]. The importance of performing a complete pathological resection has been stressed in the literature, although no standard guidelines regarding the recommended distance of clearance have been published [3, 16–18]. In the current series, those who developed local recurrence were found to have closer margins than those who did not, with only 1 of the 18 (5.6%) patients who recurred locally having more than 2 cm circumferential clearance. However, marginal status was not found to be independently prognostic of oncological outcomes in this series. This would suggest that the ability to achieve greater margins is dependent on other biological tumour factors that also determine outcome, such a size. Accordingly, no difference in local recurrence rates was noted between patients undergoing plastic reconstruction and those closed primarily. It is likely that the major determinant of outcome in RIAS is tumour biology and, although the initial surgery should aim for macroscopic clearance, it should be cautioned that achieving greater negative margins does not necessarily equate to improved patient outcomes.

Despite the majority of patients presenting with localised disease that was amenable to surgery, the rates of local and systemic relapse in RIAS are high. Tumour size was identified as the only independent prognostic factor of outcomes in this series, being associated with both DMFS and OS. A meta-analysis of patients with RIAS also identified tumour size as an important prognostic factor, being associated with LRFS and, alongside patient age, with OS [19]. As may be expected, poorer survival outcomes were noted in patients presenting with locally advanced disease unsuitable for surgical management in our series. These factors highlight the importance of early diagnosis in this patient group. Angiosarcomas often present insidiously with purple or red skin changes and may be easily mistaken for bruising or benign skin changes leading to delayed investigation and diagnosis (Fig. 2). Early detection and prompt referral may potentially reduce the number of patients presenting with irresectable disease and improve both local and distant disease control.

The role of peri-operative chemotherapy in the management of RIAS remains to be clarified. In the current series, of the 7 patients treated with neoadjuvant chemotherapy for localised irresectable disease, 3 patients achieved a sufficient response to facilitate surgery. Similar results were noted in the Phase II ANGIOTAX study, in which 30 patients with localised irresectable or metastatic angiosarcoma were treated with paclitaxel [20]. Five patients had partial responses, 3 of whom had localised irresectable lesions in the breast that were rendered resectable following treatment. On histopathological assessment of the resection specimens, 2 of these patients had achieved a complete histological response.

The use of neo/adjuvant chemotherapy was also found to be associated with improved local disease control in a large retrospective series of patients with radiation-induced sarcomas of all sites, although not associated with improved rates of systemic relapse or survival [3]. Adjuvant chemotherapy was not found to produce a benefit in terms of local control or overall survival study of high-risk soft-tissue sarcomas treated with surgery and radiation [21]. As such, there is limited evidence to suggest that neo/adjuvant chemotherapy produces a survival benefit in RIAS, although it certainly may be of use as an induction therapy prior to surgery in those presenting with locally advanced disease and may offer patients effective disease palliation in addition. Targeted therapies may offer an alternative treatment in patients with progressive disease, with the tyrosine kinase inhibitor pazopanib demonstrating activity in both locally advanced and metastatic angiosarcoma [22].

RIAS are rare, aggressive soft-tissue lesions with limited treatment options and high-rates of both local and systemic relapse. Neoadjuvant chemotherapy may have a role in downsizing locally advanced disease although has no proven effect on survival.

Authors' contributions

Study concept and design: AJH, CB, AM, IJ, RJ, KT. Acquisition, analysis and interpretation of data: RC, HS, RS, GS, OA, KK. Drafting, revising and approving manuscript: RC, HS, RS, GS, OA, KT, AM, KK, IJ, RJ, CB, AJH. All authors read and approved the final manuscript.

Competing interests

The authors declare that they have no competing interests.

Funding

No funding was received for this study.

References

1. Monroe AT, Feigenberg SJ, Mendenhall NP. Angiosarcoma after breast-conserving therapy. Cancer. 2003;97(8):1832–40.
2. Sheth GR, Cranmer LD, Smith BD, Grasso-Lebeau L, Lang JE. Radiation-induced sarcoma of the breast: a systematic review. Oncologist. 2012;17(3):405–18.
3. Torres KE, Ravi V, Kin K, Yi M, Guadagnolo BA, May CD, et al. Long-term outcomes in patients with radiation-associated angiosarcomas of the breast following surgery and radiotherapy for breast cancer. Ann Surg Oncol. 2013;20(4):1267–74.
4. West JG, Qureshi A, West JE, Chacon M, Sutherland ML, Haghighi B, et al. Risk of angiosarcoma following breast conservation: a clinical alert. Breast J. 2005;11(2):115–23.
5. Huang J, Mackillop WJ. Increased risk of soft tissue sarcoma after radiotherapy in women with breast carcinoma. Cancer. 2001;92(1):172–80.
6. Jallali N, James S, Searle A, Ghattaura A, Hayes A, Harris P. Surgical management of radiation-induced angiosarcoma after breast conservation therapy. Am J Surg. 2012;203(2):156–61.
7. Lindet C, Neuville A, Penel N, Lae M, Michels JJ, Trassard M, et al. Localised angiosarcomas: the identification of prognostic factors and analysis of treatment impact. A retrospective analysis from the French Sarcoma Group (GSF/GETO). Eur J Cancer. 2013;49(2):369–76.

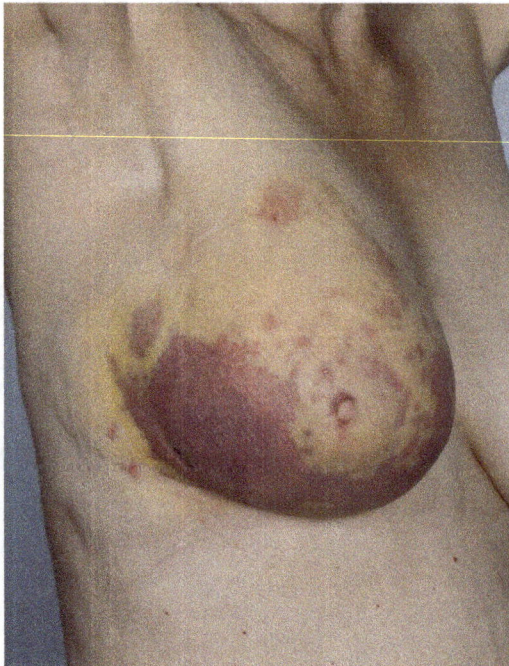

Fig. 2 The typical appearances of radiation-induced angiosarcoma of the breast

8. Alvarado-Miranda A, Bacon-Fonseca L, Ulises Lara-Medina F, Maldonado-Martinez H, Arce-Salinas C. Thalidomide combined with neoadjuvant chemotherapy in angiosarcoma of the breast with complete pathologic response: case report and review of literature. Breast Care. 2013;8(1):74–6.

9. Oxenberg J, Khushalani NI, Salerno KE, Attwood K, Kane JM 3rd. Neoadjuvant chemotherapy for primary cutaneous/soft tissue angiosarcoma: determining tumor behavior prior to surgical resection. J Surg Oncol. 2015;111(7):829–33.

10. Quadros CA, Vasconcelos A, Andrade R, Ramos RS, Studart E, Nascimento G, et al. Good outcome after neoadjuvant chemotherapy and extended surgical resection for a large radiation-induced high-grade breast sarcoma. Int Semin Surg Oncol. 2006;3:18.

11. Young RJ, Brown NJ, Reed MW, Hughes D, Woll PJ. Angiosarcoma. Lancet Oncol. 2010;11(10):983–91.

12. Zemanova M, Machalekova K, Sandorova M, Boljesikova E, Skulte-tyova M, Svec J, et al. Clinical management of secondary angiosarcoma after breast conservation therapy. Rep Pract Oncol Radiother. 2014;19(1):37–46.

13. Styring E, Fernebro J, Jonsson PE, Ehinger A, Engellau J, Rissler P, et al. Changing clinical presentation of angiosarcomas after breast cancer: from late tumors in edematous arms to earlier tumors on the thoracic wall. Breast Cancer Res Treat. 2010;122(3):883–7.

14. Seinen JM, Styring E, Verstappen V, Vult von Steyern F, Rydholm A, Suurmeijer AJ, et al. Radiation-associated angiosarcoma after breast cancer: high recurrence rate and poor survival despite surgical treatment with R0 resection. Ann Surg Oncol. 2012;19(8):2700–6.

15. Shah S, Rosa M. Radiation-associated angiosarcoma of the breast: clinical and pathologic features. Arch Pathol Lab Med. 2016;140(5):477–81.

16. Billings SD, McKenney JK, Folpe AL, Hardacre MC, Weiss SW. Cutaneous angiosarcoma following breast-conserving surgery and radiation: an analysis of 27 cases. Am J Surg Pathol. 2004;28(6):781–8.

17. Brenn T, Fletcher CD. Radiation-associated cutaneous atypical vascular lesions and angiosarcoma: clinicopathologic analysis of 42 cases. Am J Surg Pathol. 2005;29(8):983–96.

18. Lindford A, Bohling T, Vaalavirta L, Tenhunen M, Jahkola T, Tukiainen E. Surgical management of radiation-associated cutaneous breast angiosarcoma. J Plast Reconstr Aesthet Surg. 2011;64(8):1036–42.

19. Depla AL, Scharloo-Karels CH, de Jong MA, Oldenborg S, Kolff MW, Oei SB, et al. Treatment and prognostic factors of radiation-associated angiosarcoma (RAAS) after primary breast cancer: a systematic review. Eur J Cancer. 2014;50(10):1779–88.

20. Penel N, Bui BN, Bay JO, Cupissol D, Ray-Coquard I, Piperno-Neumann S, et al. Phase II trial of weekly paclitaxel for unresectable angiosarcoma: the ANGIOTAX Study. J Clin Oncol. 2008;26(32):5269–74.

21. Woll PJ, Reichardt P, Le Cesne A, Bonvalot S, Azzarelli A, Hoekstra HJ, et al. Adjuvant chemotherapy with doxorubicin, ifosfamide, and lenograstim for resected soft-tissue sarcoma (EORTC 62931): a multicentre randomised controlled trial. Lancet Oncol. 2012;13(10):1045–54.

22. Kollar A, Jones RL, Stacchiotti S, Gelderblom H, Guida M, Grignani G, et al. Pazopanib in advanced vascular sarcomas: an EORTC Soft Tissue and Bone Sarcoma Group (STBSG) retrospective analysis. Acta Oncol. 2017;56(1):88–92.

18

Low-grade central fibroblastic osteosarcoma may be differentiated from its mimicker desmoplastic fibroma by genetic analysis

Wangzhao Song[1], Eva van den Berg[2], Thomas C. Kwee[3], Paul C. Jutte[4], Anne-Marie Cleton-Jansen[5], Judith V. M. G. Bovée[5] and Albert J. Suurmeijer[1]* (ORCID)

Abstract

Background: We studied two cases of rare fibrous bone tumors, namely desmoplastic fibroma (DF) and low-grade central osteosarcoma (LGCOS) resembling desmoplastic fibroma (DF-like LGOS). As the clinical presentation, imaging features and histopathology of DF and DF-like LGOS show much overlap, the objective of this study was to investigate the value of cytogenetic analysis, molecular pathology and immunohistochemistry in discrimination of these two mimickers.

Case presentation: A mutation in *CTNNB* (S45F) and nuclear beta-catenin immunostaining were observed in DF. DF-LGCOS had amplification of *CDK4* and showed strong nuclear expression of CDK4 by IHC. Moreover, the karyotype of DF-LGCOS showed an interstitial heterozygous deletion of the long arm of chromosome 13 (q12q32), associated with loss of the *RB1* tumor suppressor gene.

Conclusions: Karyotyping and molecular genetic analysis may contribute to a conclusive diagnosis.

Keywords: Bone sarcoma, Desmoplastic fibroma, Low-grade osteosarcoma, CDK4, RB1

Background

The histopathological diagnosis of bone tumors is usually rather straightforward, since the most common bone tumors show differentiation along osteoblastic or chondroblastic lines, and form bone matrix or cartilage, which usually can be easily detected in routinely stained tissue sections.

In the past decades, advances in the field of immunohistochemistry (IHC) and molecular pathology have allowed a precise diagnosis in difficult cases. Examples are IHC for *SATB2* to confirm a tentative diagnosis of osteosarcoma, molecular DNA analysis for nonrandom gene translocations to differentiate Ewing sarcoma from other round cell sarcomas, and detection of *H3F3A* mutations to accurately diagnose giant cell tumor of bone.

However, for fibrous tumors of bone the incremental value of IHC and DNA methods over standard basic histology is rather limited. This category of fibrous tumors of bone includes the desmoplastic fibroma (DF)—a rare, locally aggressive tumor—and fibrosarcoma—a tumor once considered to be very common, but currently a diagnosis of exclusion, that one is only allowed to make after having ruled out other spindle cell tumors, e.g. low grade myofibroblastic sarcoma, myoepithelial tumors, follicular dendritic cell tumors, synovial sarcoma, and, last but not least, a rare variant of low-grade central osteosarcoma (LGCOS) resembling desmoplastic fibroma (DF-like LGCOS).

By co-incidence, two patients with these rare bone tumors (DF and DF-LGCOS) were treated in our

*Correspondence: a.j.h.suurmeijer@umcg.nl
[1] Department of Pathology and Medical Biology, University Medical Center Groningen, University of Groningen, P.O. Box 30.001, 9700 RB Groningen, The Netherlands
Full list of author information is available at the end of the article

sarcoma center in the same week. In addition to IHC, we decided to apply classic cytogenetics and next generation sequencing (NGS), which proved to be very helpful in discriminating these two morphologic mimickers.

Case presentation

Case 1: a 10-year-old girl, with a history of distal radius fracture 3 years earlier, presented with a firm, nontender swelling in the same right distal forearm. Her wrist function was unimpaired. As shown in Fig. 1, X-ray examination revealed a large lobulated, compartmentalized, osteolytic, expansive tumor mass in the metadiaphysis of the distal radius. On MRI, the tumor measured $35 \times 46 \times 47$ mm and had a well-defined boundary, but no sclerotic margin. Starting from the distal radius, there was cortical destruction, an extensive soft tissue component, and impression and bowing of the distal ulna. There were no imaging signs of invasive growth, necrosis or fluid-liquid mirrors. Bone scintigraphy did not show increased uptake at the location of the lesion. These imaging features were consistent with a destructive tumor that originated from the distal radius, grew slowly, and then broke through the cortex of the radius into the adjacent soft tissue. The tumor was excised intralesionally. Grossly, the largest tumor fragment measured $6 \times 5 \times 3$ cm. On cut surface the tumor tissue was pale and fibrous.

Tumor histology was reminiscent of desmoid fibromatosis and consistent with desmoplastic fibroma, as it showed a lesion composed of bundles of moderately cellular, collagenous tumor tissue with fibroblastic spindle cells with oval, monomorphic nuclei with bland, finely granular chromatin, small nucleoli and ample cytoplasm. Mitoses were not found (Fig. 2a).

Cytogenetic analysis revealed a normal female karyotype in 18 cells, with trisomy 8 detected in 2 cells (Fig. 2b).

The cancer hotspot NGS analysis revealed a CTNNB1 hotspot class 5 pathogenic variant in exon 3: p.Ser45Phe and, using IHC, the fibroblastic tumor cells showed more than focal nuclear staining for beta-catenin (Fig. 2c), in support of a diagnosis of desmoplastic fibroma.

Case 2: a 24-year-old woman presented with progressive pain in the right hip region that had existed for 1 year. X-ray images showed an osteolytic tumor in the metadiaphysis of the right distal femur with cortical bone destruction on the dorsolateral side. The central part of the tumor had no matrix calcification. On MRI, the tumor destroyed the cortex and extended to the surrounding soft tissues. There was strong tumor enhancement after administration of intravenous gadolinium (Fig. 3a). A resection of the right distal femur was performed. The tumor in the distal femur measured 12×4 cm. On cut surface the tumor was pale and fibrous. There was extension to surrounding soft tissue (Fig. 3b).

Tumor histology strongly resembled the desmoplastic fibroma diagnosed in case 1, however, with some differences. As shown in Fig. 4a, this tumor also consisted of bundles of moderate cellular tissue, with fibroblast-like, spindle cells in abundant collagenous stroma. However, there was evidence of invasive growth in trabecular bone and surrounding skeletal muscle tissue. Although nuclear chromatin was bland, few normal mitoses were found. Osteoid or trabecular bone was absent.

As depicted in Fig. 4b, cytogenetic analysis showed an abnormal karyotype: 47~49,XX,del(13) (q12q32),+ 1~2r,+1~2mar,1dmin [cp17]/46,XX [2]. This encompasses an interstitial deletion of the long arm of chromosome 13 (q12q32), consistent with heterozygous loss of the RB1 tumor suppressor gene. With cancer hotspot NGS analysis we found amplification of CDK4 (NM_000075.3) and an imbalance of the RB1 gene on chromosome 13.

With IHC, tumor cells exhibited strong nuclear staining for CDK4 (Fig. 4c) and moderate nuclear staining for SATB2. RB1 expression was heterogeneous, not completely lost.

In this case a conclusive diagnosis of DF-LGOS could be made, based on histologic features (an invasive fibroblastic tumor with mitotic activity), karyotyping (heterozygous loss of RB1) and molecular genetics/IHC (CDK4 amplification).

Discussion and conclusions

We have presented the clinical presentation, imaging studies, gross and microscopic pathology, IHC, cytogenetics and molecular genetics (cancer hotspot analysis) of DF and DF-LCOS, two very rare bone tumors, which closely resemble each other.

DF is very rare indeed. Among 4692 benign bone tumors treated in the Birmingham Royal Orthopedic Hospital, Evans et al. [1] identified 13 cases of DF, an incidence of 0.003%. Böhm et al. [2] reviewed 189 cases of DF reported in the literature up to 1996 and observed that, although DF occurs at all ages, children and young adults are most commonly affected, three-quarter of patients being younger than 31 years. Sex distribution is almost equal. DF most commonly presents in the mandible (22%), but also in pelvic bones (13%), and long bones—femur (15%), radius (12%), and tibia (9%). Notably, pathologic fracture of a long bone was reported in 12% of patients. Thus, the clinical presentation of our DF case as a tumor in the distal radius of a 10-year-old girl, who had experienced a radius fracture 3 years earlier, matches data from the literature.

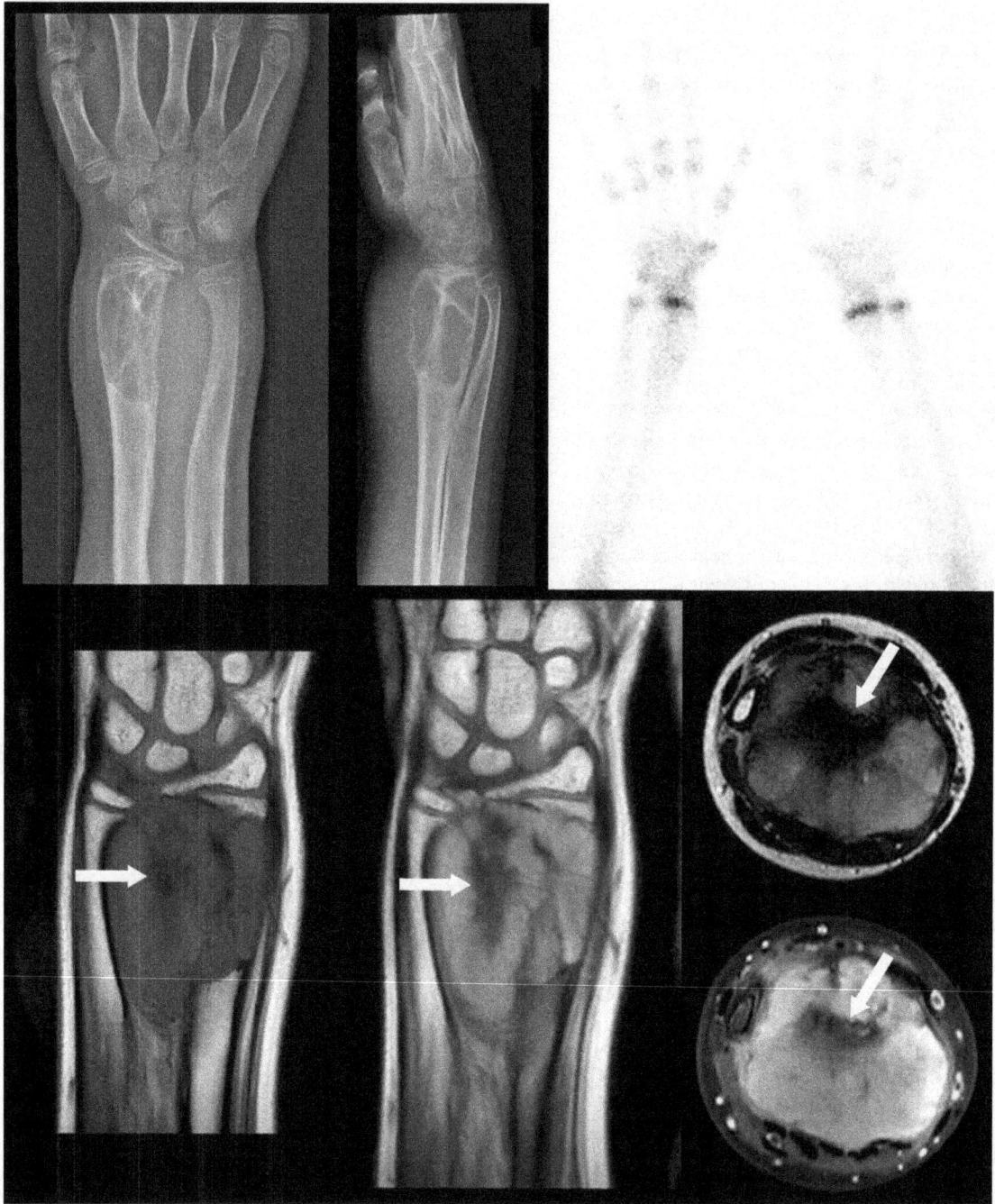

Fig. 1 Conventional AP and lateral radiographs (top left and top middle) show an expansive bubbly lytic bone lesion in the diaphysis-metaphysis of the right distal radius with a narrow zone of transition, nonsclerotic margins, cortical thinning and destruction, and an accompanying large soft-tissue mass which appears to compress the distal ulna with bowing of the latter. Bone scintigraphy (top right) shows no increased uptake at the location of the lesion. MRI with coronal T1-weighted (bottom left) and gadolinium-enhanced T1-weighted (bottom middle) images, and axial T2-weighted and gadolinium-enhanced fat-suppressed T1-weighted images (bottom right) are in keeping with the conventional radiographic findings, and also demonstrate no signs of invasion in surrounding muscles or ulna. Remarkably, in the center of the lesion there is low signal on all sequences (arrows), most strikingly on the T2-weighted sequence. Because the combined imaging features suggest a slow-growing (most likely benign) process with fibrotic components, the differential diagnostic considerations include desmoplastic fibroma, and (less likely) giant-cell tumor or fibrous dysplasia

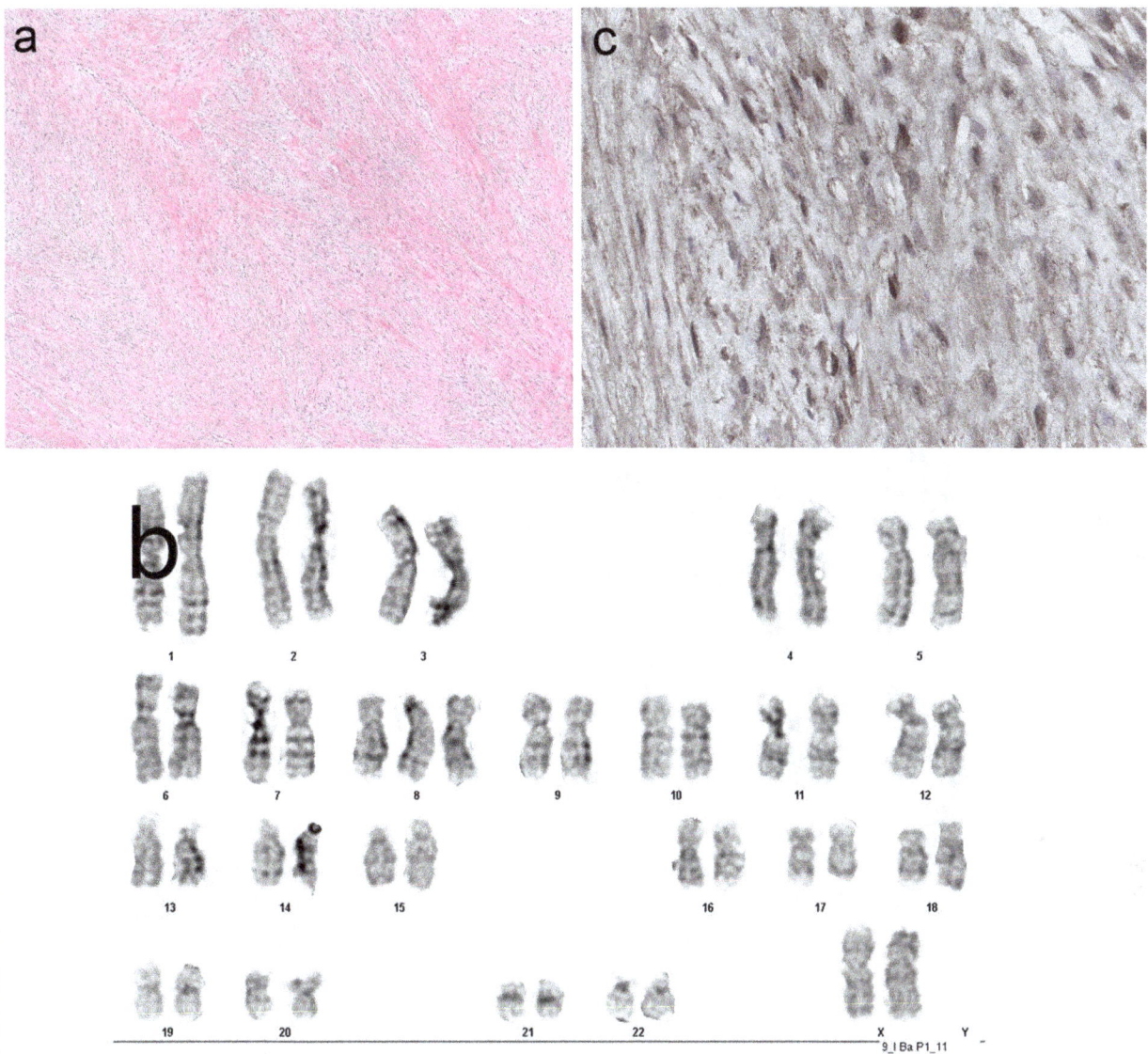

Fig. 2 Histology, karyotype and beta-catenin nuclear expression in DF. **a** Histology showing a fibroblastic tumor with little or no nuclear atypia or mitotic activity (H&E, original magnification × 200). As such, the histology of DF resembles that DF-LGCOS shown in Fig. 4a. **b** DF karyotype: 47,XX,+8[2]/46,XX[18]. **c** IHC expression of beta-catenin in several tumor cell nuclei of DF (original magnification × 400)

It is well appreciated that DF has a high recurrence rate after intralesional excision [1, 2], but since DF is a benign tumor that does not metastasize, we choose to remove the radius tumor of this young girl intralesionally, in order to preserve arm and wrist function. Unfortunately, a recurrence has occurred 12 months after surgery.

As our case illustrates, DF may present as a slowly progressive but locally aggressive tumor. As reviewed by Nedopil et al. [3] by imaging studies, DF can show cortical breakthrough and extension in surrounding soft tissue.

Moreover, infiltrative tumor growth may be seen by microscopy. Mitoses are only rarely found, an important criterion to discriminate DF from DF-LCOS or low-grade fibrosarcoma [4].

Cytogenetic analysis of our DF case revealed a normal female karyotype in 18 cells, with a trisomy 8 detected in 2 cells. To our knowledge, only two papers have been published on the cytogenetics and molecular genetics of DF. Bridge et al. [5] found trisomies 8 and 20 in a single case of DF, but again, these cytogenetic abnormalities were also detected in other fibro-osseous bone tumors,

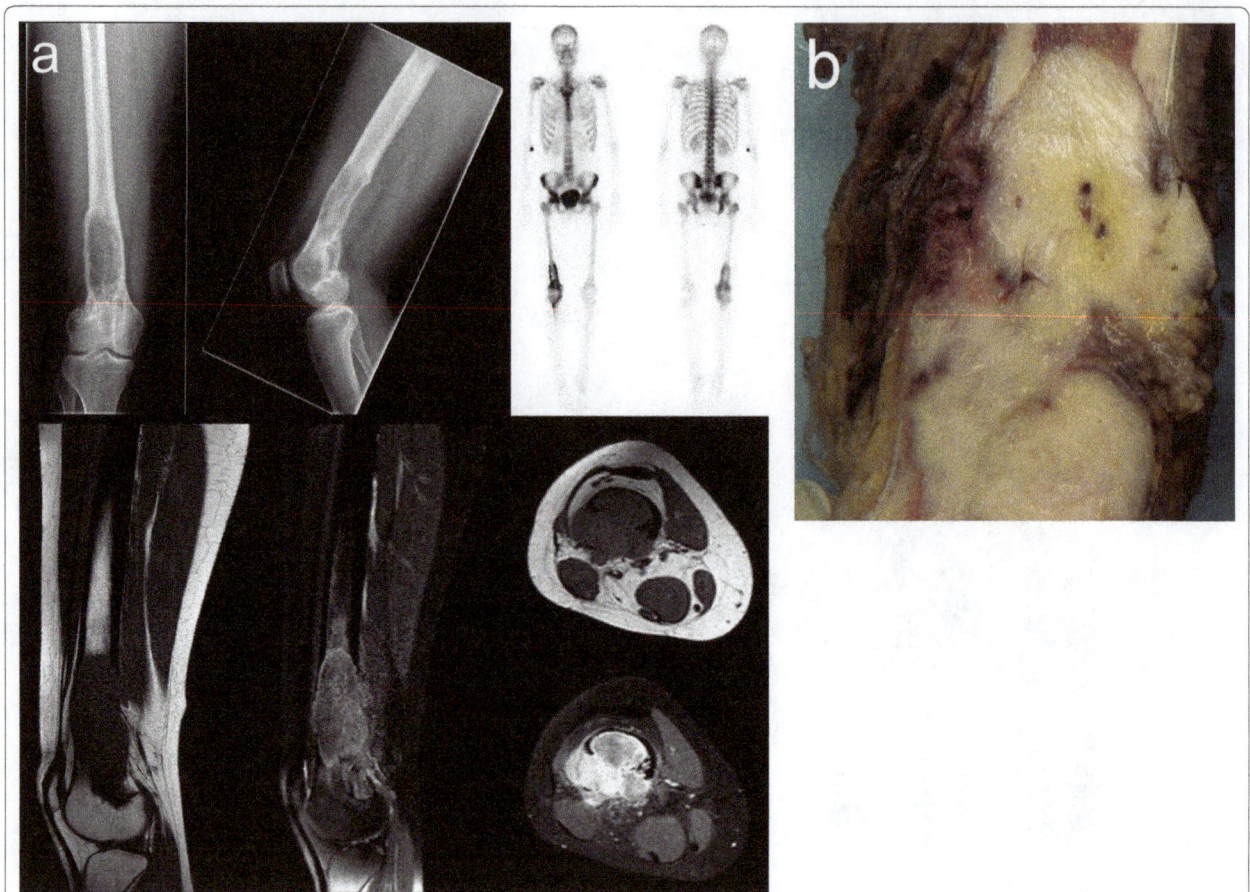

Fig. 3 Conventional AP, lateral radiographs and gross morphology of DF-LGCOS. **a** Conventional AP, lateral radiographs (top left and top middle) show an expansive osteolytic lesion in the diaphysis-metaphysis of the right distal femur with an ill-defined border and cortical destruction. Bone scintigraphy (top right) demonstrates increased uptake at the location of the lesion, but no suspicious uptake elsewhere. MRI with sagittal T1-weighted (bottom left) and fat-suppressed proton density-weighted (bottom middle) images, and axial T1-weighted and gadolinium-enhanced fat-suppressed T1-weighted images (bottom right) show the T1 hypointense, T2 hyperintense, and vividly enhancing lesion in the right distal femur as a large soft-tissue mass with cortical breakthrough and extra-osseous expansion. The combined imaging features are highly suggestive of an aggressive malignant lesion, with osteosarcoma, Ewing sarcoma, and chondrosarcoma being the main differential diagnostic considerations. **b** Gross specimen of DF-LGCOS, showing a white, fibrous tumor of the distal femur with cortical breakthrough and invasion of soft tissue. As such, the gross appearance of DF-LGCOS resembles DF

by which these are noncontributory to a certain DF diagnosis.

An abnormal karyotype 46,XX,del(11)(q13q23),der(19) t(11;19)(q13;p13)del(11)(q23) was reported by Trombetta et al. [6] in a DF occurring in the femur of a 20-year-old female patient. It was hypothesized that loss of a genomic region in 11q, an area containing the genes *RBM14, RBM4, RBM4B, SPTBN2,* and *C11orf80* may be of pathogenic significance.

Using IHC, others and we have noticed nuclear staining of beta-catenin in DF [3, 4, 7–11]. However, although nuclear expression of beta-catenin supports a diagnosis of DF, one has to be aware that nuclear immunostaining of beta-catenin also occurs in other fibro-osseous bone

tumors [9] or fibrous soft tissue tumors [12]. Moreover, IHC for beta-catenin is not specific for *APC/CTNNB1* mutations in fibro-osseous bone tumors. *CTNNB1* mutations are a rare molecular event in the few cases of DF that have been analyzed [7–9]. In fact, Flucke et al. [8] found a p.T41A *CTNNB1* mutation in 1 out of 2 cases of DF arising in the mandible, Horvai and Jordan [9] found an *APC* mutation, but no *CTNNB1* mutation in a single DF analyzed, and Hauben et al. [7] found no *CTNNB1* mutation in six DF cases. Using NGS, we detected a *CTNNB1* hotspot class 5 pathogenic variant in exon 3: p.S45F, which is a gain of function mutation. Clearly, to be able to estimate the real frequency of *CTNNB1* mutations in DF, more cases have to be studied, preferably

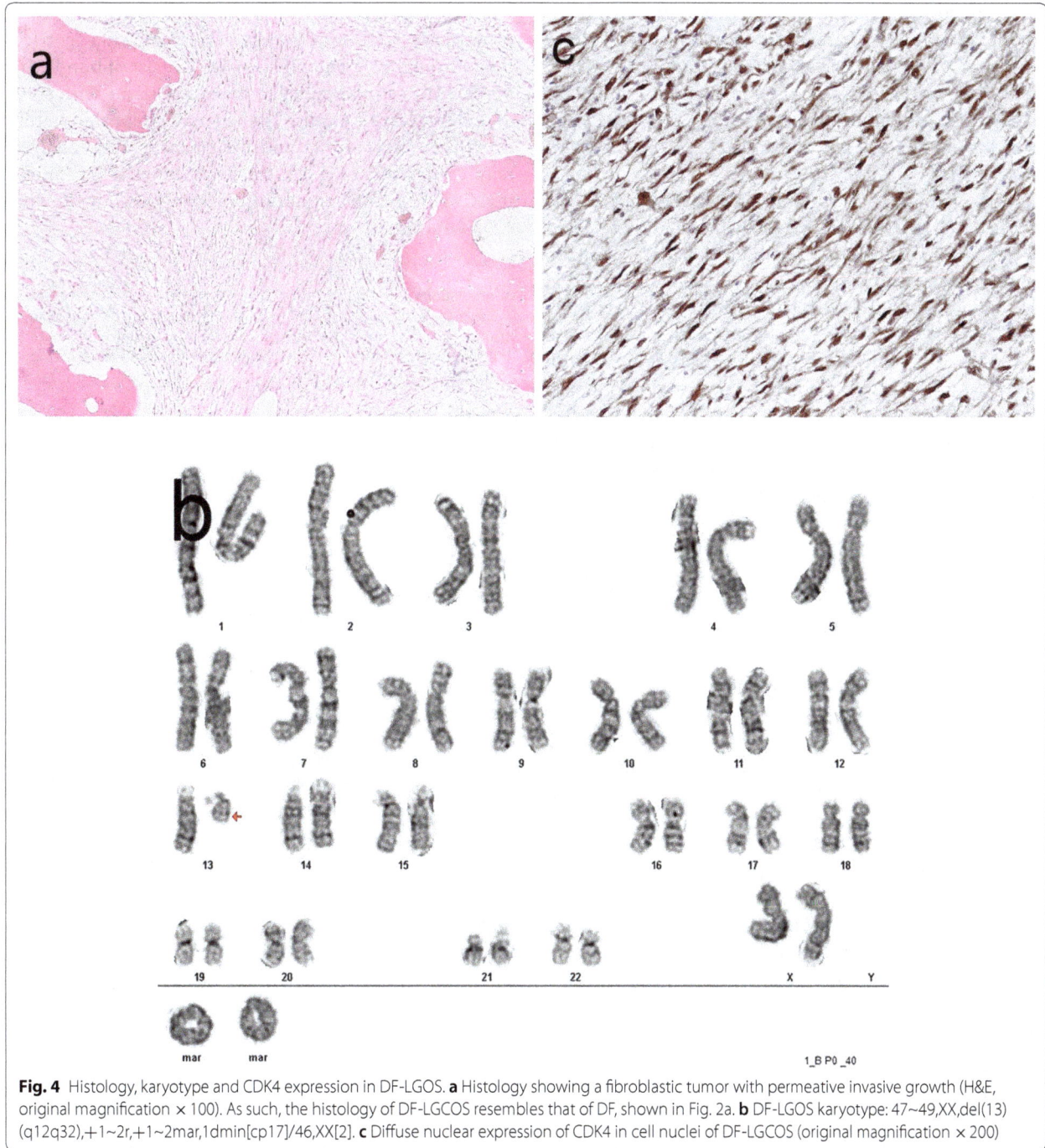

Fig. 4 Histology, karyotype and CDK4 expression in DF-LGOS. **a** Histology showing a fibroblastic tumor with permeative invasive growth (H&E, original magnification × 100). As such, the histology of DF-LGCOS resembles that of DF, shown in Fig. 2a. **b** DF-LGOS karyotype: 47~49,XX,del(13)(q12q32),+1~2r,+1~2mar,1dmin[cp17]/46,XX[2]. **c** Diffuse nuclear expression of CDK4 in cell nuclei of DF-LGCOS (original magnification × 200)

using NGS, since NGS has a higher sensitivity compared with traditional DNA sequencing methods in picking up *CTNNB1* mutations [13] Interestingly, the S45F *CTNNB* mutation also occurs in desmoid fibromatosis, in particular in aggressive and recurrent lesions [14]. However, it remains to be proven that DF is the bony counterpart of desmoid fibromatosis of soft tissue. In this respect, one may argue whether our case 1 represents a soft tissue tumor that had invaded bone. However, given the imaging features, in particular the bubbly compartmentalized appearance of the radius tumor and the bowing of the distal ulna without bone invasion (see Fig. 1), we regarded the radius tumor in this girl as a slow growing primary bone tumor with soft tissue extension, a clinical presentation consistent with a histopathologic diagnosis of desmoplastic fibroma of bone.

The majority of central osteosarcomas are high-grade conventional osteosarcomas, in which the tumor cells show severe nuclear atypia and produce a variable amount of cartilaginous or osteoid matrix. High grade osteosarcomas with severe nuclear atypia, but little or no matrix formation can be confirmed by SATB2 immuno-histochemistry [15, 16].

Our DF-LGCOS case is part of another subset of low grade central osteosarcomas namely the ones that resemble DF and have little or no osteoid matrix deposition. So far, this very rare OS subtype has only been described in case reports and small series [17, 18]. Most likely these rare DF-LCOS have been included in the histological spectrum of fibrosarcomas of bone [4]. We agree with Horvai and Jordan [9], who stated that it seems logical that at least a subset of fibrosarcomas of bone are actually osteosarcomas with little or no osteoid or bone formation. Surprisingly, in the 2013 WHO classification of tumors of soft tissue and bone, fibrosarcomas of bone are defined as intermediate to high grade spindle cell tumors that lack any line of differentiation other than fibroblastic, leaving little room for the recognition of low grade variants, also excluding DF- LGCOS.

Strong and diffuse SATB2 nuclear IHC staining reflects an osteoblastic line of differentiation. To date, only one Chinese study investigated SATB2 expression in low grade osteosarcoma and desmoplastic fibroma. These authors found that low-grade osteosarcoma and fibrous dysplasia are positive for SATB2, while desmoplastic fibroma, low-grade fibrosarcoma and other fibrous tumors are negative [19].

The notion that DF-LGCOS is an osteosarcoma variant is also supported by the cytogenetics and molecular genetics of our second case. DF-LGCOS had a karyotype with interstitial deletion of the long arm of chromosome 13 (q12q32), consistent with loss of the *RB1* tumor suppressor gene, a genetic abnormality found in a substantial number of osteosarcomas. Notably, cancer hotspot NGS analysis revealed amplification of *CDK4* and IHC showed overexpression of CDK4.

The prototypical LGCOS (which resembles parosteal osteosarcoma) usually produces abundant bone matrix and contains trabecular woven bone. The fibroblastic stromal cells of the prototypical LGCOS show slight nuclear atypia and mitosis are not easily discerned. This subset of LGCOS often has gain or amplification of the *MDM2* and/or *CDK4* genes, which can be visualized by their nuclear expression by IHC [19]. By IHC, CDK4 is positive in the majority of LGOS, and, when combined with MDM2 immunostaining, the sensitivity and specificity for LGOS is 100% and 97.5%, respectively [20].

The clinical presentation, imaging studies and gross morphology of DF-LGCOS shows much overlap with

DF. Both are fibrous tumors of bone with are slowly progressive and locally aggressive showing cortical breakthrough. DF and DF-LGCOS consist of bundles of moderately cellular collagenous tumor tissue with spindled fibroblast-like cells. The two cases reported herein show that karyotyping and molecular genetic analysis may contribute to a conclusive diagnosis, DF showing *CTNNB1* S45F mutation and DF-LGCOS showing *CDK4* amplification.

Abbreviations

DF: desmoplastic fibroma; DF-like LGCOS: low-grade central osteosarcoma (LGCOS) resembling desmoplastic fibroma; NGS: next generation sequencing; IHC: immunohistochemistry; LGCOS: low-grade central osteosarcoma; CC1: cell conditioning buffer 1.

Authors' contributions

WS observed pathology specimens, participated in the study design and drafted the manuscript. EB and AMCJ performed classic cytogenetics and next generation sequencing, respectively. TCK interpreted imaging features. PCJ performed the surgery, managed the patient and completed the clinical data collection. JVMGB conceived of the study, participated in its design. AJS conceived, designed and supervised this article. All authors read and approved the final manuscript.

Author details

[1] Department of Pathology and Medical Biology, University Medical Center Groningen, University of Groningen, P.O. Box 30.001, 9700 RB Groningen, The Netherlands. [2] Department of Genetics, University Medical Center Groningen, University of Groningen, P.O. Box 30.001, 9700 RB Groningen, The Netherlands. [3] Department of Radiology, Nuclear Medicine and Molecular Imaging, University Medical Center Groningen, University of Groningen, P.O. Box 30.001, 9700 RB Groningen, The Netherlands. [4] Department of Orthopedic Surgery, University Medical Center Groningen, University of Groningen, P.O. Box 30.001, 9700 RB Groningen, The Netherlands. [5] Department of Pathology, Leiden University Medical Center, Leiden, The Netherlands.

Acknowledgements

We want to acknowledge Tom van Wezel and Dina Ruano Neto (Pathology, LUMC) for setting up the NGS pipeline.

Competing interests

The authors declare that they have no competing interests.

Funding

Wangzhao Song receives funding from the China Scholarship Council (CSC) program (Grant No: 201606940023).

References

1. Evans S, Ramasamy A, Jeys L, et al. Desmoplastic fibroma of bone: a rare bone tumour. J Bone Oncol. 2014;3:77–9.
2. Bohm P, Krober S, Greschniok A, et al. Desmoplastic fibroma of the bone. A report of two patients, review of the literature, and therapeutic implications. Cancer. 1996;78:1011–23.
3. Nedopil A, Raab P, Rudert M. Desmoplastic fibroma: a case report with three years of clinical and radiological observation and review of the literature. Open Orthop J. 2013;8:40–6.
4. Saito T, Oda Y, Tanaka K, et al. Low-grade fibrosarcoma of the proximal humerus. Pathol Int. 2003;53:115–20.
5. Bridge JA, Swarts SJ, Buresh C, et al. Trisomies 8 and 20 characterize a subgroup of benign fibrous lesions arising in both soft tissue and bone. Am J Pathol. 1999;154:729–33.
6. Trombetta D, Macchia G, Mandahl N, et al. Molecular genetic characterization of the 11q13 breakpoint in a desmoplastic fibroma of bone. Cancer Genet. 2012;205:410–3.

7. Hauben E, Jundt G, Cleton-Jansen AM, et al. Desmoplastic fibroma of
    bone: an immunohistochemical study including beta-catenin expression
    and mutational analysis for beta-catenin. Hum Pathol. 2005;36:1025–30.
8. Flucke U, Tops BB, van Diest PJ, et al. Desmoid-type fibromatosis of the
    head and neck region in the paediatric population: a clinicopathological
    and genetic study of seven cases. Histopathology. 2014;64:769–76.
9. Horvai A, Jordan R. Fibro-osseous lesions of the craniofacial bones:
    β-catenin immunohistochemical analysis and CTNNB1 and APC mutation
    analysis. Head Neck Pathol. 2014;8(3):291–7.
10. Woods TR, Cohen DM, Islam MN, et al. Desmoplastic fibroma of the man-
    dible: a series of three cases and review of literature. Head Neck Pathol.
    2015;9:196–204.
11. Okubo T, Saito T, Takagi T, et al. Desmoplastic fibroma of the rib with
    cystic change: a case report and literature review. Skeletal Radiol.
    2014;43:703–8.
12. Carlson JW, Fletcher CD. Immunohistochemistry for beta-catenin in the
    differential diagnosis of spindle cell lesions: analysis of a series and review
    of the literature. Histopathology. 2007;51:509–14.
13. Colombo C, Urbini M, Astolfi A, et al. Novel intra-genic large deletions
    of CTNNB1 gene identified in WT desmoid-type fibromatosis. Genes
    Chromosomes Cancer. 2018. https://doi.org/10.1002/gcc.22644.
14. van Broekhoven DL, Verhoef C, Grünhagen D, et al. Prognostic value of
    CTNNB1 gene mutation in primary sporadic aggressive fibromatosis. Ann
    Surg Oncol. 2015;22:1464–70.
15. Conner JR, Hornick JL. SATB2 is a novel marker of osteoblastic differentia-
    tion in bone and soft tissue tumours. Histopathology. 2013;63:36–49.
16. Davis JL, Horvai AE. Special AT-rich sequence-binding protein 2 (SATB2)
    expression is sensitive but may not be specific for osteosarcoma as com-
    pared with other high-grade primary bone sarcomas. Histopathology.
    2016;69:84–90.
17. Kurt AM, Unni KK, McLeod RA, et al. Low-grade intraosseous osteosar-
    coma. Cancer. 1990;65:1418–28.
18. Bertoni F, Bacchini P, Fabbri N, et al. Osteosarcoma. Low-grade
    intraosseous-type osteosarcoma, histologically resembling parosteal
    osteosarcoma, fibrous dysplasia, and desmoplastic fibroma. Cancer.
    1993;71:338–45.
19. Chen CY, Zhang HZ, Jiang ZM, et al. Value of MDM2, CDK4 and SATB2
    immunohistochemistry in histologic diagnosis of low-grade osteosar-
    coma. Zhonghua Bing Li Xue Za Zhi. 2016;45:387–92.
20. Yoshida A, Ushiku T, Motoi T, et al. Immunohistochemical analysis of
    MDM2 and CDK4 distinguishes low-grade osteosarcoma from benign
    mimics. Mod Pathol. 2010;23:1279–88.

Different quality of treatment in retroperitoneal sarcomas (RPS) according to hospital-case volume and surgeon-case volume

Sergio Sandrucci[1][*], Agostino Ponzetti[2], Claudio Gianotti[1], Baudolino Mussa[3], Patrizia Lista[2], Giovanni Grignani[4], Marinella Mistrangelo[2], Oscar Bertetto[5], Daniela Di Cuonzo[6] and Giovannino Ciccone[6]

Abstract

Background: Retroperitoneal sarcomas (RPS) should be surgically managed in specialized sarcoma centers. However, it is not clearly demonstrated if clinical outcome is more influenced by Center Case Volume (CCV) or by Surgeon Case Volume (SCV). The aim of this study is to retrospectively explore the relationship between CCV and SCV and the quality of surgery in a wide region of Northern Italy.

Methods: We retrospectively collected data about patients M0 surgically treated for RPSs in 22 different hospitals from 2006 to 2011, dividing them in two hospital groups according to sarcoma clinical activity volume (HCV, high case volume or LCV, low case volume hospitals). The HCV group (> 100 sarcomas observed per year) included a Comprehensive Cancer Center (HVCCC) with a high sarcoma SCV (> 20 cases/year), and a Tertiary Academic Hospital (HVTCA) with multiple surgeon teams and a low sarcoma SCV (≤ 5 cases/year for each involved surgeon). All other hospitals were included in the LCV group (< 100 sarcomas observed per year).

Results: Data regarding 138 patients were collected. Patients coming from LCV hospitals (66) were excluded from the analysis as prognostic data were frequently not available. Among the 72 remaining cases of HCV hospitals 60% of cases had R0/R1 margins, with a more favorable distribution of R0/R1 versus R2 in HVCCC compared to HVTCA.

Conclusions: In HCV hospitals, sarcoma SCV may significantly influence RPS treatment quality. In low-volume centers surgical reports can often miss important prognostic issues and surgical quality is generally poor.

Keywords: Retroperitoneal sarcomas, Multidisciplinary management, Hospital case volume, Surgeon case volume, Quality of surgery, Retrospective analysis

Background

Retroperitoneal sarcomas (RPS) account for 10–15% of soft tissue sarcomas (STS) with an expected annual incidence of nearly 1500 cases in Europe and an expected 5-year overall survival (OS) of 30–35% [1]. Histopathological analysis can reveal multiple histotypes with liposarcoma and leiomyosarcoma as the most common [2].

The mainstay of treatment is surgical resection due to its survival advantage over nonsurgical treatments [3]. The intent of surgery is complete tumor resection with negative margins, which may require en bloc removal of adjacent involved organs or tissues. Of course, a wide margin per se may not be enough to guarantee an improved prognosis especially in specific histotypes (e.g. leiomyosarcoma) thus making it crucial to balance between wider excision and multimodal treatments [4]. Given the low incidence of RPS, individual hospitals and

---

*Correspondence: sergio.sandrucci@unito.it
[1] Visceral Sarcoma Unit, University of Turin, Cso Dogliotti 14, 10126 Turin, Italy
Full list of author information is available at the end of the article

surgeons generally observe very few cases; for this reason available guidelines and consensus-papers state that, as a complex and rare disease, every case of RPS should be referred to a specialized sarcoma center and managed by a multidisciplinary team [5–7]. However, it is unclear what factor(s), for example, case volume, surgeon activity volume, hospital type, or the availability of adjuvant therapies, is/are the principal driver(s) of improved outcomes.

It is not clearly demonstrated if for STS, and specifically for RPS, clinical outcome is more influenced by center case volume (CCV) or by surgeon case volume (SCV). In the literature, the effect of surgeon versus hospital volume on outcomes after complex oncological surgery is poorly characterized [8]. Published retroperitoneal sarcoma series are mostly collected from high volume centers, in which the multidisciplinary aspect is most relevant rather than the surgeon's caseload. The lack of surgeon-specific identifiers makes impossible to explore the interplay between hospital and surgeon volume and their impact on oncological outcomes. Therefore, it is unclear whether the principal determinant of oncological outcomes is high hospital case volume or high surgeon case volume. Providing care for RPS patients frequently requires a multidisciplinary team approach, and the team itself may be just as important than the surgeon in producing favorable outcomes.

NICE guidelines state that a surgeon with specific expertise in these tumors, who is a core member of the multidisciplinary team (MDT), is needed within a reference center; they also consider the number of new cases per year as an important quality evaluation item for sarcoma multidisciplinary teams. A sarcoma MDT should be expected to manage at least 100 new STS patients per year, and this caseload should be based either in a single hospital or in several geographically close and closely affiliated hospitals, which would constitute a sarcoma treatment network [9].

Due to the rarity of these diseases, it is difficult for a general surgeon to reach an adequate case volume. The only paper dealing with the problem of adequate surgical volumes in STS proposed a ≥ 5 sarcoma surgeries/year cut off, after an analysis of 4205 STS cases registered in the Florida Cancer Data System (FCDS) in which medical facilities above the 67th percentile for volume were defined as high-volume centers [10].

Concerning the treatment of retroperitoneal sarcomas, the aim of this study is to retrospectively explore the relationship between the hospital or surgeon case volume and the quality of surgery in a region of Northern Italy.

Methods

We retrospectively collected data concerning two regions of northern Italy, Piedmont and Aosta Valley (with a total amount of 4.5 million of inhabitants), to identify RPS patients, without distant metastases at diagnosis, operated during the period from 2006 to 2011 in order to analyze care center characteristics (according to high or low CCV and SCV) and quality of surgical treatment. Data collection was authorized by a partnership between the Department « Rete Oncologica del Piemonte e della Valle d'Aosta » (Piedmont and Aosta Valley Oncologic Network) and Italian Pathologist Association (SIAPEC) stipulated in June 2012; all data were recorded anonymously respecting Italian privacy rules.

Data of histopathological reports from January 2006 to December 2011 were collected from local databases of 22 different hospitals. According to the type of electronic database available in every single hospital, site-specific search strings were prepared using keywords able to describe the site and the morphology (i.e. "retroperitoneum" and/or "sarcoma") and SNOMED codes used for sarcomas morphology [11].

All extracted cases were screened by a skilled medical oncologist and collected in an encrypted database, which contained clinical and histopathological data, with particular attention to ESMO guidelines main prognostic items such as tumor size, grading, surgical margins (according to the R0, 1 and 2 ranking), preoperative biopsy and tumor integrity.

In our study patients data retrieved from different hospitals were split in two groups according to their yearly sarcoma caseload, adopting the 100 cases/year cut-off rule suggested by NICE [9] (Fig. 1).

In the "high volume" group two institutions were included:

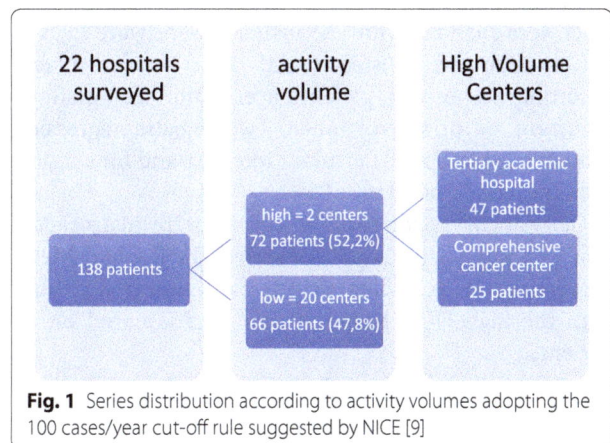

Fig. 1 Series distribution according to activity volumes adopting the 100 cases/year cut-off rule suggested by NICE [9]

- "Candiolo Cancer Center, a high volume Comprehensive Cancer Center (HVCCC) with nearly 150 STS cases observed per year.
- "Città della Salute e della Scienza" San Giovanni Battista hospital, a high volume Tertiary Care Academic hospital (HVTCA) with more than 100 STS cases observed per year.

In the "low volume" group all other hospitals were included (low volume secondary care hospitals, LVSCH).

In this series three different approaches to RPS are represented:

- HVCCC, a high-volume cancer center with a sarcoma-committed surgical team (high CCV and SCV > 20 surgeries per year) and a regular RPS-multidisciplinary board (RMB);
- HVTCA, a high-volume tertiary care academic hospital without a sarcoma-committed surgical team (high CCV and SCV ≤ 5 cases per year for each involved surgeon) and a formalized RMB;
- LVSCH, a group of low volume hospitals (low CCV and SCV < 5 RPS surgeries per year) without a formalized RMB.

Missing clinical informations concerning the "high volume" group were sorted from the institutional internal electronic chart database of each institution.

Missing data about the patients in charge to LVSCH were not obtained, due to the absence of a reliable database or, in case of an existing one, to access restrictions for external investigators.

Follow up was available only for the HV hospital patients; the median value was of 85 months (range 72–100).

Statistical analysis

Data were analyzed with SAS system 9.2 software.

The crude and adjusted hazard ratios were calculated according to hospital, patient's age, tumor size, grading, recurrent or primitive tumor. Two logistic regression models were adopted: for tumor integrity and for surgical margins (confidence limits 95%).

The Kaplan–Meier survival curve for primary/recurrent RPS was calculated on HV series. The Kaplan–Meier survival curve according to surgical margins was built with the high HCV hospitals data, and is based on 57 patients.

Results

Data from 22 hospitals were available: 138 patients (55% males and 45% females) were identified with a diagnosis of RPS from 2006 to 2011.

According to care center volume 47 cases (34.1%) were treated in HVTCA, 25 (18.1%) in HVCCC: 66 cases (47.8%) were treated in LVSCH.

As regards this latter group of patients, the lack of essential information impaired any statistical analysis. In particular, no useful informations were available concerning tumor diameter, preoperative biopsy, margins evaluation and FNLCLCC grading. For this reason, data from this latter group was not considered in the subsequent analysis, which has been conducted only on HTVCA and HVCCC patients.

The main characteristics of this series are summarized in Table 1.

Seventeen different histotypes were observed. The most frequent was liposarcoma (55.5%), followed by leiomyosarcoma (14%), sarcoma NOS (11%) and other histotypes. The difference between the two groups was not significant.

The tumor was primitive in 63.8% and recurrent in 36.2%: in HVCCC primaries were 56% and recurrences 44%; in HVTCA 68 and 32%. (Chi Squared test, P = 0.30).

According to FNCLCC grading, 14% of tumors were G1, 31% were G2 and 37.5% G3. In 17.5% of cases, this information was not recorded. The subdivision of grades G1/G2–3 in HVCCC and HVTCA was 31/52 and 53/30 (Chi Squared test, P = 0.91), respectively.

Tumor diameter was smaller than 10 cm in 30.5% of cases (32% for HVTCA and 28% for HVCCC), greater than 10 cm in 69.5% (68% for HVTCA and 72% for HVCCC) (Chi Squared test, P = 0.2622).

A preoperative biopsy was performed in 63.8% of patients, of which 66.5% coming from HVTCA and 60% from HVCCC.

According to previous experiences [12, 13] surgical resections were classified as macroscopically complete (R0 or R1) or incomplete (R2). 60% of RPS had a R0/R1 resection, 25% had R2 resection. In 15% of cases the status of surgical margins was not recorded. In HVCCC group the distribution R0/R1 versus R2 was 80 and 12%; in HVTCA, 49 and 32% (Chi Squared test, P = 0.0133; Fig. 2).

Tumors were removed intact in 50% of cases. In HVCCC group the rate of fragmented/intact specimens was 24 and 76%, and in HVTCA, 63.8 and 36.2% (Chi Squared test, P = 0.01, Fig. 2), respectively.

Table 1 patients from high volume centers (HCV) main characteristics

	Global HVC	%	HVTCA	%	HVCCC	%	HVTCA versus HVCCC
Age							
< 60	15	21.0	11	23.5	4	19.0	P = 0.81
≥ 60	57	79.0	36	76.5	21	81.0	
Sex							
M	43	59.7	24	51.0	19	76.0	P = 0.62
F	29	40.3	23	49.0	6	24.0	
Primary/recurrent							
Primary	46	63.8	32	68.0	14	56.0	P = 0.30
Recurrent	26	36.2	15	32.0	11	44.0	
Diameter							
< 10 cm	22	30.5	15	32.0	7	28.0	P = 0.26
≥ 10 cm	50	69.5	32	68.0	18	72.0	
Histotype							
Liposarcoma	40	55.5	24	51.0	16	64.0	P = ns
Leiomyosarcoma	10	14.0	9	19.0	1	4.0	
Sarcoma NOS	8	11.0	1	2.0	7	28.0	
Others	14	19.5	13	28.0	1	4.0	
Grading							
1	10	14.0	7	14.8	3	12.0	P = 0.9
2	22	31.0	18	38.2	4	19.0	
3	27	37.5	14	30.0	13	52.0	
Unknown	13	17.5	8	17.0	5	17.0	
Preoperative biopsy							
Yes	46	63.8	31	66.5	15	60.0	P = 0.45
No	26	36.2	16	33.5	10	40.0	
Margins							
R0	20	28.0	10	21.0	10	40.0	R0 + R1 versus R2 P = 0.013
R1	23	32.0	13	28.0	10	40.0	
R2	18	25.0	15	32.0	3	12.0	
Unknown	11	15.0	9	19.0	2	8.0	
Fragmentation							
Yes	36	50.0	30	63.8	6	24.0	P = 0.01
No	36	50.0	17	36.2	19	76.0	

Statistically significant P values are in italic

HVTCA high volume Tertiary Care Academic Hospital, *HVCCC* high volume Comprehensive Cancer Center

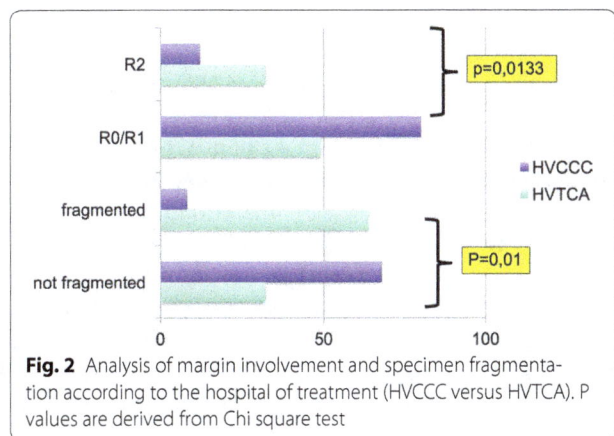

Fig. 2 Analysis of margin involvement and specimen fragmentation according to the hospital of treatment (HVCCC versus HVTCA). P values are derived from Chi square test

We compared HVTCA and HVCCC groups with the Chi squared test for grading, surgical margins, tumor size and intact specimen removal. In both logistic regression models concerning intact specimen and surgical margins (Table 2), only the "care center" item demonstrated a statistically significant correlation (i.e. HVCCC versus HVTCA) (P = 0.03, adjusted effects).

5 years survival according to the quality of margins was 65% for R0–R1 and 31% for R2 patients (Chi Squared test, P < 0.001) without differences between HVCCC and HVTCA cases (Chi Squared test, P = 0.06 Fig. 3).

Table 2 Logistic regression model about the factors potentially affecting the quality of surgical margins (R0/1 versus R2)

Covariates	Rough effects	P	IC95%	Adjusted effects	P	IC95%
HVCCC[a]	–	–	–	–	–	–
HVTCA	5.262	0.0192	1.311–21.115	8.335	0.0306	1.220–57.242
Liposarcoma	–	–	–	–	–	–
Leiomyosarcoma	1.094	0.9059	0.248–4.829	1.193	0.8388	0.218–6.543
Others	1.176	0.8551	0.206–6.731	0.470	0.5620	0.037–6.034
Age	0.970	0.3390	0.912–1.032	0.973	0.4823	0.903–1.049
Primary	–	–	–	–	–	–
Recurrent	1.450	0.5490	0.430–4.889	3.252	0.1608	0.626–16.897
< 10 cm	–	–	–	–	–	–
> 10 cm	1.107	0.8830	0.285–4.297	0.808	0.8104	0.141–4.617
G1	–	–	–	–	–	–
G2/G3	0.288	0.0797	0.071–1.159	0.365	0.3485	0.045–2.999
Unknown	3.718	0.2369	0.422–32.759	1.687	0.7363	0.080–35.384

[a] *HVCCC* high volume Comprehensive Cancer Center, *HVTCA* high volume Tertiary Care Academic Hospital

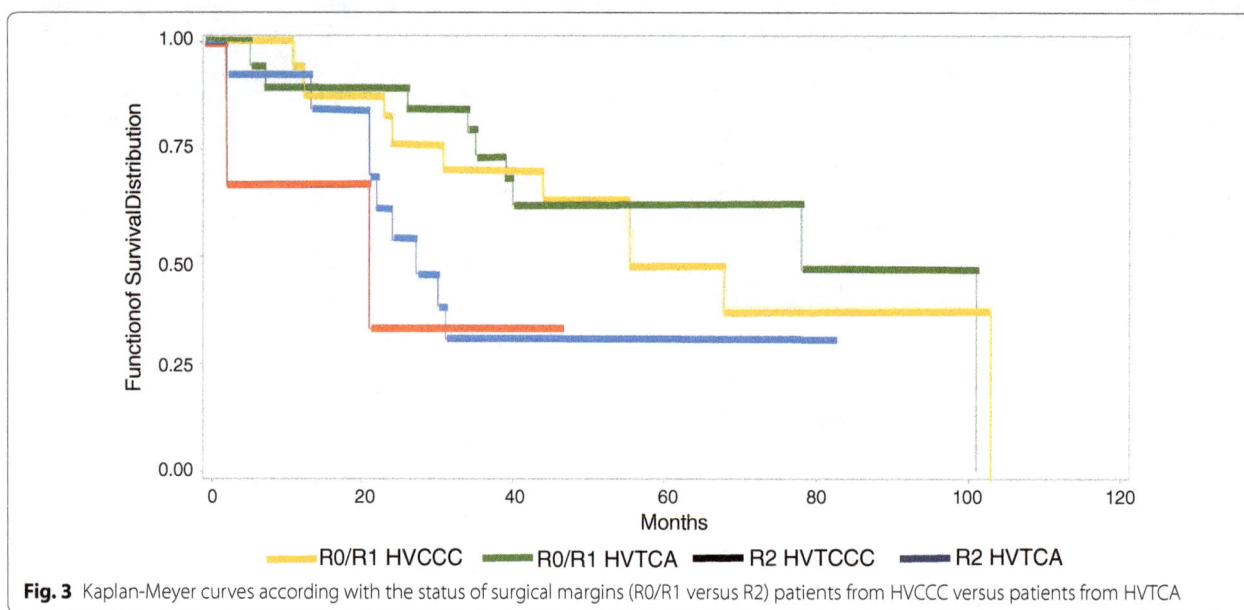

Fig. 3 Kaplan-Meyer curves according with the status of surgical margins (R0/R1 versus R2) patients from HVCCC versus patients from HVTCA

Discussion

The outcome of surgical treatment of many common tumors (as for example rectal cancer, breast cancer, lung cancer, prostate cancer, head and neck cancers and esophageal cancer) are clearly influenced by both center case volume (CCV) and surgeon case volume (SCV) [14, 15].

In STS, several studies state that HCV hospital may assure higher survival rate [10, 16].

Some retrospective data show that the management of RPS in sarcoma-specialized centers is associated with a lower loco-regional relapse rate and a 5-year OS of nearly 60–65% [17, 18] and that high-volume centers perform surgery more adherently to clinical STS guidelines than low-volume ones [19, 20].

In real life, up to 63% of STS in UK are referred to non-specialized centers [16]; up to 50% of non-oncology committed surgeons perform extremity soft tissue sarcoma resections in California [21]. In a recent survey the German Interdisciplinary Sarcoma Group [22] analyzed university medical centers plus those ones treating more than 10 RPS per year in comparison to centers following less than 10 RPS per year, finding relevant differences regarding tumor biopsy policy, resection strategies and multimodal therapies. Only 11 surgical departments on 191 surveyed treated more than 10 RPS patients per year;

in only 19 hospitals a multidisciplinary sarcoma board was active and in 54% of the departments pretreatment tumor biopsy was a standard procedure. These results suggest the need for dedicated RPS education programs and centralized registration for RPS treatment.

Berger et al. [23] identified 2762 patients from the US National Cancer Database treated for retroperitoneal sarcoma. The majority (59.4%, n = 1642) underwent resection at an academic cancer center. Resection for retroperitoneal sarcoma performed at academic cancer center was an independent predictor of margin-negative resection but was not a statistically significant risk factor for survival, suggesting that site of care may contribute to the quality of retroperitoneal sarcoma surgery.

The management of soft tissue sarcomas requires integrated care at a referral center, as suggested by existing guidelines and consensus statements. Diagnosis of the primary lesion, distant metastasis, or subsequent local recurrence require the use of advanced imaging as well as the expertise of appropriately trained teams. Experts involved in soft tissue sarcoma care suggest treatment with respect to using, dosing, and timing of radiation and chemotherapy tailored for every individual patient [5, 24].

Surgery of RPS, especially for wide re-excision after unplanned primary excision of a mass, requires specific multidisciplinary teamwork [25, 26]. There are data concerning RPS which show that patients treated in sarcoma reference centers can achieve better oncological outcomes [17, 18].

In this study, we collected data concerning the treatment of RPS from 22 hospitals, of which 20 (90%) treated less than 5 cases per year; the low quality of retrieved information from this low volume activity hospitals (LVSCH), mirrors the incidental character of this type of surgery.

We considered margins as macroscopically negative (R0/R1) or macroscopically positive (R2), as available literature shows that this margin classification has a definite prognostic value without great differences between R0 and R1 in the retrospective setting; is often difficult to correctly assess microscopic margins in big retroperitoneal masses in absence of a real compartment or of the possibility of a wide excision [6, 12, 13, 27–30]. The multivariate analysis confirmed that, within high CCV centers, the one with a dedicated surgical team and a RMB (HVCCC) had a better quality of macroscopic margins and a higher rate of intact tumor resection. Keung et al. [31] highlights the importance of maintaining tumor specimen integrity during surgery because tumor fragmentation is independently associated with worse PFS and OS. Bonvalot and colleagues [32] similarly reported that tumor rupture was associated with worse OS.

Maintaining tumor specimen integrity is often a daunting challenge given the large size, location, and adjacent organ involvement of many of these tumors, and therefore, tumor integrity can be considered a proxy of surgical quality.

It is expected that outcomes directly under the surgeon's control, that is, the completeness of resection, are more strongly associated with surgeon volume, a marker of surgical expertise, rather than by hospital volume, which is a somewhat imprecise marker of surgeon experience as well as hospital structure and process characteristics.

Important limitations of this study are its retrospective nature, based on histopathological reports, the omission of non-surgically treated patients, the retrieval of missing data from different databases and the absence of clinical history and follow-up information, particularly about RFS, in patients treated in LVSCH.

Conclusion

Outside reference or tertiary care centers, the quality of RPS management may be lower because the relevance of both tumor integrity and surgical margin quality are not completely understood and therefore, documented.

In light of the persistent association between improved surgical oncology outcomes and high-volume activity, the centralization of high-risk cancer surgery has been proposed [26–28]. A volume-outcome relationship exists for RPS so, centralization may improve outcomes for RPS keeping in mind that surgical experience plays a larger role for these outcomes than structural/process characteristics.

Authors' contributions

SS: study design, manuscript editing. AP, CG, PL, GG data input and completion, MM, OB data collection. DDC, GC. Statistic workout. BM manuscript revision. All authors read and approved the final manuscript.

Author details

[1] Visceral Sarcoma Unit, University of Turin, Cso Dogliotti 14, 10126 Turin, Italy. [2] Medical Oncology 1 Division, Città della Salute e della Scienza, Turin, Italy. [3] Department of Surgical Sciences, University of Turin, Turin, Italy. [4] Department of Medical Oncology, Candiolo Cancer Institute-FPO, IRCCS, Candiolo, Italy. [5] Regional Oncologic Network Department, Turin, Italy. [6] Cancer Epidemiology Unit, Città della Salute e della Scienza, Turin, Italy.

Acknowledgements

Not applicable.

Competing interests

The authors confirm that there are no known competing interests associated with this publication and there has been no significant financial support for this work that could have influenced its outcome.

Funding
Not applicable.

References

1. Gatta G, van der Zwan JM, Casali PG, et al. Rare cancers are not so rare: the rare cancer burden in Europe. Eur J Cancer. 2011;47:2493–511.
2. Vijay AA, Ram L. Retroperitoneal liposarcoma. A comprehensive review. Am J Clin Oncol. 2015;2015(38):213–9.
3. Bonvalot S, Raut CP, Pollock RE, et al. Technical considerations in surgery for retroperitoneal sarcomas: position paper from E-surge, a master class in sarcoma surgery, and EORTC-STBSG. Ann Surg Oncol. 2012;19:2981–91.
4. Callegaro D, Fiore M, Gronchi A. Personalizing surgical margins in retroperitoneal sarcomas. Exp Rev Anticancer Ther. 2015;15:553–67.
5. The ESMO/European Sarcoma Network Working Group. Soft tissue and visceral sarcomas: ESMO clinical practice guidelines for diagnosis, treatment and follow-up. Ann Oncol. 2014;25(Supplement 3):iii102–12.
6. Trans-Atlantic RPS Working Group. Management of primary retroperitoneal sarcoma (RPS) in the adult: a consensus approach from the transatlantic RPS working group. Ann Surg Oncol. 2015;22:256–63.
7. Tan MC, Yoon SS. Surgical Management of retroperitoneal and pelvic sarcomas. J Surg Oncol. 2015;111:553–61.
8. Maurice MJ, Yih JM, Ammori JB, Abouassaly R. Predictors of surgical quality for retroperitoneal sarcoma: volume matters. J Surg Oncol. 2017. https://doi.org/10.1002/jso.24710.
9. National Institute for Health Care and Excellence. Manual for cancer services. sarcoma measures. Version 1.0; 2014. p. 9. http://www.cquins.nhs.uk/?menu=resources. Accessed 1 Dec 2016.
10. Gutierrez JC, Perez EA, Moffat FL, et al. Should soft tissue sarcomas be treated at high-volume centers? Ann Surg. 2007;245:952–8.
11. Fritz A, Percy C, Jack A, et al. International classification of diseases for oncology. 3rd ed. Geneva: World Health Organization; 2000.
12. Gronchi A, Strauss DC, Miceli V, et al. Variability in patterns of recurrence after resection of primary retroperitoneal sarcoma (RPS) a report on 1007 patients from the multi-institutional collaborative RPS working group. Ann Surg. 2016;263:1002–9.
13. Raut CP, Swallow CJ. Are radical compartmental resections for retroperitoneal sarcomas justified? Ann Surg Oncol. 2010;17(6):1481–4.
14. Chan CM, Huang KY, Hsu TW, et al. Multivariate analyses to assess the effects of surgeon and hospital volume on cancer survival rates: a nationwide population-based study in Taiwan. PLoS ONE. 2012;7:e40590.
15. Halm EA, Lee C, Chassin MR. Is volume related to outcome in health care? a systematic review and methodologic critique of the literature. Ann Intern Med. 2002;137:511–20.
16. Bhangu AA, Beard JAS, Grimer RJ. Should soft tissues sarcomas be treated at a specialist centre? Sarcoma. 2004;8:1–16.
17. Bonvalot S, Miceli R, Berselli M, et al. Aggressive surgery in retroperitoneal soft tissue sarcoma carried out at high-volume centers is safe and is associated with improved local control. Ann Surg Oncol. 2010;17:1507–14.
18. Toulmonde M, Bonvalot S, Méeus P, et al. Retroperitoneal sarcomas: pattern of care at diagnosis, prognostic factors and focus on main histological subtypes: a multicenter analysis of the French Sarcoma Group. Ann Oncol. 2014;25:735–42.
19. Ray-Cocquard I, Thiesse P, Ranchère-Vince D, et al. Conformity to clinical practice guidelines, multidisciplinary management nad outcome if treatment for soft tissues sarcomas. Ann Oncol. 2004;15:307–15.
20. Mathoulin-Pellissier S, Chevreau C, Bellera C, et al. Adherence to consensus-based diagnosis and treatment guidelines in adult soft-tissue sarcoma patients: a French prospective population-based study. Ann Oncol. 2014;25:225–31.
21. Canter RJ, Smith CA, Martinez SR, et al. Extremity soft tissue tumor surgery by surgical specialty: a comparison of case volume among oncology and non-oncology-designated surgeons. J Surg Oncol. 2013;108:142–7.
22. Jakob J, Gerres A, Ronellenfitsch U, et al. Treatment of retroperitoneal sarcoma in Germany: results of a survey of the German society of general and visceral surgery, the German interdisciplinary sarcoma study group and the advocacy group Das Lebenshaus. Chirurg. 2017. https://doi.org/10.1007/s00104-017-0504-2.
23. Berger NG, Silva JP, Mogal H, et al. Overall survival after resection of retroperitoneal sarcoma at academic cancer centers versus community cancer centers: an analysis of the national cancer data base. Surgery. 2017;163:318–23.
24. Papagelopoulos PJ, Mavrogenis AF, Mastorakos DP, et al. Current concepts for management of soft tissue sarcomas of the extremities. J Surg Orthop Adv. 2008;17:204–15.
25. Umer HM, Umer M, Qadir I, et al. Impact of unplanned excision on prognosis of patients with extremity soft tissue sarcoma. Sarcoma. 2013; Article ID 498604.
26. Wasif N, Smith CA, Tamurian RM, et al. Influence of physician specialty on treatment recommendations in the multidisciplinary management of soft tissue sarcoma of the extremities. JAMA Surg. 2013;148:632–9.
27. Cho SY, Moon KC, Cheong MS, et al. Significance of microscopic margin status in completely resected retroperitoneal sarcoma. J Urol. 2011;186:59–65.
28. Doepker M, Hanna KH, Thompson ZJ, et al. Recurrence and survival analysis of resected soft tissue sarcomas of pelvic retroperitoneal structures. J Surg Oncol. 2016;113:103–7.
29. Abdelfatah E, Guzzetta AA, Nagarajan N, et al. Long-term outcomes in treatment of retroperitoneal sarcomas: a 15 year single-institution evaluation of prognostic features. J Surg Oncol. 2016;114:56–64.
30. Klooster B, Rajeev R, Chrabaszcz S, et al. Is long-term survival possible after margin-positive resection of retroperitoneal sarcoma (RPS)? J Surg Oncol. 2016;113:823–7.
31. Keung EZ, Hornick JL, Bertagnolli MM, Baldini EH, Raut CP. Predictors of outcomes in patients with primary retroperitoneal dedifferentiated liposarcoma undergoing surgery. J Am Coll Surg. 2014;218(2):206–17.
32. Bonvalot S, Rivoire M, Castaing M, et al. Primary retroperitoneal sarcomas: a multivariate analysis of surgical factors associated with local control. J Clin Oncol. 2009;27:31–7.

20

Survival is influenced by approaches to local treatment of Ewing sarcoma within an international randomised controlled trial: analysis of EICESS-92

Jeremy Whelan[1,3]*, Allan Hackshaw[2], Anne McTiernan[1], Robert Grimer[4], David Spooner[5], Jessica Bate[1], Andreas Ranft[6], Michael Paulussen[7], Herbert Juergens[8], Alan Craft[3,9] and Ian Lewis[3,10]

Abstract

Background: Two national clinical trial groups, United Kingdom Children's Cancer and Leukaemia Group (CCLG) and the German Paediatric Oncology and Haematology Group (GPOH) together undertook a randomised trial, EICESS-92, which addressed chemotherapy options for Ewing's sarcoma. We sought the causes of unexpected survival differences between the study groups.

Methods: 647 patients were randomised. Cox regression analyses were used to compare event-free survival (EFS) and overall survival (OS) between the two study groups.

Results: 5-year EFS rates were 43% (95% CI 36–50%) and 57% (95% CI 52–62) in the CCLG and GPOH patients, respectively; corresponding 5-year OS rates were 52% (95% CI 45–59%) and 66% (95% CI 61–71). CCLG patients were less likely to have both surgery and radiotherapy (18 vs. 59%), and more likely to have a single local therapy modality compared to the GPOH patients (72 vs. 35%). Forty-five percent of GPOH patients had pre-operative radiotherapy compared to 3% of CCLG patients. In the CCLG group local recurrence (either with or without metastases) was the first event in 22% of patients compared with 7% in the GPOH group. After allowing for the effects of age, metastases, primary site, histology and local treatment modality, the risk of an EFS event was 44% greater in the CCLG cohort (95% CI 10–89%, p = 0.009), and the risk of dying was 30% greater, but not statistically significant (95% CI 3–74%, p = 0.08).

Conclusions: Unexpected differences in EFS and OS occurred between two patient cohorts recruited within an international randomised trial. Failure to select or deliver appropriate local treatment modalities for Ewing's sarcoma may compromise chances of cure.

Keywords: Ewing sarcoma, Local therapy

*Correspondence: jeremy.whelan@nhs.net
[1] Department of Oncology, University College Hospitals London NHS Foundation Trust, 250 Euston Road, London NW1 2PG, UK
Full list of author information is available at the end of the article

Background

Collaboration between national clinical study groups to run large randomised trials is advantageous, especially in rare disease settings. It allows rapid accrual of larger numbers of patients to provide sufficient power for robust analyses. Indeed, joint studies may be the only means of effectively answering randomised questions in rare cancers [1, 2]. EICESS-92, a trial developed and completed by the Children's Cancer and Leukaemia Group (CCLG, formerly United Kingdom Children's Cancer Study Group, UKCCSG) and the Cooperative Ewing's Sarcoma Studies (CESS) group of the German Paediatric Oncology and Haematology Group (GPOH) with associated institutions in Austria, Switzerland and the Netherlands, addressed two chemotherapy questions in patients with Ewing sarcoma (ES). It remains one of the largest randomised studies conducted in this cancer.

The primary aims of the trial were to demonstrate an increase in event-free survival (EFS), and decreased treatment-related morbidity for patients with standard risk disease. The overall results of the trial have been reported [3]. However, we found evidence that EFS and overall survival (OS) differed between the CCLG and GPOH study groups. Although these data have been reported in abstract form, this more detailed analysis retains relevance and influence on practice [4].

Patients and methods

The trial design of EICESS-92 is outlined in Fig. 1, and details are described elsewhere [3]. The study was confined to patients with primary tumours of bone.

Patients with localised tumours of < 100 ml were classified as standard risk (SR), patients with large localised tumours (≥ 100 ml), or with metastatic disease, were classified as high risk (HR). Patients were randomly assigned to one of two treatment arms. SR-patients received four VAIA courses (vincristine, doxorubicin, ifosfamide, actinomycin D) followed by ten courses of

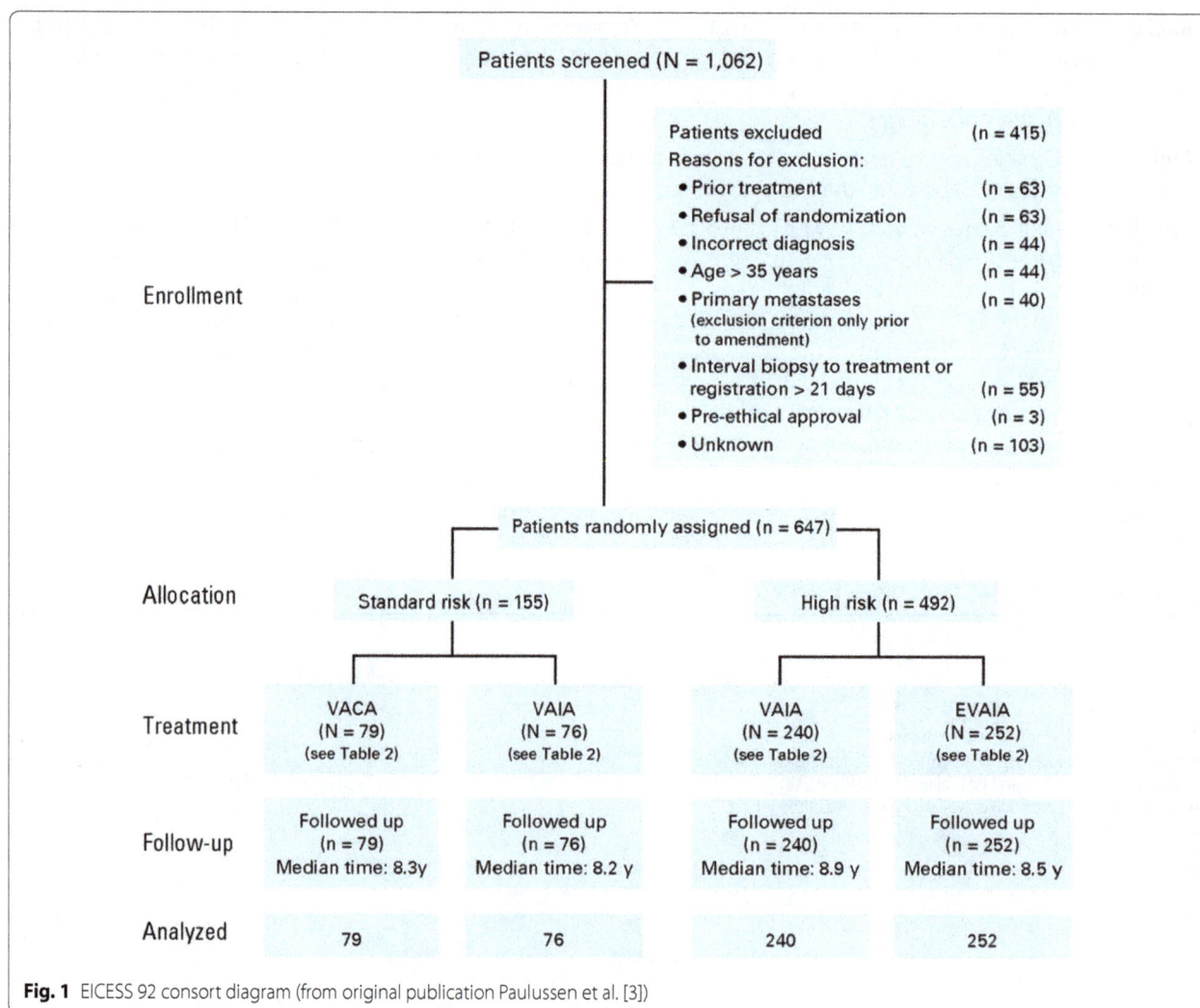

Fig. 1 EICESS 92 consort diagram (from original publication Paulussen et al. [3])

either VAIA or VACA (cyclophosphamide instead of ifos-famide) whilst HR-patients were randomised to either fourteen courses of VAIA or fourteen courses of VAIA with etoposide (EVAIA) [3].

Surgery and/or radiotherapy to the primary tumour ('local therapy') were scheduled to occur after four cycles of chemotherapy, at week 12. The choice of local therapy was made by clinicians for individual patients. The proto-col was permissive but indicated that surgery should be undertaken whenever possible. Preoperative radiother-apy (44.8 Gy) was recommended when there was < 50% reduction of a soft tissue component, evident on repeat imaging after 2 chemotherapy courses. Radiotherapy (54.4 Gy) replaced surgery for tumours deemed inoper-able. Post-operative radiotherapy (54.4 Gy) was recom-mended after intralesional surgery or marginal surgery with poor response (< 90% necrosis). Postoperative radiotherapy (44.8 Gy) was to be considered for marginal resections with good response (≥ 90% necrosis) or wide resections with poor response. Hyperfractionated irra-diation was recommended in these cases.

In the CESS group, the practice for treating clinical teams of routinely seeking advice from clinicians in the central trials office is well established including detailed guidance about radiotherapy planning [5]. No similar process was in place in the UK although the majority of patients selected for surgery by local clinicians were operated on at four centres only.

Statistical methods

The EICESS database was frozen in March 2007. EFS was calculated from the date of randomisation until the date of relapse, death or second malignancy, whichever occurred first. OS was calculated from the date of ran-domisation until date of death. Patients alive at last fol-low-up were censored at date last seen. Kaplan–Meier survival curves were examined, and Cox regression mod-elling was used to investigate differences after adjust-ing for multiple factors, producing hazard ratios (HR). Results are also presented separately for patients with only localised disease.

Results

Between 1992 and 1998, 647 patients were randomised: 210 CCLG and 437 GPOH (CONSORT diagram Fig. 1). The median follow-up was 8.5 years.

Patient characteristics

These were largely similar between the trial groups, except that CCLG patients tended to have more extrem-ity tumours (Table 1; 55 vs. 45%), fewer central tumours (40 vs. 54%), and fewer with atypical Ewing's sarcoma (4 vs. 16%), compared to GPOH patients.

Table 1 Comparison of patient characteristics between CCLG and GPOH

	Number of patients (percentage)		p value
	CCLG	GPOH	
	N = 210	N = 437	
Gender			
Female	84 (40)	177 (40)	0.90
Male	126 (60)	260 (60)	
Age (approx quartiles) (years)			
0–9	34 (16)	94 (22)	0.17
10–14	74 (35)	123 (28)	
15–19	58 (28)	115 (26)	
20–35	44 (21)	105 (24)	
Primary site			
Central axis	84 (40)	236 (54)	< 0.001 (0.004)
Extremity	115 (55)	197 (45)	
Unknown	11 (5)	4 (1)	
Axial skeletal	26 (12)	89 (20)	
Spine	7 (3	30 (7)	
Pelvis	51 (24)	117 (27)	
Limb proximal	61 (29)	103 (23)	
Limb distal	54 (26)	94 (22)	
Unknown	11 (5)	4 (1)	
Volume			
< 100 ml	57 (27)	117 (27)	0.48 (0.97)
≥ 100 ml	149 (71)	304 (69)	
Unknown	4 (2)	16 (4)	
Metastases			
No	150 (71)	329 (75)	0.27 (0.41)
Yes[d]	56 (27)	105 (24)	
Unknown	4 (2)	3 (1)	
Histology			
Ewing's sarcoma	140 (67)	261 (60)	< 0.001 (< 0.001)
Atypical Ewing's	8 (4)	70 (16)	
PNET	43 (20)	101 (23)	
Other[a]	6 (3)	5 (1)	
Unknown	13 (6)	0 (0)	
Risk group			
Standard (SR)	53 (25)	102 (23)	0.60
High (HR)	157 (75)	335 (77)	
Trial treatment			
SR-VACA	27 (13)	52 (12)	0.96
SR-VAIA	26 (12)	50 (11)	
HR-VAIA	76 (36)	164 (38)	
HR-EVAIA	81 (39)	171 (39)	
Histological response[c]			
Good	52 (25) [58]	78 (18) [65]	< 0.001 [0.33]
Poor	37 (18) [42]	42 (10) [35]	
No surgery	103 (49)	111 (25)	
NA[b]	3 (1)	200 (46)	
Unknown	15 (7)	6 (1)	

Table 1 continued

	Number of patients (percentage)		p value
	CCLG	GPOH	
	N = 210	N = 437	
No. of chemotherapy cycles received			
1–4	18 (8.6)	26 (6.0)	0.32
5–9	22 (10.5)	62 (14.2)	
10–13	36 (17.10)	83 (19.0)	
14	131 (62.4)	254 (58.2)	
Unknown	3 (1.4)	12 (2.8)	

p values including unknown data; the p values in brackets exclude unknown data

[a] Osteosarcoma or soft tissue

[b] NA not applicable, i.e. patients with early radiotherapy before surgery

[c] The numbers in square brackets are based only on patients with a good or poor response

[d] The proportions of patients with bone or bone marrow metastases were similar: 8% GPOH and 5% CCLG

Where histological response data were available for patients who did not receive pre-operative radiotherapy, there was no significant difference in the proportion of patients from the two study groups with either a good or poor histological response (Table 1, p = 0.33).

Chemotherapy and local therapy

There was no evidence of a difference in the delivery of chemotherapy between groups. The number of chemotherapy cycles received (Table 1) and the median total dose for each cytotoxic drug administered per patient were similar. A similar proportion completed all 14 cycles; 62% vs. 58% in the CCLG and GPOH groups, respectively (p = 0.30).

Table 2 shows the type of local therapy used in CCLG and GPOH patients. Most CCLG patients (72%) had a single therapy (surgery alone or radiotherapy alone); whilst most GPOH patients had both radiotherapy and surgery (59%), which was mainly radiotherapy followed by surgery (45%). Only 18% of CCLG patients had both radiotherapy and surgery. A similar pattern was seen for patients without metastatic disease.

Patient characteristics were examined which might influence the selection of local treatment (Table 3). Many patients with metastatic disease were treated with radiotherapy alone in both trial groups, though the percentage was higher in CCLG patients. A substantial proportion of CCLG patients with central axis tumours had radiotherapy alone (62%), while those with extremity tumours tended to have surgery alone. CCLG patients were more likely to have both radiotherapy and surgery if they had extremity tumours compared

Table 2 Comparison of local treatment modality in CCLG and GPOH

	Number of patients (percentage)		p value
	CCLG	GPOH	
	N = 210	N = 437	
Local treatment modality			
Surgery alone	70 (33)	71 (16)	< 0.001[a]
Radiotherapy alone	81 (39)	85 (19)	
Radiotherapy then surgery	6 (3)	195 (45)	
Surgery then radiotherapy	32 (15)	60 (14)	
None (progressive disease)	18 (9)	7 (2)	
Unknown	3 (1)	19 (4)	
Localised disease only			
Surgery alone	59 (39)	63 (19)	< 0.001
Radiotherapy alone	53 (35)	55 (17)	
Radiotherapy then surgery	5 (3)	147 (45)	
Surgery then radiotherapy	24 (16)	47 (14)	
None (progressive disease)	9 (6)	3 (1)	
Unknown	0	14 (4)	

[a] p value for the association between type of local treatment and study group. The p value is also < 0.001 if 'none' or 'unknown' are excluded

to central axis tumours (23 vs. 11%). A similar pattern was seen in GPOH patients, though there was much less of a difference in the proportion who had both therapies depending on whether they had extremity or central axis tumours (64% vs. 54%). While there was no evidence of an association between choice of local treatment and either tumour volume (p = 0.44) or age (p = 0.12) in GPOH patients, there was evidence of this in CCLG patients. Those with a volume < 100 ml were more likely to have surgery alone (47%), and those with a volume ≥100 ml tended to have radiotherapy alone. Proportionally more patients with volume ≥100 ml received both therapies compared to those with volume < 100 ml (21 vs. 10%). In the CCLG group there was a clear trend with age; the proportions receiving single modality treatment were 94% (age 0–9 years), 75% (age 10–14 years), 68% (age 15–19 years) and 59% (age 20–35 years), indicating that older patients tended to be given both therapies.

Overall outcome

Appendix Table 6 shows the distribution of events and deaths by trial group. The CCLG cohort had more local relapses (with or without metastatic disease) than GPOH; 22 vs. 7%. Appendix Tables 7, 8 show the distribution of events according to local therapy. Figure 2 shows EFS and OS according to trial group. Both outcomes were poorer in the CCLG patients.

Table 3 Association between the choice of local modality treatment and specified patient characteristics

| | Number of patients (percentage), excluding missing data | | | | | | | | | |
| | CCLG | | | | | GPOH | | | | |
	N	None	RT alone	Surgery alone	RT and surgery	N	None	RT alone	Surgery alone	RT and surgery
Disease										
Localised	150	9 (6)	53 (35)	59 (39)	29 (19)	315	3 (1)	55 (17)	63 (20)	194 (62)
Metastatic	56	9 (16)	27 (48)	11 (20)	9 (16)	101	4 (4)	30 (30)	8 (8)	59 (58)
Localised extremity disease	91	5 (5)	18 (20)	46 (50)	22 (24)	155	1 (1)	8 (5)	44 (28)	102 (66)
Localised pelvic disease	31	0	24 (77)	6 (19)	1 (3)	79	1 (1)	27 (36)	7 (9)	39 (53)
Primary site										
Central axis	84	9 (11)	52 (62)	14 (17)	9 (11)	226	4 (2)	73 (32)	22 (10)	127 (56)
Extremity	115	7 (6)	28 (24)	54 (47)	26 (23)	189	3 (2)	11 (6)	48 (25)	127 (67)
Volume (ml)										
< 100	57	5 (9)	19 (33)	27 (47)	6 (10)	111	3 (3)	26 (23)	16 (14)	66 (59)
≥ 100	146	13 (9)	61 (42)	40 (27)	32 (22)	292	4 (1)	54 (18)	52 (18)	182 (62)
Age (years)										
0–9	34	0	10 (29)	22 (65)	2 (6)	92	1 (1)	18 (20)	22 (24)	51 (55)
10–14	74	5 (7)	32 (43)	24 (32)	13 (18)	118	0	30 (25)	11 (9)	77 (65)
15–19	56	5 (9)	25 (45)	13 (23)	13 (23)	111	3 (3)	21 (19)	21 (19)	66 (59)
20–35	43	8 (19)	14 (33)	11 (26)	10 (23)	97	3 (3)	16 (16)	17 (18)	61 (63)

Chi square tests were used to examine the association between each factor and choice of local therapy, excluding those who received no local treatment ('None' in the table)

CCLG: disease (p = 0.04); primary site (p < 0.001); volume (p = 0.01); age (p = 0.01)

GPOH: disease (p = 0.002); primary site (p < 0.001); volume (p = 0.44); age (p = 0.12)

N total number of patients *RT* radiotherapy

Differences in survival between the trial groups allowing for specified factors

The risk of having an event or dying for CCLG patients compared to GPOH was examined using Cox regression modelling. Overall, the chance of having an event (relapse, death or second malignancy) was increased by 42% (HR 1.42, 95% CI 1.13–1.77, p = 0.002) in the CCLG group compared to the GPOH group. The CCLG group had an increased risk of dying of 45% (HR 1.45, 95% CI 1.14–1.86, p = 0.003) in comparison to the GPOH group (Appendix Table 9). The table also shows that the excess risk (42% EFS, and 45% OS) did not materially change, even after allowing for several prognostic factors: age, metastatic disease status, primary site or histology. The association between outcome and study group was very similar when only examining patients with non-metastatic disease. Combined local treatment seemed to have an effect on OS (reducing the excess risk from 45 to 30%) but not EFS. When several prognostic factors were allowed for together, there was still an increased risk among CCLG patients: 44% for EFS (HR 1.44, p = 0.009) and 30% for OS (HR 1.30, p = 0.08, which was not statistically significant). We further examined the effect separately among patients with localised disease only and those with metastatic disease. The EFS and OS hazard

ratios were: 1.47 (95% CI 1.11–1.96) and 1.52 (95% CI 1.11–2.07) for those with localised disease only. For those with metastatic disease, the HRs for EFS and OS were: 1.20 (95% CI 0.82–1.74) and 1.22 (95% CI 0.82–1.80) based on all patients, and 0.98 (95% CI 0.65–1.48) and 1.01 (0.66–1.57) based on those who had local therapies.

In an analysis in which only patients that had a local recurrence (with or without distant recurrence) were counted as an event (all other events censored at the time when they occurred), an excess risk was still found in CCLG patients compared to GPOH. The hazard ratios were: 3.46 (95% CI 2.19–5.47) unadjusted, and 3.47 (95% CI 2.00–6.01), allowing for age, primary site, histology and local treatment.

Appendix Table 9 also shows hazard ratios for CCLG compared to GPOH patients only among those who received local treatment. The HRs were 1.22 and 1.28 for EFS and OS, respectively. These estimates were somewhat lower than those in all patients (and only just missed statistical significance, due to being based on a smaller number of patients), indicating that the difference between the HRs based on all patients and those based only on those who had local treatment is largely due to excluding those with progressive disease or missing data on local therapy. The EFS HR of 1.22 reduced

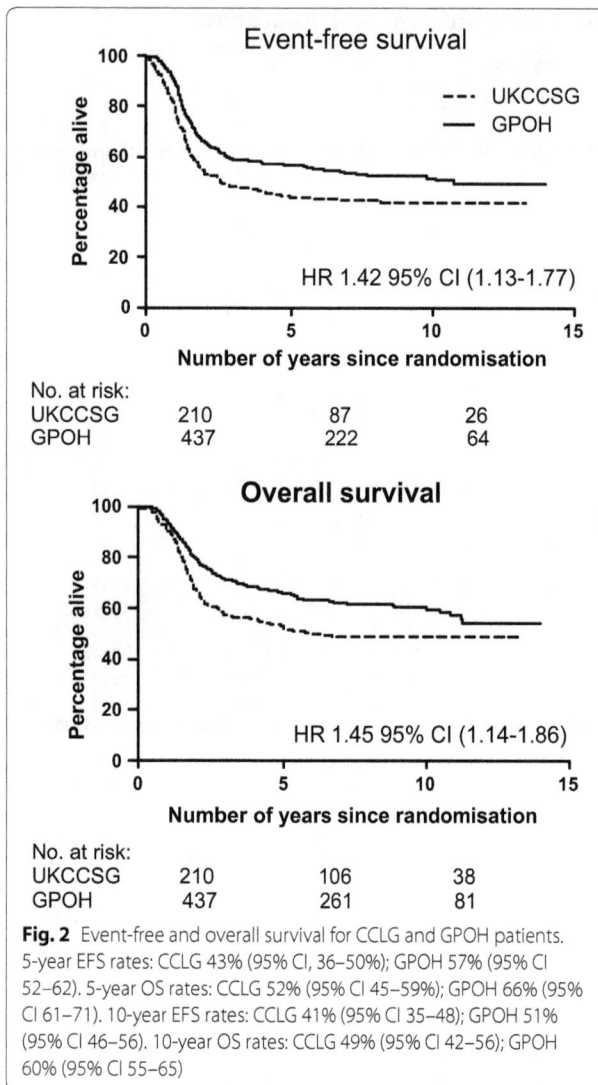

Fig. 2 Event-free and overall survival for CCLG and GPOH patients. 5-year EFS rates: CCLG 43% (95% CI, 36–50%); GPOH 57% (95% CI 52–62). 5-year OS rates: CCLG 52% (95% CI 45–59%); GPOH 66% (95% CI 61–71). 10-year EFS rates: CCLG 41% (95% CI 35–48); GPOH 51% (95% CI 46–56). 10-year OS rates: CCLG 49% (95% CI 42–56); GPOH 60% (95% CI 55–65)

to 1.14 after allowing for the type of local treatment, i.e. it is partly explained by differences in the local therapy administered (consistent with Table 2) further indicating the influence of local treatments on survival outcomes.

When we examined the effect of different local treatment modalities on outcomes, there was no evidence of a difference between CCLG and GPOH patients for either EFS or OS among those who received radiotherapy alone (Table 4). This is not surprising given that the proportions with a local relapse (with or without metastases) were not very different: 22% CCLG vs. 16% GPOH (Appendix Table 7, 8). The risk of an event or death was moderately higher in the CCLG group among patients who had surgery alone (excess risk: EFS 31% and OS 50%, though neither were statistically significant). However, among patients who had both radiotherapy and surgery

(Table 4), CCLG patients were 67% more likely to have an event (p = 0.03) and 65% more likely to die (p = 0.05). The adjusted point estimates were similar but were not statistically significant (p = 0.07 for both EFS and OS). To further consider different numbers of CCLG and GPOH patients who received radiotherapy then surgery or vice versa, Table 4 shows HRs within in each subgroup: there was still evidence of an excess risk among CCLG patients. Appendix Table 10 is only based on patients without metastatic disease: the conclusions were similar to Table 4. Appendix Table 11 is based only on patients with metastatic disease: it is difficult to make any reliable conclusions because of the smaller patient numbers.

Local treatment and timing of treatment

GPOH patients were more likely to have "early" local therapy, i.e. within 12 weeks of starting chemotherapy, compared to CCLG patients: 43% (176/407) vs. 9% (17/180), p < 0.001. This is consistent with the greater use of pre-operative radiotherapy. GPOH patients were also less likely to have "late" local therapy, i.e. more than 15 weeks from start of chemotherapy; 20% (82/407), vs. 32% (57/180) p = 0.004. There was an association between clinical outcome and the length of time from the start of chemotherapy to the start of local therapy (considered as a continuous variable). For every increase of 4 weeks, the risk of an (EFS) event increased by 27% (HR 1.27, 95% CI 1.05–1.53) among patients who had pre-operative radiotherapy; 14% (HR 1.14, 95% CI 1.02–1.27) among those who had surgery, with or without subsequent radiotherapy; and 7% (HR 1.07, 95% CI 0.96–1.19) among those who had radiotherapy alone.

Appendix Table 12 examines the influence of type of local treatment and its timing (in all patients and only those with localised disease). Either factor reduced the HRs for EFS and OS to a similar extent. In the multivariate model they were each independent prognostic factors. However, Table 4 and Appendix Table 10 show that when the data were presented by type of treatment, the timing had some effect but it still did not largely explain the difference between CCLG and GPOH outcomes (surgery with or without radiotherapy).

Localised extremity tumours

Table 5 shows the hazard ratios comparing CCLG with GPOH, according to primary site. When 253 patients with localised extremity tumours were examined, statistically significant survival differences remained between the two study groups. There was a 68% increase in the death rate among CCLG patients compared to those in GPOH, after allowing for local therapy and other factors (Table 5, p = 0.05). The 5-year survival rates were: GPOH 81% (95% CI 75–87%), and CCLG 62% (95% CI 52–72%).

Table 4 Hazard ratios (CCLG vs. GPOH) according to local treatment modality

	Local treatment modality				Subdivision of RT and surgery group	
	None N = 23	Radiotherapy (RT) alone N = 164	Surgery alone N = 138	RT and surgery N = 289	RT then surgery N = 201	Surgery then RT N = 88
No. events						
EFS	21	105	53	131	93	38
OS	19	92	41	109	79	30
Unadjusted						
EFS	20 (2.64–161)	0.86 (0.58–1.26)	1.31 (0.76–2.25)	1.67 (1.05–2.66)	2.22 (0.81–6.07)	1.99 (1.05–3.78)
OS	1.50 (0.56–3.96)	0.95 (0.63–1.44)	1.50 (0.81–2.80)	1.65 (1.00–2.74)	1.96 (0.72–5.37)	2.10 (1.02–4.30)
Adjusted for age, metastatic disease, primary site and histology						
EFS	53 (4.0–477)	0.92 (0.62–1.38)	1.24 (0.70–2.20)	1.82 (1.12–2.94)	2.40 (0.84–6.84)	2.50 (1.24–5.06)
OS	2.09 (0.64–6.79)	1.06 (0.69–1.63)	1.41 (0.73–2.74)	1.81 (1.07–3.05)	2.21 (0.77–6.35)	2.76 (1.26–6.05)
Adjusted for age, metastatic disease, primary site, histology and time between the start of chemotherapy and starting local treatment						
EFS		0.91 (0.60–1.38)	1.24 (0.70–2.19)	1.61 (0.96–2.70)	1.98 (0.70–5.60)	2.83 (1.30–6.16)
OS		1.04 (0.67–1.63)	1.43 (0.73–2.78)	1.68 (0.97–2.91)	1.94 (0.68–5.58)	3.39 (1.42–8.06)

Hazard ratios greater than 1 indicate that CCLG patients had a higher risk of having an event or dying compared to GPOH patients

Based on data excluding patients with unknown primary site because there were so few

EFS event-free survival; *OS* overall survival

Table 5 Hazard ratios (CCLG vs. GPOH) according to primary site and localised disease

	No. events	Unadjusted		Adjusted for age, metastatic disease, histology and local treatment	
		Hazard ratio 95% CI	p value	Hazard ratio 95% CI	p value
Central axis					
All (n = 320)					
EFS	177	1.48 (1.08–2.03)	0.02	1.27 (0.89–1.82)	0.19
OS	154	1.47 (1.05–2.06)	0.03	1.20 (0.82–1.75)	0.36
Localised (n = 220)					
EFS	102	1.47 (0.97–2.24)	0.07	1.33 (0.82–2.16)	0.24
OS	87	1.46 (0.93–2.30)	0.10	1.15 (0.69–1.92)	0.58
Extremity					
All (n = 312)					
EFS	140	1.56 (1.12–2.18)	0.009	1.75 (1.18–2.60)	0.005
OS	112	1.69 (1.17–2.45)	0.006	1.59 (1.02–2.46)	0.04
Localised (n = 253)					
EFS	99	1.68 (1.13–2.50)	0.01	1.56 (1.00–2.43)	0.05
OS	75	1.86 (1.18–2.93)	0.007	1.68 (1.00–2.81)	0.05
Pelvic disease					
All (n = 168)					
EFS	100	1.36 (0.90–2.05)	0.14	1.05 (0.65–1.70)	0.84
OS	90	1.32 (0.85–2.04)	0.21	0.98 (0.60–1.62)	0.94
Localised (n = 107)					
EFS	56	1.22 (0.69–2.15)	0.51	0.98 (0.51–1.89)	0.96
OS	51	1.17 (0.64–2.14)	0.61	1.01 (0.51–2.03)	0.97

Hazard ratios greater than 1 indicate that CCLG patients had a higher risk of having an event or dying compared to GPOH patients

Hazard ratios for localised disease were not adjusted for metastatic disease

EFS event-free survival; *OS* overall survival

There were no differences in the baseline patient characteristics or number of chemotherapy cycles received, except a slight excess of atypical ES in GPOH; 15% (24/162) vs. 5% (5/91) in CCLG. For patients with localised extremity tumours, combined modality treatment was used more frequently in GPOH patients than CCLG patients (66% vs. 24%) whereas a greater proportion of CCLG patients were treated with radiotherapy alone (20% vs. 5%). More CCLG patients had a local recurrence, with or without metastatic disease (16% vs. 3%).

Central axis and pelvic tumours

Among patients with central axis tumours, the HRs for both EFS and OS reduced after allowing for several factors, and most of the reduction was due to adjusting for local treatment, indicating that this does have a role. A more pronounced reduction was seen for patients with pelvic disease (HRs: EFS 1.05, OS 0.98). Patients with localised pelvic tumours had a similar survival whether treated in the CCLG or GPOH: the 5-year OS rates were 52 and 56%, respectively (p = 0.65), and the adjusted OS HR was 1.01, 95% CI 0.51–2.03 (Table 5), allowing for the different local treatment modalities used between the two cohorts. Radiotherapy alone was the local treatment modality used in 77% (24/31) CCLG patients compared to 34% (27/79) GPOH patients. Surgery combined with radiotherapy was only used for 3% of CCLG patients (1/31) compared to 49% of GPOH patients (39/79). A survival advantage seemed evident for patients with localised pelvic tumours selected for surgery, compared to those who had radiotherapy alone (hazard ratio 0.50, 95% CI 0.28–0.88, p = 0.016).

Discussion

The EICESS-92 clinical trial revealed unexpected differences in survival between cohorts of ES patients from two countries. Differences in mortality from cancer between countries are well documented in Europe, especially for common cancers [6, 7]. These differences in outcome have also been reported for rare cancers [8, 9]. Survival in the UK is lower for some cancers than in other Western European and Nordic countries. Explanations for these differences may include: registry data being unrepresentative or containing artefact; differences in population health or use of health resources; differences in stage of cancer at diagnosis and variable access to optimal treatment or expertise [10]. Within EURO-CARE 3, which examined registry data for 20 European countries, 5-year survival from ES ranged from 31 to 86% for the period 1990–1994 [11]. The EUROCARE-5 study investigated whether survival differences among European countries had changed further from 1999 to 2007 and found persisting inequalities both for children and adolescents and young adults [12, 13]. The main influences on continued survival disparity are attributable to lack of health-care resources and access to modern treatments, lack of specialised centres with multidisciplinary teams, delayed diagnosis and treatment and poor management of treatment, and drug toxicity. However, this is unlikely to fully account for the wide range in survival from ES reported here.

Given that all patients were treated according to a common protocol, the substantial survival differences between national study groups in this randomised trial are striking. Survival for the entire group of 647 patients exceeded 60% but this disguises the 14% inferior 5 year survival of the cohort of patients recruited through the CCLG. The inferior outcome was not obviously accounted for by differences in baseline characteristics, delivery of chemotherapy or follow up. Differences were found in management of the primary tumour and in the rates of local recurrence associated with different treatment modalities. We believe that this evidence provides support that variations in local therapy influence survival.

It is possible that inherent differences in health care delivery systems between the two study groups may have contributed to survival differences. No differences were found in the tumour volume and the frequency of presentation with metastases between the two study groups, factors which might indicate systematic delays in diagnosis in one study group compared to the other. Likewise, there was no indication of a systematic difference in the way chemotherapy was delivered.

Approaches to local tumour control were clearly different between the two groups, including the timing of local treatments, but they did not explain all of the difference, particularly when patients had surgery. Primary tumour control in ES can be achieved with surgery, radiotherapy or a combination of both. The choice is based on balancing the differing morbidities of the two modalities for each individual patient. The optimal approach for local control remains a topic of debate. The relative merits of surgery and radiotherapy have been debated but conclusions are often obscured by patient selection which biases comparison [5, 14–17]. Tumours that are inoperable and thus treated by radiotherapy alone are often associated with other adverse features such as large volume [18–21]. The greater incidence of local relapse in CCLG patients indicates that both selection of patients for, and delivery of, surgery and radiotherapy may have been sub-optimal.

While not specific to Ewing sarcoma, there is a general consensus on the relevance of centralization to high volume centres and networks for sarcoma, especially for diagnosis and surgery [22, 23]. The degree of centralisation and the process of decision-making about local therapy differed between the two study groups in EICESS-92.

Ideally, the optimal local treatment for an individual patient should be decided through consideration of patient characteristics, the potential benefit and harm of the treatment options, and patient preference. In the CESS group, treatment took place in three hundred or more centres, most of which treat relatively few patients. However, each centre was familiar with accessing specialist guidance from the trial headquarters. This extended to a centralised system of advice for local therapy planning [5]. A consequence is likely to have been considerable consistency of local treatment approach within the majority of the GPOH cohort. In contrast, although surgery for bone sarcomas took place mainly in four centres in the UK, advice about local tumour management was only sought on an ad hoc basis and there was no similar system for any degree of central treatment planning.

The EICESS-92 trial is an example of how collaboration between national clinical study groups is required to run large randomised trials with sufficient power for robust analyses in rare cancers. It is acknowledged that the work has been delayed in its publication but it has been revisited to coincide with a strong current focus and drive for international consensus on the role of surgery and radiotherapy in ES.

The low rates of local recurrence evident with patients undergoing combined modality treatment and the enhanced survival for a cohort of patients, more of whom underwent surgical resection and received radiotherapy, indicates that clinicians should always consider this option. Nevertheless, this must be balanced against the additional late effects, including second malignancies, which are associated with the use of radiotherapy in ES.

Conclusion

In summary, unexpected differences in survival between cohorts of patients within the same randomised trial have been identified and are national in origin. It appears that less aggressive methods of local control have resulted in a higher rate of local recurrence and this was associated with a higher risk of metastatic disease and subsequent death. These data reinforce the importance of careful planning of treatment for local tumour control in ES and that radiotherapy alone should be discouraged when sur-

gical resection can be undertaken. International clinical trials may offer opportunities to explore the impact of different treatment approaches. As a consequence of the results from this trial, the UK has initiated a system for centralised national review and guidance on local treatment decision making for ES. This system is currently undergoing evaluation.

Authors' contributions
JW, AMCT, AH, RG, AC, DS, JB, IL and MP contributed to discussion, interpretation and appraisal of the presented data. All but AH and JB participated in the EICESS 92 study. AH undertook the statistical analysis. JW and AH drafted the manuscript. HJ and AC critically appraised the manuscript and were joint chairman of the EICESS 92 study. All authors read and approved the final manuscript.

Author details
[1] Department of Oncology, University College Hospitals London NHS Foundation Trust, 250 Euston Road, London NW1 2PG, UK. [2] Cancer Research UK and UCL Clinical Trials Centre, University College London, London, UK. [3] Children's Cancer and Leukaemia Group Data Centre, Cancer Studies and Molecular Medicine, University of Leicester, Leicester, UK. [4] The Royal Orthopaedic Hospital, Birmingham, UK. [5] Queen Elizabeth II Hospital, Birmingham, UK. [6] University Hospital Essen, Essen, Germany. [7] Vestische Kinder- und Jugendklinik Datteln, University Witten/Herdecke, Datteln, Germany. [8] Department of Pediatric Hematology and Oncology, University Children's Hospital Münster, Münster, Germany. [9] Northern Institute for Cancer Research, Newcastle University, Newcastle upon Tyne, UK. [10] University of Leeds and Leeds Community Healthcare Trust, Leeds, UK.

Acknowledgements
We are grateful for the support given to this project by staff at the CCLG Data Centre in Leicester, especially Claire Weston and Carolyn Douglas. This work was undertaken in part at UCLH/UCL who received a proportion of funding from the Department of Health's NIHR Biomedical Research Centres funding scheme. Presented in part at ASCO Annual Meeting, Atlanta, June 2006.

Competing interests
The authors declare they have no competing interests.

Funding
Supported by Deutsche Krebshilfe (Grants No. DKH M43/92/Jü2 and DKH 70-2551 Jü3), and European Union Biomedicine and Health Programme (Grants No. BMH1-CT92-1341 and BMH4-983956), and Cancer Research United Kingdom.

Appendix
See Tables 6, 7, 8, 9, 10, 11 and 12.

Table 6 Number of patients and events according to trial group

	Number of patients (percentage)		Total
	CCLG N = 210	GPOH N = 437	
First events (total)	119 (57)	204 (47)	323
Death-treatment related	1 (0.5)	3 (1)	4
Disease progression	3 (1)	12 (3)	15
Unknown cause	3 (1)	1 (0.2)	3
Distant metastases	66 (31)	148 (34)	214
[Distant metastases in those with metastatic disease at baseline]	[25 (12%)]	[57 (13%)]	[82]
Local relapse	29 (14)	13 (3)	42
Local and distant relapse	16 (8)	18 (4)	34
Relapse (unspecified site)	0	4 (1)	4
Second malignancy	2 (1)	5 (1)	7
All deaths	105 (50)	168 (38)	273

As a percentage of the number of patients from either CCLG or GPOH

Table 7 Distribution of first events by treatment modality: CCLG patients

	Local treatment modality, N (%)						Total
	Surgery alone N = 70	RT alone N = 81	RT then surgery N = 6	Surgery then RT N = 32	None N = 18	Unknown N = 3	
No event	41 (59)	31 (38)	2 (33)	14 (44)	0	2 (67)	90
Local recurrence	5 (7.1)	12 (15)	1 (17)	1 (3.1)	10 (56)	0	29
Distant recurrence	18 (26)	28 (35)	1 (17)	13 (41)	5 (28)	1 (33)	66
Local and distant	3 (4.3)	6 (7.4)	2 (33)	3 (9.4)	2 (11)	0	13
Relapse-unspecified	0	0	0	0	0	0	0
Second malignancy	1 (1.4)	1 (1.2)	0	0	0	0	2
Death—no relapse	2 (2.9)	3 (3.7)	0	1 (3.1)	1 (5.6)	0	7
All deaths	24 (34)	45 (56)	4 (67)	15 (47)	16 (89)	1 (33)	105

RT radiotherapy

Table 8 Distribution of first events by treatment modality: GPOH patients

	Local treatment modality, N (%)						Total
	Surgery alone N = 71	RT alone N = 85	RT then surgery N = 195	Surgery then RT N = 60	None N = 7	Unknown N = 19	
No event	46 (65)	30 (35)	106 (54)	38 (63)	1 (14)	12 (63)	233
Local recurrence	3 (4.2)	3 (3.5)	3 (1.5)	4 (6.7)	0	0	13
Distant recurrence	19 (27)	36 (42)	71 (36)	16 (27)	2 (29)	4 (21)	148
Local and distant	2 (2.8)	10 (12)	4 (2.0)	1 (1.7)	0	1 (5.3)	18
Relapse-unspecified	0	1 (1.2)	2 (1.0)	0	0	1 (5.3)	4
Second malignancy	1 (1.4)	2 (2.4)	2 (1.0)	0	0	0	5
Death—no relapse	0	3 (3.5)	7 (3.6)	1 (1.7)	4 (57)	1 (5.3)	16
All deaths	18 (25)	47 (55)	75 (38)	17 (28)	6 (86)	5 (26)	158

To one decimal place if < 10%

RT radiotherapy

Table 9 Hazard ratios for comparing CCLG and GPOH patients

	EFS		OS	
	HR (95% CI)	p value	HR (95% CI)	p value
All patients				
Unadjusted	1.42 (1.13–1.77)	0.002	1.45 (1.14–1.86)	0.003
Unadjusted HR, in localised disease only	1.47 (1.11–1.96)	0.007	1.52 (1.11–2.07)	0.009
Adjusted for risk group and trial treatment	1.43 (1.14–1.79)	0.002	1.49 (1.17–1.91)	0.001
Adjusted for each of the following factors separately[a]				
Age	1.45 (1.15–1.81)	0.001	1.47 (1.15–1.88)	0.002
Metastatic disease	1.38 (1.10–1.73)	0.005	1.42 (1.11–1.81)	0.005
Primary site	1.48 (1.18–1.86)	<0.001	1.52 (1.19–1.95)	0.001
Histology	1.41 (1.12–1.77)	0.004	1.44 (1.12–1.85)	0.004
Local treatment modality[b]	1.45 (1.12–1.89)	0.006	1.30 (0.98–1.72)	0.07
Adjusted for age, metastatic disease, primary site, histology and local treatment[a]	1.44 (1.10–1.89)	0.009	1.30 (0.97–1.74)	0.08
Adjusted HR, in localised disease only	1.48 (1.05–2.09)	0.026	1.29 (0.88–1.89)	0.19
Only patients who had local therapy; excluding progressive disease (n = 25) and where it was not known whether local therapy was given or not n = 22)				
Unadjusted	1.22 (0.96–1.55)	0.11	1.28 (0.99–1.67)	0.06
Adjusted for type of local treatment[c]	1.14 (0.87–1.51)	0.34	1.25 (0.92–1.68)	0.15
Adjusted for time between the start of chemotherapy and starting local treatment	1.12 (0.87–1.44)	0.37	1.18 (0.90–1.55)	0.22
Adjusted for age, metastatic disease, primary site, histology, local treatment, and time between the start of chemotherapy and starting local treatment	1.13 (0.84–1.50)	0.42	1.25 (0.91–1.71)	0.17

Hazard ratios greater than 1 indicate that CCLG patients had a higher risk of having an event or dying compared to GPOH patients

EFS event-free survival; *OS* overall survival

[a] Using Cox regression modelling (age as a continuous variable). Missing data for the other variables were included as a separate category, but excluding these from the analyses did not materially change the hazard ratio estimates in the table

[b] Includes categories for no local therapy and missing data

[c] Surgery alone, radiotherapy alone, surgery then radiotherapy, radiotherapy then surgery

Table 10 Hazard ratios (CCLG vs. GPOH) according to local treatment modality, among patients with localised disease only

	Local treatment modality			Subdivision of RT and surgery group	
	Radiotherapy (RT) alone N = 108	Surgery alone N = 119	RT and surgery N = 221	RT then surgery N = 152	Surgery then RT N = 69
No. events					
EFS	62	42	83	61	22
OS	53	33	66	49	17
Unadjusted					
EFS	0.89 (0.54–1.46)	1.44 (0.78–2.64)	1.66 (0.94–2.96)	2.44 (0.76–7.81)	2.36 (1.02–5.45)
OS	0.99 (0.56–1.64)	1.74 (0.86–3.51)	1.60 (0.84–3.06)	2.70 (0.84–8.73)	2.03 (0.78–5.28)
Adjusted for age, primary site and histology					
EFS	0.98 (0.58–1.66)	1.51 (0.78–2.94)	1.65 (0.91–2.99)	2.39 (0.71–8.05)	2.12 (0.83–5.40)
OS	1.10 (0.62–1.95)	1.94 (0.89–4.25)	1.50 (0.77–2.93)	3.10 (0.90–10.70)	1.74 (0.60–5.08)
Adjusted for age, primary site, histology and time between the start of chemotherapy and starting local treatment					
EFS	0.95 (0.54–1.67)	1.48 (0.76–2.89)	1.48 (0.81–2.69)	1.69 (0.50–5.68)	2.10 (0.82–5.41)
OS	1.03 (0.55–1.90)	1.92 (0.87–4.24)	1.39 (0.71–2.74)	2.49 (0.72–8.58)	1.74 (0.59–5.10)

Hazard ratios greater than 1 indicate that CCLG patients had a higher risk of having an event or dying compared to GPOH patients

Based on data excluding patients with unknown primary site because there were so few

EFS event-free survival; *OS* overall survival

Table 11 Hazard ratios (CCLG vs. GPOH) according to local treatment modality, among patients with metastatic disease only

	Local treatment modality		
	Radiotherapy (RT) alone N = 56	Surgery alone N = 19	RT and surgery N = 66
No. events			
EFS	43	11	48
OS	39	8	43
Unadjusted			
EFS	0.79 (0.43–1.44)	0.79 (0.24–2.61)	2.01 (0.89–4.54)
OS	0.92 (0.49–1.74)	0.71 (0.18–2.85)	1.98 (0.88–4.47)
Adjusted for age, primary site, histology and time between the start of chemotherapy and starting local treatment			
EFS	0.81 (0.44–1.67)	Too few patients to allow for other factors reliably	2.51 (0.89–7.06)
OS	1.01 (0.50–2.01)		2.54 (0.90–7.20)

Hazard ratios greater than 1 indicate that CCLG patients had a higher risk of having an event or dying compared to GPOH patients

Based on data excluding patients with unknown primary site because there were so few

EFS event-free survival; *OS* overall survival

Table 12 Hazard ratios for comparing CCLG and GPOH patients, after examining local treatment and time to local treatment

	EFS		OS	
	HR (95% CI)	p value	HR (95% CI)	p value
All patients				
Unadjusted	1.22 (0.96–1.56)	0.10	1.29 (0.99–1.68)	0.055
Adjusted for local treatment[a]	1.14 (0.87–1.51)	0.34	1.25 (0.93–1.68)	0.15
Adjusted for between the start of chemotherapy and starting local treatment	1.13 (0.88–1.45)	0.34	1.19 (0.91–1.56)	0.20
Adjusted for both local treatment and timing	1.11 (0.84–1.47)	0.46	1.21 (0.90–1.65)	0.21
Localised disease only				
Unadjusted	1.31 (0.97–1.76)	0.08	1.39 (1.00–1.93)	0.048
Adjusted for local treatment[a]	1.22 (0.87–1.72)	0.25	1.30 (0.89–1.90)	0.17
Adjusted for between the start of chemotherapy and starting local treatment	1.18 (0.87–1.60)	0.30	1.24 (0.88–1.74)	0.21
Adjusted for local treatment and the time between the start of chemotherapy and starting local treatment	1.14 (0.81–1.62)	0.45	1.20 (0.82–1.77)	0.35
Metastatic disease only				
Unadjusted	0.98 (0.65–1.48)	0.93	1.01 (0.66–1.57)	0.94
Adjusted for local treatment[a]	0.98 (0.61–1.56)	0.93	1.11 (0.68–1.81)	0.69
Adjusted for between the start of chemotherapy and starting local treatment	0.95 (0.62–1.45)	0.81	1.00 (0.64–1.57)	0.98
Adjusted for both local treatment and timing	0.99 (0.61–1.60)	0.97	1.14 (0.69–1.89)	0.60

Type of local treatment and time to local treatment seem to be independent factors. In the Cox regression which contains both of them, the p values for each variable are: All patients EFS: local treatment ($p < 0.0001$); time to local treatment ($p < 0.001$)

All patients OS: local treatment ($p < 0.0001$); time to local treatment ($p < 0.001$)

Patients with localised disease only, EFS: local treatment ($p = 0.002$); time to local treatment ($p = 0.002$)

Patients with localised disease only OS: local treatment ($p = 0.002$; time to local treatment ($p = 0.004$)

[a] Surgery alone, radiotherapy alone, surgery then radiotherapy, radiotherapy then surgery

References

1. Gaspar N, Hawkins DS, Dirksen U, Lewis IK, Ferrari S, Le Deley MC, Kovar J, Grimer R, Whelan J, Claude L, Delattre O, Paulussen M, Picci P, Sundby Hall K, van den Berg H, Ladenstein R, Michon J, Hiorth L, Judson I, Luksch R, Bernstein ML, Marec-Berard P, Brennan B, Craft AW, Womer RB, Juergens H, Oberlin O. Ewing sarcoma: current management and future approaches through collaboration. J Clin Oncol. 2015;20:3036–46.
2. Bolling T, Braun-Munzinger G, Burdach S, Calaminus G, Craft A, Delattre O, Delege MC, Dirksen U, Dockhorn-Dworniczak B, Dunst J, Engel S, Faldum A, Frohlich B, Gadner H, Gobel U, Gosheger G, Hardes J, Hawkins DS, Hiorth L, Hoffmann C, Kovar H, Kruseova J, Ladenstein R, Leuschner I, Lewis IJ, Oberlin O, Paulussen M, Potratz J, Ranft A, Rossig C, Rube C, Sauer R, Schober O, Schuck A, Timmermann B, Tirode F, van den Berg H, van Valen F, Vieth V, Willich N, Winkelmann W, Whelan J, Womer RB. Development of curative therapies for Ewing sarcomas by interdisciplinary cooperative groups in Europe. Klin Padiatr. 2015;227:108–15.
3. Paulussen M, Craft AW, Lewis I, Hackshaw A, Douglas C, Dunst J, Schuck A, Winkelmann W, Kohler G, Poremba C, Zoubek A, Ladenstein R, van den Berg H, Hunold A, Cassoni A, Spooner D, Grimer R, Whelan J, McTiernan A, Jurgens H, European Intergroup Cooperative Ewing's Sarcoma Study 92. Results of the EICESS-92 Study: two randomized trials of Ewing's sarcoma treatment—cyclophosphamide compared with ifosfamide in standard-risk patients and assessment of benefit of etoposide added to standard treatment in high-risk patients. J Clin Oncol. 2008;26:4385–93.
4. Whelan JS, McTiernan A, Weston C, Douglas C, Grimer R, Cassoni A, Spooner D, Paulussen M, Jurgens H, Craft A, Lewis I. Consequences of different approaches to local treatment of Ewing's sarcoma within an international randomised controlled trial: analysis of EICESS-92. J Clin Oncol. 2006;24(18_suppl):9533.
5. Dunst J, Schuck A. Role of radiotherapy in Ewing tumors. Pediatr Blood Cancer. 2004;42:465–70.
6. Sant M, Capocaccia R, Coleman MP, Berrino F, Gatta G, Micheli A, Verdecchia A, Faivre J, Hakulinen T, Coebergh JW, Martinez-Garcia C, Forman D, Zapoone A, EUROCARE Working Group. Cancer survival increases in Europe, but international differences remain wide. Eur J Cancer. 2001;37:1659–67.
7. Karim-Kos HE, de Vries S, Soeriomataram I, Lemmens V, Siesling S, Coebergh JW. Recent trends of cancer in Europe: a combined approach of incidence, survival and mortality for 17 cancer sites since the 1990s. Eur J Cancer. 2008;44:1345–89.
8. Gatta G, Trama A, Capacaccia R, RARECARENet Working Group. Epidemiology of rare cancers and inequalities in oncologic outcomes. Eur J Surg Oncol. 2017;19:685–6.
9. Gatta G, Capocaccia R, Botta L, Mallone S, De Angelis R, Ardanaz E, Comber H, Dimitrova N, Leinonen MK, Siesling S, van der Zwan JM, Van Eycken L, Visser O, Zakelj MP, Anderson LA, Bella F, Kaire I, Otter R, Stiller CA, Trama A, RARECAREnet Working Group. Burden and centralised treatment in Europe of rare tumours: results of RARECAREnet—a population-based study. Lancet Oncol. 2017;18:1022–39.
10. Coleman MP, Gatta G, Verdecchia A, Esteve J, Sant M, Storm H, Allemani C, Ciccolallo L, Santaguilani M, Berrino F, EUROCARE Working Group. EUROCARE-3 summary: cancer survival in Europe at the end of the 20th century. Ann Oncol. 2003;14:128–49.
11. Gatta G, Capocaccia R, De Angelis R, Stiller C, Coebergh JW, EUROCARE Working Group. Cancer survival in European adolescents and young adults. Eur J Cancer. 2003;39:2600–10.
12. Gatta G, Botta L, Rossi S, Aareleid T, Bielska-Lasota M, Clavel J, Dimitrova N, Jakab Z, Kaatsch P, Lacour B, Mallone S, Marcos-Gragera R, Minicozzi P, Sánchez-Pérez MJ, Sant M, Santaquilani M, Stiller C, Tavilla A, Trama A, Visser O, Peris-Bonet R, EUROCARE Working Group. Childhood cancer survival in Europe 1999–2007: results of EUROCARE-5–a population-based study. Lancet Oncol. 2014;15:35–47.
13. Trama A, Botta L, Foschi R, Ferrari A, Stiller C, Desandes E, Maule MM, Merletti F, Gatta G, EUROCARE-5 Working Group. Survival of European adolescents and young adults diagnosed with cancer in 2000–07: population-based data from EUROCARE-5. Lancet Oncol. 2016;17:896–906.
14. Schuck A, Ahrens S, Paulussen M, Kuhlen M, Konemann S, Rube C, Winkelmann W, Kotz R, Dunst J, Willich N, Jurgens H. Local therapy in localized Ewing tumors: results of 1058 patients treated in the CESS 81, CESS 86, and EICESS 92 trials. Int J Radiat Oncol Biol Phys. 2003;55:168–77.
15. Miller BJ, Gao Y, Duchman KR. Does surgery or radiation provide the best overall survival in Ewing Sarcoma? A review of the National Cancer Data Base. J Surg Oncol. 2017;116:384–90.
16. DuBois SG, Krailo MD, Gebhardt MC, Donaldson SS, Marcus KJ, Dormans J, Shamberger RC, Sailer S, Nicholas RW, Healey JH, Tarbell NJ, Randall RL, Devidas M, Meyer JS, Granowetter L, Womer RB, Bernstein M, Marina N, Grier HE. Comparative evaluation of local control strategies in localized Ewing sarcoma of bone: a report from the Children's Oncology Group. Cancer. 2015;121:467–75.
17. Bacci G, Ferrari S, Mercuri M, Longhi A, Giacomini S, Forni C, Bertoni F, Manfrini M, Barbieri E, Lari S, Donati D. Multimodal therapy for the treatment of nonmetastatic Ewing sarcoma of pelvis. J Pediatr Hematol Oncol. 2003;25:118–24.
18. Foulon S, Brennan B, Gaspar N, Dirksen U, Jeys L, Cassoni A, Claude L, Seddon B, Marec-Berard P, Whelan J, Paulussen M, Streighbuerger A, Oberlin O, Juergens H, Grimer R, Le Deley MC. Can postoperative radiotherapy be omitted in localised standard risk Ewing sarcoma? An observation study of the Euro-E.W.I.N.G group. Eur J Cancer. 2016;61:128–36.
19. Cotterill SJ, Ahrens S, Paulussen M, Jurgens HF, Voute PA, Gadner H, Craft AW. Prognostic factors in Ewing's tumor of bone: analysis of 975 patients from the European Intergroup Cooperative Ewing's Sarcoma Study Group. J Clin Oncol. 2000;18:3108–14.
20. Ning MS, Perkins SM, Borinstein SC, Holt GE, Stavas MJ, Shinohara ET. Role of radiation in the treatment of non-metastatic osseous Ewing Sarcoma. J Med Imaging Radiat Oncol. 2016;60:119–28.
21. Werier J, Yao X, Caudrelier JM, Di Primio G, Ghert M, Gupta AA, Kandel R, Verma S. A systematic review of optimal treatment strategies for localised Ewing's sarcoma of bone after neo-adjuvant chemotherapy. Surg Oncol. 2016;25:16–23.
22. Blay J-Y, Stoeckle E, Italiano, A, Rochwerger RA, Duffaud F, Bonvalot S, Honore C, Decanter G, Maynou C, Anract P, Ferron G, Guillemin F, Gouin F, Rios M, Kurtz JE, Meeus P, Coindre JM, Ray-Coquard I, Penel N, Le Cesne A. Improved overall and progression free survival after surgery in expert sites for sarcoma patients: a nationwide study of FSG-GETO/NETSARC. Ann Oncol. 2017;28(suppl_5):v521–38. https://doi.org/10.1093/annonc/mdx387.001.
23. Pasquali S, Bonvalot S, Tzanis D, Casali PG, Trama A, Gronchi A, RARE-CARENet Working Group. Treatment challenges in and outside a network setting: soft tissue sarcomas. Eur J Surg Oncol. 2017;19:30705–9.

21

Reversible rituximab-induced rectal Kaposi's sarcoma misdiagnosed as ulcerative colitis in a patient with HIV-negative follicular lymphoma

Emilien Billon[1], Anne-Marie Stoppa[2], Lena Mescam[3], Massimo Bocci[4], Audrey Monneur[1], Delphine Perrot[1,6] and François Bertucci[1,5,6]*

Abstract

Background: Kaposi's sarcoma is a low-grade mesenchymal angioproliferative tumor, most commonly observed in immunocompromised individuals, such as HIV-infected patients. Iatrogenic Kaposi's sarcoma occurs in patients undergoing immunosuppressive therapies. Rituximab is a chimeric monoclonal antibody targeted against the pan B cell marker CD20. Because of its immunosuppressive effects through reduction of mature B-cells, it may exacerbate Kaposi's sarcoma in HIV-positive patients. Rituximab-related Kaposi's sarcomas have been previously reported in only two HIV-negative patients and were treated surgically.

Case presentation: Here, we report on a Kaposi's sarcoma that developed under rituximab treatment in a HIV-negative 55-year-old patient treated for follicular lymphoma. The lesion developed during the maintenance rituximab therapy at the rectal level with an aspect of apparent ulcerative colitis, without any cutaneous lesion. The premature stop of rituximab led to the complete regression of Kaposi's sarcoma, without any additional specific treatment.

Conclusions: To our knowledge, this is the third case of Kaposi's sarcoma diagnosed under rituximab in a HIV-negative patient, the first one at the rectal level and the first one that completely regresses after stop of rituximab. This case raises awareness of iatrogenic Kaposi's sarcoma in HIV-negative patients treated with rituximab, and further highlights the importance of immunosuppression in the pathophysiology of disease.

Keywords: Follicular lymphoma, Immune suppression, Kaposi sarcoma, Rituximab

Background

Kaposi's sarcoma is a low-grade mesenchymal angioproliferative tumor caused by the lytic replication of human herpesvirus type 8 (HHV8), identified with Polymerase Chain Reaction (PCR) in 95% of cases. The lesions predominantly present at muco-cutaneous sites, but may involve all organs and anatomic locations. Kaposi's sarcoma occurs most commonly in immunocompromised individuals such as HIV-infected patients. Iatrogenic

Kaposi's sarcoma occurs in patients undergoing immunosuppressive therapies for autoimmune disorders or after organ transplantation [1].

Rituximab is a chimeric murine/human monoclonal antibody (mAb) targeted against the pan B-cell marker CD20. It was the first mAb to receive approval by the Food and Drug Administration for use in cancer treatment. Since its approval for relapsed/refractory non-Hodgkin's lymphoma in 1997, rituximab has been licensed for use in the treatment of numerous other B-cell malignancies, including the follicular lymphoma [2], as well as autoimmune conditions, including rheumatoid arthritis. Because of its immunosuppressive effects through action on CD20 and reduction of mature B-cells,

---

*Correspondence: bertuccif@ipc.unicancer.fr
[1] INSERM UMR1068, CNRS UMR725, Department of Medical Oncology, Centre de Recherche en Cancérologie de Marseille (CRCM), Institut Paoli-Calmettes, 232 Bd de Sainte-Marguerite, 13009 Marseille, France
Full list of author information is available at the end of the article

rituximab therapy may exacerbate Kaposi's sarcoma in HIV-positive patients [3]. Rituximab-related Kaposi's sarcomas have been previously reported in two HIV-negative patients, without multicentric Castelman's disease [4, 5], and were treated surgically.

We herein report a rectal Kaposi's sarcoma that developed under rituximab treatment in a HIV-negative patient treated for follicular lymphoma, and that completely regressed upon cessation of rituximab, without any additional specific treatment.

Case presentation

In July 2014, a 55-year-old Caucasian man with cervical and mediastinal polyadenopathies was diagnosed with a non-Hodgkin follicular lymphoma (WHO grade 2) in our institution (Fig. 1A, B). There was no clinical general symptom, and the disease stage was II. He had no specific personal or familial medical history. Because of the low malignancy grade and the low tumor mass, no treatment was introduced, and a monitoring was set up. In June 2015, because of increase in size of cervical adenopathies, therapy combining rituximab (375 mg/m^2) and bendamustine (90 mg/m^2) was initiated. Six monthly cycles were delivered, with good tolerance and complete metabolic response (PET-scan of October 2015), then followed by maintenance rituximab (375 mg/m^2, 1 injection every 2 months) started in December 2015 and planned for 2 years (Fig. 2) [6].

In June 2016, before the fourth maintenance injection, the patient developed diarrhea alternating with

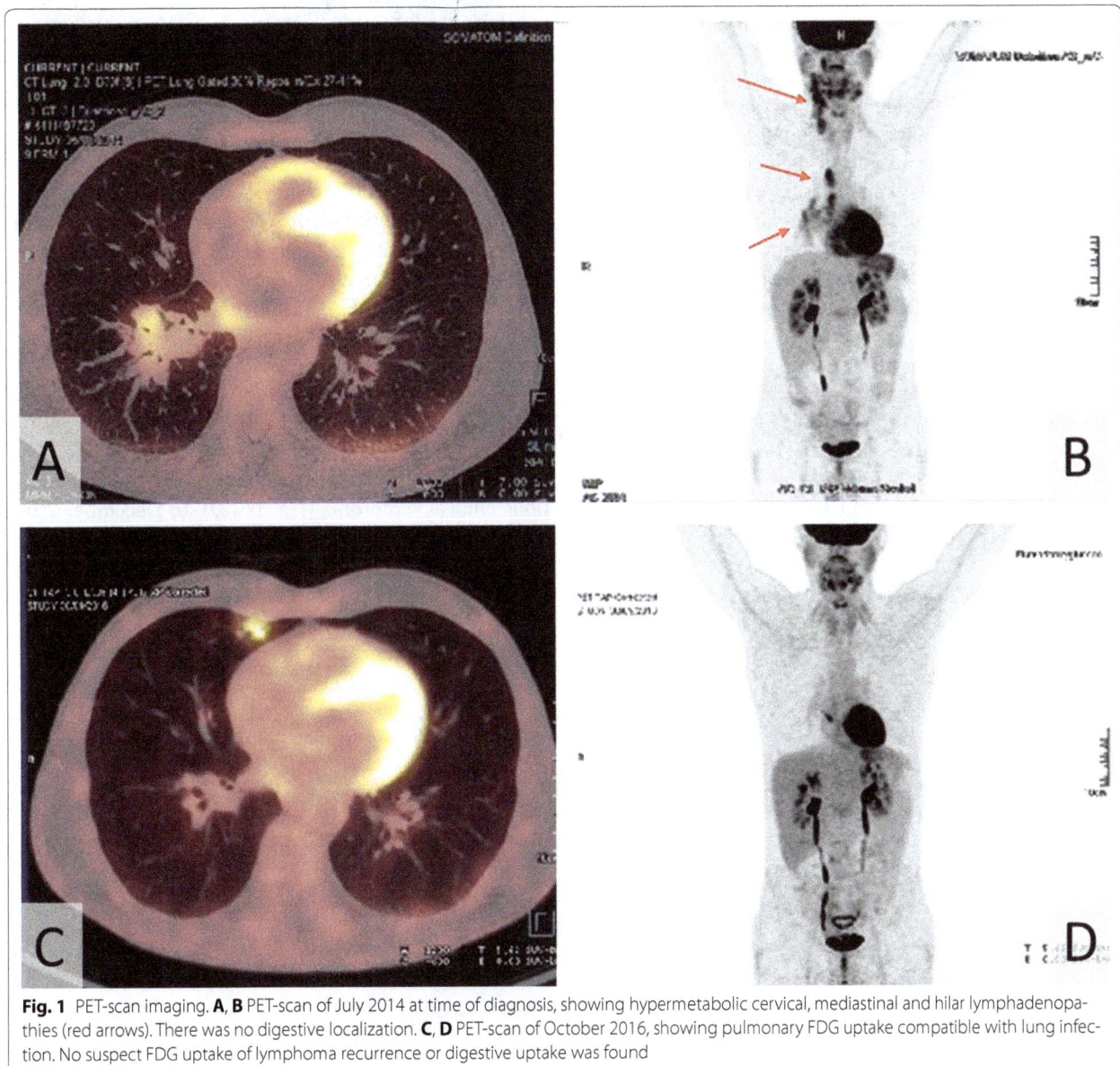

Fig. 1 PET-scan imaging. **A, B** PET-scan of July 2014 at time of diagnosis, showing hypermetabolic cervical, mediastinal and hilar lymphadenopathies (red arrows). There was no digestive localization. **C, D** PET-scan of October 2016, showing pulmonary FDG uptake compatible with lung infection. No suspect FDG uptake of lymphoma recurrence or digestive uptake was found

constipation, nausea, associated with weight loss. Colonoscopy showed sigmoiditis, with a 4-mm-depth rectal ulceration at 20 cm of the anal canal (Fig. 3), compatible with ulcerative colitis. Multiple biopsies were performed, and the provisional diagnosis of ulcerative colitis was retained before availability of pathological results. No fecal calprotectin measurement was done. Mesalazine therapy (2 g/day) was introduced in September 2016. Pathological analysis of the colic biopsies showed aspects of non-specific subacute colitis. However, the rectal biopsy showed a spindle-cell proliferation with high cell density. Cell atypia were moderate, the cytoplasm was scarce, and the nuclei were slightly dyscaryotic, with rare mitoses. There was no necrosis. Immunohistochemistry (IHC) revealed positive staining of cancer cells for CD34 and negative for CD117. The diagnosis of Kaposi's sarcoma was suspected, and the samples were sent to our Department of Pathology for reviewing by expert pathologist within the French Sarcoma Network (Réseau de Référence en Pathologie des Sarcomes, RRePS). The diagnosis of rectal Kaposi's sarcoma was confirmed in October 2016: there was an ill-defined, fasciculated to diffuse proliferation of spindle cells with little to moderate nuclear atypia and few mitoses, outlining vascular slots; IHC showed positive staining of tumor cells for CD31 and ERG endothelial markers and for HHV8, and negative staining for CD117, DOG1, and STAT6 (Fig. 4). No cutaneous lesion was present. The patient stopped mesalazine after 1 month treatment because of relief of digestive symptoms and the diagnosis of ulcerative colitis was not finally retained because of pathological results Blood tests did not detect HHV-8 viremia, and the patient was serologically negative for HIV-1 and HIV-2, hepatitis B and C, and HTLV1 viruses. The circulating CD4+ T-cell count was 387/mm^3.

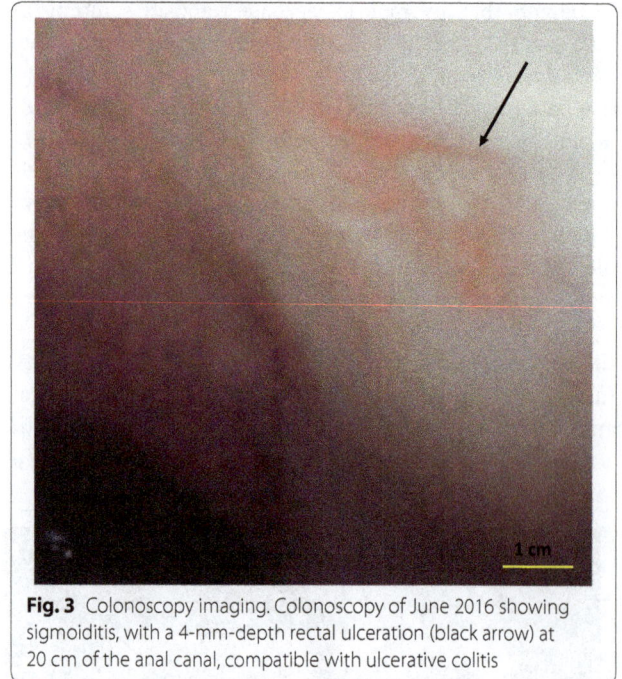

Fig. 3 Colonoscopy imaging. Colonoscopy of June 2016 showing sigmoiditis, with a 4-mm-depth rectal ulceration (black arrow) at 20 cm of the anal canal, compatible with ulcerative colitis

Given the description in the literature of rituximab-induced Kaposi's sarcoma in HIV-positive patients, rituximab was prematurely discontinued in October 2016 after the sixth maintenance injection. At this time, PET-scan showed neither suspect hypermetabolism of lymphomatous recurrence, nor digestive FDG uptake likely because of the disappearance of colitis after mesalazine treatment and the low proliferation rate of sarcoma. We noted only the appearance of lung lesions of infectious appearance without concomitant respiratory and infectious clinical symptoms (Fig. 1C, D). In December 2016, after complete disappearance of digestive symptoms, the patient underwent a colonoscopy, which was strictly

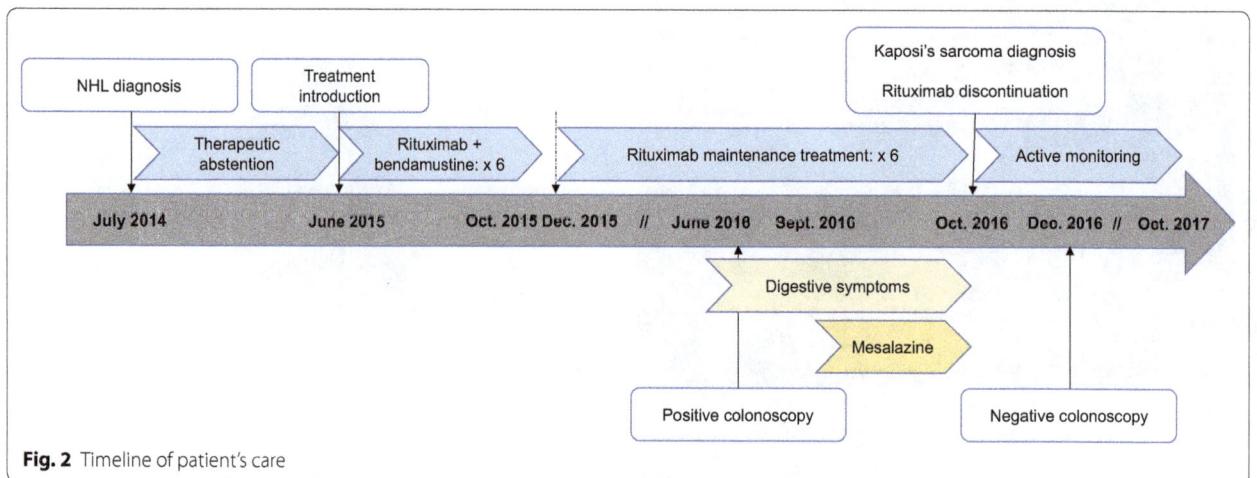

Fig. 2 Timeline of patient's care

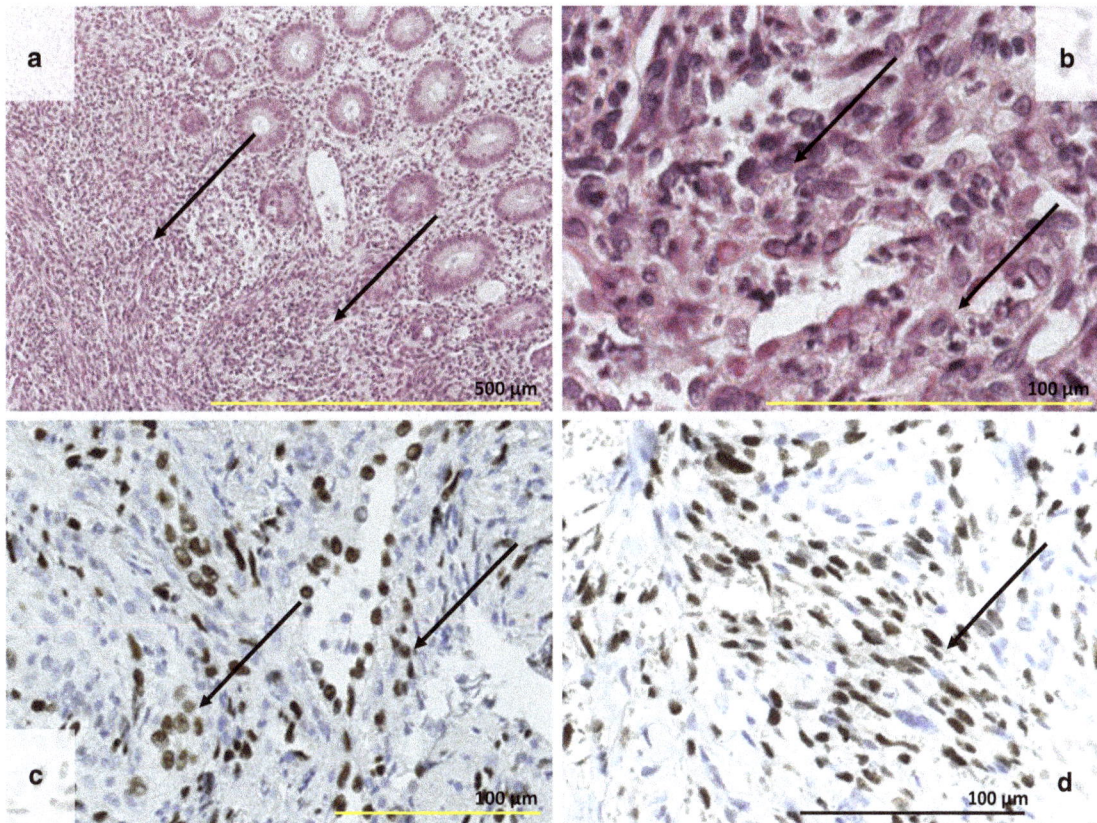

Fig. 4 Pathological aspect of the rectal Kaposi's sarcoma. **a** Microscopic aspect of the biopsy of rectal ulceration: the rectal mucosa is infiltrated by an ill-defined cellular fasciculated to diffuse proliferation (HES ×10). **b** Microscopic aspect showing spindle cells with little to moderate nuclear atypia surround vascular clefts. Few mitoses are noted. Lymphocytes and plasma cells are admixed (HES ×40). **c** IHC with ERG antibody: the lining cells of vascular structures and spindle cells express the ERG endothelial marker (×20). **d** IHC with HHV8 antibody: see the nuclear positive immunostaining of spindle tumor cells (×40)

normal without any sign of rectal Kaposi's sarcoma or colitis. Because of the infectious images on the PET-scan, explorations were carried out with pneumocystis PCR, and CMV, HSV, and HTLV1 serologies. All these explorations remained negative, as well as a bronchoscopy. Of note, in July 2017, the colonoscopy was normal, notably at the rectal level. In October 2017, 12 months after the last dose of rituximab maintenance, our patient was still in complete remission of his lymphoma.

Discussion and conclusions

We report a case of rectal Kaposi's sarcoma likely induced by rituximab therapy in a HIV-negative patient treated for a follicular lymphoma. The lesion developed while being treated with maintenance rituximab, leading to prematurely stop the treatment. Interestingly, stopping rituximab allowed the complete regression of Kaposi's sarcoma. To our knowledge, this is the first description of such case in the literature.

Two other cases of rituximab-induced Kaposi's sarcoma in HIV-negative patients have been reported in the literature. One case of cutaneous Kaposi's sarcoma was described in a patient treated with rituximab for thrombotic thrombocytopenic purpura. The lesion was treated with cryodestruction [4]. Another case was reported in an 84-year-old patient after undergoing rituximab-containing chemotherapy (R-CHOP regimen) for the treatment of a diffuse large B-cell lymphoma (DLBCL); after the seventh cycle, the patient developed a severe bacterial pneumonia and subsequent CMV viremia. The cutaneous

Kaposi's sarcoma developed after the complete resolution of pneumonia and was treated with surgical resection [5]. Our case is the first rituximab-induced Kaposi's sarcoma that developed at the mucosa level. The diagnosis of Kaposi's sarcoma of the bowel was difficult to establish immediately in the absence of skin and oral lesions, and a provisional diagnosis of ulcerative colitis was made before availability of pathological results. We suppose that the inflammation present in the mucosa was secondary to the underlying submucosal Kaposi's sarcoma ulceration. Kaposi's sarcoma of the bowel presenting as apparent ulcerative colitis has already been reported in HIV-positive patients several years ago, when the pathological diagnosis used antibodies for IHC less sensitive and specific than now [7, 8]. But, intestinal Kaposi's sarcoma has also been reported during the last decades in HIV-negative patients treated with immunosuppressive drugs for ulcerative colitis or Crohn disease, mimicking acute flare of colitis. Table 1 summarizes the cases reported since 2000 [9–22], as well as the other cases diagnosed in HIV-negative patients treated with immunosuppressive drugs after organ transplantation or for another inflammatory disease. In our case, we observed the complete resolution of Kaposi's sarcoma 2 months after rituximab discontinuation without the use of any specific treatment. To our knowledge, this is the first case of reversible rituximab-induced KS described in the literature. In their review, Antman and Chang [23] reported several examples of Kaposi's sarcoma regressions in renal transplant recipients after cessation, reduction or modification of immunosuppressive therapy. However, such modification led to graft rejection in approximately half of the patients. Similarly, in a HIV-negative patient treated with corticosteroid for idiopathic thrombocytopenic purpura, the skin Kaposi' tumors regressed soon after discontinuation of corticosteroid therapy, and no recurrence was observed during the 30-month follow-up period [24]. In our case, we suppose that the rituximab cessation permitted immune restitution and regression of Kaposi's sarcoma.

The role of CD4 T-cells in the Kaposi's sarcoma pathophysiology is suspected [25], especially in HIV-positive patients who usually present Kaposi's sarcoma when circulating CD4+ T-cell count is under $350/mm^3$ under highly active antiretroviral therapy [26]. In our case as well as in Ureshino's case, the CD4+ T-cell count was higher than $350/mm^3$ [5], suggesting that cellular immunodeficiency played only a minor role in the development of Kaposi's sarcoma in these patients. As B-cells are the HHV8's main human reservoir, another hypothesis may be that B-cell depletion induced by rituximab can expose endothelial cells to high HHV8 level, causing latent viral infection, and promoting Kaposi's sarcoma development [23]. In HIV-positive patients, lower B-cell counts are associated with the risk of Kaposi's sarcoma development [27], suggesting a role of humoral immune system in disease etiopathogenesis. One study, which investigated the pathological findings in a HIV-positive patient with rituximab-related Kaposi's sarcoma who was treated for multicentric Castleman's disease, showed depletion of intralesional B-lymphocytes accompanied with an upregulation of the HHV8 gene product K5 [28]. These authors also postulated that the diminished B-lymphocyte count interfered with the normal immune response to HHV8, allowing for viral activation. Unfortunately, the circulating CD20+ cell count and the Ig levels were not available for our patient, but they were low in the Ureshino's case [5]. Despite the widespread use of rituximab, there has been only one case of rituximab-related Kaposi's sarcoma in HIV-negative patients with DLBCL [5], and it was suggested that additional factors causing systemic inflammation, such as an infection, might contribute to the development of Kaposi's sarcoma in addition to rituximab. In our patient, lung infection may have triggered Kaposi's sarcoma progression.

In conclusion, we report the case of Kaposi's sarcoma diagnosed under rituximab in a HIV-negative patient, the first one at the rectal level, and the first one that completely regressed after cessation of rituximab. This case further highlights the importance of immunosuppression in the pathophysiology of Kaposi's sarcoma and how immune restitution takes part in its management. It also suggests awareness of iatrogenic Kaposi's sarcoma in patients treated with rituximab. Even if the occurrence of Kaposi's sarcoma is a very rare event, vigilance is needed, particularly for cancer patients often immunocompromised by disease and treatments. Patients at risk of HHV8 infection (ethnicity with high Fitzpatrick skin phototype, Mediterranean or equatorial African geographic origin, male gender, homosexuality or multiple sexual partners, immune deficiency) should be carefully screened for HHV8 before rituximab and closely monitored during treatment. Even if efforts to develop a HHV8 vaccine are ongoing [29], no prophylaxis for Kaposi's sarcoma is available today. Finally, given the risk of lymphoma progression after rituximab cessation, further

Table 1 Published cases of intestinal Kaposi's sarcoma in HIV-negative patients after 2000

First author	Year	Sex	Age at diagnosis (years)	Clinical conditions	Visceral KS localizations	Immunosuppression therapy	Tumor HHV8 status	Blood HHV8 status	KS management
Cohen	2001	F	67	Crohn disease	Ileum	Prednisone	ND	ND	Discontinuation of immunosuppressive therapy
Kang	2004	F	60	Ulcerative colitis	Colon	Prednisone	+	ND	ND
Nepomniashchaia	2004	M	41	Allogenic kidney transplantation	Stomach, intestinal mesentery, cerebral	ND	ND	ND	ND
Bursics	2005	M	49	Ulcerative colitis	Colon	Methylprednisolone	–	–	Discontinuation of immunosuppressive therapy and coloproctectomy
Svrcek	2009	M	62	Ulcerative colitis	Rectum	Steroid, azathioprine	+	+	Discontinuation of immunosuppressive therapy and coloproctectomy
Girelli	2009	M	43	Ulcerative colitis	Descending colon	Prednisone, mesalazine, ciclosporin	+	–	Discontinuation of immunosuppressive therapy and coloproctectomy
Rodriguez	2010	M	65	Ulcerative colitis	Colon	Prednisone, methotrexate	+	+	Discontinuation of immunosuppressive therapy and coloproctectomy
Tas	2012	F	77	Chronic anemia	Colon, lymph nodes	None	+	ND	Etoposide
Pioche	2013	M	49	Ulcerative colitis	Colon	Corticosteroids, azathioprine, ciclosporin, infliximab	+	+	Coloprotectomy
Hamzaoui	2013	M	30	Ulcerative colitis	Colorectal	Prednisone, mesalazine, azathioprine, infliximab	+	ND	Subtotal colectomy
Herculano	2014	M	63	Ulcerative colitis	Sigmoid colon	Prednisolone, mesalazine	+	–	Discontinuation of immunosuppressive therapy
Windon	2017	M	21	Crohn disease	Colon	Prednisone, infliximab	–	–	Discontinuation of immunosuppressive therapy
Duh	2017	M	48	Ulcerative colitis	Rectum	Prednisone	+	ND	Discontinuation of immunosuppressive therapy followed by subtotal colectomy
Kumar	2017	M	70	Ulcerative colitis	Ascending colon	None	+	ND	ND

KS Kaposi's sarcoma, F female, M male, ND not determined

studies are needed to better understand the immunological mechanisms involved in rituximab-induced Kaposi's sarcoma and to define optimal treatment.

Abbreviations

CMV: cytomegalovirus; DLBCL: diffuse large B-cell lymphoma; HHV8: human herpes virus type 8; HIV: human immunodeficiency virus; HSV: herpes simplex virus; HTLV1: human T-cell lymphotropic virus de type I; IHC: immunohistochemistry; mAb: monoclonal antibody; PCR: polymerase chain reaction; PET-scan: positron emission tomography scan; RRePS: Réseau de Référence en Pathologie des Sarcomes; WHO: World Health Organization.

Authors' contributions

Conception and design: FB; Manuscript writing: FB and EB; Final approval: FB, EB, AMS, LM, MB, AM, DP; Pathological explorations: LM; Patient's management: AMS, MB, LM, FB. All authors read and approved the final manuscript.

Author details

[1] INSERM UMR1068, CNRS UMR725, Department of Medical Oncology, Centre de Recherche en Cancérologie de Marseille (CRCM), Institut Paoli-Calmettes, 232 Bd de Sainte-Marguerite, 13009 Marseille, France. [2] Department of Hematology, Institut Paoli-Calmettes, Marseille, France. [3] Department of Pathology, Institut Paoli-Calmettes, Marseille, France. [4] Department of Digestive Endoscopy Centre Hospitalier Edmond Garcin, Aubagne, France. [5] Faculty of Medicine, Aix-Marseille University, Marseille, France. [6] French Sarcoma Group, Paris, France.

Acknowledgements

Our work is supported by Institut Paoli-Calmettes.

Competing interests

The authors declare that they have no competing interests.

Funding

Not applicable.

References

1. Geraminejad P, Memar O, Aronson I, Rady PL, Hengge U, Tyring SK. Kaposi's sarcoma and other manifestations of human herpesvirus 8. J Am Acad Dermatol. 2002;47:641–55.
2. Fisher RI, LeBlanc M, Press OW, Maloney DG, Unger JM, Miller TP. New treatment options have changed the survival of patients with follicular lymphoma. J Clin Oncol Off J Am Soc Clin Oncol. 2005;23:8447–52.
3. Gérard L, Michot J-M, Burcheri S, Fieschi C, Longuet P, Delcey V, et al. Rituximab decreases the risk of lymphoma in patients with HIV-associated multicentric Castleman disease. Blood. 2012;119:2228–33.
4. Jerdan K, Brownell J, Singh M, Braniecki M, Chan L. A case report of iatrogenic cutaneous Kaposi sarcoma due to rituximab therapy for thrombotic thrombocytopenic purpura. Acta Oncol. 2017;56:111–3.
5. Ureshino H, Ando T, Kojima K, Itamura H, Jinnai S, Doi K, et al. Rituximab containing chemotherapy (R-CHOP)-induced Kaposi's sarcoma in an HIV-negative patient with diffuse large B cell lymphoma. Intern Med. 2015;54:3205–8.
6. Salles G, Seymour JF, Offner F, López-Guillermo A, Belada D, Xerri L, et al. Rituximab maintenance for 2 years in patients with high tumour burden follicular lymphoma responding to rituximab plus chemotherapy (PRIMA): a phase 3, randomised controlled trial. Lancet. 2011;377:42–51.
7. Biggs BA, Crowe SM, Lucas CR, Ralston M, Thompson IL, Hardy KJ. AIDS related Kaposi's sarcoma presenting as ulcerative colitis and complicated by toxic megacolon. Gut. 1987;28:1302–6.

Weber JN, Carmichael DJ, Boylston A, Munro A, Whitear WP, Pinching AJ. Kaposi's sarcoma of the bowel-presenting as apparent ulcerative colitis. Gut. 1985;26:295–300.
Cohen RL, Tepper RE, Urmacher C, Katz S. Kaposi's sarcoma and cytomegaloviral ileocolitis complicating long-standing Crohn's disease in an HIV-negative patient. Am J Gastroenterol. 2001;96:3028–31.

10. Kang MJ, Namgung KY, Kim MS, Ko BS, Han CS, Ahn HT, et al. A case of Kaposi's sarcoma associated with ulcerative colitis. Korean J Gastroenterol Taehan Sohwagi Hakhoe Chi. 2004;43:316–9.
11. Nepomniashchaia EM, Gusarev SA, Kirichenko IG. Generalized Kaposi's sarcoma after allogenic transplantation of cadaver kidney. Arkh Patol. 2004;66:55–7.
12. Bursics A. HHV-8 positive, HIV negative disseminated Kaposi's sarcoma complicating steroid dependent ulcerative colitis: a successfully treated
8. case. Gut. 2005;54:1049–50.
13. Svrcek M, Tiret E, Bennis M, Guyot P, Fléjou J-F. KSHV/HHV8-associated intestinal Kaposi's sarcoma in patient with ulcerative colitis receiv-
9. ing immunosuppressive drugs: report of a case. Dis Colon Rectum. 2009;52:154–8.
14. Girelli CM, Serio G, Rocca E, Rocca F. Refractory ulcerative colitis and iatrogenic colorectal Kaposi's sarcoma. Dig Liver Dis. 2009;41:170–4.
15. Rodríguez-Peláez M, Fernández-García MS, Gutiérrez-Corral N, de Francisco R, Riestra S, García-Pravia C, et al. Kaposi's sarcoma: an opportunistic infection by human herpesvirus-8 in ulcerative colitis. J Crohns Colitis. 2010;4:586–90.
16. Tas F, Yegen G, Keskin S, Gozubuyukoglu N. Classic Kaposi's sarcoma with colonic involvement: a rare presentation with successful treatment with oral etoposide. J Cancer Res Ther. 2012;8:112.
17. Pioche M, Boschetti G, Cotte E, Graber I, Moussata D, François Y, et al. Human herpesvirus 8-associated colorectal Kaposi's sarcoma occurring in a drug-induced immunocompromised patient with refractory ulcerative colitis: report of a new case and review of the literature. Inflamm Bowel Dis. 2013;19:E12–5.
18. Hamzaoui L, Kilani H, Bouassida M, Mahmoudi M, Chalbi E, Siai K, et al. Iatrogenic colorectal Kaposi sarcoma complicating a refractory ulcerative colitis in a human immunodeficiency negative-virus patient. Pan Afr Med J. 2013;15. https://doi.org/10.11604/pamj.2013.15.154.2988.
19. Herculano R, Barreiro P, Hann A, Chapim I, Bispo M, Santos S, et al. Drug-induced colonic Kaposi's sarcoma in a HIV-negative patient with ulcerative colitis: a case report and review of the literature. Int J Colorectal Dis. 2014;29:1441–2.
20. Windon AL, Shroff SG. Iatrogenic Kaposi's sarcoma in an HIV-negative young male with Crohn's disease and IgA nephropathy: a case report and brief review of the literature. Int J Surg Pathol. 2017. https://doi.org/10.1177/1066896917736610.
21. Duh E, Fine S. Human herpesvirus-8 positive iatrogenic Kaposi's sarcoma in the setting of refractory ulcerative colitis. World J Clin Cases. 2017;5:423–7.
22. Kumar V, Soni P, Garg M, Abduraimova M, Harris J. Kaposi sarcoma mimicking acute flare of ulcerative colitis. J Investig Med High Impact Case Rep. 2017;5:232470961771351.
23. Antman K, Chang Y. Kaposi's sarcoma. N Engl J Med. 2000;342:1027–38.
24. Toyohama T, Nagasaki A, Miyagi J, Takamine W, Sunagawa K, Uezato H, et al. Kaposi's sarcoma in a human immunodeficiency virus-negative patient treated with corticosteroid for idiopathic thrombocytopenic purpura. Intern Med Tokyo Jpn. 2003;42:448–9.
25. Robey RC, Mletzko S, Gotch FM. The T-cell immune response against Kaposi's sarcoma-associated herpesvirus. Adv Virol. 2010;2010:1–9.
26. Lupia R, Wabuyia PB, Otiato P, Fang C-T, Tsai F-J. Risk factors for Kaposi's sarcoma in human immunodeficiency virus patients after initiation of antiretroviral therapy: A nested case–control study in Kenya. J Microbiol Immunol Infect. 2017;50:781–8.
27. Stebbing J, Gazzard B, Newsom-Davis T, Nelson M, Patterson S, Gotch F, et al. Nadir B cell counts are significantly correlated with the risk of Kaposi's sarcoma. Int J Cancer. 2004;108:473–4.
28. Pantanowitz L, Früh K, Marconi S, Moses AV, Dezube BJ. Pathology of rituximab-induced Kaposi sarcoma flare. BMC Clin Pathol. 2008;8:7.
29. Wu TT, Qian J, Ang J, Sun R. Vaccine prospect of Kaposi sarcoma-associated herpesvirus. Curr Opin Virol. 2012;2:482–8.

22

A retrospective cohort study of treatment patterns among patients with metastatic soft tissue sarcoma in the US

Victor M. Villalobos[1], Stacey DaCosta Byfield[2]* ⓘ, Sameer R. Ghate[3] and Oluwakayode Adejoro[2]

Abstract

Background: Since treatment patterns in metastatic soft tissue sarcoma (mSTS) have not been studied subsequent to US approval of pazopanib in 2012, this study sought to examine mSTS treatment patterns by line of therapy, including regimen and duration of therapy.

Methods: This retrospective study employed administrative claims from a large US health plan from 1/2006–9/2015. Adult mSTS patients were required to have an NCCN-recommended therapy and be continuously enrolled in the health plan during the study period. The most frequent regimens for distinct lines of therapy (LOT) were assessed. Sensitivity analyses evaluated changes to study findings using two alternate medical and pharmacy claims diagnostic algorithms to define the STS study population.

Results: Among 555 patients with mSTS, mean age was 59 years and 54% were male. During the study period, 41% of patients initiated ≥ 2 LOTs; 16% had ≥ 3 LOTs and 5% had ≥ 4 LOTs. Docetaxel + gemcitabine was most common in LOT1, pazopanib in LOT2 and LOT3, and doxorubicin in LOT4. The five most common LOT1 regimens represented 53% of patients; among the remaining 47%, the most common regimen represented < 6% of patients. Among patients with pazopanib in LOT2 and LOT3, the most common prior regimen was docetaxel + gemcitabine (47% and 30% respectively). Kaplan–Meier estimation of median treatment duration overall for LOT1 was 3.5 months, while for LOT2 and LOT3, median treatment duration was 2.9 and 3.3 months, respectively. For both sensitivity analyses, patient demographic and clinical characteristics were similar to the original study population, and the five most frequently used regimens in LOT1 and LOT2 were similar among the three populations regardless of the population selection criteria employed.

Conclusion: Choice of regimen by LOT among patients with mSTS is varied; < 65% of patients in any LOT received the five most common regimens. Pazopanib, the only approved targeted therapy, is primarily used in second and later lines of therapy and is mostly given post docetaxel + gemcitabine.

Keywords: Metastatic soft tissue sarcoma, Treatment patterns, Pazopanib

Background

Soft tissue sarcoma (STS) is a heterogeneous group of uncommon tumors that arise from mesenchymal cells at connective tissue body sites which differ by various inherent features including histology, molecular genetic profiles, site predilection, and outcomes of care [1]. STS includes approximately 40 malignant histological subtypes, and is most prominent in the extremities (50%), trunk and retroperitoneum (40%), and head and neck (10%). STS represent ~ 1% of all adult malignancies [2]. An estimated 11,930 new cases of STS were diagnosed in 2015 in the US [3]. STS is associated with high mortality; an estimated 4870 deaths due to STS were estimated to occur in the US in 2015 [3].

The choice of chemotherapy in metastatic STS (mSTS) should be individualized based on empirical knowledge

*Correspondence: Stacey.DacostaByfield@optum.com
[2] Optum, MN101-E300, 11000 Optum Circle, Eden Prairie, MN 55344, USA
Full list of author information is available at the end of the article

of the chemosensitivity of various histologic subtypes and biology of the tumor [4–6]. Most sarcomas are sensitive to gemcitabine/docetaxel and doxorubicin; angiosarcomas are sensitive to taxanes, liposarcomas are sensitive to doxorubicin-based regimens, synovial sarcomas are sensitive to ifosfamide and leiomyosarcomas are sensitive to gemcitabine, doxorubicin, ifosfamide, and trabectedin [4, 7, 8]. Pazopanib, the first targeted therapy for STS, was approved by the US Food and Drug Administration (FDA) in April 2012 for mSTS among patients with prior chemotherapy [9]; subsequently, olaratumab was approved in the US in October 2016 for treatment of soft tissue sarcomas [10]. National Comprehensive Cancer Network (NCCN) treatment recommendations include single agents (including dacarbazine, doxorubicin and ifosfamide), anthracycline-based combination regimens, or targeted therapy with pazopanib for relapsed or advanced/metastatic disease [2]. Choice of chemotherapy is influenced by both the stage of disease and practitioner preference. Single agent therapies are typically used in the metastatic setting, whereas chemotherapy combinations are generally used in the neoadjuvant/adjuvant setting or in settings where response is favored.

Several studies evaluating treatment patterns in STS have been published which precede pazopanib's availability in the US. The retrospective Sarcoma Treatment and Burden of Illness in North America and Europe (SABINE) study of treatment patterns in North America and Europe found that doxorubicin monotherapy or an anthracycline plus ifosfamide were the most common first-line treatments in metastatic/relapsed STS, and the most common second-line treatment was gemcitabine plus docetaxel [11]. A second US-based study found doxorubicin plus ifosfamide or docetaxel plus gemcitabine accounted for a combined 53% of first-line treatment in mSTS, and docetaxel plus gemcitabine accounted for 52% of second-line treatment [12]. Finally, a study conducted in the US of patients with metastatic/relapsed STS found that 44% received anthracycline-based and 28% received gemcitabine-based first-line regimens; gemcitabine-based (28%) and anthracycline-based (24%) regimens were most commonly used second-line, and no consistent regimens were used beyond second line of therapy (LOT) [13].

Large medical and pharmacy claims databases, which are used for billing and payment purposes, are useful to examine "real-world" practice patterns across different treatment settings within the US. Due to the large numbers of patients covered within these databases, they are particularly valuable to evaluate treatment for relatively rare conditions. Since prior published evaluations of treatment patterns in mSTS preceded pazopanib's US approval date, current treatment patterns among patients with mSTS are unknown. The primary objective of our study was to examine treatment patterns by LOT, including regimen and duration of therapy, in a large US administrative claims database. The secondary objective of this study was to identify and describe characteristics of patients who initiated therapy for mSTS.

Methods

This was a retrospective cohort study which employed medical and pharmacy claims from the Optum Research Database (ORD). The ORD contains inpatient, outpatient, and pharmacy claims for commercial enrollees with both medical and pharmacy benefit coverage from a health plan affiliated with Optum from 1993 to the present. For 2013, data relating to approximately 12.7 million individuals (~ 4% of the US population in 2013) with both medical and pharmacy benefit coverage are available. In addition, ORD also contains inpatient, outpatient, and pharmacy claims for approximately 4.2 million enrollees in Medicare Part C (commonly referred as Medicare Advantage program) since 2006. Social Security Administration (SSA) Death Master Files were also used to supplement patient death information, if applicable.

Cohort selection criteria

The study included data from January 1, 2006 through September 30, 2015. Eligible patients had commercial or Medicare Advantage insurance with both medical and pharmacy benefits. Patients were required to have had at least one prescription for NCCN-recommended systemic anticancer therapy (Appendix 1: Table 3) for mSTS management during the study identification period (May 1, 2012 through August 31, 2015). The index date was the start date of the first LOT for treatment of mSTS during the identification period. All available patient baseline data from January 1, 2006 through the index date was extracted to ascertain initial treatment and evidence of metastatic disease. Patients were required to have had at least two non-diagnostic medical claims in any position for STS [non-gastrointestinal stromal tumors (GIST)] [International Classification of Diseases, 9th revision, Clinical Modification (ICD-9-CM) 171.xx], at least 30 days apart, during the identification period. The study population was limited to patients 18 years of age or older as of the index date. Patients were required to be newly treated for metastasis, defined as follows: (1) at least one claim with a diagnosis code for metastasis (ICD-9-CM 196.x, 197.x, 198.x, 199.0) in any position during the variable baseline through follow-up period; the date of the first claim with a metastasis diagnosis was termed the 'met date', (2) the 'met date' was required to be prior to or on the index date (the start of the first LOT during the identification period) with no claims for systemic anticancer therapy between the 'met date' and the index date, (3) no LOTs with claims for metastatic disease prior to the index date, (4) patients were continuously benefit-eligible from at least 6 months preceding the 'met date', through the index date and for one or more months after the index date, and (5) at least one claim for STS was required prior to or on the 'met date'. A cohort identification timeline is included in Appendix 2: Fig. 4. To exclude GIST, patients with one or more claims for imatinib during the study identification period were eliminated from the final study population. Patient treatment cohorts were determined based on the most common regimens received during the first LOT.

Independent study variables

Baseline patient demographic and clinical characteristics were evaluated for the study population based on health plan administrative claims and enrollment data. Demographic characteristics such as age as of index year, gender, and geographic region of health plan were assessed. Baseline clinical characteristics included Quan-Charlson comorbidity score [14], a composite comorbidity score (higher score = greater comorbidity burden) calculated based on assignment of a point value for specific diagnosis codes on medical claims during the pre-index period corresponding to chronic disease states. For example, a 'healthy' patient with no comorbid conditions would have a total composite score of 0.0. Metastatic disease is associated with a point value of 6.0; a patient with claims history consistent with metastatic disease but no other comorbid conditions would have a composite score of 6.0. Radiation during the baseline period was evaluated using procedure codes [Current Procedural Terminology (CPT), Healthcare Common Procedure Coding System (HCPCS), Medicare diagnosis-related group (MS-DRG), revenue, and ICD-9-CM procedure codes]. History of surgical procedure(s) during baseline was captured using CPT, HCPCS, and ICD-9-CM procedure codes.

Study endpoints

Primary outcomes included specific anticancer medication regimens by LOT and duration of therapy. Up to four LOT regimens were assessed. A specific LOT began on the date of the first infusion or fill for a systemic anticancer agent, and the regimen associated with this LOT included all anti-cancer agents received within 45 days following the first infusion or fill date. This specific LOT continued until the earliest of any of the following: (1) addition or substitution of a new agent after the initial agent(s) (LOT end date defined as the day prior to the start of the new agent, but discontinuation of one agent from a multidrug regimen did not qualify as ending LOT); (2) a treatment gap ≥ 60 days after the runout

date of all agents in the LOT [LOT end date was the runout date prior to the gap; runout date was defined for infused/injected drugs as the latest date of administration + 29 days, and for drugs obtained through pharmacy benefit runout date was fill date + (days supply − 1)]; (3) death; or (4) disenrollment or end of the study period. A LOT was considered censored if the LOT ended due to end of study period or disenrollment. Second through fourth LOTs were identified by the initiation of anticancer therapy after the end of the previous LOT. Note that a re-initiation of a previous regimen would be considered a new LOT as long as criterion #2 above (a treatment gap of ≥ 60 days) was met. The algorithm described above applied to the other LOTs and the number of LOTs examined was dependent on available sample size. The most common regimens by LOT were identified, and a count of LOTs was computed.

Statistical methods

Descriptive statistics of all variables were calculated for the mSTS population, including means and 95% confidence intervals (CI) for continuous variables, and frequency tables and percentages for categorical variables. Global comparisons of patient characteristics were made across LOT1 regimens and included Chi square testing for frequency tables and analysis of variance for continuous variables. Duration of therapy for each LOT was summarized with arithmetic means and using Kaplan–Meier methods.

Sensitivity analyses

To investigate the potential impact of the inadvertent inclusion of patients without mSTS in our study population due to limitations associated with using medical claims to identify patients with mSTS, two sensitivity analyses evaluated changes to study findings when more restrictive claims diagnostic criteria were applied to STS population identification. The first sensitivity analysis excluded patients who received atypical anticancer agents (bevacizumab, carboplatin, paclitaxel) during the study period. The second sensitivity analysis excluded both patients who used atypical anticancer agents (bevacizumab, carboplatin, paclitaxel) and patients with one or more claims with a non-STS cancer diagnosis in the first or second position in conjunction with a code for an injectable systemic anticancer therapy on the same claim. Descriptive analyses were performed on both study subpopulations.

Results

A total of 138,859 patients were prescribed an STS drug during the study identification period, and 1740 (1.3%) had at least two claims for STS at least 30 days apart during continuous enrollment (Fig. 1). Subsequent to application of all other cohort inclusion and exclusion criteria, 555 patients with mSTS were identified for the final study cohort. Mean age overall was 58.8 (SD 16.3) years and 46.3% were female (Table 1). Among the mSTS study cohort, 41.3% had 2 LOTs, 15.9% had 3 LOTs, and 5.0% had 4 LOTs during the study period. Across all LOTs, the most frequently prescribed agent (in either mono- or combination therapy) was gemcitabine (43%), followed by doxorubicin (36%), docetaxel (35%), and pazopanib (21%) (Appendix 3: Fig. 5).

The most frequent LOT1 regimen was docetaxel + gemcitabine (22.3%), followed by doxorubicin (13.0%) (Fig. 2a). There was considerable variation in LOT1 regimens, as almost half (47%) of patients had 'other' first-line therapies, and among these patients, each specific regimen accounted for < 6% of all patients (Appendix 4: Table 4). There were significant differences

in mean age and gender by LOT1 regimen (Table 1). About 2 in 3 patients (65.4%) were covered by commercial insurance, while 34.6% were covered by Medicare Advantage. Geographic distribution of the mSTS cohort was consistent with the overall distribution of all health plan enrollees. Mean Quan-Charlson comorbidity score was 7.6 for the mSTS cohort and was similar regardless of LOT1 regimen. Almost half (45.2%) of patients overall had radiation during the variable baseline period, and 71.5% had evidence of a surgical procedure. Overall mean duration of follow-up was 325.8 days (SD 265.3).

The most common therapeutic regimens by LOT are shown in Fig. 2. Fewer than 65% of patients in any LOT received one of the top 5 most common regimens. In LOT2 (Fig. 2b), pazopanib (19%) was the most frequent regimen, followed by docetaxel + gemcitabine (17%). Pazopanib (31%) was also the most common LOT3

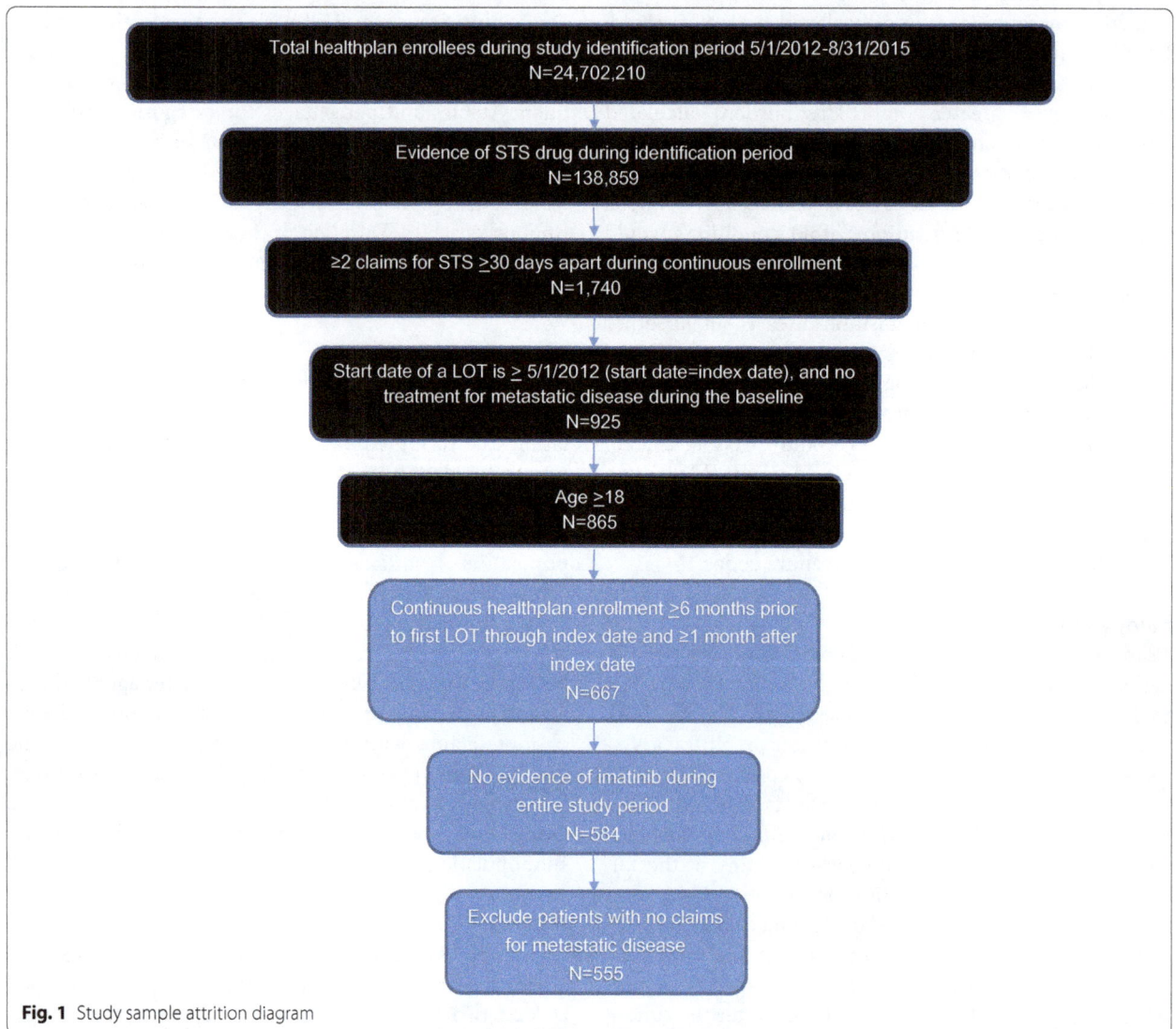

Fig. 1 Study sample attrition diagram

Table 1 Patient baseline demographic and clinical characteristics

	Total	First LOT						Overall p value
		GEM + DOC	DOX	PAZO	DOX + IFO	GEM	Others	
N (%)	555 (100)	124 (22.3)	72 (13.0)	38 (6.8)	31 (5.6)	29 (5.2)	261 (47.0)	
Age, mean (95% CI)	58.8 (57.5–60.2)	57.1 (54.9–59.3)	65.9 (62.5–69.3)	59.0 (53.3–64.7)	54.7 (48.9–60.4)	66.3 (61.5–71.1)	57.4 (55.2–59.5)	< 0.001
Age categories, n (%)								
18–44	108 (19.5)	17 (13.7)	6 (8.3)	11 (29.0)	10 (32.3)	1 (3.5)	63 (24.1)	< 0.001
45–54	91 (16.4)	30 (24.2)	9 (12.5)	3 (7.9)	3 (9.7)	4 (13.8)	42 (16.1)	0.091
55–64	132 (23.8)	42 (33.9)	16 (22.2)	8 (21.1)	7 (22.6)	6 (20.7)	53 (20.3)	0.104
65–74	128 (23.1)	28 (22.6)	19 (26.4)	8 (21.1)	10 (32.3)	8 (27.6)	55 (21.1)	0.708
75+	96 (17.3)	7 (5.7)	22 (30.6)	8 (21.1)	1 (3.2)	10 (34.5)	48 (18.4)	< 0.001
Female, n (%)	257 (46.3)	75 (60.5)	36 (50.0)	21 (55.3)	10 (32.3)	13 (44.8)	102 (39.1)	0.001
Coverage type, n (%)								
Commercial	363 (65.4)	90 (72.6)	38 (52.8)	28 (73.7)	22 (71.0)	15 (51.7)	170 (65.1)	0.036
Aged < 65 years	318 (87.6)	85 (94.4)	30 (79.0)	22 (78.6)	20 (90.9)	10 (66.7)	151 (88.8)	0.010
Aged 65+ years	45 (12.4)	5 (5.6)	8 (21.1)	6 (21.4)	2 (9.1)	5 (33.3)	19 (11.1)	0.010
Medicare advantage	192 (34.6)	34 (27.4)	34 (47.2)	10 (26.3)	9 (29.0)	14 (48.3)	91 (34.9)	0.036
Geographic region, n (%)								
Northeast	92 (16.6)	17 (13.7)	11 (15.3)	7 (18.4)	8 (25.8)	6 (20.7)	43 (16.5)	0.672
Midwest	151 (27.2)	32 (25.8)	24 (33.3)	10 (26.3)	8 (25.8)	9 (31.0)	68 (26.1)	0.860
South	228 (41.1)	57 (46.0)	25 (34.7)	17 (44.7)	9 (29.0)	9 (31.0)	111 (42.5)	0.313
West	84 (15.1)	18 (14.5)	12 (16.7)	4 (10.5)	6 (19.4)	5 (17.2)	39 (14.9)	0.931
Quan-Charlson comorbidity score, mean (95% CI)	7.6 (7.4–7.7)	7.4 (7.1–7.7)	7.7 (7.4–8.1)	7.6 (6.9–8.3)	6.9 (6.5–7.4)	8.0 (7.3–8.6)	7.6 (7.4–7.8)	0.166
≥ 1 Radiation claim, n (%)	251 (45.2)	37 (29.8)	44 (61.1)	18 (47.4)	9 (29.0)	14 (48.3)	129 (49.4)	< 0.001
≥ 1 Surgery claim, n (%)	397 (71.5)	96 (77.4)	53 (73.6)	28 (73.7)	20 (64.5)	20 (69.0)	180 (69.0)	0.544
Length of follow-up (days), mean (95% CI)	325.8 (303.6–347.9)	363.6 (313.9–413.3)	316.0 (261.8–370.2)	317.8 (234.6–401.0)	365.4 (254.9–475.8)	186.1 (121.3–251.0)	322.4 (289.6–355.3)	0.043

DOC docetaxel, *DOX* doxorubicin, *GEM* gemcitabine, *IFO* ifosfamide, *PAZO* pazopanib, *SD* standard deviation

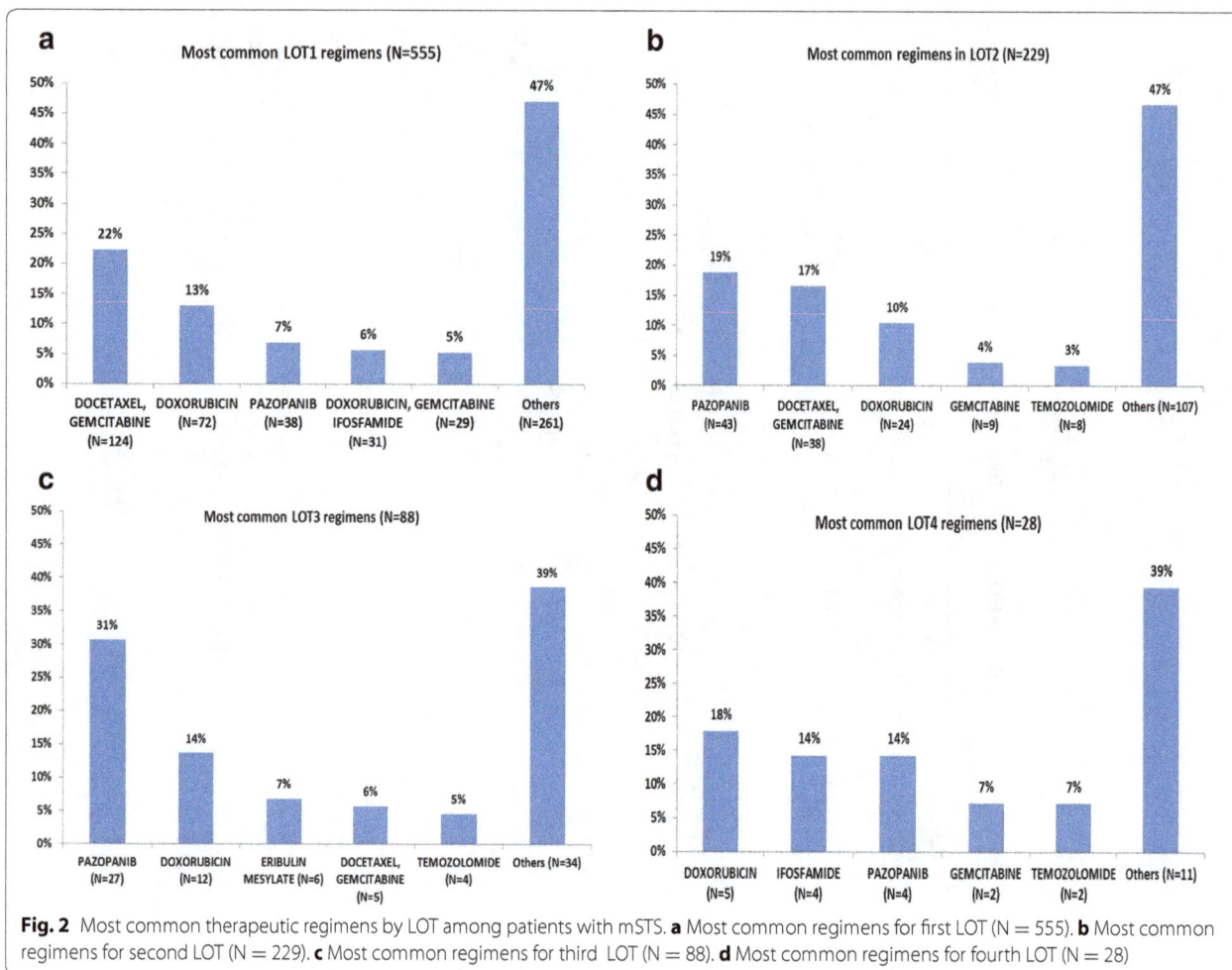

Fig. 2 Most common therapeutic regimens by LOT among patients with mSTS. **a** Most common regimens for first LOT (N = 555). **b** Most common regimens for second LOT (N = 229). **c** Most common regimens for third LOT (N = 88). **d** Most common regimens for fourth LOT (N = 28)

regimen, followed by doxorubicin (14%), while doxorubicin (18%) was most common in LOT4, followed by ifosfamide (14%) and pazopanib (14%) (Fig. 2c). A list of medications included in the 'other' category for LOT1–LOT3 is included in Appendix 4: Table 4.

Mean (median) treatment duration overall for LOT1 was 3.7 months (2.9 months), while for LOT2 and LOT3, mean treatment duration was 2.8 (2.3) and 3.0 (2.6) months, respectively. Mean (median) duration of therapy for patients initially treated with pazopanib was 5.2 (3.1) months. Figure 3 depicts Kaplan–Meier estimates for LOT1, LOT2, and LOT3; Kaplan–Meier estimation of median duration of therapy for LOT1, LOT2 and LOT3 were 3.5, 2.9 and 3.3 months, respectively. There was a significant difference in the duration of LOT1 by regimen (global p value = 0.014) (Fig. 3a) while for LOT2 and LOT3, median treatment durations by respective LOT regimens were similar (Fig. 3b, c).

Among patients with more than one LOT during the study period (n = 229), the most frequently prescribed LOT2 regimen was pazopanib (n = 43; 19% of 229

patients) (Table 2). Most patients treated with pazopanib in LOT2 used docetaxel + gemcitabine (n = 20; 47% of 43 patients) in LOT1. Among patients with more than 2 LOTs during the study period (n = 88), of the patients who received pazopanib as their LOT3 regimen (n = 27; 31% of 88 patients), 30% used docetaxel + gemcitabine for LOT2 (n = 8), and 15% each (n = 4) used pazopanib or doxorubicin. A small number of patients received the same medication regimen for sequential LOTs; for example, five patients were treated with docetaxel + gemcitabine for both LOT1 and LOT2 (Table 2).

Sensitivity analyses

Patient demographic and clinical characteristics were similar across the original population and both sensitivity I and sensitivity II populations (data not shown); minor differences can be explained by new exclusionary criteria used to restrict the study population. The five most frequently used regimens in LOT1 and LOT2 were similar among the three populations regardless of the population selection criteria.

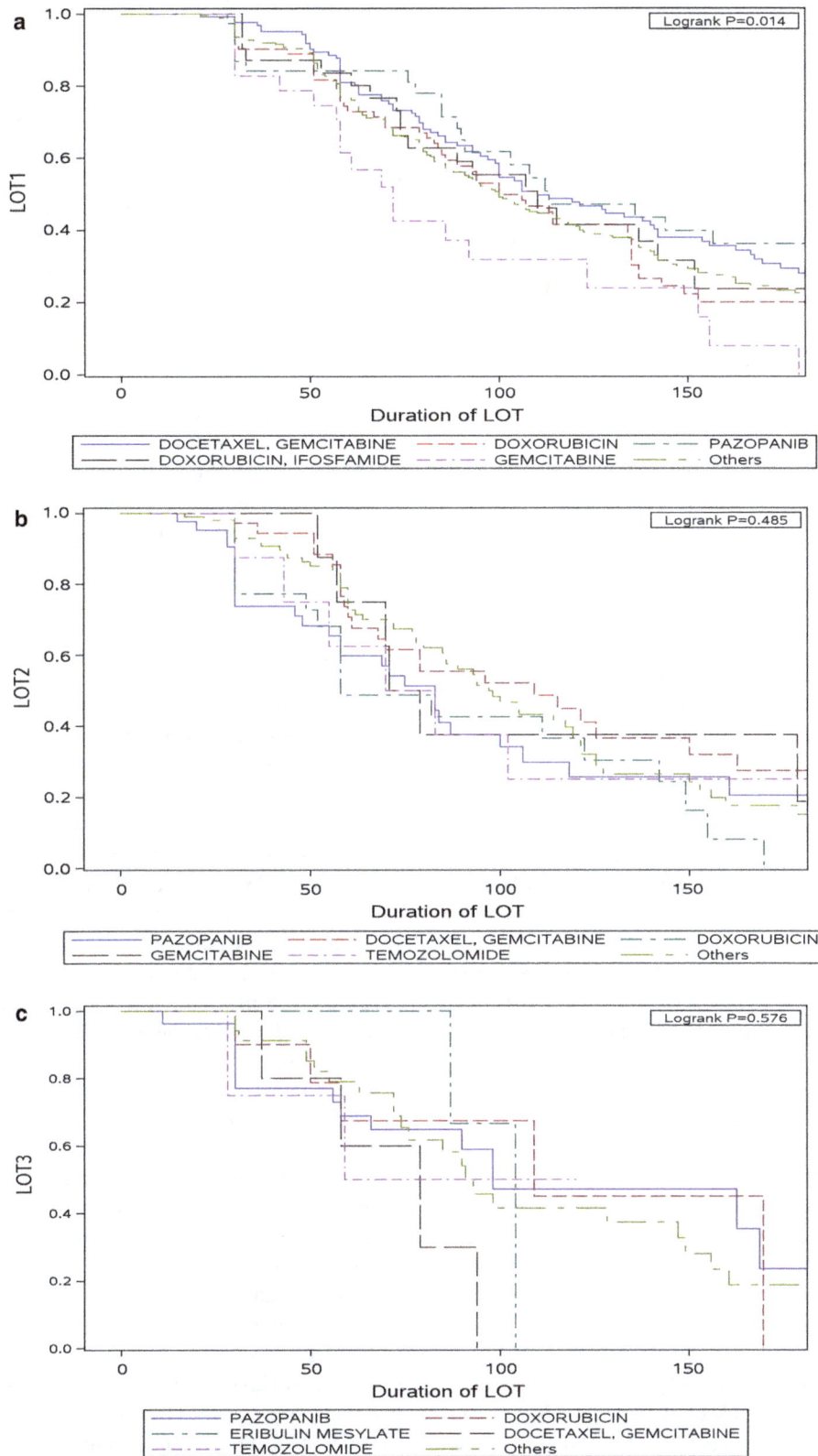

Fig. 3 Duration of first, second and third LOTs. **a** Duration of therapy for LOT1 by treatment regimen. **b** Duration of therapy for LOT2 by treatment regimen. **c** Duration of therapy for LOT3 by treatment regimen

Across all three study populations, the lowest percentage of patients (32%) were classified in the 'other' medications category in the sensitivity I population.

Discussion

We found wide variation in the regimens used across all LOTs for the treatment of mSTS. In LOT1, only 53% of patients combined were treated with the 5 most common LOT1 regimens, and about 47% of patients received a regimen other than these regimens. The most commonly used regimen within the 'other' category accounted for < 6% of the STS population. Our findings may, in part, be explained by the numerous histological types (> 40) of STS, varying chemosensitivity of histological types, disease progression, and the lack of evidence on the optimal treatment and sequence of treatment of each histology. It is also possible that our results reflect variable clinician expertise with and adherence to recommended chemotherapy treatment guidelines [2]. Consistent with the findings of Wagner et al. [13], no consistent regimens were used beyond second-line treatment in the current study. Docetaxel + gemcitabine, followed by doxorubicin and pazopanib, were the top three regimens in LOT1, and docetaxel + gemcitabine was the first line regimen in 47% of patients who received pazopanib as LOT2 and 58% of patients who received doxorubicin as LOT2. Doxorubicin has generally been the mainstay of first line therapy for most mSTS, due to its lower toxicity and relative ease of administration [15, 16]. The recent GeDDiS trial compared first line treatment of doxorubicin to docetaxel + gemcitabine among patients with advanced or metastatic STS in the United Kingdom and Switzerland. Study investigators concluded that doxorubicin is appropriate as the standard first line treatment for most patients with advanced STS, as compared to docetaxel + gemcitabine, it is less difficult to administer, perceived by patients as less toxic, and less expensive, despite comparable survival outcomes [15]. The addition of olaratumab to first line therapy is likely to solidify the use of doxorubicin in the first line [17]. Prior studies of first-line treatment have found that the most common regimens were doxorubicin monotherapy (34%) or an anthracycline + ifosfamide (30%) [11], anthracycline-based (44%) or gemcitabine-based (28%) [13], doxorubicin (± ifosfamide) (46%) [12], or doxorubicin (± ifosfamide) (66%) [18]. Docetaxel + gemcitabine may be preferred for certain mSTS including leiomyosarcomas and undifferentiated pleomorphic sarcomas (UPS) [16]. Since histology was not captured in the claims data used for the current study, we have no knowledge of whether our study's results were driven by histologic subtype, and it is unclear whether inconsistent findings between studies, even for preferred first-line regimens, is more related to histologic subtypes represented by the individual study populations or true differences in practice patterns. Doxorubicin alone was

more popular than doxorubicin + ifosfamide while docetaxel + gemcitabine were more popular than gemcitabine alone. Published evidence suggests that the therapeutic effect of doxorubicin + ifosfamide is additive with no statistically significant overall survival benefit and is associated with more adverse effects compared to the synergistic relationship between gemcitabine and docetaxel [16, 19, 20].

In the current study, pazopanib, followed by docetaxel + gemcitabine, were the leading regimens in LOT2. Compared to other regimens used in mSTS, pazopanib may be preferred by patients due to its oral route of administration. Clinical trials of pazopanib have found lower rates of certain adverse events (anemia, neutropenia, nausea/vomiting, and elevated AST/ALT) than reported for clinical trials of trabectedin, though anorexia was more common with pazopanib [7, 21, 22]. However, the lack of head-to-head clinical trials comparing these agents and the use of different patient populations to evaluate event rates makes direct comparisons problematic. Trabectedin was not available in the US until late 2015, though it has been commonly used as a second-line treatment in Europe since 2007. Prior to pazopanib's availability in the US, Wagner et al. (2000–2011) found that gemcitabine-based (28%) and anthracycline-based (24%) regimens were used most often in LOT2 [13]. The most common second-line treatment was docetaxel + gemcitabine (18%) in the SABINE study by Leahy et al. [11]. Also, Chen et al. found that docetaxel + gemcitabine (52%) was the most common regimen in LOT2 [12]. These results suggest widespread use of gemcitabine in LOT2 prior to pazopanib's US availability, either alone or in combination with docetaxel, and less variation in LOT2 regimen preference across different study populations. In contrast, Bae and colleagues found that 53% used ifosfamide in LOT2 in an Australian advanced STS population, although pazopanib was sporadically used as subsequent LOTin Bae's study population following its availability in Australia in March of 2014 [18].

To our knowledge, the current study is the first published study of treatment patterns in mSTS since pazopanib became available in the US in 2012. A somewhat unexpected finding of our study was that ~ 7% of patients received pazopanib as initial therapy, as pazopanib is approved as second or later line of management for mSTS in the US. This may represent off-label use of pazopanib, possibly related to early clinical trial results suggesting a role for pazopanib in first-line treatment of soft tissue sarcomas, including solitary fibrous tumor (SFT) and clear cell sarcoma [23–25]. However, it may be that physicians may be more comfortable with this drug early on and consider it to be a more tolerable treatment than other first-line options, such as high dose doxorubicin. Additionally, it is possible that the use of pazopanib as first LOT in our study may be a misclassification of LOT2 as

Table 2 LOT transition among patients with > 1 LOT

LOT1	LOT2 (N = 229)										
	Pazopanib		Docetaxel, gem-citabine		Doxorubicin		Gemcitabine		Temozolomide		Others
	(N = 43, 18.8%)		(N = 38, 16.6%)		(N = 24, 10.5%)		(N = 9, 3.9%)		(N = 8, 3.5%)		(N = 107, 46.7%)
	n	%	n	%	n	%	n	%	n	%	n	%
Docetaxel, gemcitabine	20	46.5	5	13.2	14	58.3	0	0.0	0	0.0	19	17.8
Doxorubicin	4	9.3	12	31.6	1	4.2	1	11.1	2	25.0	13	12.2
Pazopanib	3	7.0	4	10.5	1	4.2	3	33.3	2	25.0	4	3.7
Doxorubicin, ifosfamide	3	7.0	5	13.2	0	0.0	1	11.1	0	0.0	2	1.9
Gemcitabine	2	4.7	0	0.0	0	0.0	0	0.0	0	0.0	6	5.6
Others	11	25.6	12	31.6	8	33.3	4	44.4	4	50.0	63	58.9

LOT2	LOT3 (N = 88)										
	Pazopanib		Doxorubicin		Eribulin mesylate		Docetaxel, gemcitabine		Temozolomide		Others
	(N = 27, 30.7%)		(N = 12, 13.6%)		(N = 6, 6.8%)		(N = 5, 5.7%)		(N = 4, 4.5%)		(N = 34, 38.6%)
	n	%	n	%	n	%	n	%	n	%	n	%
Pazopanib	4	14.8	5	41.7	0	0.0	0	0.0	2	50.0	5	14.7
Docetaxel, gemcitabine	8	29.6	2	16.7	0	0.0	1	20.0	0	0.0	2	5.9
Doxorubicin	4	14.8	1	8.3	1	16.7	1	20.0	0	0.0	4	11.8
Gemcitabine	1	3.7	2	16.7	0	0.0	0	0.0	0	0.0	2	5.9
Temozolomide	2	7.4	0	0.0	0	0.0	1	20.0	0	0.0	3	8.8
Others	8	29.6	2	16.7	5	83.3	2	40.0	2	50.0	18	52.9

LOT1 regimens using administrative claims data to ascertain LOT. Additionally, another unexpected finding of our analysis was significant usage of carboplatin in our mSTS cohort, since this drug has very limited efficacy in sarcoma. These observations may reflect the somewhat fragmented oncology care for sarcoma within the American health system. While in Europe, most sarcoma patients are referred as standard practice to high-volume referral centers, many patients in the United States are treated in private, non-academic practices. Lack of experience with sarcomas may result in therapeutic choices that do not align with evidence-based best practices and therefore receiving care under the guidance of a high-volume referral center may be important for patients' receipt of optimal recommendations for therapy.

Treatment with new drugs (different agents from LOT1) was the common strategy during disease progression/subsequent LOTs. Drug rechallenge, the repeat administration of the same regimen which may occur following drug holiday, disease progression or relapse, was low in general, but higher among docetaxel + gemcitabine-treated patients than pazopanib-treated patients, and in later LOTs than earlier LOTs. This may reflect fewer regimen options for subsequent therapy to choose from after selection of initial treatment regimen. Shorter duration of therapy for later LOTs relative to LOT1 as observed in our study could be multifactorial and be suggestive of worsening disease or resistant disease. Longer duration of therapy on pazopanib may suggest ease of use, relative effectiveness, and/or tolerability of pazopanib. Finally, results of sensitivity analyses in more rigorously defined mSTS patient subsets confirmed our overall results.

Limitations

Our study's results should be interpreted in the context of several important study limitations. This study relied on identification codes on administrative claims data to determine STS, disease metastasis and the earliest date of pharmacy claims for identifying the initial patient population. The reporting of metastatic disease through the listing of its ICD code on claims by the treating physician may not be done consistently, and it was not possible for us to independently verify via pathological diagnosis; hence there is possibility for misclassification of patients with mSTS. Administrative claims data also do not contain clinical prognostic information (e.g. histologic subtype, clinical stage and extent of disease) of patients. The codification of sarcomas is particularly problematic, since most of the diagnostic subtypes utilize the same ICD-9-CM code. Conducting sub-analyses on patients with prevalent histologic subtypes would have provided better information applicable to patients with similar histologic subtype, but this was not possible using medical claims data. A regimen change may not always be due to disease progression but also other events like adverse events or drug toxicities, which may not be ascertainable using claims data. We used information from the public view of the SSA death files for cohort selection, and these files do not comprehensively capture all deaths. Finally, a medical-claims based algorithm was developed to classify LOT1-4, and may not accurately identify specific LOTs. The LOT algorithm reflects gaps in therapy but, due to the nature of claims data, the reason for these gaps is unknown, and therapy lapses due to tolerability issues, medication persistence and adherence, drug rechallenge, and other clinically relevant therapy gaps may have been classified as distinct LOTs; this may explain why a small number of patients were treated with the same regimens for two sequential LOTs. Furthermore, our LOT algorithm considered all anti-cancer agents administered within 45 days following the first infusion as the initial regimen received, and it is possible that a true subsequent LOT may start within 45 days and represent a distinct LOT but not correctly be classified as such.

Conclusions

While our study lacked clinical diagnostic information to enable investigation of treatment patterns by histologic subtypes, this is the first study of treatment patterns in mSTS to be conducted since the US approval of pazopanib in 2012, and our findings provide direction for future research in mSTS treatment patterns. We found wide variations in the regimens used in all LOTs for the treatment of mSTS. Fewer than 65% of patients in any LOT received the five most common regimens. In LOT1, approximately 47% of patients received 'other' chemotherapy, and the most commonly used regimen within the 'other' category accounted for less than 5% of the STS population. Docetaxel + gemcitabine, followed by doxorubicin and pazopanib, were the top three regimens in LOT1, while pazopanib, followed by docetaxel + gemcitabine, were the leading regimens in LOT2.

Treatment with new drugs (different agents from LOT1) was the common strategy during disease progression. Pazopanib, the only approved targeted therapy for mSTS, is frequently administered second-line post docetaxel + gemcitabine, was used by 7% of patients in LOT1, and is being adopted in second and later LOTs since its availability in 2012.

Abbreviations

mSTS: metastatic soft tissue sarcoma; NCCN: National Comprehensive Cancer Network; LOT: line of therapy; STS: soft tissue sarcoma; FDA: Food and Drug Administration; SABINE: Sarcoma Treatment and Burden of Illness in North America and Europe; ORD: Optum Research Database; SSA: Social Security Administration; GIST: gastrointestinal stromal tumors; ICD-9-CM: International Classification of Diseases, 9th revision, Clinical Modification; CPT: Current Procedural Terminology; HCPCS: Healthcare Common Procedure Coding System; MS-DRG: Medicare Diagnosis-Related Group; CI: confidence interval.

Authors' contributions

SDB and OA participated in study design, analyzed and interpreted study data and contributed to manuscript writing and editing for content. SG and VV contributed to study design, interpreted study data and contributed to manuscript content editing. All authors read and approved the final manuscript.

Author details

[1] University of Colorado Anschutz Medical Campus, 1665 Aurora Ct ACP 5329 Mail Stop F704 Aurora, Denver, CO 80045, USA. [2] Optum, MN101-E300, 11000 Optum Circle, Eden Prairie, MN 55344, USA. [3] Novartis, One Health Plaza 345/5130B, East Hanover, NJ 07936, USA.

Acknowledgements

The authors would like to acknowledge Jen Wogen, MedMentis Consulting LLC, for medical writing assistance on this manuscript. Portions of this study were presented at 2016 Annual Meeting of the Connective Tissue Oncology Society, November 9–12, 2016, in Lisbon, Portugal.

Competing interests

SDB is a full-time employee of Optum and owns company stock. At the time the study was conducted, OA was a full-time employee of Optum. SG is a full-time employee of Novartis Pharmaceuticals Corporation, the source of funding for this study, and also owns Novartis stock. VV has received consulting fees from Novartis Pharmaceuticals Corporation and Eli Lilly & Co., and serves on advisory boards for Bayer AG and Janssen Pharmaceuticals, Inc.

Funding

This study was funded by Novartis Pharmaceuticals Corporation.

Appendix 1
See Table 3.

Table 3 List of NCCN-recommended systemic anticancer therapies

NCCN-recommended systemic cancer therapy
Bevacizumab
Carboplatin
Cyclophosphamide
Dacarbazine
Dactinomycin
Docetaxel
Doxorubicin/pegylated liposomal doxorubicin
Epirubicin
Eribulin
Etoposide
Gemcitabine
Ifosfamide
Irinotecan
Paclitaxel
Pazopanib
Sorafenib
Sunitinib
Temozolomide
Topotecan
Trabectedin
Vincristine
Vinorelbine

Appendix 2

See Fig. 4.

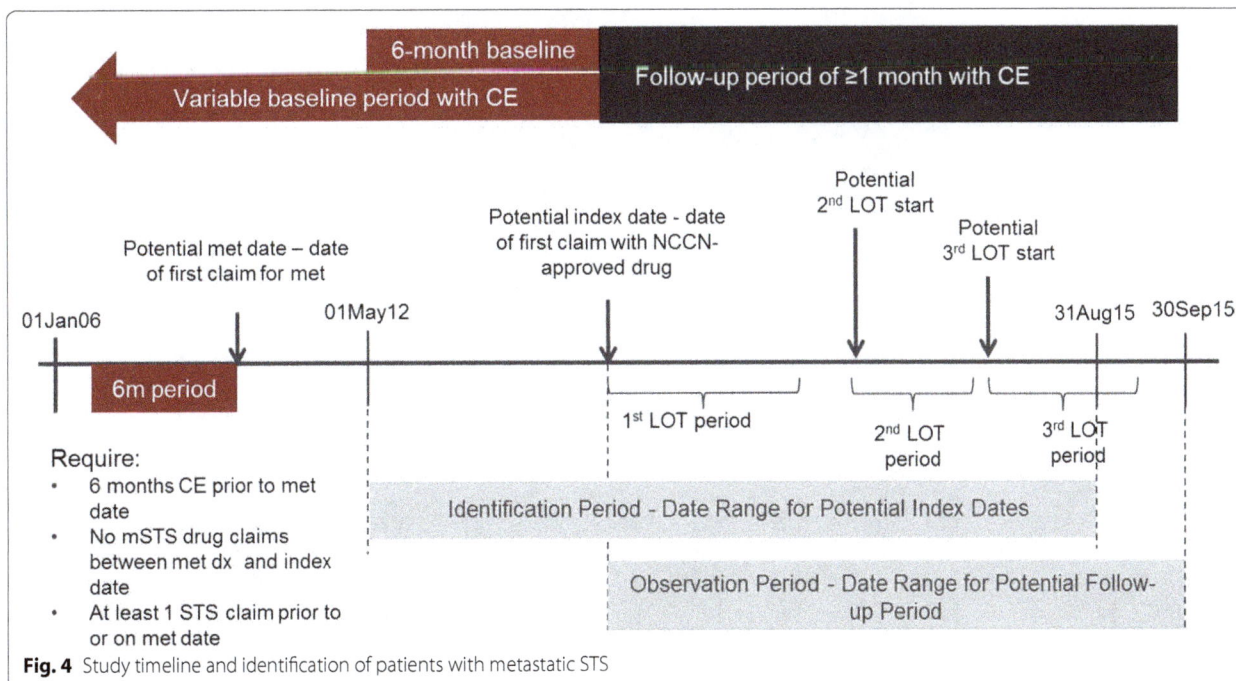

Fig. 4 Study timeline and identification of patients with metastatic STS

Appendix 3

See Fig. 5.

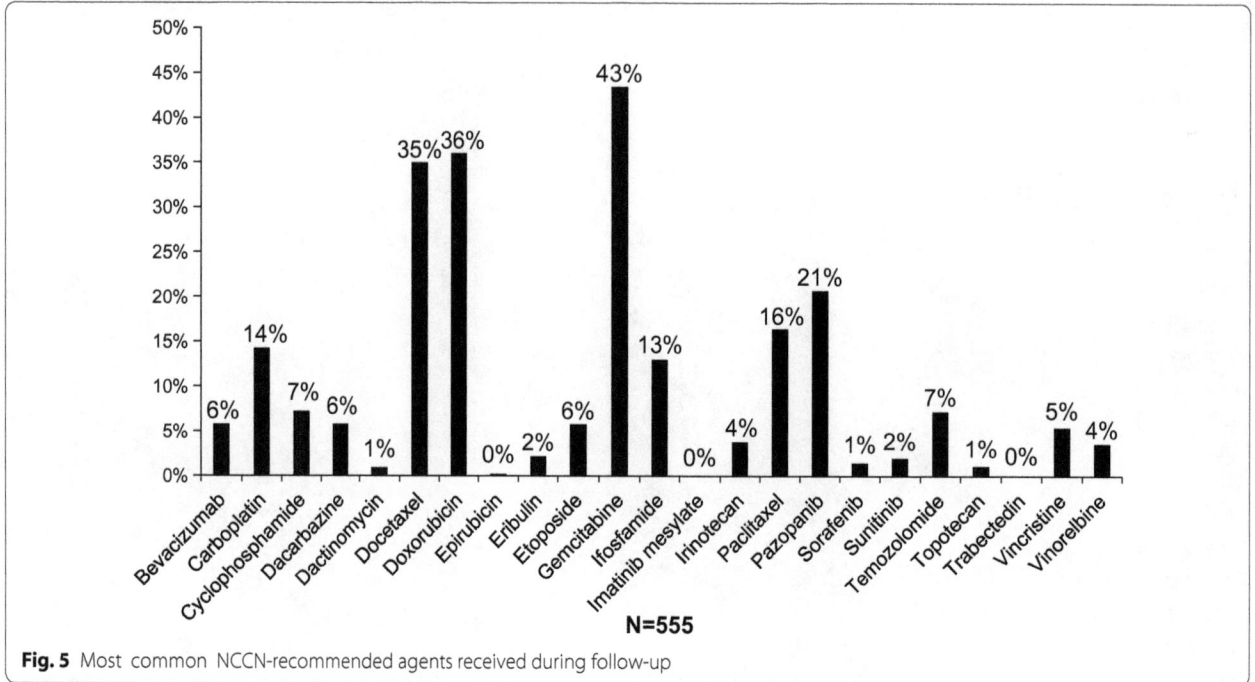

Fig. 5 Most common NCCN-recommended agents received during follow-up

Appendix 4

See Table 4.

Table 4 Frequency of use of specific medications included in 'Other' category for LOT1-LOT3

	Frequency	Percent (%)
LOT 1 regimen		
Carboplatin, paclitaxel	29	5.2
Paclitaxel	28	5.0
Carboplatin	18	3.2
Temozolomide	14	2.5
Bevacizumab	12	2.2
Cyclophosphamide, doxorubicin, vincristine	9	1.6
Sunitinib	8	1.4
Docetaxel	8	1.4
Etoposide	7	1.3
Ifosfamide	7	1.3
Etoposide, ifosfamide	6	1.1
Carboplatin, docetaxel	6	1.1
Irinotecan, temozolomide	5	0.9
Sorafenib	5	0.9
Gemcitabine, paclitaxel	4	0.7
Carboplatin, etoposide	4	0.7
Cyclophosphamide	4	0.7
Dacarbazine	4	0.7
Docetaxel, doxorubicin, gemcitabine	4	0.7
Bevacizumab, temozolomide	3	0.5
Bevacizumab, carboplatin, paclitaxel	3	0.5
Vincristine	3	0.5
Vinorelbine	3	0.5
Carboplatin, gemcitabine	3	0.5
Cyclophosphamide, dactinomycin, vincristine	3	0.5
Cyclophosphamide, doxorubicin, etoposide, ifosfamide, vincristine	3	0.5
Dacarbazine, doxorubicin	3	0.5
Eribulin	3	0.5
Gemcitabine, vinorelbine	2	0.4
Irinotecan	2	0.4
Irinotecan, temozolomide, vincristine	2	0.4
Carboplatin, irinotecan	2	0.4
Cyclophosphamide, etoposide	2	0.4
Cyclophosphamide, vinorelbine	2	0.4
Cyclophosphamide, dacarbazine, doxorubicin	2	0.4
Cyclophosphamide, doxorubicin, irinotecan, vincristine	2	0.4
Docetaxel, gemcitabine, pazopanib	2	0.4
Doxorubicin, gemcitabine	2	0.4
Doxorubicin, pazopanib	2	0.4
Etoposide, ifosfamide, methotrexate	1	0.2
Gemcitabine, ifosfamide	1	0.2

Table 4 continued

	Frequency	Percent (%)
Gemcitabine, sunitinib	1	0.2
Ifosfamide, paclitaxel	1	0.2
Methotrexate	1	0.2
Pazopanib, sorafenib	1	0.2
Bevacizumab, irinotecan	1	0.2
Bevacizumab, irinotecan, temozolomide, vincristine	1	0.2
Bevacizumab, paclitaxel	1	0.2
Bevacizumab, docetaxel	1	0.2
Bevacizumab, doxorubicin	1	0.2
Temozolomide, topotecan, vincristine	1	0.2
Carboplatin, etoposide, irinotecan	1	0.2
Carboplatin, gemcitabine, paclitaxel	1	0.2
Carboplatin, methotrexate, paclitaxel	1	0.2
Carboplatin, epirubicin, paclitaxel	1	0.2
Cyclophosphamide, dacarbazine, doxorubicin, vincristine	1	0.2
Cyclophosphamide, doxorubicin	1	0.2
Cyclophosphamide, doxorubicin, etoposide, vincristine	1	0.2
Cyclophosphamide, doxorubicin, paclitaxel	1	0.2
Dacarbazine, gemcitabine	1	0.2
Dacarbazine, pazopanib	1	0.2
Dacarbazine, doxorubicin, gemcitabine	1	0.2
Dacarbazine, doxorubicin, ifosfamide	1	0.2
Dacarbazine, doxorubicin, methotrexate	1	0.2
Docetaxel, paclitaxel	1	0.2
Docetaxel, doxorubicin, gemcitabine, ifosfamide	1	0.2
Doxorubicin, gemcitabine, vinorelbine	1	0.2
Doxorubicin, ifosfamide, pazopanib	1	0.2
Doxorubicin, ifosfamide, vincristine	1	0.2
LOT 2 regimen		
Methotrexate	7	3.1
Paclitaxel	7	3.1
Carboplatin, paclitaxel	7	3.1
Doxorubicin, ifosfamide	5	2.2
Gemcitabine, paclitaxel	4	1.7
Ifosfamide	4	1.7
Sorafenib	4	1.7
Vinorelbine	4	1.7
Dacarbazine, doxorubicin	4	1.7
Docetaxel	4	1.7
Bevacizumab	3	1.3
Carboplatin	3	1.3
Dacarbazine	3	1.3
Etoposide	2	0.9
Bevacizumab, paclitaxel	2	0.9
Bevacizumab, temozolomide	2	0.9
Bevacizumab, docetaxel, gemcitabine	2	0.9

Table 4 continued

	Frequency	Percent (%)
Carboplatin, gemcitabine	2	0.9
Doxorubicin, gemcitabine	2	0.9
Eribulin	2	0.9
Etoposide, ifosfamide	1	0.4
Etoposide, ifosfamide, irinotecan, vincristine	1	0.4
Gemcitabine, irinotecan	1	0.4
Gemcitabine, pazopanib	1	0.4
Gemcitabine, vinorelbine	1	0.4
Irinotecan, temozolomide	1	0.4
Irinotecan, temozolomide, vincristine	1	0.4
Paclitaxel, pazopanib	1	0.4
Pazopanib, sunitinib	1	0.4
Sunitinib	1	0.4
Bevacizumab, dacarbazine	1	0.4
Bevacizumab, doxorubicin	1	0.4
Topotecan	1	0.4
Carboplatin, methotrexate, paclitaxel	1	0.4
Cyclophosphamide, etoposide	1	0.4
Cyclophosphamide, methotrexate	1	0.4
Cyclophosphamide, temozolomide, topotecan	1	0.4
Cyclophosphamide, topotecan	1	0.4
Cyclophosphamide, vincristine	1	0.4
Cyclophosphamide, dacarbazine, doxorubicin	1	0.4
Cyclophosphamide, dacarbazine, doxorubicin, vincristine	1	0.4
Cyclophosphamide, docetaxel	1	0.4
Cyclophosphamide, doxorubicin, etoposide, ifosfamide	1	0.4
Cyclophosphamide, doxorubicin, etoposide, ifosfamide, vincristine	1	0.4
Cyclophosphamide, doxorubicin, vincristine	1	0.4
Dacarbazine, gemcitabine	1	0.4
Dacarbazine, ifosfamide	1	0.4
Dacarbazine, doxorubicin, ifosfamide	1	0.4
Docetaxel, gemcitabine, paclitaxel	1	0.4
Docetaxel, gemcitabine, pazopanib	1	0.4
Docetaxel, doxorubicin, gemcitabine	1	0.4
Doxorubicin, gemcitabine, vinorelbine	1	0.4
Doxorubicin, paclitaxel	1	0.4
Doxorubicin, pazopanib	1	0.4
LOT 3 regimen		
Vinorelbine	4	4.5
Gemcitabine	3	3.4
Paclitaxel	2	2.3
Cyclophosphamide, dactinomycin, vincristine	2	2.3
Cyclophosphamide, doxorubicin, vincristine	2	2.3

Table 4 continued

	Frequency	Percent (%)
Docetaxel	2	2.3
Etoposide, ifosfamide	1	1.1
Etoposide, ifosfamide, irinotecan	1	1.1
Gemcitabine, irinotecan	1	1.1
Gemcitabine, methotrexate	1	1.1
Ifosfamide	1	1.1
Irinotecan, temozolomide	1	1.1
Irinotecan, vincristine	1	1.1
Sorafenib	1	1.1
Bevacizumab, gemcitabine, paclitaxel	1	1.1
Bevacizumab, cyclophosphamide, sorafenib	1	1.1
Carboplatin	1	1.1
Topotecan	1	1.1
Cyclophosphamide, topotecan	1	1.1
Cyclophosphamide, doxorubicin	1	1.1
Cyclophosphamide, doxorubicin, irinotecan, vincristine	1	1.1
Dacarbazine	1	1.1
Dacarbazine, pazopanib	1	1.1
Dacarbazine, vinorelbine	1	1.1
Dacarbazine, doxorubicin	1	1.1

References

1. Tuna M, Ju Z, Amos CI, Mills GB. Soft tissue sarcoma subtypes exhibit distinct patterns of acquired uniparental disomy. BMC Med Genom. 2012;5:60.
2. National Comprehensive Cancer Network. NCCN clinical practice guidelines in oncology. Soft Tissue Sarcoma V1. 2015.
3. American Cancer Society. Cancer facts and figures 2015. Atlanta: American Cancer Society; 2015.
4. Casali PG. Histology- and non-histology-driven therapy for treatment of soft tissue sarcomas. Ann Oncol. 2012;23(Suppl 10):x167–9.
5. Pang A, Carbini M, Maki RG. Contemporary therapy for advanced soft-tissue sarcomas in adults: a review. JAMA Oncol. 2016;2(7):941–7.
6. Brennan MF, Antonescu CR, Maki RG. Management of soft tissue sarcoma. Berlin: Springer Science & Business Media; 2012.
7. Demetri GD, Chawla SP, von Mehren M, Ritch P, Baker LH, Blay JY, Hande KR, Keohan ML, Samuels BL, Schuetze S, et al. Efficacy and safety of trabectedin in patients with advanced or metastatic liposarcoma or leiomyosarcoma after failure of prior anthracyclines and ifosfamide: results of a randomized phase II study of two different schedules. J Clin Oncol. 2009;27(25):4188–96.
8. Demetri GD, von Mehren M, Jones RL, Hensley ML, Schuetze SM, Staddon A, Milhem M, Elias A, Ganjoo K, Tawbi H, et al. Efficacy and safety of trabectedin or dacarbazine for metastatic liposarcoma or leiomyosarcoma after failure of conventional chemotherapy: results of a phase III randomized multicenter clinical trial. J Clin Oncol. 2016;34(8):786–93.
9. FDA News Release. FDA approves Votrient for advanced soft tissue sarcoma. 2012.
10. FDA News Release. FDA grants accelerated approval to new treatment for advanced soft tissue sarcoma. October 19, 2016 edn; 2016.
11. Leahy M, Garcia Del Muro X, Reichardt P, Judson I, Staddon A, Verweij J, Baffoe-Bonnie A, Jonsson L, Musayev A, Justo N, et al. Chemotherapy treatment patterns and clinical outcomes in patients with metastatic soft tissue sarcoma. The SArcoma treatment and Burden of Illness in North America and Europe (SABINE) study. Ann Oncol. 2012;23(10):2763–70.

12. Chen C, Borker R, Ewing J, Tseng WY, Hackshaw MD, Saravanan S, Dhanda R, Nadler E. Epidemiology, treatment patterns, and outcomes of metastatic soft tissue sarcoma in a community-based oncology network. Sarcoma. 2014;2014:145764.

13. Wagner MJ, Amodu LI, Duh MS, Korves C, Solleza F, Manson SC, Diaz J, Neary MP, Demetri GD. A retrospective chart review of drug treatment patterns and clinical outcomes among patients with metastatic or recurrent soft tissue sarcoma refractory to one or more prior chemotherapy treatments. BMC Cancer. 2015;15:175.

14. Quan H, Li B, Couris CM, Fushimi K, Graham P, Hider P, Januel JM, Sundararajan V. Updating and validating the Charlson comorbidity index and score for risk adjustment in hospital discharge abstracts using data from 6 countries. Am J Epidemiol. 2011;173(6):676–82.

15. Seddon BM, Strauss SJ, Whelan J, et al. Gemcitabine and docetaxel versus doxorubicin as first-line treatment in previously untreated advanced unresectable or metastatic soft-tissue sarcomas (GeDDiS): a randomised controlled phase 3 trial. Lancet. 2017;18(10):1397–410.

16. Bramwell VH, Anderson D, Charette ML. Doxorubicin-based chemotherapy for the palliative treatment of adult patients with locally advanced or metastatic soft-tissue sarcoma: a meta-analysis and clinical practice guideline. Sarcoma. 2000;4(3):103–12.

17. Tap WD, Jones RL, Van Tine BA, Chmielowski B, Elias AD, Adkins D, Agulnik M, Cooney MM, Livingston MB, Pennock G, et al. Olaratumab and doxorubicin versus doxorubicin alone for treatment of soft-tissue sarcoma: an open-label phase 1b and randomised phase 2 trial. Lancet. 2016;388(10043):488–97.

18. Bae S, Crowe P, Gowda R, Joubert W, Carey-Smith R, Stalley P, Desai J. Patterns of care for patients with advanced soft tissue sarcoma: experience from Australian sarcoma services. Clin Sarcoma Res. 2016;6:11.

19. Bramwell VH, Anderson D, Charette ML, Sarcoma Disease Site G. Doxorubicin-based chemotherapy for the palliative treatment of adult patients with locally advanced or metastatic soft tissue sarcoma. Cochrane Database Syst Rev. 2003;3:CD003293.

20. Maki RG. Gemcitabine and docetaxel in metastatic sarcoma: past, present, and future. Oncologist. 2007;12(8):999–1006.

21. Colosia A, Khan S, Hackshaw MD, Oglesby A, Kaye JA, Skolnik JM. A systematic literature review of adverse events associated with systemic treatments used in advanced soft tissue sarcoma. Sarcoma. 2016;2016:3597609.

22. van der Graaf WT, Blay JY, Chawla SP, Kim DW, Bui-Nguyen B, Casali PG, Schoffski P, Aglietta M, Staddon AP, Beppu Y, et al. Pazopanib for metastatic soft-tissue sarcoma (PALETTE): a randomised, double-blind, placebo-controlled phase 3 trial. Lancet. 2012;379(9829):1879–86.

23. Karch A, Koch A, Grunwald V. A phase II trial comparing pazopanib with doxorubicin as first-line treatment in elderly patients with metastatic or advanced soft tissue sarcoma (EPAZ): study protocol for a randomized controlled trial. Trials. 2016;17(1):312.

24. Maruzzo M, Martin-Liberal J, Messiou C, Miah A, Thway K, Alvarado R, Judson I, Benson C. Pazopanib as first line treatment for solitary fibrous tumours: the Royal Marsden Hospital experience. Clin Sarcoma Res. 2015;5:5.

25. Outani H, Tanaka T, Wakamatsu T, Imura Y, Hamada K, Araki N, Itoh K, Yoshikawa H, Naka N. Establishment of a novel clear cell sarcoma cell line (Hewga-CCS), and investigation of the antitumor effects of pazopanib on Hewga-CCS. BMC Cancer. 2014;14:455.

23

Periostin expression in neoplastic and non-neoplastic diseases of bone and joint

Jennifer M. Brown[1], Akiro Mantoku[2], Afsie Sabokbar[1], Udo Oppermann[1], A. Bass Hassan[1], Akiro Kudo[2] and Nick Athanasou[1*]

Abstract

Background: Periostin is a matricellular protein that is expressed in bone and joint tissues. To determine the expression of periostin in primary bone tumours and to assess whether it plays a role in tumour progression, we carried out immunohistochemistry and ELISA for periostin in a range of neoplastic and non-neoplastic bone and joint lesions.

Methods: 140 formalin-fixed paraffin-embedded sections of bone tumours and tumour-like lesions were stained by an indirect immunoperoxidase technique with a polyclonal anti-periostin antibody. Periostin expression was also assessed in rheumatoid arthritis (RA) and non-inflammatory osteoarthritis (OA) synovium and synovial fluid immunohistochemistry and ELISA respectively.

Results: Periostin was most strongly expressed in osteoid/woven bone of neoplastic and non-neoplastic bone-forming lesions, including osteoblastoma, osteosarcoma, fibrous dysplasia, osteofibrous dysplasia, fracture callus and myositis ossificans, and mineralised chondroid matrix/woven bone in chondroblastoma and clear cell chondrosarcoma. Reactive host bone at the edge of growing tumours, particularly in areas of increased vascularity and fibrosis, also stained strongly for periostin. Vascular elements in RA synovium strongly expressed periostin, and synovial fluid levels of periostin were higher in RA than OA.

Conclusions: In keeping with its known role in modulating the synthesis of collagen and other extracellular matrix proteins in bone, strong periostin expression was noted in benign and malignant lesions forming an osteoid or osteoid-like matrix. Periostin was also noted in other bone tumours and was found in areas of reactive bone and increased vascularity at the edge of growing tumours, consistent with its involvement in tissue remodelling and angiogenesis associated with tumour progression.

Keywords: Periostin expression, Bone tumours, Tumour progression

Background

Periostin, a secreted extracellular matrix protein that belongs to the fasciclin family, was originally characterised in osteoblasts and first termed osteoblast-specific factor 2 [1, 2]. Periostin is a matricellular protein that does not have a specific structural role but rather interacts with cell surface receptors, proteases and other molecules that modulate cell adhesion/migration and the fibrillogenesis of collagen and other extracellular matrix (ECM) proteins [3–6]. Periostin has a multidomain structure in which particular domains bind to many proteins and enzymes that promote ECM protein crosslinking. Periostin is involved in the formation and maintenance of normal bone and teeth tissues and is highly expressed in tissue components that are subject to mechanical stress, such as the periosteum and the periodontal ligament. It has also been observed in other organs and tissues including heart, breast, lung, thyroid, skin, placenta and ovary [3–6].

Periostin is expressed at sites of injury/repair and inflammation [3, 6, 7]. It has been identified in rheumatoid arthritis (RA) and osteoarthritis (OA) joints [8, 9] with a recent study identifying periostin as a key

*Correspondence: nick.athanasou@ndorms.ox.ac.uk
[1] Nuffield Department of Orthopaedics, Rheumatology and Musculoskeletal and Sciences, Nuffield Orthopaedic Centre, University of Oxford, Oxford OX3 7HE, UK
Full list of author information is available at the end of the article

regulator in RA synoviocyte migration/invasion associated with pannus formation [10]. Periostin is also expressed in a number of cancers where it is thought, by various mechanisms, to play a role in tumour progression [3, 6, 11, 12]. Periostin has been identified in a few bone tumours, including fibrous dysplasia and osteosarcoma [13–15], but its expression in other bone neoplasms has not been fully investigated.

In this study we investigated immunophenotypic expression of periostin in a wide range of primary tumours and tumour-like lesions of bone as well as in bone secondaries and metastatic osteosarcomas. Our aims were two-fold: first, to determine whether periostin expression is increased in specific bone tumour types; and second, to examine whether periostin plays a role in tumour progression.

Methods

Neoplastic and non-neoplastic tissue samples analysed

Tissue samples from 140 biopsies or surgical resections of bone tumours and tumour-like lesions, were retrieved from the files of the Nuffield Orthopaedic Centre, Histopathology Department, Oxford (Table 1). Criteria for the histological diagnosis of bone and joint lesions investigated in this study were those of the 2013 WHO Classification of Tumours of Soft Tissue and Bone [16]. The tissues were fixed in 10% buffered formalin and, where necessary, decalcified in 5% nitric acid or EDTA. In addition, formalin-fixed paraffin-embedded sections of synovial tissue derived from patients with RA (n=21) and OA (n=19) were examined. Samples of normal bone and joint tissues from amputation specimens of individuals with no history or evidence of joint disease or neoplasia were used as controls. Synovial fluid (SF) was also aspirated from the knee joint of nine patients with OA and nine patients with RA. Ethics approval was obtained from the National Research Ethical Committee, and patient consent was acquired prior to the collection of samples.

Immunohistochemistry for periostin

Immunohistochemical staining for periostin was carried out by an indirect immunoperoxidase technique (without any antigen retrieval procedure) using a polyclonal rabbit antiserum against human periostin raised by using peptide DNLDSDIRRGLESNVN (representing aminoacids 143–158 of human periostin) as an immunogen [13, 17]. As in previous studies [17], the antibody dilution was 1:250 and sections of normal skin were employed as a positive control.

Periostin expression in OA and RA synovial fluid

A quantitative measure of the level of periostin in knee joint RA and OA synovial fluid was determined by ELISA

Table 1 Bone tumours/tumour-like lesions analysed in this study

Tissue type	Number analysed
Osteoma	2
Osteoid osteoma	4
Osteoblastoma	6
Osteosarcoma, conventional	20
Osteosarcoma, telangiectatic	2
Osteosarcoma, small cell	2
Osteosarcoma, parosteal	2
Fibrous dysplasia	10
Osteofibrous dysplasia	2
Fracture	2
Myositis ossificans	2
Enchondroma	3
Chondroblastoma	9
Chondromyxoid fibroma	3
Chondrosarcoma, conventional	20
Chondrosarcoma, clear cell	5
Giant cell tumour of bone	8
Aneurysmal bone cyst	4
Solitary bone cyst	2
Non-ossifying fibroma	3
Undifferentiated pleomorphic sarcoma	3
Ewing sarcoma	6
Adamantinoma of long bone	1
Chordoma	2
Plasma cell myeloma	2
Lymphoma	2
Langerhans cell histiocytoma	2
Metastatic breast carcinoma	3
Metastatic melanoma	1

(enzyme-linked immunosorbent assay). The periostin concentration was assessed using a Human periostin/OSF-2 ELISA kit (Adiopo bioscience, Santa Clara, CA, USA). Statistical evaluation was performed using the Mann–Whitney U test with p values less than 0.05 considered as statistically significant.

Results

Periostin expression in normal bone and joint tissues

In normal bone there was strong expression of periostin in collagenous fibrous tissue of the periosteum. At points of tendon or ligament insertion into bone, strong periostin staining was also seen within collagenous tissue. There was no staining for periostin in normal lamellar cortical and cancellous bone, and osteocytes, bone lining cells, osteoblasts and osteoclasts did not express periostin. Fatty and hematopoietic marrow was generally negative for periostin but, in some specimens, staining for periostin was noted in small sinusoidal vascular channels within the marrow. In normal joints, the synovium and hyaline articular cartilage did not stain for periostin.

Periostin expression in tumours and tumour-like lesions of bone and joint

Strong staining for periostin was seen in the osteoid matrix formed by osteoblastic cells in neoplastic and non-neoplastic bone-forming lesions. Periostin staining was noted in the osteoid matrix covering organized reactive bone in fracture callus and myositis ossificans. In osteoblastoma, newly formed osteoid stained strongly for periostin (Fig. 1a); staining for periostin was less pronounced in woven bone and was absent in lamellar bone surrounding the lesion. In osteosarcoma, there was strong staining for periostin in the osteoid matrix formed by malignant cells (Fig. 1b); staining for periostin was seen in all osteosarcomas but the extent of expression was variable with osteoid-rich tumours showing the strongest and most diffuse staining (Fig. 1c). A similar pattern of staining for periostin was noted in lung nodules of metastatic osteosarcoma (Fig. 1d). In small cell osteosarcoma, periostin was expressed in the matrix between tumor cells (Fig. 1e). In chondroblastic and telangiectatic osteosarcomas, cartilage and giant cell components of the tumor were negative. In parosteal osteosarcoma, periostin expression was noted focally in the matrix in areas of tumor cell proliferation. There was strong staining for periostin in fibrous dysplasia and osteofibrous dysplasia, predominantly in the cellular fibrous stroma between bone trabeculae (Fig. 1f).

There was no specific staining of the chondroid matrix or cartilage cells for periostin in enchondroma, osteochondroma, or low/high-grade conventional chondrosarcoma. The dense fibrous perichondrium covering osteochondromas (which is continuous with the periosteum) stained strongly for periostin (Fig. 2a). At the base of growing osteochondromas, there was focal staining of the matrix and thin-walled vessels in areas of enchondral ossification and remodeling of newly formed bone. In chondroblastoma, areas of chondroid matrix, some of which showed evidence of mineralisation, stained focally for periostin (Fig. 2b). There was also focal staining of the matrix around chondroblasts. There was no staining for periostin in chondromyxoid fibroma. In clear cell chondrosarcoma, periostin staining was seen in the mineralized osteoid-like matrix covering woven bone and cartilage formed by vacuolated tumor cells.

In aneurysmal bone cyst (ABC) and simple bone cyst, the fibrous stroma and reactive bone within the cyst wall was positive for periostin (Fig. 3a). In giant cell tumour of bone (GCTB), there was focal, occasionally strong staining for periostin in the collagenous connective tissue matrix around mononuclear cells (Fig. 3b). Giant cells in GCTB, chondroblastoma and ABC were

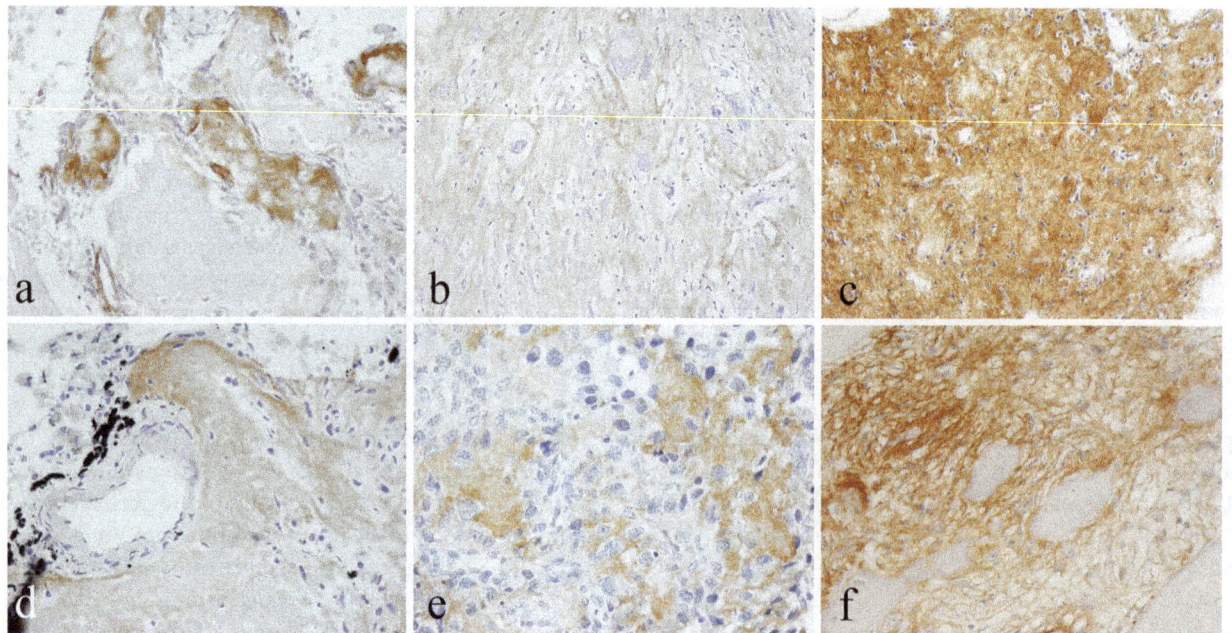

Fig. 1 Immunohistochemical staining for periostin in osteoid/newly formed bone of: **a** osteoblastoma; **b** high-grade osteoblastic osteosarcoma; **c** osteoid-rich area of high-grade osteosarcoma; **d** small cell osteosarcoma; **e** osteosarcoma metastasis in lung; **f** fibrous dysplasia

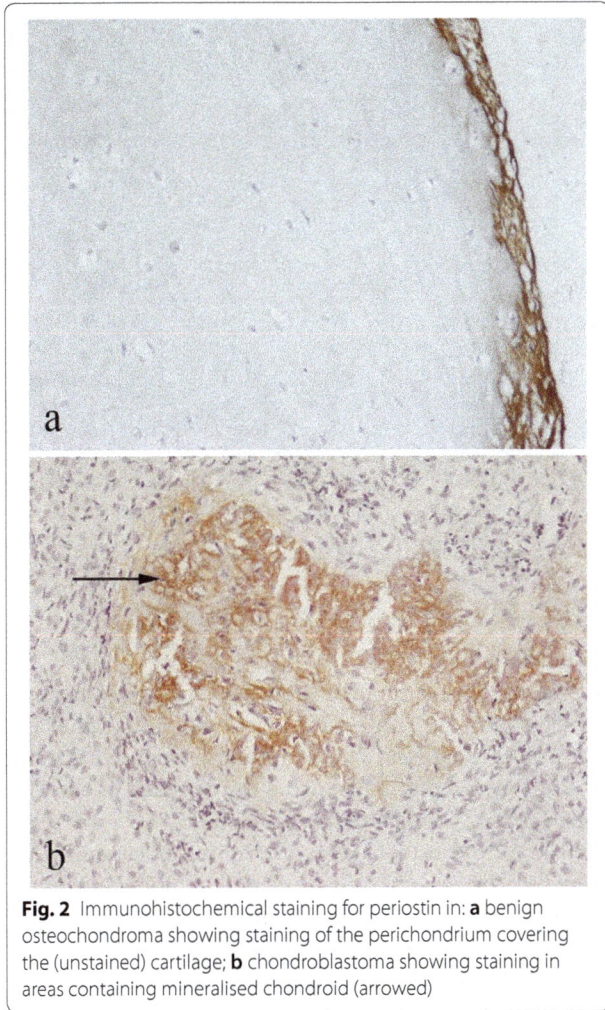

Fig. 2 Immunohistochemical staining for periostin in: **a** benign osteochondroma showing staining of the perichondrium covering the (unstained) cartilage; **b** chondroblastoma showing staining in areas containing mineralised chondroid (arrowed)

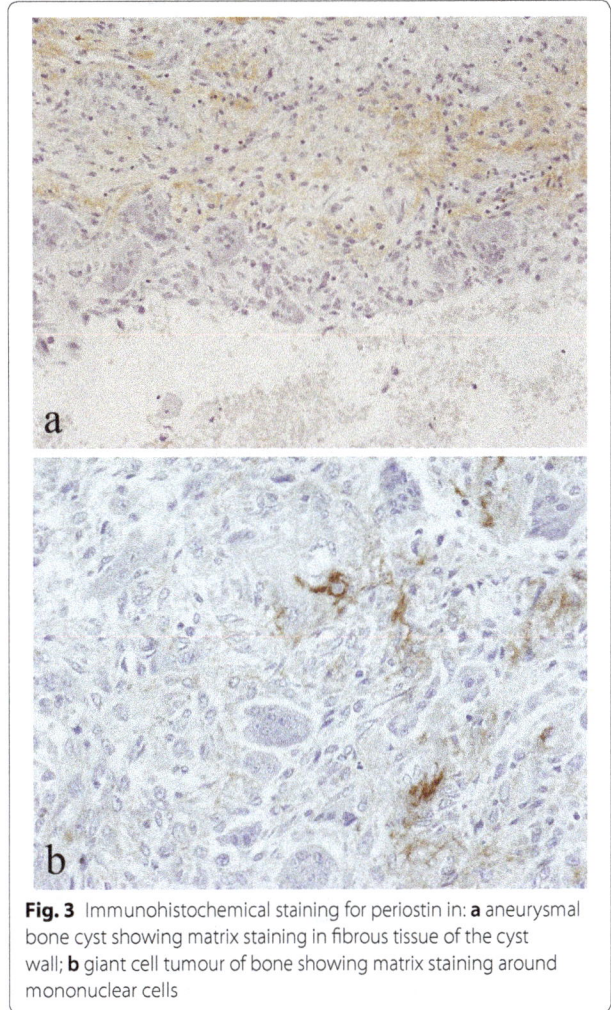

Fig. 3 Immunohistochemical staining for periostin in: **a** aneurysmal bone cyst showing matrix staining in fibrous tissue of the cyst wall; **b** giant cell tumour of bone showing matrix staining around mononuclear cells

negative for periostin. Variable focal staining for periostin was seen in cellular and collagenous connective tissue of other bone tumours, including non-ossifying fibroma and undifferentiated pleomorphic sarcoma. No specific staining for periostin was noted in Langerhans cell histiocytosis, Ewing sarcoma, lymphoma, myeloma, chordoma or adamantinoma.

Staining for periostin was noted in non-neoplastic bone at the edge of growing benign and malignant primary bone tumours (Fig. 4a); this was in areas of fatty marrow in which there was fibrosis, increased vascularity and reactive bone formation with prominent staining often noted in the smooth muscle wall of small blood vessels with lining endothelial cells unstained. Infiltrating secondary carcinomas and melanomas that had metastasised to bone showed a similar pattern of staining for periostin in surrounding non-neoplastic

bone. Strong periostin staining of vessels was also seen within metastatic tumours (Fig. 4b).

Periostin expression in OA and RA

Immunohistochemistry showed no staining for periostin of synovial lining cells in OA or RA synovium. Strong staining for periostin was noted in RA in the superficial subintima where there was staining of the fibrous tissue matrix and the smooth muscle wall of small blood vessels in areas of increased vascularity (Fig. 5a); in contrast, non-inflammatory OA synovium showed no subintimal periostin staining; (Fig. 5b). Periostin was also expressed in the matrix around large vessels in the deep subintima and capsule of RA joints. ELISA studies showed that the average human periostin concentration in synovial fluid was 107.4 ng/ml and 67.1 ng/ml in RA patients and OA patients respectively (Fig. 6). This was not of statistical significance (p=0.29), but higher periostin levels were more frequently seen in RA than OA synovial fluid.

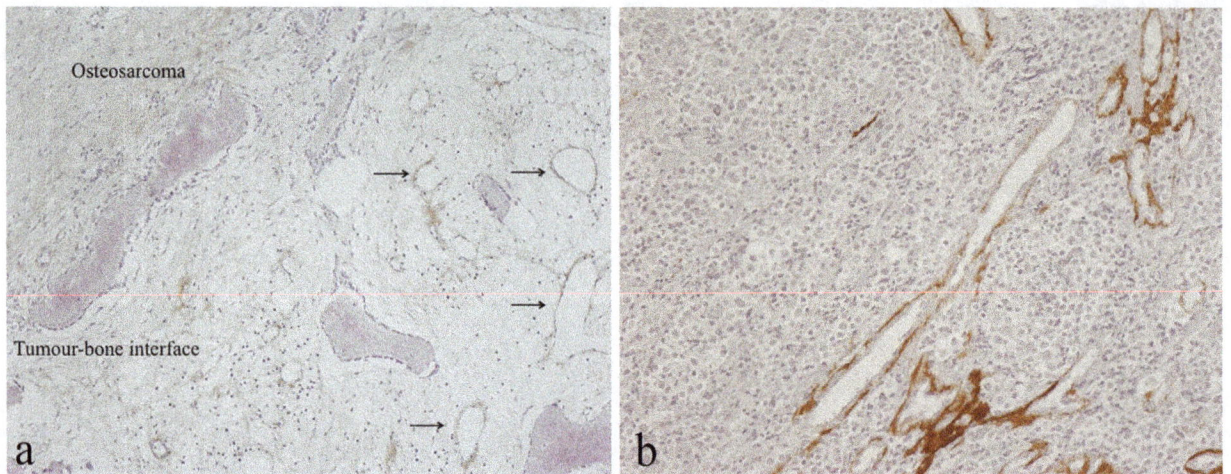

Fig. 4 Immunohistochemical staining for periostin in: **a** osteosarcoma showing staining of vessels and matrix in fatty marrow in non-neoplastic bone at the tumour margin (arrowed); **b** metastatic melanoma showing prominent staining of vessels within the tumour

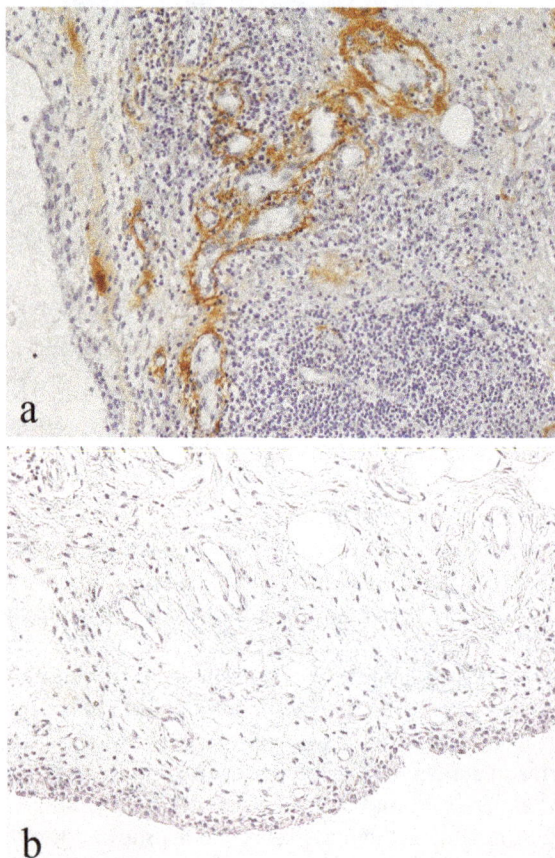

Fig. 5 Immunohistochemical staining for periostin in: **a** RA synovium showing prominent staining of vessels in the subintima; **b** OA synovium

Discussion

In this study, we have characterised periostin expression in neoplastic and non-neoplastic lesions of bone and joint. In keeping with its role in bone matrix formation, periostin was found to be strongly expressed in osteoid/bone-forming lesions; it was also noted in the mineralised chondroid/osteoid matrix of chondroblastomas and clear cell chondrosarcomas and in the connective tissue matrix of other primary bone tumours. Periostin expression was also prominent in areas of reactive host bone around infiltrating primary and secondary bone tumours, suggesting a role for this matricellular protein in tumour progression.

Periostin is a 90-kDa secreted protein which binds to type I collagen and other ECM proteins including fibronectin, Notch1, tenascin-C and BMP-1 [3–6, 18–20]; periostin acts to increase osteoblast proliferation, differentiation, adhesion and survival, and plays a key role in bone matrix formation. Periostin plays a role in bone remodelling by regulating collagen cross-linking and fibrillogenesis. In periostin-null mice, collagen fibrillogenesis is disrupted in the periosteum and mechanical loading results in a disorganised matrix formation. In addition, periostin expression is associated with reduced sclerostin and preservation of bone mass. Periostin increases ECM production by fibroblasts/myofibroblasts and promotes mesenchymal stem cell differentiation into osteoblasts, resulting in the formation of bone matrix. Periostin is known to function as a signalling molecule through integrin receptors and WNT-β-catenin pathways whereby it stimulates osteoblast function and bone formation.

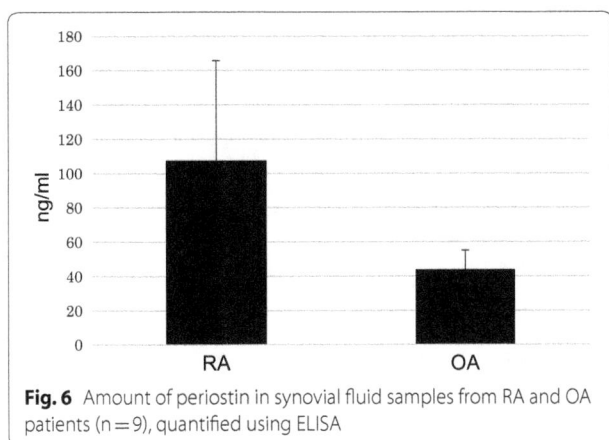

Fig. 6 Amount of periostin in synovial fluid samples from RA and OA patients (n = 9), quantified using ELISA

Periostin was originally called osteoblast specific factor-2 and in this study we have shown that periostin is highly expressed in reparative lesions associated with osteoid/woven bone formation, such as fracture callus and myositis ossificans as well as in benign and malignant bone-forming tumours. Expression of periostin in osteosarcoma has previously been reported with high expression being correlated with tumour angiogenesis and poor prognosis [14, 15]. We noted periostin expression in both low-grade parosteal osteosarcomas and high-grade conventional osteosarcomas as well as in lung metastases of osteosarcoma with the extent of periostin expression appearing to be more related to formation of an osteoid matrix than histological parameters of tumour grade. Strong periostin expression was consistently noted in fibrous dysplasia and osteofibrous dysplasia, fibro-osseous bone tumours in which there is formation of woven bone with intramembranous ossification similar to that which occurs beneath the periosteum. Periostin was also seen in cellular fibrous tissue and areas of reactive osteoid/bone formation in other bone lesions, including simple bone cyst, ABC, fracture callus and myositis ossificans. It was also noted in the connective tissue matrix around mononuclear cells in giant cell tumour of bone; these cells are known to exhibit several osteoblast markers including alkaline phosphatase, RUNX2, osterix and RANKL [21]. Focal but less prominent staining for periostin was also noted in cellular and collagenous fibrous tissue of other primary bone tumours including non-ossifying fibroma and undifferentiated pleomorphic sarcoma.

Periostin was strongly expressed in the perichondrium covering osteochondromas and in areas of endochondral ossification at the base of growing osteochondromas but there was no staining in cells or matrix of the cartilage cap. Periostin expression was absent in other cartilage tumours including enchondroma and low/high-grade conventional chondrosarcoma. Our findings contrast with those of Lai and Chen [22], who identified periostin in chondrosarcoma and enchondroma using a commercial mouse monoclonal antibody TA804575 (OriGene Technologies, Inc., Rockville, MD, USA); in our study we employed a rabbit polyclonal antibody that had been characterised in previous investigations [13, 17]. In both chondroblastoma and clear cell chondrosarcoma, strong expression of periostin was noted in areas of chondroid matrix formation. In chondroblastoma, the chondroid matrix has been described as "chondrosteoid" by some observers [23]; it has been shown that this matrix contains dentine-matrix protein-1 and sclerostin, proteins found in newly formed osteoid [24, 25]. Clear cell chondrosarcoma, which is considered by some observers to be a malignant form of chondroblastoma [23], also showed expression of periostin in areas of woven bone formed within the clear cell cartilaginous stroma.

We consistently noted increased expression of periostin in non-lesional bone at the edge of growing benign and malignant bone tumours. It has been shown that periostin plays a role in the progression of inflammatory and neoplastic lesions [6, 11, 12, 23]. Periostin is known to be expressed by fibroblasts in RA, carcinomas and other malignant tumours [26–32]. Periostin is known to stimulate cell/matrix adhesion and migration of the endothelial cells through interaction with $\alpha V\beta 3$ [33]. Endothelial cells strongly express $\alpha V\beta 3$ when stimulated by growth factors produced in inflammation, wound healing and tumours. We noted that periostin was frequently expressed in the smooth muscle wall of small blood vessels within non-lesional bone around growing tumours, both benign and malignant. Interactions between periostin and vascular endothelial growth factor (VEGF) and its receptors are thought to play a key role in physiological and pathological angiogenesis [6, 12, 29, 34–36]. Periostin is strongly expressed by vascular smooth muscle cells, particularly those which are activated and migrating from the media to the intima or proliferating and synthesising matrix proteins. It has been shown that in breast carcinoma, squamous cell carcinoma and other tumours, blood vessel density in periostin-positive tumours is higher than in periostin-negative tumours with increased tumour invasion and metastasis being reported in these periostin over-expressing tumours [28, 37–40]. We noted prominent staining of the smooth muscle wall of small blood vessels in malignant tumours that had metastasised to bone.

There were similarities in the pattern of periostin expression in inflamed RA synovium and growing bone tumours. Periostin is known to be involved in the migration of synovial fibroblasts associated with RA pannus formation and joint destruction [4, 10]. We noted strong expression of periostin in the subintimal connective tissue matrix and smooth muscle wall of small blood vessels in RA synovium, indicating that periostin-associated angiogenesis may play a role in RA disease progression. We also noted higher levels of periostin in RA compared with OA synovial fluid and little staining for periostin in OA synovium. Increased levels of periostin have been associated with tumour angiogenesis, metastatic potential and poor prognosis in osteosarcoma patients [14, 15]. It has been shown that small interfering RNA against periostin significantly reduces the migration of fibroblast-like cells in RA [10]. Analogously, inhibition of periostin gene expression suppresses the proliferation and invasion of U2OS osteosarcoma cells [41] Our immunohistochemical finding of increased expression of periostin at the edge of growing bone tumours is in keeping with a role for periostin in tumour growth and, taken with the results of previous studies, suggests that periostin could represent a potential therapeutic target to control the growth of osteosarcoma and other bone tumours.

Conclusions

In keeping with its known role in modulating the synthesis of collagen and other extracellular matrix proteins in bone, strong periostin expression was noted in benign and malignant lesions forming an osteoid or osteoid-like matrix. Periostin was also noted in other bone tumours and was found in areas of reactive bone and increased vascularity at the edge of growing tumours, consistent with its involvement in tissue remodelling and angiogenesis associated with tumour progression.

Abbreviations

ABC: aneurysmal bone cyst; BMP-1: bone morphogenetic protein-1; ECM: extracellular matrix; ELISA: enzyme linked immunosorbent assay; GCTB: giant cell tumour of bone; OA: osteoarthritis; RA: rheumatoid arthritis; RANKL: receptor activator of nuclear factor kappa-B ligand; RUNX2: Runt-related transcription factor 2; SF: synovial Fluid; VEGF: vascular endothelial growth factor.

Authors' contributions

AK, AS, JMB, OU and NAA were the major contributors in writing the manuscript. NAA made the final editing of the manuscript. JMB, AM, ABH assisted in carrying out of the study, the data collection and the preparation of the manuscript. All authors read and approved the final manuscript.

Author details

[1] Nuffield Department of Orthopaedics, Rheumatology and Musculoskeletal and Sciences, Nuffield Orthopaedic Centre, University of Oxford, Oxford OX3 7HE, UK. [2] Department of Biological Information, Tokyo Institute of Technology, Yokohama 226-8501, Japan.

Acknowledgements

We would like to thank Sarah Turton for typing the manuscript and David Mahoney and Takeshi Kashima for help with the ELISA studies.

Competing interests

The authors declare that they have no competing interests.

Funding

This study was supported by the Sasakawa Foundation and the European Union through funding of the EuroBoNet and EuroSarc consortiums. The funders played no role in the collection of data, interpretation of results or writing of the manuscript.

References

1. Takeshita S, Kikuno R, Tezuka K, Amann E. Osteoblast-specific factor 2: cloning of putative bone adhesion protein with homology with the insect protein fasciclin I. Biochem J. 1993;294:271–8.
2. Horiuchi K, Amizuka N, Takeshita S, et al. Identification and characterization of a novel protein, periostin, with restricted expression to periosteum and periodontal ligament and increased expression by transforming growth factor beta. J Bone Miner Res. 1999;14:1239–49.
3. Kudo A. Periostin in fibrillogenesis for tissue regeneration: periostin actions inside and outside the cell. Cell Mol Life Sci. 2011;68:3201–7.
4. Merle B, Garnero P. The multiple facets of periostin in bone metabolism. Osteoporos Int. 2012;23:1199–212.
5. Cobo T, Voloria CG, Solares L, Fontanil T, Gonzales-Chanorro E, De Carlos F, Cobo JM, Cal S, Obaya AJ. Role of periostin in adhesion and migration of bone remodelling cells. PLoS ONE. 2016;11:e0147837.
6. Conway SJ, Izuhara K, Kudo Y, Litvin J, Markwald R, Ouyang G, Arron JR, Holeweg CT, Kudo A. The role of periostin in tissue remodelling across health and disease. Cell Mol Life Sci. 2014;71:1279–88.
7. Shimazaki M, Nakamura K, Kii I, et al. Periostin is essential for cardiac healing after acute myocardial infarction. J Exp Med. 2008;205:295–303.
8. Kasperkovitz PV, Timmer TC, Smeets TJ, et al. Fibroblast-like synoviocytes derived from patients with rheumatoid arthritis show the imprint of synovial tissue heterogeneity: evidence of a link between an increased myofibroblast-like phenotype and high-inflammation synovitis. Arthritis Rheum. 2005;52:430–41.
9. Geyer M, Grassel S, Straub RH, et al. Differential transcriptome analysis of intra-articular lesional vs intact cartilage reveals new candidate genes in osteoarthritis pathophysiology. Osteoarthritis Cartilage. 2009;17:328–35.
10. You S, Yoo SA, Choi S, et al. Identification of key regulators for the migration and invasion of rheumatoid synoviocytes through a systems approach. Proc Natl Acad Sci USA. 2014;111(550–555):11.
11. Ye D, Shen ZS, Qiu SJ, Li Q, Wang GL. Role and underlying mechanisms of the interstitial protein periostin in the diagnosis and treatment of malignant tumours. Oncol Lett. 2017;14:5099–106.
12. Ratajczak-Wielgomas K, Dziegiel P. The role of periostin in neoplatic processes. Folia hitiochem Cytobiol. 2015;53:120–32.
13. Kashima TG, Nishiyama T, Shimazu K, et al. Periostin, a novel marker of intramembranous ossification, is expressed in fibrous dysplasia and in c-Fos-overexpressing bone lesions. Hum Pathol. 2009;40:226–37.
14. Hu F, Wang W, Zhou HC, Shang XF. High expression of periostin is dramatically associated with metastatic potential and poor prognosis of patients with osteosarcoma. World J Surg Oncol. 2014;12:287.
15. Hu F, Shang XF, Wang W, Jiang W, Fang C, Tan D, Zhou HC. High expression of periostin is significantly correlated with tumour angiogenesis and poor prognosis in osteosarcoma. Int J Exp Pathol. 2016;97(1):86–92.
16. Fletcher CDM, Bridge JA, Hogendoorn PCW, Mertens F, editors. WHO classification of tumours of soft tissue and bone. 4th ed. IARC: Lyon; 2013.
17. Kikuchi Y, Kashima TG, Nishiyama T, et al. Periostin is expressed in pericryptal fibroblasts and cancer-associated fibroblasts in the colon. J Histochem Cytochem. 2008;56:753–64.
18. Maruhasi T, Kii I, Saito M, Kudo A. Interaction between periostin and BMP-1 promotes proteolytic activation of lysl oxidase. J Biol Chem. 2010;285:13294–303.
19. Kii I, Nishiyama T, Li M, Matumoto K, Saito M, Amizuka N, Kudo A. Incorporation of tenascin-C into the extracellular matrix by periostin underlies an extracellular meshwork architecture. J Biol Chem. 2010;285:2028–39.
20. Bonnet N, Standley KN, Bianchi EN, Stadelmann V, Foti M, Conway SJ, Ferrari SL. The matricellular protein periostin is required for sost inhibition and the anabolic response to mechanical loading and physical activity. J Biol Chem. 2009;284:35939–50.
21. Athanasou NA, Bansai M, Forsyth R, Reid RP, Sapi Z. Giant cell tumour of bone. In: Fletcher CDM, Bridge JA, Hogendoorn PCW, Mertens F, editors. WHO classification of tumours of soft tissue and bone. 4th ed. Lyon: IARC; 2013. p. 321–4.

22. Lai X, Chen S. Identification of novel biomarker candidates for immuno-histochemical diagnosis to distinguish low-grade chondrosarcoma from enchondroma. Proteomics. 2015;15:2358–68.
23. Mirra JM. Bone tumors: clinical radiological and pathological correlation. Philadelphia: Lee and Febiger; 1989.
24. Kashima TG, Dongre A, Oppermann U, Athanasou NA. Dentine matrix protein (DMP-1) is a marker of bone-forming tumours. Virchows Arch. 2013;462(5):583–91.
25. Inagaki Y, Hookway ES, Kashima TG, Munemoto M, Tanaka Y, Hassan AB, Oppermann U, Athanasou NA. Sclerostin expression in bone tumours and tumour-like lesion. Histopathology. 2016;69:470–8.
26. Izuhara K, Nunomura S, Nanri Y, Ono J, Mitamura Y, Yoshihara T. Periostin in inflammation and allergy. Cell Mol Life Sci. 2017;74:4293–303.
27. Puglisi F, Puppin C, Pegolo E, Andreetta C, Pascoletti G, D'Aurizio F, Pandolfi M, Fasola G, Piga A, Damamte G, Di Loreto C. Expression of periostin in human breast cancer. J Clin Pathol. 2008;61:494–8.
28. Oh H, Bae JM, Wen XY, Chon Y, Kin JJ, Kang GH. Overexpression of periostin in tumour stroma is a poor prognostic indicator of colorectal cancer. J Pathol Trans Med. 2017;51:306–13.
29. Shao R, Bao S, Bai X, Blanchette C, Anderson RM, Dang T, Gishizky ML, Marks JR, Wang XF. Aquired expression of periostin by human breast cancer angiogenesis through up-regulation of vascular endothelial growth factor receptor 2 expression. Mol Cell Biol. 2004;24:3992–4003.
30. Fukushima N, Kikuchi Y, Nishiyama T, et al. Periostin deposition in the stroma of invasive and intraductal neoplasms of the pancreas. Mod Pathol. 2008;21:1044–53.
31. Kikuchi Y, Kunita A, Iwata C, et al. The niche component periostin is produced by cancer-associated fibroblasts, supporting the growth of gastric cancer through ERK activation. Am J Pathol. 2014;184:859–70.
32. Tilman G, Mattiussi M, Brasseur F, van Baren N, Decottignies A. Human periostin gene expression in normal tissues, tumours and melanoma: evidence for periostin production by both stromal and melanoma cells. Mol Cancer. 2007;17(6):80.
33. Gillian L, Matei D, Fisherman DA, Gerbin CS, Karlan BY, Chang DD. Periostin secreted by epithelial ovarian carcinoma is a ligand for alpha (V) beta (3) and alpha (V) beta (5) integrins and promotes cell motility. Cancer Res. 2002;62:5358–64.
34. Litvin J, Chen X, Keleman S, Zhu S, Autleri M. Expression and function of periostin-like factor in vascular smooth muscle cells. Am J Physiol Cell Physiol. 2007;292:C1672–80.
35. Kim BR, Kwon YW, Park GT, Choi EJ, Seo JK, Jang IH, Kim SC, Ko HC, Lee SC, Kim JH. Identification of a novel angiogenic peptide from periostin. PLoS ONE. 2017;12(11):e0187464.
36. Lu YI, Wang W, Jia WD, et al. High-level expression of periostin is closely related to metastatic potential and poor prognosis of hepatocellular carcinoma. Med Oncol. 2013;30:385.
37. Lindner V, Wang Q, Conley BA, Friesel RE, Vary CP. Vascular injury induces expression of periostin: implications for vascular cell differentiation and migration. Arterioscler Thromb Vasc Biol. 2005;25:77–83.
38. Kudo Y, Ogawa I, Kitajima S, et al. Periostin, a stroma-associated protein, correlates with tumour invasiveness and progression in nasopharyngeal carcinoma. Clin Exp Metastasis. 2012;29:865–77.
39. Contie S, Voorzanger-Rousselot N, Litvin J, Clezardin P, Garnero P. Increased expression and serum levels of the stromal cell protein periostin in breast cancer bone metastasis. Int J Cancer. 2011;128:352–60.
40. Bao S, Ouyang G, Bai X, et al. Perisotin potently promotes metastatic growth of colon cancer by augmenting cell survival via the AkT/PKB pathway. Cancer Cell. 2004;5:329–539.
41. Liu C, Huang SJ, Qin ZL. Inhibition of periostin gene expression via RNA suppressed the proliferation, apoptosis and invasion in U2OS cells. Chin Med J. 2010;123:3677–83.

24

Retrospective audit of 957 consecutive ¹⁸F-FDG PET–CT scans compared to CT and MRI in 493 patients with different histological subtypes of bone and soft tissue sarcoma

Ruth E. Macpherson[1,2], Sarah Pratap[1,3], Helen Tyrrell[3], Mehrdad Khonsari[2], Shaun Wilson[1,5], Max Gibbons[1,4], Duncan Whitwell[1,4], Henk Giele[1,4], Paul Critchley[1,4], Lucy Cogswell[1,4], Sally Trent[1,3], Nick Athanasou[1,4,6], Kevin M. Bradley[1,2] and A. Bassim Hassan[1,3,6]*

Abstract

Background: The use of ¹⁸F-FDG PET–CT (PET–CT) is widespread in many cancer types compared to sarcoma. We report a large retrospective audit of PET–CT in bone and soft tissue sarcoma with varied grade in a single multi-disciplinary centre. We also sought to answer three questions. Firstly, the correlation between sarcoma sub-type and grade with ¹⁸FDG SUVmax, secondly, the practical uses of PET–CT in the clinical setting of staging (during initial diagnosis), restaging (new baseline prior to definitive intervention) and treatment response. Finally, we also attempted to evaluate the potential additional benefit of PET–CT over concurrent conventional CT and MRI.

Methods: A total of 957 consecutive PET–CT scans were performed in a single supra-regional centre in 493 sarcoma patients (excluding GIST) between 2007 and 2014. We compared, PET–CT SUVmax values in relation to histology and FNCCC grading. We compared PET–CT findings relative to concurrent conventional imaging (MRI and CT) in staging, restaging and treatment responses.

Results: High-grade (II/III) bone and soft tissue sarcoma correlated with high SUVmax, especially undifferentiated pleomorphic sarcoma, leiomyosarcoma, translocation induced sarcomas (Ewing, synovial, alveolar rhabdomyosarcoma), de-differentiated liposarcoma and osteosarcoma. Lower SUVmax values were observed in sarcomas of low histological grade (grade I), and in rare subtypes of intermediate grade soft tissue sarcoma (e.g. alveolar soft part sarcoma and solitary fibrous tumour). SUVmax variation was noted in malignant peripheral nerve sheath tumours, compared to the histologically benign plexiform neurofibroma, whereas PET–CT could clearly differentiate low from high-grade chondrosarcoma. We identified added utility of PET–CT in addition to MRI and CT in high-grade sarcoma of bone and soft tissues. An estimated 21% overall potential benefit was observed for PET–CT over CT/MRI, and in particular, in 'upstaging' of high-grade disease (from M0 to M1) where an additional 12% of cases were deemed M1 following PET–CT.

Conclusions: PET–CT in high-grade bone and soft tissue sarcoma can add significant benefit to routine CT/MRI staging. Further prospective and multi-centre evaluation of PET–CT is warranted to determine the actual predictive value

*Correspondence: bass.hassan@path.ox.ac.uk
[6] NIHR Musculoskeletal Biomedical Research Unit (Sarcoma Theme), Sarcoma and TYA Unit of the NHS Oncology Department, and Sir William Dunn School of Pathology, University of Oxford, South Parks Road, Oxford OX1 3RE, UK
Full list of author information is available at the end of the article

and cost-effectiveness of PET–CT in directing clinical management of clinically complex and heterogeneous high-grade sarcomas.

Keywords: Sarcoma, Positron emission tomography, Multi-disciplinary, Staging, Therapeutic response

Background

Conventional cross-sectional imaging techniques are routinely applied to the diagnostic and staging imaging of bone and soft tissue sarcomas, e.g. CT and MRI [1–3]. Diagnostic review of biopsies and staging scans in supra-regional multi-disciplinary teams (MDT), aims to inform clinical management in line with national and international sarcoma guidelines. MRI is also generally performed to guide local staging and restaging following neo-adjuvant therapy, whereas in subsequent post-treatment follow-up, high resolution CT is primarily used for the detection of distant metastases, particularly in the lung. As primary curative treatment for sarcoma is mostly surgical, accurate staging is essential in order to minimize inappropriate interventions in the presence of metastatic disease.

Combined ^{18}F-FDG Positron Emission Tomography with CT (PET–CT) offers potential advantages with respect to sarcoma, as it provides both metabolic and anatomical imaging combined in a single examination. Sarcomas are frequently large tumours (>5 cm) with intra-tumour regional and cellular heterogeneity, and frequently in larger tumours, central necrosis associated with hypoxia. As mesenchymal derived cancers, sarcomas may be detected by ^{18}FDG uptake because of the general high metabolic activity and insulin sensitivity of these tissues. The maximum standardized uptake value (SUVmax) of ^{18}FDG into higher-grade sarcoma appears to correlate with mitotic count and grade in some reported series [4, 5], and potentially with overall prognosis [6–10]. Reporting response assessment to oncological therapies using SUVmax before and after treatment, may also better correlate with histological response compared to dimensions alone [11]. With the advent of new systemic therapies that are either cytostatic or immune-modulatory, PET–CT has additional potential advantages in assessing responses depending on the therapeutic mechanism.

Despite these potential advantages, there have been relatively few reported series, with low cases numbers, providing information on which to base the routine application of functional PET–CT in specialist sarcoma clinical practice [12–20]. Moreover, in rare (<6 per 100,000 population) sarcoma subtypes (approximately 80 different molecular based diagnostic subtypes in the WHO classification 2013), there appears even less 'real world' reported evidence for the application of PET–CT. Here,

we retrospectively audit consecutively performed PET–CT scans in a supra-regional sarcoma centre. We initially attempted to address three questions; the correlation between histological sub-type and grade with ^{18}FDG uptake; the use of PET–CT in the clinical setting of staging (during initial diagnosis), restaging (new baseline prior to definitive intervention) and treatment response, and the potential additional benefit obtained from PET–CT over concurrent conventional CT and MRI imaging in these settings.

Methods

Patient database

Retrospective audit of consecutive ^{18}FDG PET–CT scans from one supra-regional UK sarcoma centre (Multi-disciplinary team, Oxford Sarcoma Service, Oxford University Hospitals Foundation Trust, UK) occurred between 1st February 2007 and 25th June 2014. The radiology search for scans was independently cross-referenced with the Oxford Sarcoma Service (OxSarc) sarcoma database (2006–2014) for diagnosis and outcome, to ensure that patients had been captured on both systems. The histological subtype and grade of each sarcoma was confirmed by pathology review and accessed via the local EPR system. Grade I sarcoma were regarded as low-grade, and grade II and III sarcoma as high-grade. All imaging (MRI, CT and PET–CT) were performed as directed either by the MDT, or were performed just prior to referral by an external clinician, with the information obtained used for consensus MDT agreement for subsequent clinical management. Thus, all scans performed and reported here were approved by the MDT specialist sarcoma team, and were therefore driven either as a result of the initial histology result of the biopsy, or appearances of local imaging of the presenting mass etc.

Imaging procedures

PET–CT imaging from June 2007 to 2nd November 2009 was performed on a GE Discovery (STE BGO 16 slice CT, 400 MBq ^{18}FDG, 60 min uptake period, fixed 80 mA/140 kV for CT, 4 min per bed position) and from 3rd November 2009, on a GE Discovery 690 (LYSO time of flight) 64 slice CT, 4 MBq/kg ^{18}FDG, 90 min uptake period, modulated mA based on noise index (n=25) 120 kV, 4 min per bed position). All scans included the skull base to either the upper thigh, or at least the joint below primary disease in the lower limbs where required, and included the head in skull or head and neck disease. Patients were fasted with a standard procedure for at least 6 h prior to the PET–CT. All the PET–CT examinations were independently reported by two consultant radiologists subspecializing in nuclear medicine and PET–CT, and were re-reviewed by a post CCT radiologist subspecializing in nuclear medicine/PET (RM) as part of this evaluation alongside the verified reports.

For the purpose of assessing the correlation between sarcoma grade and disease avidity, the FDG avidity calculated as standardized uptake value (SUVmax) on each PET–CT was recorded. SUVmax is simply the decay corrected maximum tracer activity (^{18}FDG) within a volume of interest (VOI) and is available on all PET–CT scans. The standardized uptake value is (SUV) = [VOI activity concentration]/[injected activity/Weight g/mL], and if 1 mL of tissue volume is taken to weigh 1 g, then it becomes unit-less. The most FDG avid focus site of disease, whether primary or metastatic, was utilized as the SUVmax. In those cases where the SUVmax was not documented, this was re-calculated using standard GE supplied PET–CT analysis software. If there was CT evidence of a disease site however, with the FDG uptake at or below background (mediastinal blood pool) levels i.e. sites that are FDG essentially negative, the FDG avidity was documented as equal to 1.

Imaging evaluation

All ^{18}FDG PET–CT and conventional imaging modalities (CT and MRI) were re-analyzed with respect to sarcoma diagnostic sub-type, the timing and purpose of the scan with respect to staging, restaging or treatment response. The differences in sarcoma disease distribution between the ^{18}FDG PET–CT and conventional MRI/CT scans were documented if scans were performed within 4 weeks of each other, otherwise any differences were not reported for the purpose of this evaluation. Not all patients had all types of scan within 4 weeks of each other, and so comparisons are necessarily retrospective and cannot be formally evaluated beyond descriptive reporting. For bone and pulmonary metastatic sites that were identified by PET–CT, the non-contrast enhanced CT components of the scan were examined separately and considered as the 'conventional' CT imaging modality. For soft tissue sites, including abdominal and pelvic sites, comparisons were made between ^{18}FDG PET–CT and either separate contrast enhanced CT scans or MRI scans where possible. The specific ^{18}FDG PET–CT advantages over conventional imaging were also determined for occult and solitary disease in either visceral, bone, muscular, sub-cutaneous and nodal sites. Histopathology was undertaken using standard diagnostic pathway with UK sarcoma reference pathologist (NA), using

conventional WHO international guidelines (2012) and French based staging system (FNCCC). For the assessment of additional potential advantages of PET–CT, this was only conferred once histological data was reviewed to determine whether 'PET positive' disease had been histologically proven, or, if sampling had not been undertaken, where there was imaging evidence of progression over time confirming the presence of malignant disease, except for the common incidental unrelated sites in the colon, thyroid, prostate and breast.

Statistical analysis

Descriptive statistics using Prism 7.0a were applied, including ANOVA and non-parametric Mann–Whitney tests. Sensitivity, specificity, positive predictive value and negative predictive values were calculated by standard means.

Results

Over the 7-year period of the audit evaluation, a total of 493 patients (age range 15–91, median 55 years) referred to the Oxford MDT with histologically confirmed sarcoma, underwent a total of 957 PET–CT scans during their course of management. The number of patients within sarcoma sub-types, the number of PET–CT studies performed and the clinical indications for performing PET–CT are shown (Table 1, Fig. 1). Most PET–CT scans were performed in high-grade (n = 930) versus low-grade sarcoma (n = 27, e.g. low grade chondrosarcoma and low grade soft tissue sarcoma), with a wide distribution of histological subtypes that reflect the distribution of referred cases (shown are where there were > 4 cases per histological subtype, Fig. 1). PET–CT scans were usually performed as a result of MDT decisions, usually in the context of patients that were being planned to undergo radical treatments, such as radical surgery, and where the scan was for initial staging and exclusion of metastatic disease (36% of scans). All of these cases had concurrent MRI and CT imaging already, mainly for local staging and exclusion of lung metastasis. In this staging population, a further 12% (42/344) then had detectable metastatic disease overall by PET–CT that was not detected by conventional CT/MRI. Re-staging with a new baseline scan occurred in cases with suspected later relapse, prior to potential further radical and salvage treatment (39% of scans), and assessment of treatment response to therapeutics in the remaining (35% of scans, see Table 1).

A statistically significant difference was observed between mean SUVmax of high and of low-grade sarcoma independent of histological subtype (p value < 0.0001, Fig. 2). Most high-grade sarcomas had mean SUVmax values greater than 10, with wide distribution of SUVmax activity rather than a defined cut-off,

Table 1 Number of patients, PET–CTs and indication for PET–CTs according to sarcoma subtype

Sarcoma pathological diagnosis	Number of patients	Number of PET–CT scans			
		Total	Staging[a] (with metastasis)	Restaging	Treatment response
Undifferentiated pleomorphic[b]	81	166	64 (6)	62	40
Angiosarcoma[c]	8	11	7 (1)	3	1
Leiomyosarcoma	89	166	43 (8)	84	39
Rhabdomyosarcoma	16	53	13 (4)	15	25
Myxofibrosarcoma	21	30	14 (2)	8	8
Epithelioid sarcoma	10	23	7 (1)	15	1
Osteosarcoma	48	98	39 (7)	28	31
Clear cell sarcoma	6	8	5 (1)	3	0
Ewing sarcoma/DSRCT	31	120	20 (6)	47	53
Synovial sarcoma	26	44	17 (3)	24	3
De-differentiated liposarcoma	18	36	11 (1)	17	8
Solitary fibrous tumour	14	25	8 (1)	9	8
Chondrosarcoma grade 2/3	24	45	18 (1)	17	10
Myxoid/round cell liposarcoma	26	36	18 (4)	12	6
Alveolar soft part sarcoma	4	4	4 (1)	0	0
MPNST	37	65	33 (4)	21	11
Low grade soft tissue sarcoma	25	17	17 (0)	0	0
Chondrosarcoma grade 1	9	10	6 (0)	4	0
Total	493	957	344 (51)	369	244

DSRCT desmoplastic small round cell sarcoma, *MPNST* malignant peripheral nerve sheath tumour, includes low-grade

[a] Note this is overall detection of metastatic disease at initial CT and MRI staging only, 'added value' comparison is reported in Table 3

[b] Includes high grade 'spindle cell sarcoma'

[c] Includes 'high grade epitheloid haemangioendothelioma'

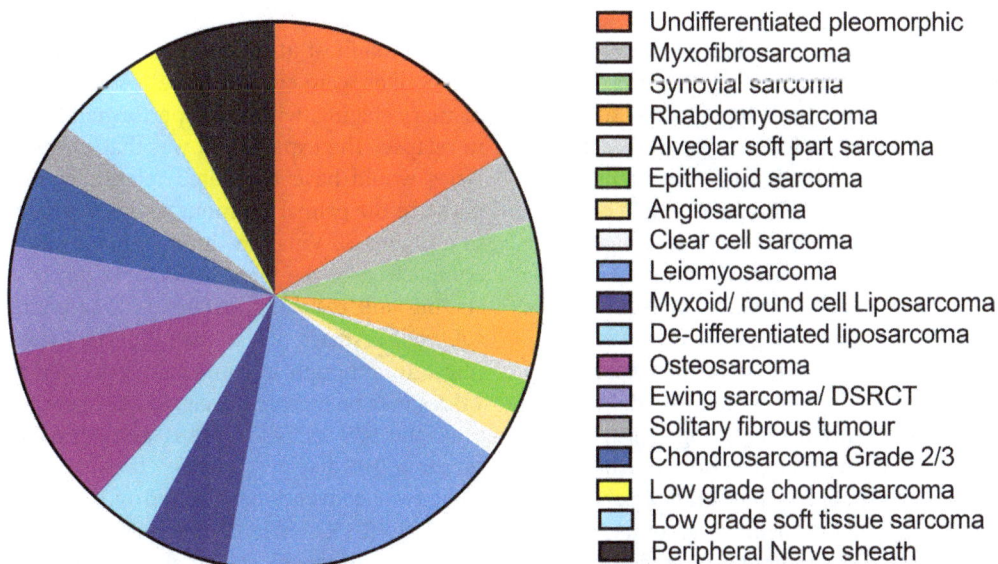

Fig. 1 Distribution of molecular-histological subtypes of the 493 sarcoma cases reported that underwent a ^{18}F-FDG PET–CT between 2007 and 2014. Following diagnostic biopsy (core needle or excision biopsy), the molecular and histological subtypes of sarcoma were identified. A total of 493 cases of sarcoma were diagnosed and were distributed into the following listed sub-types (minimum 4 cases per subtype, pie chart runs clockwise)

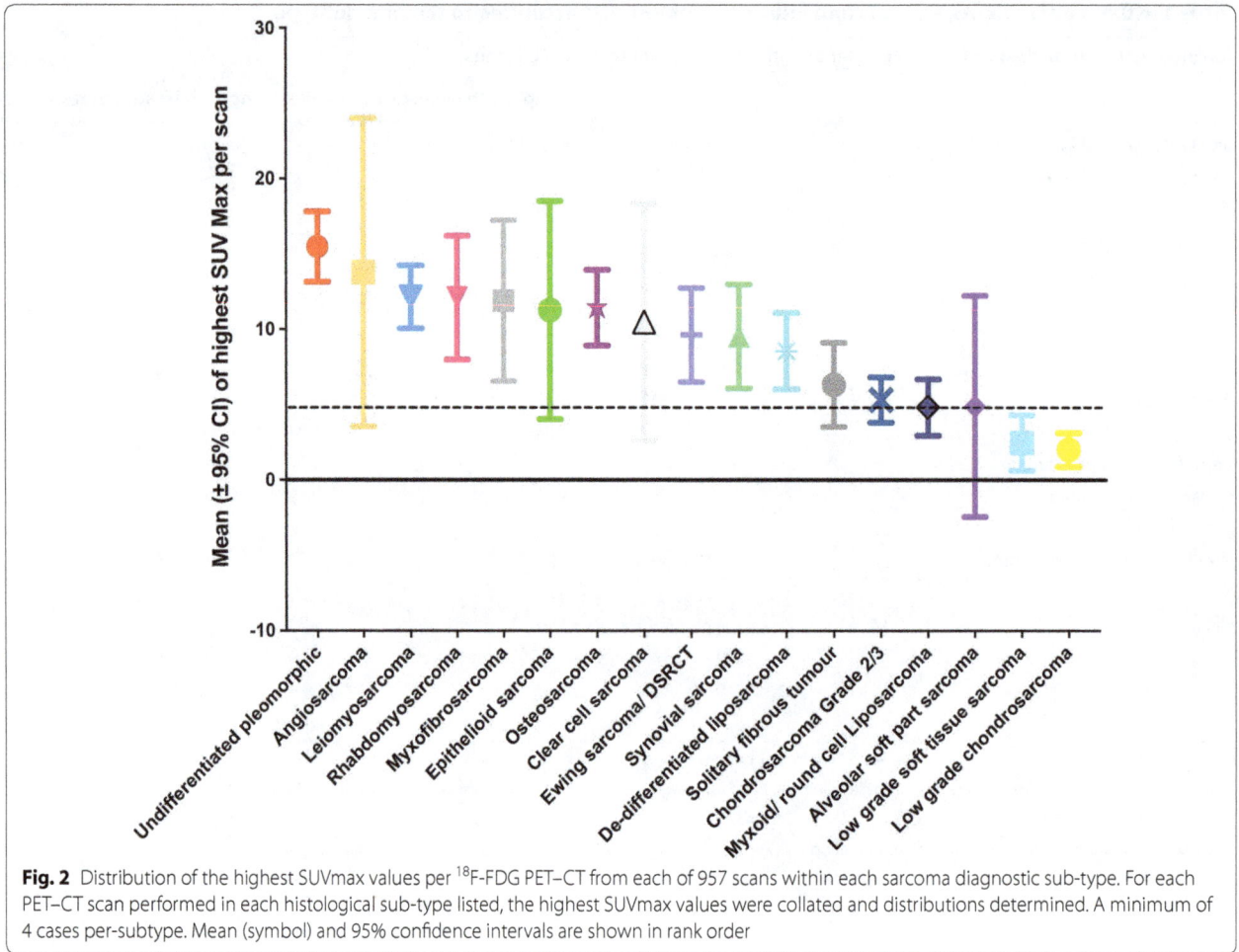

Fig. 2 Distribution of the highest SUVmax values per ^{18}F-FDG PET–CT from each of 957 scans within each sarcoma diagnostic sub-type. For each PET–CT scan performed in each histological sub-type listed, the highest SUVmax values were collated and distributions determined. A minimum of 4 cases per-subtype. Mean (symbol) and 95% confidence intervals are shown in rank order

making the distinction within grade and between histological subtypes more subtle (Fig. 2). Importantly, between the specific low and high-grade subtypes, there appeared significant differences in SUVmax that presumably reflects the differential mechanisms of cellular derangement (Fig. 3a). For the example of chondrosarcoma, the differences between low and high-grade defined histologically also appeared to threshold at the SUVmax value of 4 (Fig. 3b), whereas in MPNST, the spectrum of SUVmax values significantly overlapped depending on the histological classification, making any distinction of grade based on SUVmax less discriminative and less correlative with histology (Fig. 3c). A further factor in relation to SUVmax distribution and histology also includes the anatomical origin of otherwise indentical histologies, exemplified by leiomyosarcoma, with an apparent higher SUVmax observed in gynaecological compared to non-gynaecological (vascular) origin leiomyosarcoma (Fig. 3d).

As a result of intra-tumoural heterogeneity, differences in SUVmax between sarcoma sites within each patient

may be manifest at different stages of the disease. SUVmax values were compared between scans performed at primary staging, with those performed later in follow-up in relapse. The expectation was that more aggressive cell types would have populated relapse disease sites compared to the primary tumour, and potentially be reflected in a higher SUVmax in those relapsed sites. Subsequent comparison of the highest SUVmax per scan at primary staging and restaging, grouped by sarcoma histological subtype, revealed no statistically significant differences (Figs. 4), although in some subtypes, trends in SUVmax values may be increasing, e.g. in leiomyosarcoma.

Of the 930 PET–CT scans performed in high-grade sarcoma, 193 displayed features considered to have added value over conventional CT and/or MRI performed concurrently (21%, Table 2). Of these 193 PET–CT scans, 56 were performed at initial sarcoma diagnostic staging, 78 at re-staging (new baselines) and 59 in treatment (chemotherapy) responses (Table 2). Here, 'added value' refers to any additional specific features offered by PET–CT. Specifically, added value does not only relate to the

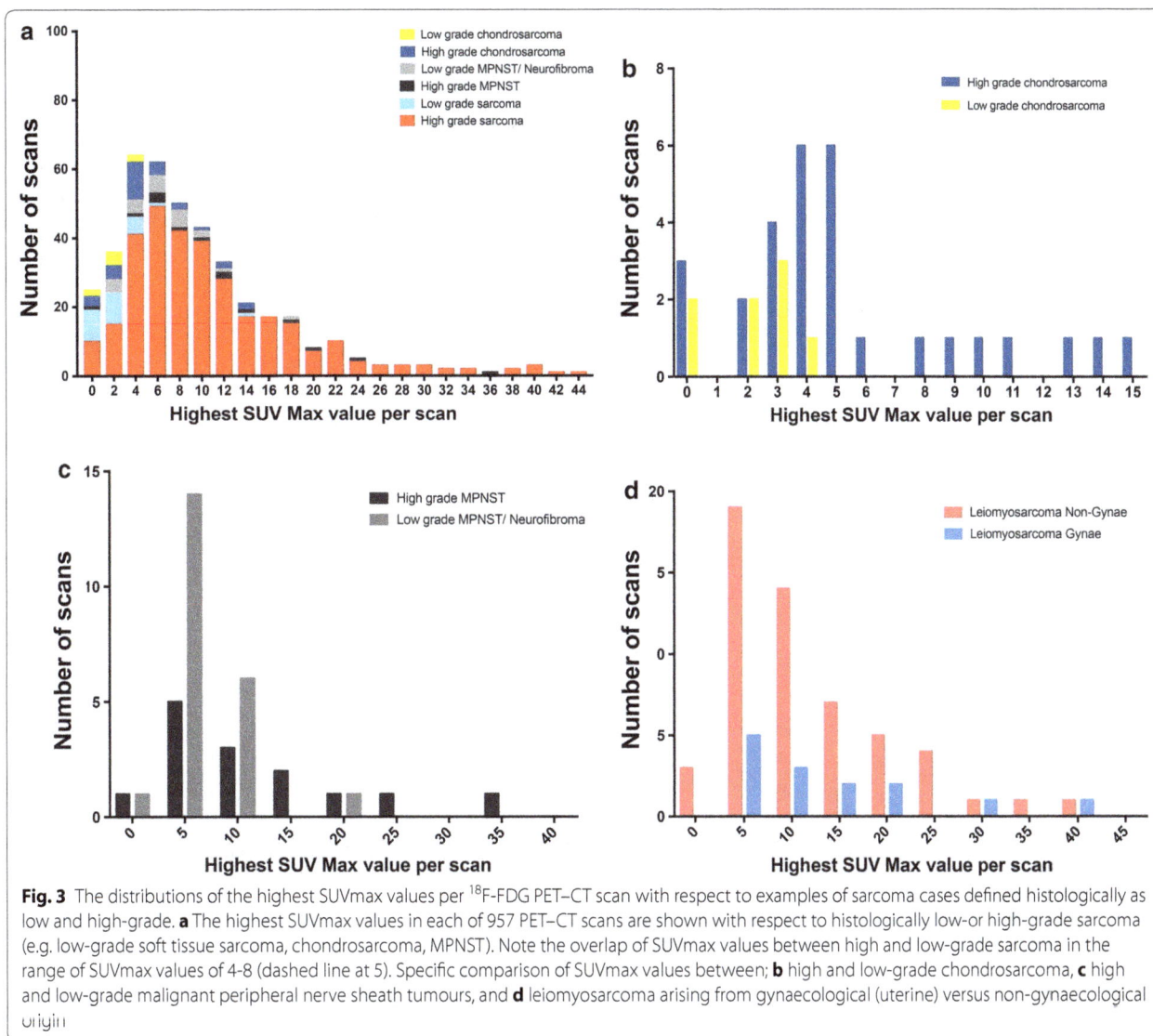

Fig. 3 The distributions of the highest SUVmax values per ^{18}F-FDG PET–CT scan with respect to examples of sarcoma cases defined histologically as low and high-grade. **a** The highest SUVmax values in each of 957 PET–CT scans are shown with respect to histologically low-or high-grade sarcoma (e.g. low-grade soft tissue sarcoma, chondrosarcoma, MPNST). Note the overlap of SUVmax values between high and low-grade sarcoma in the range of SUVmax values of 4-8 (dashed line at 5). Specific comparison of SUVmax values between; **b** high and low-grade chondrosarcoma, **c** high and low-grade malignant peripheral nerve sheath tumours, and **d** leiomyosarcoma arising from gynaecological (uterine) versus non-gynaecological origin

identification of further metastatic disease sites in addition to those already identified by the conventional CT and MRI imaging, but to those features resulting in so-called 'upstaging' of disease. For example, PET–CT specific detection of either occult muscular and soft tissue metastases, small peritoneal or other visceral metastases not visualized by conventional non-contrast enhanced CT (as part of PET–CT) and MRI imaging (Table 3, see examples in Fig. 5). Thus, 'added value' of PET–CT reflects detection of metastatic disease (M1) in patients who would be otherwise staged as M0 by conventional imaging approaches. In patients with high-grade sarcoma, it was possible to compare a total of 284 PET–CT scans with the conventional CT and MRI specifically during the initial diagnostic staging. In terms of the presence or absence of metastatic disease (M0 versus M1),

of these, 232 patients were true negatives for metastatic disease (negative in both PET–CT and the conventional imaging), 24 were true positive (positive in both PET–CT and the conventional imaging), 23 were false negatives (positively identified disease in PET–CT) and 1 was a false positive (non-disease associated FDG uptake). This retrospective data results in an overall metastatic disease rate of 10% based on conventional CT and MRI, and 22% for detection with dual modality PET–CT. As both CT and PET should both be able to detect the predominant sites of pulmonary metastatic disease, this additional benefit might be expected to be mainly because of detection of non-pulmonary metastatic disease sites. Following scrutiny of these staging PET–CTs, 'added value' was indeed associated with detection of occult metastatic sites in bone, muscle and visceral sites, accounting for the

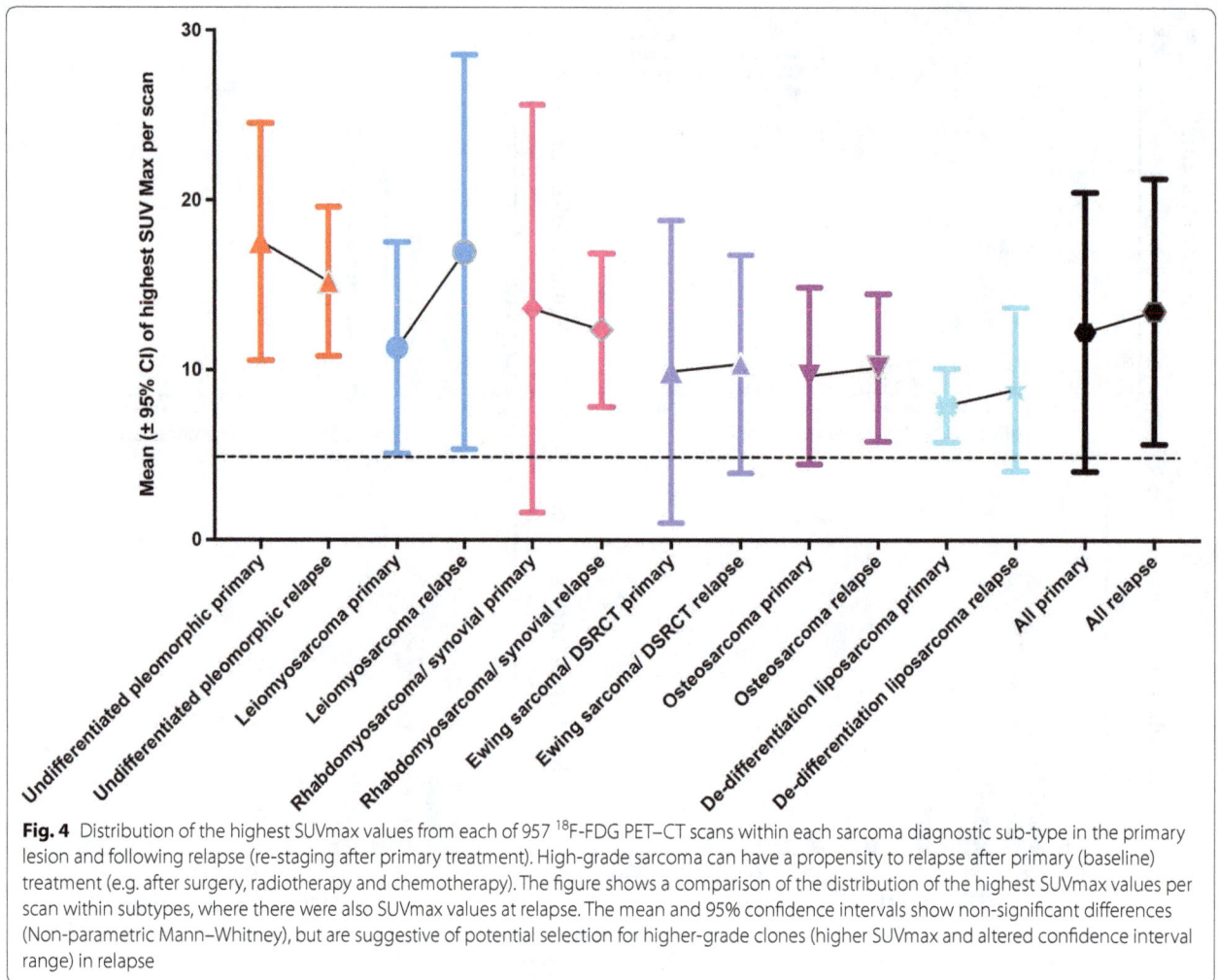

Fig. 4 Distribution of the highest SUVmax values from each of 957 ^{18}F-FDG PET–CT scans within each sarcoma diagnostic sub-type in the primary lesion and following relapse (re-staging after primary treatment). High-grade sarcoma can have a propensity to relapse after primary (baseline) treatment (e.g. after surgery, radiotherapy and chemotherapy). The figure shows a comparison of the distribution of the highest SUVmax values per scan within subtypes, where there were also SUVmax values at relapse. The mean and 95% confidence intervals show non-significant differences (Non-parametric Mann–Whitney), but are suggestive of potential selection for higher-grade clones (higher SUVmax and altered confidence interval range) in relapse

PET–CT upstaging (Table 3). Overall, given the prevalence of sarcoma sub-types in this bone and soft tissue sarcoma series, and compared to conventional MRI/CT, PET–CT appeared to have a greater sensitivity (96% vs 54%), positive predictive value (96%) and negative predictive value (99%), even though these sensitivity and specificity values were not prospectively evaluated.

Moreover, 'added value' also relates to altered FDG avidity in static sized lesions, either indicating increased SUVmax suggesting disease presence or progression, and decreased SUVmax, as a reflection of responses to oncological treatment. In this context, PET–CT specifically might have 'added value' in the characterization of enlarged FDG negative loco-regional lymph nodes that are likely reactive rather than sarcoma containing, and in the detection of FDG avid lesions near prostheses following reconstructive surgery, where MRI and CT artifacts preclude accurate assessment (Table 3). These findings

overall are therefore relevant both to achieving accurate TNM staging, but also to directly influence clinical decision-making for subsequent radical surgical, radiotherapy and chemotherapy interventions.

In terms of histological sub-types, the highest overall 'added value' appeared in the context of malignant peripheral nerve sheath tumour subtype of sarcoma (41.6%), whereas in most cases of myxofibrosarcoma and solitary fibrous tumour, the advantages of PET–CT were manifest during follow-up re-staging and treatment response assessment (Table 2). For chemo-sensitive sarcoma, 'added value' was skewed towards the chemotherapy treatment response assessment scans (e.g. in chemotherapy responsive rhabdomyosarcoma and Ewing sarcoma), and following trabectedin chemotherapy, such as in leiomyosarcoma (Table 2) [21]. For diagnostic staging and re-staging, significant 'added value' reasons also included identification of local recurrence sites at and

Fig. 5 Examples of ^{18}F-FDG PET and fused PET–CT images with added value detection of disease sites in sarcoma. All images are on an SUV scale of 0–6. **a** Case of a 57 year-old female with hilar lung metastatic leiomyosarcoma, but with occult metastatic sites (arrows; right buttock and left para-aortic region) not clearly evident on conventional CT scans. **b** Case of a 54 year-old female with undifferentiated pleomorphic sarcoma (UPS) with primary right axillary disease, but with an occult bone secondary in the pelvis (arrow) on PET–CT. **c** Case of a 23 year-old male with distal femur osteosarcoma post MAP chemotherapy (pre-op) and after reconstructive surgery and prosthetic replacement with a local recurrence (post-op). Arrow indicates FDG avid nodule of local recurrence close to the prosthetic margin not visible on CT

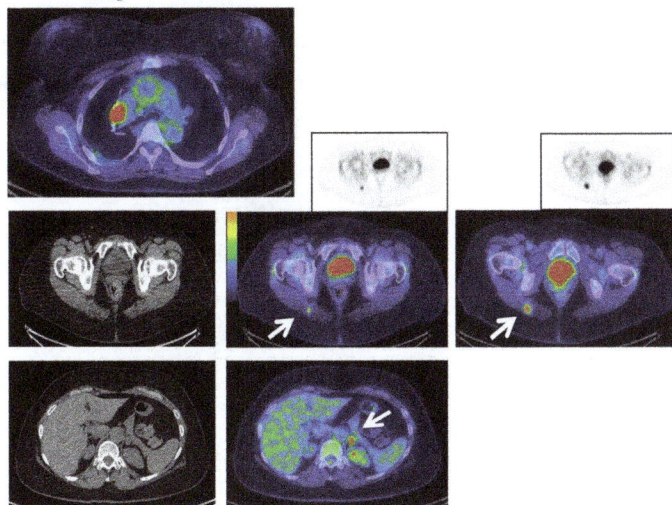

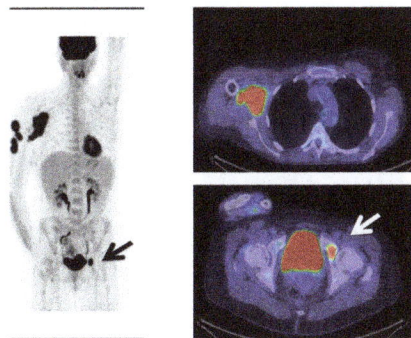

near prostheses (18/138), during the follow up of FDG positive lesions (17/138), for all lesions missed (not easily visible) by conventional imaging (16/138), for intralesional heterogeneity to guide diagnostic biopsies (16/138), and for occult (not previously visible) bone metastasis (13/138).

Discussion

Here we report a retrospective audit and evaluation of PET–CT clinical use in a single tertiary UK sarcoma center. The data represents one of the largest reported series of PET–CT use in routine sarcoma clinical practice, but this does not represent a definitive, prospective, clinical and cost effective evaluation. Despite these caveats, the use of PET–CT in this report does appear in line with evolving guidelines, including the most recent 2016

Royal College of Radiologists, UK guidelines for PET–CT in sarcoma [22]. As such, it provides valuable preliminary evidence on which to base future multi-center evaluation in a routine clinical practice, as a clinical research tool, and in the development of evidence suitable for supporting appropriate reimbursement.

In sarcoma, oncogenic drivers frequently result in up-regulation of glucose transporters, such as GLUT4 [23], resulting in higher ^{18}FDG SUVmax levels associated with aggressive cell behavior, and when there is associated immune cell infiltration, such as in giant cell tumour of bone [24]. As expected, we observed statistically significant differences of mean SUVmax between low-grade and high-grade sarcoma histological sub-types. Moreover, significant variation in SUVmax was observed between different patients who had the same sarcoma

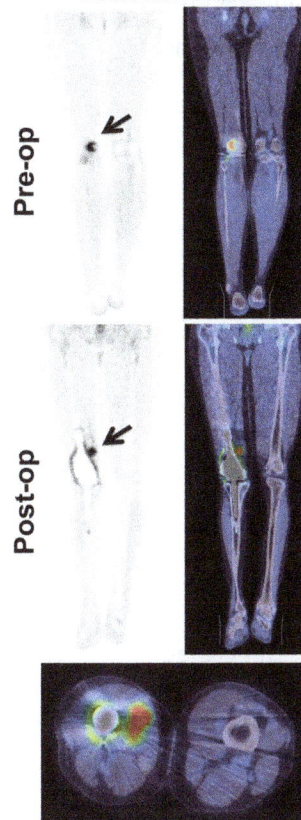

Table 2 Number of PET–CTs in which 'added value' was detected compared to conventional imaging (MRI/CT) according to sarcoma subtype

Sarcoma pathological diagnosis	Percentage of PET–CT with added value	Number of PET–CT with added value over MRI/CT		
		Staging	Restaging	Treatment response
Undifferentiated pleomorphic[a]	13.3% (22/166)	6	11	5
Angiosarcoma[b]	9% (1/11)	1	0	0
Leiomyosarcoma	18% (30/166)	7	14	9
Rhabdomyosarcoma	24.6% (13/53)	3	2	8
Myxofibrosarcoma	26.7% (8/30)	0	5	3
Epithelioid sarcoma	13% (3/23)	1	2	0
Osteosarcoma	23.5% (23/98)	6	9	8
Clear cell sarcoma	12.5% (1/8)	1	0	0
Ewing sarcoma/DSRCT	27.5% (33/120)	7	12	14
Synovial sarcoma	13.6% (6/44)	3	2	1
De-differentiated liposarcoma	8.3% (3/36)	1	1	1
Solitary fibrous tumour	28% (7/25)	0	5	2
Chondrosarcoma grade 2/3	24.4% (11/45)	3	5	3
Myxoid/round cell liposarcoma	11.1% (4/36)	2	1	1
Alveolar soft part sarcoma	25% (1/4)	1	0	0
MPNST	41.6% (27/65)	14	9	4
Low grade soft tissue sarcoma	0% (0/17)	0	0	0
Chondrosarcoma grade 1	0% (0/10)	0	0	0
Total	21% (193/930)	56	78	59

DSRCT desmoplastic small round cell sarcoma, *MPNST* malignant peripheral nerve sheath tumour, includes low-grade

[a] Includes high grade 'spindle cell sarcoma'

[b] Includes 'high grade epitheloid haemangioendothelioma'

sub-type. The latter probably reflects the functional heterogeneity within the tumour and its associated microenvironment, indicating that between sarcoma subtypes, primary and metastatic disease, there are differences in SUVmax that reflect those at the molecular, cellular and micro-environment level. PET–CT appeared useful in identifying sarcoma sites that contained both high and low- grade elements (the extremes of heterogeneity), for example in de-differentiated liposarcoma, de-differentiated chondrosarcoma and in MPNST. SUVmax values > 5 were consistent with higher-grade disease, except in the case of MPNST, where there was much less correlation of SUVmax with histological assessment of grade. Thus, low-grade soft tissue sarcoma and low-grade bone sarcoma (e.g. chondrosarcoma) do not probably warrant routine PET–CT estaging valuation, unless there is clinical suspicion of high-grade transformation, such as in either large axial or pelvic chondrosarcoma.

The additional benefits ("added value") of PET–CT appeared to be in a range of clinical contexts, making specific comparisons and overall evaluation more complex. Here we attempted to simply compare conventional CT and MRI scans performed concurrently with the PET–CT, in order to scope the scenarios that might

justify PET–CT as a routine dual scanning modality, and that impacts on potentially clinically important features. What we have not been able to fully assess in all circumstances, is to prospectively prove that direct and important changes to subsequent clinical management of patients ensued as a result of the PET–CT results, and the PET–CT results alone. For example, there can be no doubt from the radiological and clinical point of view, that the 'added value' of PET–CT in upstaging of disease from M0 to M1 would have had clinical impact that might make the difference between either reconstructing a limb, resecting a tumour or amputation. In this regard, our evidence suggests that whole body PET–CT has particular utility in detection of occult non-pulmonary disease not visible on conventional CT and MRI. As both CT and PET should both be able to detect the predominant sites of pulmonary metastatic disease, scrutiny of these staging PET–CTs for 'added value' was indeed associated with detection of occult metastatic sites in bone, muscle and visceral sites, accounting for the PET–CT upstaging. Moreover, 'added value' to guiding biopsies to active and viable areas of the tumour, thereby avoiding regions of necrosis, and in the post-operative setting, where MRI artifacts near metallic prostheses prevents

Table 3 Summary of the 'added value' features of PET–CT compared to conventional imaging (MRI and CT)

Reasons for added value of PET–CT over conventional imaging	Number of PET–CT scans per indication		
	Staging[b]	Restaging[a]	Treatment response
Occult bone metastases	10	3	1
Recurrence at local site or adjacent to metallic prosthesis not definitive on conventional imaging	0	18	2
Follow up of occult bone metastases	0	8	10
Occult muscular metastases	3	0	0
Follow up of occult muscular metastases	0	3	2
Cardiac metastases (muscular) not detected on conventional imaging	2	1	0
Subcentimetre FDG avid nodes	5	2	1
Static tumoural size, reduced FDG avidity	0	7	16
Static tumoural size, increased FDG avidity	6	2	6
Solitary FDG avid pulmonary nodule, indeterminate on CT	7	3	0
Missed visceral disease on CT/MRI	11	5	5
Metastasis outside the fields of conventional imaging	1	0	0
FDG negative suspected recurrence adjacent to prosthesis or locally in patient with prior markedly avid disease	0	3	2
Intra-lesional heterogeneity—guided biopsy to avoid underestimation of grade	10	6	0
Enlarged FDG negative nodes with moderately FDG avid primary	1	2	0
Increase in tumoural size but reduced avidity	0	0	7
Recurrence at an ablation or surgical site, indeterminate on MRI	0	2	0
Follow up of FDG positive disease adjacent to prosthesis or local surgical site	0	13	7
Total	56	78	59

[a] Restaging = new baseline imaging prior to new clinical management intervention

[b] Actual number of M0 to M1 upstaging = 25

adequate visualization of potential local recurrence, are also bona fide reasons to adopt PET–CT [8, 25, 26]. Conversely, inflammation related [18]FDG avid foci in PET–CT studies immediately following surgery, chemotherapy and radiotherapy, can be mistaken for tumour deposits, and can be miss-interpreted by inexperienced reporting, resulting in false positives.

The choice of imaging is therefore a significant consideration when determining the timing of assessment, and may bias the subsequent reporting of results in this study. In the treatment response assessment, PET–CT addresses the discrepancy between the change in lesion size and metabolic response, and was the commonest reason for "added value" of PET–CT over conventional imaging in our series. In the staging and re-staging groups, occult metastatic disease and FDG avid nodal disease, which were not enlarged by CT criteria, may have led to improved TNM staging accuracy overall. Likewise, the presence of new sites of disease (occult disease) in the standardized dimension assessment of oncological treatment response, also indicates the need to stop current treatment and to re-evaluate alternative strategies. Whilst the staging and later findings related to 'added value' are based on comparison of imaging modalities performed within a few weeks, and whilst some

sarcomas may rapidly grow over such a time frame, these cases are very rare, and so we believe that the comparison period is valid.

The heterogeneity of the behavior of sarcoma cells points to the potential for high-grade cell types with more aggressive features to populate recurrent sites of disease detected at restaging. SUVmax alone does not, however, constitute a complete analysis of heterogeneity, and this question requires further analyses, as the overall [18]FDG distribution within tumours has not been assessed. Further prospective validation of PET–CT in sarcoma is justified, as 'added value' components may also reflect differences in reporting experience and protocols. To eliminate future bias, the prospective evaluation of conventional imaging compared with PET–CT across institutions will require standardized reporting (independent double blind reporting) for both modalities. Moreover, quantification of patient outcomes with respect to changes in clinical management would need to be prospectively compared, as well as staging accuracy and cost effectiveness for the patient pathway. In summary, PET–CT in high-grade sarcoma offers the prospect additional benefit in routine staging of high-grade sarcoma at baseline, and specific staging situations during relapse and treatment.

Conclusion

We report a large retrospective audit of PET–CT in bone and soft tissue sarcoma with varied grade in a single multi-disciplinary centre. A total of 957 consecutive PET–CT scans were performed in a single supra-regional centre in 493 sarcoma patients (excluding GIST) between 2007 and 2014. High-grade (II/III) bone and soft tissue sarcoma correlated with high SUVmax, especially undifferentiated pleomorphic sarcoma, leiomyosarcoma, translocation induced sarcomas (Ewing, synovial, alveolar rhabdomyosarcoma), de-differentiated liposarcoma and osteosarcoma. We identified added utility of PET–CT in addition to MRI and CT in high-grade sarcoma of bone and soft tissues. An estimated 21% overall potential benefit was observed for PET–CT over CT/MRI, and in particular, in 'upstaging' of high-grade disease (from M0 to M1) where an additional 12% of cases were deemed M1 following PET–CT. This large study suggests PET–CT in high-grade bone and soft tissue sarcoma can add significant benefit to routine CT/MRI staging. Further prospective and multi-centre evaluation of PET–CT is warranted to determine the actual predictive value and cost-effectiveness of PET–CT in directing clinical management of clinically complex and heterogeneous high-grade sarcomas.

Authors' contributions

REM, SP, KMB and ABH conceived the study. REM performed data analysis of PET–CT comparison with CT/MRI, REM, SP, HT and NA assessed databases and confirmed diagnostic subtypes/grade. REM, MK and KMB reported and evaluated PET–CT scans. SP, SW, MG, DW, PC, LC, ST, KMB and ABH evaluated PET–CT as part of the Oxford Sarcoma MDT. REM, KMB and ABH wrote the paper, all authors made comments. All authors read and approved the final manuscript.

Author details

[1] Oxford Sarcoma Service (OxSarc), Oxford University Hospitals Foundation Trust, Oxford OX3 7LE, UK. [2] Department of Radiology, Oxford University Hospitals Foundation Trust, Oxford OX3 7LE, UK. [3] Department of Oncology, Churchill Hospital, Oxford University Hospitals Foundation Trust, Oxford OX3 7LE, UK. [4] Nuffield Orthopaedic Centre, Oxford University Hospitals Foundation Trust, Oxford OX3 7LE, UK. [5] Department of Paediatric Oncology, Oxford University Hospitals Foundation Trust, Oxford OX3 7LE, UK. [6] NIHR Musculoskeletal Biomedical Research Unit (Sarcoma Theme), Sarcoma and TYA Unit of the NHS Oncology Department, and Sir William Dunn School of Pathology, University of Oxford, South Parks Road, Oxford OX1 3RE, UK.

Acknowledgements

We thank all sarcoma patients and staff at Oxford University Hospitals Trust and Oxford Sarcoma Service.

Competing interests

The authors have no competing interests with respect to this publication. KB and ABH have worked with GE healthcare in PET–CT image analysis and MDT pilot software, respectively.

Funding

We thank OUHT and NIHR BRC2 for support (SP, ABH).

References

1. Holzapfel K, Regler J, Baum T, Rechl H, Specht K, Haller B, von Eisenhart-Rothe R, Gradinger R, Rummeny EJ, Woertler K. Local staging of soft-tissue sarcoma: emphasis on assessment of neurovascular encasement-value of MR imaging in 174 confirmed cases. Radiology. 2015;275:501–9.
2. Tzeng CW, Smith JK, Heslin MJ. Soft tissue sarcoma: preoperative and postoperative imaging for staging. Surg Oncol Clin N Am. 2007;16:389–402.
3. Bloem JL, Taminiau AH, Eulderink F, Hermans J, Pauwels EK. Radiologic staging of primary bone sarcoma: MR imaging, scintigraphy, angiography, and CT correlated with pathologic examination. Radiology. 1988;169:805–10.
4. Rakheja R, Makis W, Skamene S, Nahal A, Brimo F, Azoulay L, Assayag J, Turcotte R, Hickeson M. Correlating metabolic activity on 18F-FDG PET/CT with histopathologic characteristics of osseous and soft-tissue sarcomas: a retrospective review of 136 patients. AJR Am J Roentgenol. 2012;198:1409–16.
5. Charest M, Hickeson M, Lisbona R, Novales-Diaz JA, Derbekyan V, Turcotte RE. FDG PET/CT imaging in primary osseous and soft tissue sarcomas: a retrospective review of 212 cases. Eur J Nucl Med Mol Imaging. 2009;36:1944–51.
6. Schwarzbach MH, Hinz U, Dimitrakopoulou-Strauss A, Willeke F, Cardona S, Mechtersheimer G, Lehnert T, Strauss LG, Herfarth C, Buchler MW. Prognostic significance of preoperative [18-F] fluorodeoxyglucose (FDG) positron emission tomography (PET) imaging in patients with resectable soft tissue sarcomas. Ann Surg. 2005;241:286–94.
7. Adler LP, Blair HF, Makley JT, Williams RP, Joyce MJ, Leisure G, Al-Kaisi N, Miraldi F. Noninvasive grading of musculoskeletal tumors using PET. J Nucl Med. 1991;32:1508–12.
8. Ioannidis JP, Lau J. 18F-FDG PET for the diagnosis and grading of soft-tissue sarcoma: a meta-analysis. J Nucl Med. 2003;44:717–24.
9. Fuglo HM, Jorgensen SM, Loft A, Hovgaard D, Petersen MM. The diagnostic and prognostic value of (18)F-FDG PET/CT in the initial assessment of high-grade bone and soft tissue sarcoma. A retrospective study of 89 patients. Eur J Nucl Med Mol Imaging. 2012;39:1416–24.
10. Herrmann K, Benz MR, Czernin J, Allen-Auerbach MS, Tap WD, Dry SM, Schuster T, Eckardt JJ, Phelps ME, Weber WA, Eilber FC. 18F-FDG-PET/CT Imaging as an early survival predictor in patients with primary high-grade soft tissue sarcomas undergoing neoadjuvant therapy. Clin Cancer Res. 2012;18:2024–31.
11. Evilevitch V, Weber WA, Tap WD, Allen-Auerbach M, Chow K, Nelson SD, Eilber FR, Eckardt JJ, Elashoff RM, Phelps ME, Czernin J, Eilber FC. Reduction of glucose metabolic activity is more accurate than change in size at predicting histopathologic response to neoadjuvant therapy in high-grade soft-tissue sarcomas. Clin Cancer Res. 2008;14:715–20.
12. Sheikhbahaei S, Marcus C, Hafezi-Nejad N, Taghipour M, Subramaniam RM. Value of FDG PET/CT in patient management and outcome of skeletal and soft tissue sarcomas. PET Clin. 2015;10:375–93.
13. Quartuccio N, Fox J, Kuk D, Wexler LH, Baldari S, Cistaro A, Schoder H. Pediatric bone sarcoma: diagnostic performance of (1)(8)F-FDG PET/CT versus conventional imaging for initial staging and follow-up. AJR Am J Roentgenol. 2015;204:153–60.
14. Skamene SR, Rakheja R, Dahlstrom KR, Roberge D, Nahal A, Charest M, Turcotte R, Hickeson M, Freeman C. Metabolic activity measured on PET/CT correlates with clinical outcomes in patients with limb and girdle sarcomas. J Surg Oncol. 2014;109:410–4.
15. Combemale P, Valeyrie-Allanore L, Giammarile F, Pinson S, Guillot B, Goulart DM, Wolkenstein P, Blay JY, Mognetti T. Utility of 18F-FDG PET with a semi-quantitative index in the detection of sarcomatous transformation in patients with neurofibromatosis type 1. PLoS ONE. 2014;9:e85954.
16. Casey DL, Wexler LH, Fox JJ, Dharmarajan KV, Schoder H, Price AN, Wolden SL. Predicting outcome in patients with rhabdomyosarcoma: role of [(18)f]fluorodeoxyglucose positron emission tomography. Int J Radiat Oncol Biol Phys. 2014;90:1136–42.
17. Nose H, Otsuka H, Otomi Y, Terazawa K, Takao S, Iwamoto S, Harada M. Correlations between F-18 FDG PET/CT and pathological findings in soft tissue lesions. J Med Investig. 2013;60:184–90.

18. Choi ES, Ha SG, Kim HS, Ha JH, Paeng JC, Han I. Total lesion glycolysis by 18F-FDG PET/CT is a reliable predictor of prognosis in soft-tissue sarcoma. Eur J Nucl Med Mol Imaging. 2013;40:1836–42.

19. Al-Ibraheem A, Buck AK, Benz MR, Rudert M, Beer AJ, Mansour A, Pomykala KL, Haller B, Juenger H, Scheidhauer K, Schwaiger M, Herrmann K. (18) F-fluorodeoxyglucose positron emission tomography/computed tomography for the detection of recurrent bone and soft tissue sarcoma. Cancer. 2013;119:1227–34.

20. Roberge D, Vakilian S, Alabed YZ, Turcotte RE, Freeman CR, Hickeson M. FDG PET/CT in initial staging of adult soft-tissue sarcoma. Sarcoma. 2012;2012:960194.

21. Payne MJ, Macpherson RE, Bradley KM, Hassan AB. Trabectedin in advanced high-grade uterine leiomyosarcoma: a case report illustrating the value of (18)FDG-PET–CT in assessing treatment response. Case Rep Oncol. 2014;7:132–8.

22. The Royal College Of R, Royal College Of Physicians Of L, Royal College Of P, Surgeons Of G, Royal College Of Physicians Of E, British Nuclear Medicine S, Administration Of Radioactive Substances Advisory C. Evidence-based indications for the use of PET–CT in the United Kingdom 2016. Clin Radiol. 2016;71:e171–88.

23. Rowland AF, Fazakerley DJ, James DE. Mapping insulin/GLUT4 circuitry. Traffic. 2011;12:672–81.

24. Thomas D, Henshaw R, Skubitz K, Chawla S, Staddon A, Blay JY, Roudier M, Smith J, Ye Z, Sohn W, Dansey R, Jun S. Denosumab in patients with giant-cell tumour of bone: an open-label, phase 2 study. Lancet Oncol. 2010;11:275–80.

25. Dimitrakopoulou-Strauss A, Strauss LG, Schwarzbach M, Burger C, Heichel T, Willeke F, Mechtersheimer G, Lehnert T. Dynamic PET 18F-FDG studies in patients with primary and recurrent soft-tissue sarcomas: impact on diagnosis and correlation with grading. J Nucl Med. 2001;42:713–20.

26. Bredella MA, Caputo GR, Steinbach LS. Value of FDG positron emission tomography in conjunction with MR imaging for evaluating therapy response in patients with musculoskeletal sarcomas. AJR Am J Roentgenol. 2002;179:1145–50.

25

Preoperative radiotherapy of soft-tissue sarcomas: surgical and radiologic parameters associated with local control and survival

Panagiotis Tsagozis[1,2]* 🔟, Otte Brosjö[1,2] and Mikael Skorpil[2,3]

Abstract

Background: Preoperative radiotherapy is often used to facilitate excision of soft-tissue sarcomas. We aimed define factors that affect local tumour control and patient survival.

Methods: A single institution registry study of 89 patients with non-metastatic soft-tissue sarcomas having preoperative radiotherapy between 1994 and 2014. Radiologic (presence of peritumoural oedema and volume change following radiotherapy) and histopathologic (tumour volume, grade and surgical margin) parameters were recorded. Outcomes were the events of local recurrence, amputation, metastasis and death.

Results: Local recurrence rate was low (12%) and marginal excision gave equal local control to wide excision. Pelvic localization was associated with a higher risk for amputation. The absence of peritumoural oedema on MRI defined a subgroup of tumours with more favourable oncologic outcome. Reduction of tumour volume following radiotherapy was also associated with better patient survival. Both these radiologic parameters were associated with lower tumour grade. Tumour necrosis was not significant for patient survival. The local complication rate, mainly wound healing problems and infection, was high (40%), but did not lead to any amputation.

Conclusion: Preoperative radiotherapy of high-risk soft-tissue sarcomas allows for good local control rate at the expense of local wound complications, which are however manageable. Marginal excision is sufficient for local control. Absence of peritumoural oedema on MRI, as well as tumour size reduction following radiotherapy are associated to superior patient survival and can be used ass early prognostic factors.

Background

Treatment of soft-tissue sarcomas is mainly surgical. Radiotherapy is indicated as an adjuvant treatment in all deep-seated tumours and in superficial tumours when a wide surgical margin is not achieved [1, 2]. It is usually given post-operatively, but may be given prior to surgery in order to facilitate tumour resection, allowing for limb-sparing surgery. Furthermore, the up-front use of radiotherapy reduces the volume of irradiated tissue, and is thought to result in a better functional outcome, but on the other hand carries a higher risk for wound complications [3]. The decision to give preoperative radiotherapy

is thus individualized, taking into consideration the localization and size of the tumour, its relationship to important anatomical structures, the expected radiotherapy response and size of the radiotherapy field.

There is limited amount of data regarding the outcome of surgery preceded by radiotherapy for soft-tissue sarcomas, and there is still a debate on the factors that may determine patient prognosis. Tumour necrosis may be an objective measure of the effect of preoperative radiotherapy but there is no proof of its validity as a prognostic factor [4]. The use of radiologic measures is also questionable [5–7].

We set out to investigate the outcome of patients with soft-tissue sarcomas who were treated with radiotherapy prior to surgery, and define clinical, histologic and

*Correspondence: panagiotis.tsagkozis@sll.se
[1] Department of Orthopaedic Surgery, Karolinska University Hospital, Solna, Sweden
Full list of author information is available at the end of the article

radiologic prognostic factors associated with survival and local control of the disease in a large retrospective series.

Patients and methods

Description of the cohort

This is a single-institution registry study. Inclusion criteria for participation were the diagnosis of a soft-tissue sarcoma of the trunk or the extremities, the administration of radiotherapy treatment prior to surgery and the absence of metastases at diagnosis. Exclusion criteria were chemotherapy given in a neo-adjuvant setting and a follow-up of less than 2 years for living patients. The study confirmed to Institutional Review Board requirements. The prospective database of our department was reviewed and 121 consecutive patients with a diagnosis of soft-tissue sarcoma who had preoperative radiotherapy treatment between 1994 and 2014 were identified, out of 1005 patients who had surgery for a soft-tissue sarcoma in the same time period (12%). Of these, 89 did not have any preoperative chemotherapy (usually given in the context of the SSG-XX protocol) and were finally included in this study. Patient demographics and characteristics of the cohort are presented in Table 1. Median follow-up was 5 years.

Diagnosis, treatment and surveillance

Diagnosis was set in a multidisciplinary team meeting with the participation of orthopaedic surgeons, musculoskeletal radiologists, pathologists and oncologists. The decision to give preoperative radiotherapy was taken in the same meeting, with an indication to facilitate surgical resection of the tumour with an adequate surgical margin, taking into consideration the size and anatomical location of the tumour and its relationship to important structures such as the neurovascular bundle, its expected

radiosensitivity and the expected morbidity related to radiotherapy and surgery. These criteria remained constant throughout the study period. Standard radiology was magnetic resonance imaging (MRI) prior to radiotherapy with another examination after given radiotherapy but prior to excision of the tumour, and a complete data set with comparable sequences prior and post radiotherapy was available for 76 patients. All MRIs were reviewed by a radiologist with many years of experience in musculoskeletal tumor imaging. Tumour dimensions (maximum dimensions in 3 axes) were measured in cm and tumour response was evaluated either as a change in tumour volume, calculated by multiplication of the maximum dimension in 3 axes, or according to the RECIST criteria using the change in the maximum diameter of the tumour, where partial response was any reduction in tumour volume $\geq 30\%$ but with measurable tumour left, progressive disease any increase $\geq 20\%$, and anything else was stable disease. The degree of peritumoural oedema was subjectively evaluated in 3-grade scale (absent, moderate or heavy) using STIR and/or T2-sequences. Chest X-ray or computed tomography was used for the detection of lung metastases. Fine-needle aspiration cytology was done for diagnosis.

Radiotherapy was given as external beam photon treatment. The most common mode of radiotherapy, given in 81% of the patients, was 50 Gy given in 25 sessions of 2 Gy (5 weeks of treatment). 13% of the patients had less than 50 Gy (36–46 Gy), as a rule given in an intensity modulated treatment and 7% were treated with a dose exceeding 50 Gy (52–70 Gy). Operations were performed by consultant grade surgeons. Median time between radiotherapy and surgery was 6 weeks (range 2–28).

Surgical specimens were reviewed by a dedicated musculoskeletal pathologist. The median tumour size, as measured in the excision specimen, was 11 cm. 57% of the tumours were undifferentiated pleomorfic sarcomas, 25% liposarcomas, 8% malignant peripheral nerve sheath tumours, 7% synovial sarcomas and 3% other sarcomas.

Postoperative surveillance was according to the ESMO guidelines [8], with clinical examination and chest X-ray every 3 months for the first 2 years, every 6 months up to the 5th year after surgery, and then annually for another 5 years.

Statistical methods

Statistics were done in the SPSS software (version 20, SPSS Inc, Chicago, IL) and the STATA (version 13). Survival analyses and comparisons were done using the Kaplan–Meier method and comparisons were done using log-rank test. Hazard ratios between groups were calculated using a Cox regression analysis (proportional hazards model), where possible prognostic factors were

Table 1 Patient demographics

Age	Median: 67 years
	Range: 20–95 years
Gender	51 male
	38 female
Location	60% lower extremity
	18% upper extremity
	12% trunk
	10% pelvis
Stage (Enneking)	51% stage IIB
	31% stage IIA
	10% stage IB
	8% stage IA
Local invasion	96% deep-seated (subfacial)
	4% superficial (subcutaneous)

age (dichotomized around the median), gender, tumour grade (high or low), tumour volume (dichotomized around the median), surgical margin (wide/marginal vs intralesional), tumour necrosis (0–50%: poor response, 51–90% average response, 91–99% good response and 100% complete necrosis), and radiotherapy dose (dichotomized around the median). Competitive risk analysis was done using the method of Pepe and Mori. Chi square tests (χ^2) were used for comparisons between groups. All tests were double-sided, and a p value of ≤ 0.05 was considered significant. 95% confidence intervals are presented in brackets. The core facility of the Statistics Department of the Karolinska Institute was consulted for the analysis of the data.

Results
Radiologic and histologic evaluation of the effect of radiotherapy

We first analyzed the effect that radiotherapy had on tumour volume, measured on MRI prior to radiotherapy as well as after radiotherapy (prior to surgical excision). We found that the tumour volume decreased after radiotherapy in 51% of the cases, increased in 40% and remained stable in 9%. Using RECIST criteria, stable disease was noted in 67% of cases, progressive disease in 18% and partial regression in 15%. Another radiologic parameter that could be evaluated with accuracy was the presence of peritumoural oedema. We observed that prior to radiotherapy 77% of the tumours had peritumoural oedema (67% moderate and 10% heavy), whilst after radiotherapy 82% of the tumours had peritumoural oedema (58% moderate and 24% heavy). The absence of peritumoural oedema, both prior to as well as after radiotherapy, was associated with reduction of tumour volume as evaluated by MRI (p = 0.005). However, there was no association of peritumoural oedema with partial regression according to RECIST criteria (not shown). Furthermore, tumour grade (p = 0.001), but not tumour volume (p = 0.897) was inversely correlated to the degree of peritumoural oedema. Likewise, tumour grade (p = 0.016), but not tumour volume (p = 0.089) was also inversely correlated to reduction in tumour volume after given radiotherapy. There was no correlation between the degree of volume change and the time period between given radiotherapy and the last MRI (data not shown).

Next, the degree of tumour necrosis was quantified, based on microscopic findings after excision of the tumour, since we found post-radiotherapy MRI too unreliable regarding an accurate interpretation of tissue necrosis. In 27% of the specimens necrosis was poor, in 33% average, in 24% good and in 16% complete.

Additionally, we found that the change in tumour volume had no correlation to tissue necrosis (p = 0.638). The

presence or absence of peritumoural oedema prior to or after radiotherapy did not significantly correlate with the degree of tissue necrosis (p = 0.365 and p = 0.098 respectively).

Local control rate, surgical complications and limb survival

R0 surgical margins were achieved in 89% of the patients (wide in 49% and marginal in 40%, as per Enneking), whereas R1 (intralesional) margins were noted in 11%. No patients had R2 margins (intralesional with macroscopic tumour left). Local recurrence was noted in 12% of the patients. A R0 surgical margin (p = 0.014) was important for local control (Fig. 1), but there was no difference between a wide and a marginal margin. The association between clear margins and superior local control rate did not reach statistical significance during separate analysis of local recurrence with death as a competing factor (Additional file 1: Figure S1).

Complications were noted in 40% of the cases, with infections and/or wound healing problems in 36%. There were 6 grade I, 9 grade II, 19 grade III and 2 grade V complications according to the Clavien–Dindo classification. The time span between radiotherapy and surgery had no effect on local recurrence rate (p = 0.214) or the rate of wound complications. Radiotherapy dose was not associated to the rate of wound complications (p = 0.313) or local control rate (p = 0.605).

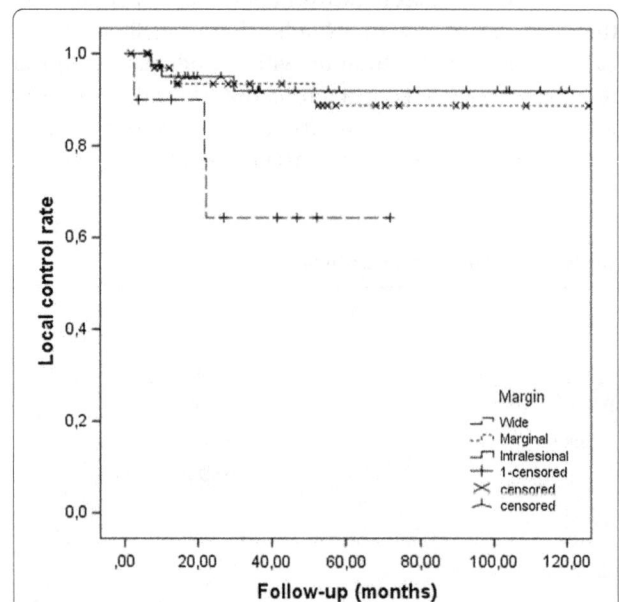

Fig. 1 Kaplan-Meier curve of local control rate depending on the surgical margin, of patients with non-metastatic soft-tissue sarcoma of the trunk and extremities, treated with preoperative radiotherapy. Excision with clear margin provides superior local control (p = 0.014), but there is no difference between wide excisions and marginal ones

There were 9 amputations (in 5 patients the tumour excision was converted to amputation during their primary operation due to technical difficulty in achieving an adequate surgical margin, and 4 had secondary amputation due to local recurrence). The 5 patients who underwent a primary amputation had comparable overall survival to the rest of the patients (p = 0.099). There were no amputations due to wound healing problems and infection. Limb salvage rate was 84% at 5 years and 10 years for upper extremity tumours and 89% at 5 years and 82% at 10 years for lower extremity tumours. Pelvic location was associated with a higher risk for amputation (Fig. 2).

Oncologic outcome and prognostic factors

Metastases were noted in 38% of the cases. The lungs were the most common localization for primary metastatic disease, as documented in 22% of the patients, whilst other atypical locations for primary metastastic disease (lymph node, skeletal and soft-tissue metastases) were relatively common in this series, as they were documented in 16% of the cases. Of the 89 patients, 31 are still alive (one with persisting tumour, the rest not having evidence of disease). Overall survival (OS) was 55% at 5 years and 44% at 10 years.

As presented in Table 2, tumour necrosis, location and surgical margin had no effect on OS. Tumour grade, tumour size and patient age were important for

Table 2 Overall survival

	Hazard ratio (95% CI)	p
Age	1.295–3.821	0.003
Gender	0.556–1.570	0.798
Volume	1.292–3.989	0.003
Grade	1.488–15.300	0.004
Surgical margin	0.442–2.788	0.823
Radiotherapy dose	0.543–2.303	0.762
Tumour necrosis	0.715–1.184	0.517

Effect of possible prognostic factors on the local recurrence rate as well as overall survival of patients with soft-tissue sarcomas of the trunk and the extremities that were treated with radiotherapy prior to surgery. Results gives as hazard rated with 95% confidence intervals and significance values (p)

OS. Tumour size (p = 0.002), grade (p = 0.028) and age (p = 0.023) retained their significance on multivariate analysis. A graphical presentation of the effect of grade and size on OS is given in Fig. 3.

We finally tested the radiologic parameters regarding their prognostic significance (Table 2). Reduction of tumour volume, in response to radiotherapy, evaluated in absolute value, was associated with a superior oncologic outcome (Fig. 4a). In contrast, tumour response using the RECIST criteria was not prognostic for overall survival (p = 0.626). Furthermore, the absence of peritumoural oedema, best evaluated at post-radiotherapy MRI, was also a favourable prognostic factor (Fig. 4b).

Discussion

The decision to give preoperative radiotherapy is mainly based on the intention to downsize the tumour and make it more easily resectable. Volume reduction may result in less morbidity by sparing important anatomical structures, whereas limb-sparing surgery in cases of close proximity of the tumour to the neurovascular bundle may sometimes be feasible only when preoperative radiotherapy is successful.

Our results support the notion that preoperative radiotherapy is a successful strategy in cases of high-risk tumours, such as large-volume ones and those in close proximity to the neurovascular bundle. In our cohort, average tumour size was larger than in published cohorts [1, 9], indicating that the case mix was in favour of large, high-risk tumours. R0 (wide/marginal) surgical margins were nonetheless achieved in a percentage comparable to routine sarcoma surgery [10]. Irradiated sarcomas often displayed clear anatomical margins during excision and were easy to dissect from nearby structures. This demonstrates the value of preoperative radiotherapy which is in accordance to an observed higher rate of resections with clear surgical margins in this setting [11]. The limb salvage rate was also good, although patients should be

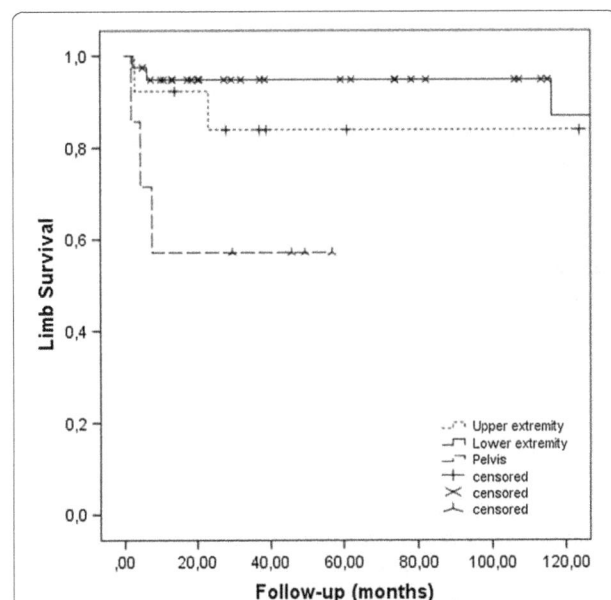

Fig. 2 Kaplan-Meier curve of limb salvage rate regarding the upper and lower extremity, of patients with non-metastatic soft-tissue sarcoma of the extremities, treated with preoperative radiotherapy. Pelvic localization is associated with a higher risk for amputation (p = 0.029)

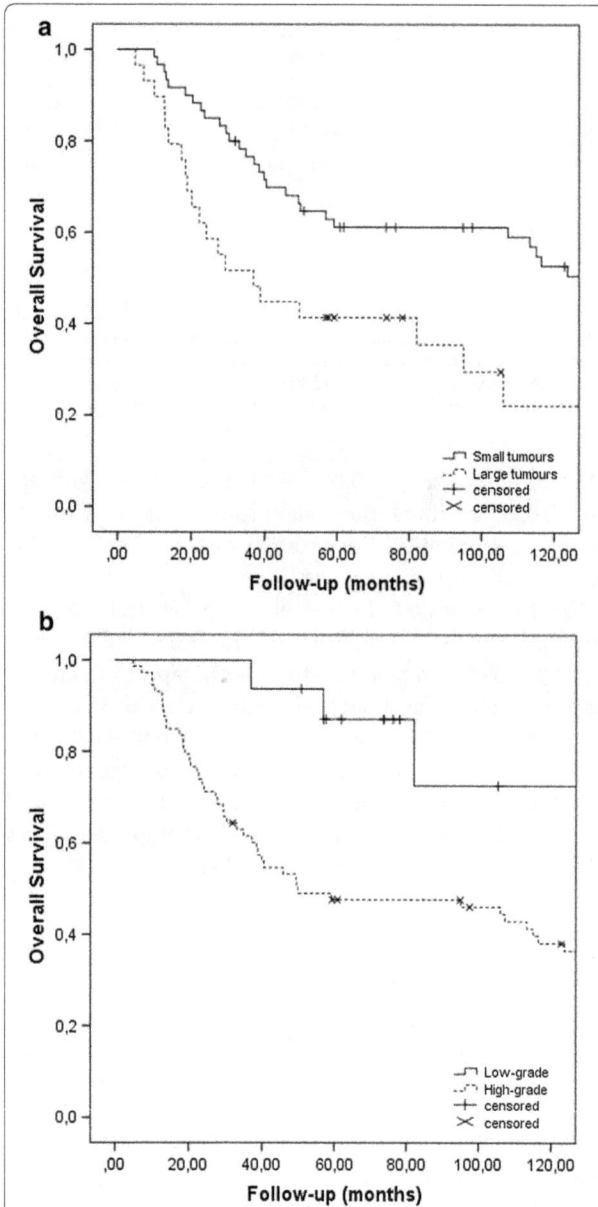

Fig. 3 Kaplan-Meier curve of overall survival depending on tumour size (**a**) and grade (**b**), of patients with non-metastatic soft-tissue sarcoma of the extremities, treated with preoperative radiotherapy. Patients with large tumours (dichotomized around the median volume) have inferior survival to the ones having smaller tumours (p = 0.003). Higher grade is also correlated to inferior overall survival (p = 0.004)

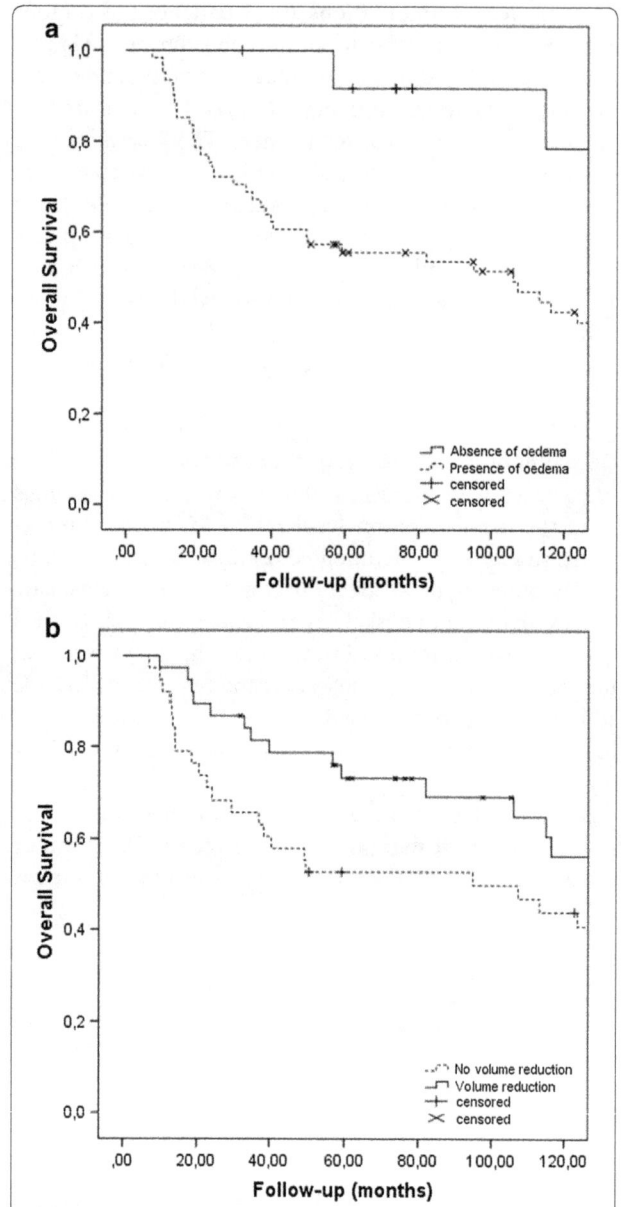

Fig. 4 Kaplan-Meier curve of overall survival depending on the presence or absence of peri-tumoural oedema on MRI (**a**), as well as on the reduction or not of tumour size (**b**), of patients with non-metastatic soft-tissue sarcoma of the extremities, treated with preoperative radiotherapy. Absence of peri-tumoural oedema after radiotherapy (p = 0.040) and reduction of tumour volume (p = 0.015) are associated with superior overall survival

aware that in some cases the surgeon has to convert a planned limb-sparing surgery to an amputation. Pelvic localization is also an important risk factor for amputation. Importantly, there was no need to strive after wide surgical margins, since close marginal excision of the tumour gave equal local control to wide surgical excision, which is in agreement with one previous study [12].

Whereas there is no consensus regarding how radical an excision of a soft-tissue sarcoma should be [13, 14], with conflicting evidence [1, 15, 16], it appears that in the case of pre-irradiated sarcomas a close R0 surgical margin is safe.

We identified two radiologic prognostic factors that are associated with a favourable oncologic outcome, namely the absence of peritumoural oedema and the reduction of tumour volume following radiotherapy. We believe that they represent independent phenomena: The absence of oedema probably marks a more indolent biological behaviour, since there was an inverse correlation between tumour grade and the absence of oedema. Since tumour grade is, as a rule, determined with sufficient accuracy only after examination of the resection specimen, absence of peritumoural oedema can be used as an early marker to predict the oncologic outcome. Reduction of tumour volume on the other hand obviously reflects the response to treatment, although intratumoural bleeding may contribute to a stable or increasing volume and MRI sequences specific for the detection of tissue haemorrhage may be useful in this setting. Two previous studies failed to show any significance of tumour volume increase on survival [5, 6], and tumour volume reduction may be a more accurate marker. Tumour response using the RECIST criteraia was not prognostic, most probably because they are more blunt and minor volume changes are not recorded as a response. Notably, the degree of necrosis at histologic examination, another parameter which may reflect response to radiotherapy, did not correlate to the oncologic outcome, corroborating recent findings [4]. This is probably because tumour necrosis is a more complex phenomenon, which depends both on the biological aggressiveness of the neoplasm (the more aggressive and fast growing, the more necrotic) and response to treatment.

Preoperative radiotherapy was accompanied by a very high risk for local complications, often wound infections, healing problems and dehiscence, which does not depend on the time to surgery or dose. This is in line with previous publications [17–20] and should be communicated to the patient during the process of shared decision-making. The use of modern radiotherapy techniques may lower the risk of local complications [21–23]. Yet, complications were manageable and did not lead to amputations of the extremity.

We recognize the retrospective nature of this study as its main limitation. However, since our aim was not a comparison of preoperative with postoperative radiotherapy, a question which has been addressed in other studies [3, 24, 25], we consider that our study provides valuable new findings regarding preoperative radiotherapy treatment of soft-tissue sarcomas, and encourage further research in this direction so that they are validated in separate large cohorts.

Conclusions

Preoperative radiotherapy allows for good local control of high-risk tumours and excellent limb salvage rates. This is at the expense of a considerable wound complication rate, which however does not pose a threat to limb survival. Simple marginal excision is safe and mutilating surgery to achieve a wide margin thus unnecessary. The absence of peritumoural oedema on MRI as well as volume reduction of the tumour after radiotherapy defines a subgroup of patients with favourable prognosis.

Additional file

Additional file 1: Figure S1. Local relapse rate depending on the quality of surgical margins (clear or intralesional) of patients with non-metastatic soft-tissue sarcoma of the extremities, treated with preoperative radiotherapy, calculated in a competitive risk model with death as a competing factor. Clear surgical margins are not associated to local control rate in a competitive risk model ($p = 0.173$).

Authors' contributions
Study conception and data retrieval: OB, PT, MS. Data analysis: PT, MS. Manuscript preparation: PT, MS. All authors read and approved the final manuscript.

Author details
[1] Department of Orthopaedic Surgery, Karolinska University Hospital, Solna, Sweden. [2] Department of Molecular Medicine and Surgery, Karolinska Institutet, Stockholm, Sweden. [3] Department of Neuroradiology, Karolinska University Hospital, Solna, Sweden.

Acknowledgements
None.

Competing interests
The authors declare that they have no competing interests.

Funding
No funding was received for this study.

References
1. Jebsen NL, Trovik CS, Bauer HCF, Rydholm A, Monge OR, Hall KS, et al. Radiotherapy to improve local control regardless of surgical margin and malignancy grade in extremity and trunk wall soft tissue sarcoma: a Scandinavian sarcoma group study. Int J Radiat Oncol Biol Phys. 2008;71(4):1196–203.
2. Albertsmeier M, Rauch A, Roeder F, Hasenhütl S, Pratschke S, Kirschneck M, et al. External beam radiation therapy for resectable soft tissue sarcoma: a systematic review and meta-analysis. Ann Surg Oncol. 2018;25:754–67.
3. Al-Absi E, Farrokhyar F, Sharma R, Whelan K, Corbett T, Patel M, et al. A systematic review and meta-analysis of oncologic outcomes of pre- versus postoperative radiation in localized resectable soft-tissue sarcoma. Ann Surg Oncol. 2010;17(5):1367–74.
4. Schaefer I-M, Hornick JL, Barysauskas CM, Raut CP, Patel SA, Royce TJ, et al. Histologic appearance after preoperative radiation therapy for soft tissue sarcoma: assessment of the European Organization for Research and Treatment of Cancer-Soft Tissue and Bone Sarcoma Group Response Score. Int J Radiat Oncol Biol Phys. 2017;98(2):375–83.
5. Delisca GO, Alamanda VK, Archer KR, Song Y, Schwartz HS, Holt GE. Tumor size increase following preoperative radiation of soft tissue sarcomas does not affect prognosis. J Surg Oncol. 2013;107(7):723–7.
6. Miki Y, Ngan S, Clark JCM, Akiyama T, Choong PFM. The significance of size change of soft tissue sarcoma during preoperative radiotherapy. Eur J Surg Oncol. 2010;36(7):678–83.
7. Einarsdottir H, Wejde J, Bauer HC. Pre-operative radiotherapy in soft tissue tumors. Assessment of response by static post-contrast MR imaging compared to histopathology. Acta Radiol. 2001;42(1):1–5.
8. ESMO/European Sarcoma Network Working Group. Soft tissue and visceral sarcomas: ESMO Clinical Practice Guidelines for diagnosis, treatment and follow-up. Ann Oncol. 2014;25(Suppl 3):102–12.

9. Coindre JM, Terrier P, Bui NB, Bonichon F, Collin F, Le Doussal V, et al. Prognostic factors in adult patients with locally controlled soft tissue sarcoma. A study of 546 patients from the French Federation of Cancer Centers Sarcoma Group. J Clin Oncol. 1996;14(3):869–77.

10. Strander H, Turesson I, Cavallin-Ståhl E. A systematic overview of radiation therapy effects in soft tissue sarcomas. Acta Oncol. 2003;42(5–6):516–31.

11. Gingrich AA, Bateni SB, Monjazeb AM, Darrow MA, Thorpe SW, Kirane AR, et al. Neoadjuvant radiotherapy is associated with R0 resection and improved survival for patients with extremity soft tissue sarcoma undergoing surgery: a National Cancer Database Analysis. Ann Surg Oncol. 2017;24(11):3252–63.

12. Dagan R, Indelicato DJ, McGee L, Morris CG, Kirwan JM, Knapik J, et al. The significance of a marginal excision after preoperative radiation therapy for soft tissue sarcoma of the extremity. Cancer. 2012;118(12):3199–207.

13. Hoefkens F, Dehandschutter C, Somville J, Meijnders P, Van Gestel D. Soft tissue sarcoma of the extremities: pending questions on surgery and radiotherapy. Radiat Oncol. 2016;11(1):136.

14. Kandel R, Coakley N, Werier J, Engel J, Ghert M, Verma S, et al. Surgical margins and handling of soft-tissue sarcoma in extremities: a clinical practice guideline. Curr Oncol. 2013;20(3):e247–54.

15. Harati K, Goertz O, Pieper A, Daigeler A, Joneidi-Jafari H, Niggemann H, et al. Soft tissue sarcomas of the extremities: surgical margins can be close as long as the resected tumor has no ink on it. Oncologist. 2017;22(11):1400–10.

16. Gundle KR, Kafchinski L, Gupta S, Griffin AM, Dickson BC, Chung PW, et al. Analysis of margin classification systems for assessing the risk of local recurrence after soft tissue sarcoma resection. J Clin Oncol. 2018;JCO2017746941.

17. Griffin AM, Dickie CI, Catton CN, Chung PWM, Ferguson PC, Wunder JS, et al. The influence of time interval between preoperative radiation and surgical resection on the development of wound healing complications in extremity soft tissue sarcoma. Ann Surg Oncol. 2015;22(9):2824–30.

18. Baldini EH, Lapidus MR, Wang Q, Manola J, Orgill DP, Pomahac B, et al. Predictors for major wound complications following preoperative radiotherapy and surgery for soft-tissue sarcoma of the extremities and trunk: importance of tumor proximity to skin surface. Ann Surg Oncol. 2013;20(5):1494–9.

19. Rosenberg LA, Esther RJ, Erfanian K, Green R, Kim HJ, Sweeting R, et al. Wound complications in preoperatively irradiated soft-tissue sarcomas of the extremities. Int J Radiat Oncol Biol Phys. 2013;85(2):432–7.

20. Tseng JF, Ballo MT, Langstein HN, Wayne JD, Cormier JN, Hunt KK, et al. The effect of preoperative radiotherapy and reconstructive surgery on wound complications after resection of extremity soft-tissue sarcomas. Ann Surg Oncol. 2006;13(9):1209–15.

21. Shah C, Verma V, Takiar R, Vajapey R, Amarnath S, Murphy E, et al. Radiation therapy in the management of soft tissue sarcoma: a Clinician's guide to timing, techniques, and targets. Am J Clin Oncol. 2016;39(6):630–5.

22. Haas RLM, Miah AB, LePechoux C, DeLaney TF, Baldini EH, Alektiar K, et al. Preoperative radiotherapy for extremity soft tissue sarcoma; past, present and future perspectives on dose fractionation regimens and combined modality strategies. Radiother Oncol J. 2016;119(1):14–21.

23. Kubicek GJ, LaCouture T, Kaden M, Kim TW, Lerman N, Khrizman P, et al. Preoperative radiosurgery for soft tissue sarcoma. Am J Clin Oncol. 2018;41(1):86–9.

24. Sampath S, Schultheiss TE, Hitchcock YJ, Randall RL, Shrieve DC, Wong JYC. Preoperative versus postoperative radiotherapy in soft-tissue sarcoma: multi-institutional analysis of 821 patients. Int J Radiat Oncol Biol Phys. 2011;81(2):498–505.

25. O'Sullivan B, Davis AM, Turcotte R, Bell R, Catton C, Chabot P, et al. Preoperative versus postoperative radiotherapy in soft-tissue sarcoma of the limbs: a randomised trial. Lancet. 2002;359(9325):2235–41.

Permissions

The contributors of this book come from diverse backgrounds, making this book a truly international effort. This book will bring forth new frontiers with its revolutionizing research information and detailed analysis of the nascent developments around the world.

We would like to thank all the contributing authors for lending their expertise to make the book truly unique. They have played a crucial role in the development of this book. Without their invaluable contributions this book wouldn't have been possible. They have made vital efforts to compile up to date information on the varied aspects of this subject to make this book a valuable addition to the collection of many professionals and students.

This book was conceptualized with the vision of imparting up-to-date information and advanced data in this field. To ensure the same, a matchless editorial board was set up. Every individual on the board went through rigorous rounds of assessment to prove their worth. After which they invested a large part of their time researching and compiling the most relevant data for our readers.

The editorial board has been involved in producing this book since its inception. They have spent rigorous hours researching and exploring the diverse topics which have resulted in the successful publishing of this book. They have passed on their knowledge of decades through this book. To expedite this challenging task, the publisher supported the team at every step. A small team of assistant editors was also appointed to further simplify the editing procedure and attain best results for the readers.

Apart from the editorial board, the designing team has also invested a significant amount of their time in understanding the subject and creating the most relevant covers. They scrutinized every image to scout for the most suitable representation of the subject and create an appropriate cover for the book.

The publishing team has been an ardent support to the editorial, designing and production team. Their endless efforts to recruit the best for this project, has resulted in the accomplishment of this book. They are a veteran in the field of academics and their pool of knowledge is as vast as their experience in printing. Their expertise and guidance has proved useful at every step. Their uncompromising quality standards have made this book an exceptional effort. Their encouragement from time to time has been an inspiration for everyone.

The publisher and the editorial board hope that this book will prove to be a valuable piece of knowledge for researchers, students, practitioners and scholars across the globe.

List of Contributors

Thorsten Hillenbrand, Franka Menge, Peter Hohenberger and Bernd Kasper
Sarcoma Unit, Interdisciplinary Tumor Center Mannheim, Mannheim University Medical Center, University of Heidelberg, Theodor-Kutzer-Ufer 1-3, 68167 Mannheim, Germany

Anna Paioli, Emanuela Palmerini, Marilena Cesari, Alessandra Longhi, Abate Massimo Eraldo, Emanuela Marchesi and Stefano Ferrari
Chemotherapy Unit, Istituto Ortopedico Rizzoli, via Pupilli, 1, 40136 Bologna, Italy

Michele Rocca
General Surgery Unit, Istituto Ortopedico Rizzoli, via Pupilli, 1, 40136 Bologna, Italy

Luca Cevolani
Department of Orthopaedic Oncology, Istituto Ortopedico Rizzoli, via Pupilli, 1, 40136 Bologna, Italy

Eugenio Rimondi and Daniel Vanel
Diagnostic and Interventional Radiology, Istituto Ortopedico Rizzoli, via Pupilli, 1, 40136 Bologna, Italy

Piero Picci
Department of Pathology, Istituto Ortopedico Rizzoli, via di Barbiano, 1/10, 40136 Bologna, Italy

Joan Maurel
Department of Medical Oncology, Hospital Clinic, CIBERehd, Translational Genomics and Targeted Therapeutics in Solid Tumors (IDIBAPS), Barcelona, Spain

Antonio López-Pousa
Department of Medical Oncology, Hospital Universitario Sant Pau, Barcelona, Spain

Silvia Calabuig
Molecular Oncology Laboratory, Fundación de Investigación del Hospital General Universitario de Valencia, Valencia, Spain

Javier Martinez-Trufero
Department of Medical Oncology, Hospital Universitario Miguel Servet, Saragossa, Spain

Xabier García-Albéniz
Harvard T.H. Chan School of Public Health, Boston, MA, USA

Adam Dangoor
Bristol Cancer Institute, Bristol Haematology & Oncology Centre, University Hospitals Bristol NHS Trust, Bristol BS2 8ED, UK

Beatrice Seddon and Jeremy Whelan
Department of Oncology, University College London Hospital NHS Trust, London NW1 2PG, UK

Craig Gerrand
The Newcastle upon Tyne Hospitals NHS Foundation Trust, Freeman Hospital, Newcastle-upon-Tyne NE7 7DN, UK

Robert Grimer
Royal Orthopaedic Hospital NHS Trust, Birmingham B31 2AP, UK

Ian Judson
Royal Marsden NHS Foundation Trust, London SW3 6JJ, UK

L. Paoluzzi, A.Cacavio, J. Weber and G. Rosen
Department of Medicine, NYU Langone Medical Center, New York, NY, USA

M. Ghesani and A. Karambelkar
Department of Radiology, NYU Langone Medical Center, New York, NY, USA

A. Rapkiewicz
Department of Pathology, New York University School of Medicine, Laura and Isaac Perlmutter Cancer Center, 10th floor, Room 1041, 160 East 34th street, New York, NY, USA

Lars M. Wagner
Division of Pediatric Hematology/Oncology, Kentucky Clinic Suite, University of Kentucky, J-457, Lexington, KY 40536, USA

K. Behi, M. Ayadi, E. Mezni, K. Meddeb, A. Mokrani, Y. Yahyaoui, F. Ksontini, H. Rais, N. Chrait and A. Mezlini
Medical Oncology Department, Salah Azaeiz Institute, Tunis, Tunisia

Ivar Hompland and Øyvind Sverre Bruland
Department of Oncology, Norwegian Radium Hospital, Oslo University Hospital, Nydalen, 0424 Oslo, Norway
Institute of Clinical Medicine, University of Oslo, Oslo, Norway

Kjetil Boye
Department of Oncology, Norwegian Radium Hospital, Oslo University Hospital, Nydalen, 0424 Oslo, Norway
Department of Tumor Biology, Norwegian Radium Hospital, Oslo University Hospital, Oslo, Norway

Kumari Ubhayasekhera and Jonas Bergquist
Department of Chemistry, Biomedical Center, Analytical Chemistry and Science for Life Laboratory, Uppsala University, Uppsala, Sweden

Arjen H. G. Cleven, Johnny Suijker, Inge H. Briaire-de Bruijn, Pauline M. Wijers-Koster, Anne-Marie Cleton-Jansen and Judith V. M. G. Bovée
Department of Pathology, Leiden University Medical Center, L1-Q, 2300 RC Leiden, The Netherlands

Georgios Agrogiannis
1st Department of Pathology, Laikon General Hospital, Athens University School of Medicine, Athens, Greece

Norma Frizzell
Department of Pharmacology, Physiology & Neuroscience, School of Medicine, University of South Carolina, Columbia, USA

Attje S. Hoekstra
Department of Human Genetics, Leiden University Medical Center, Leiden, The Netherlands

E. Hookway, K. A. Williams, A. B. Hassan, U. Oppermann, E. Soilleux and N. A. Athanasou
Nuffield Department of Orthopaedics, Rheumatology and Musculoskeletal and Sciences, University of Oxford, Nuffield Orthopaedic Centre, Oxford OX3 7HE, UK

Y. Inagaki
Nuffield Department of Orthopaedics, Rheumatology and Musculoskeletal and Sciences, University of Oxford, Nuffield Orthopaedic Centre, Oxford OX3 7HE, UK
Department of Orthopaedic Surgery, Nara Medical University, Kashihara, Japan

Y. Tanaka
Department of Orthopaedic Surgery, Nara Medical University, Kashihara, Japan

Sumitra Shantakumar
Worldwide Epidemiology, Research and Development, GlaxoSmithKline, 150 Beach Road, #26-00 Gateway West, Singapore 189720, Singapore

Alexandra Connelly-Frost
Frost Consulting, Epidemiologic Research and Grant Writing, Charlotte, NC, USA

Monica G Kobayashi and Robert Allis
Worldwide Epidemiology, Research and Development, GlaxoSmithKline, Research Triangle Park, NC, USA

Li Li
Center for Observational Data Analytics, Amgen, Thousand Oaks, CA, USA

Cassian Yee
Department of Melanoma Medical Oncology, The University of Texas MD Anderson Cancer Center, 1515 Holcombe Blvd., Houston, TX 77030, USA

Jason Roszik
Department of Melanoma Medical Oncology, The University of Texas MD Anderson Cancer Center, 1515 Holcombe Blvd., Houston, TX 77030, USA
Department of Genomic Medicine, The University of Texas MD Anderson Cancer Center, 1515 Holcombe Blvd., Houston, TX 77030, USA

Patrick Hwu
Department of Melanoma Medical Oncology, The University of Texas MD Anderson Cancer Center, 1515 Holcombe Blvd., Houston, TX 77030, USA
Department of Sarcoma Medical Oncology, The University of Texas MD Anderson Cancer Center, 1515 Holcombe Blvd., Houston, TX 77030, USA

Andrew Futreal
Department of Genomic Medicine, The University of Texas MD Anderson Cancer Center, 1515 Holcombe Blvd., Houston, TX 77030, USA

Wei-Lien Wang and Alexander J. Lazar
Department of Pathology, The University of Texas MD Anderson Cancer Center, 1515 Holcombe Blvd., Houston, TX 77030, USA

John A. Livingston, Vinod Ravi, Shreyaskumar R. Patel and Anthony P. Conley
Department of Sarcoma Medical Oncology, The University of Texas MD Anderson Cancer Center, 1515 Holcombe Blvd., Houston, TX 77030, USA

Christina L. Roland
Department of Surgical Oncology, The University of Texas MD Anderson Cancer Center, 1515 Holcombe Blvd, Houston, TX 77030, USA

Sha Lou
Center for Proteomics and Metabolomics, Leiden University Medical Center, Albinusdreef 2, Postzone L1-Q, Postbus 9600, 2300 RC Leiden, The Netherlands

Liam A. McDonnell
Center for Proteomics and Metabolomics, Leiden University Medical Center, Albinusdreef 2, Postzone L1-Q, Postbus 9600, 2300 RC Leiden, The Netherlands
Department of Pathology, Leiden University Medical Center, Leiden, The Netherlands
Fondazione Pisana per la Scienza ONLUS, Pisa, Italy

Arjen H. G. Cleven, Marieke de Graaff, Marie Kostine, Inge Briaire-de Bruijn and Judith V. M. G. Bovée
Department of Pathology, Leiden University Medical Center, Leiden, The Netherlands

Benjamin Balluff
Maastricht MultiModal Molecular Imaging Institute (M4I), Maastricht University, Maastricht, The Netherlands

Alberto Righi, Marco Gambarotti and Piero Picci
Department of Pathology, Rizzoli Institute, Via di Barbiano 1/10, 40136 Bologna, Italy

Angelo Paolo Dei Tos
Department of Pathology, Rizzoli Institute, Via di Barbiano 1/10, 40136 Bologna, Italy

Department of Pathology, Treviso Regional Hospital, Treviso, Italy

Anna Paioli, Emanuela Palmerini, Manuela Cesari, Emanuela Marchesi and Stefano Ferrari
Department of Oncology, Rizzoli Institute, Bologna, Italy

Davide Maria Donati
Department of Orthopaedic Oncology, Rizzoli Institute, Bologna, Italy

Michiel C. Verboom, Jan Ouwerkerk and Hans Gelderblom
Department of Medical Oncology, Leiden University Medical Center, Postbus 9600, 2300 RC Leiden, The Netherlands

Neeltje Steeghs and J. Martijn Kerst
Department of Medical Oncology, Antoni van Leeuwenhoek-Netherlands Cancer Institute, Postbus 90203, 1006 BE Amsterdam, The Netherlands

Jacob Lutjeboer
Department of Radiology, Interventional Radiology Section, Leiden University Medical Center, Postbus 9600, 2300 RC Leiden, The Netherlands

Winette T. A. van der Graaf
Department of Medical Oncology, Radboud University Medical Center, Postbus 9101, 6500 HB Nijmegen, The Netherlands
The Institute of Cancer Research and the Royal Marsden NHS Foundation Trust, 123 Old Brompton Road, London SW7 3RP, UK

Anna K. L. Reyners
Department of Medical Oncology, University of Groningen, University Medical Center Groningen, Postbus 30.001, 9700 RB Groningen, The Netherlands

Stefan Sleijfer
Department of Medical Oncology, Erasmus MC Cancer Institute, Postbus 2040, 3000 CA Rotterdam, The Netherlands

Kicuhoa T. Vo and Katherine K. Matthay
Department of Pediatrics, UCSF School of Medicine, San Francisco School of Medicine, UCSF Benioff Children's Hospital, University of California, 550 16th Street, 4th Floor, San Francisco, CA 94158, USA

Steven G. DuBois
Dana-Farber/Boston Children's Cancer and Blood Disorders Center, 450 Brookline Avenue, Dana 3, Boston, MA 02215, USA

R. B. Cohen-Hallaleh,   H. G. Smith,   R. C. Smith,   G. F. Stamp,   O. Al-Muderis,   K. Thway,   A. Miah,   K. Khabra,   I. Judson,   R. Jones,   C. Benson   and   A. J. Hayes
The Sarcoma Unit, The Royal Marsden Hospital NHS Foundation Trust, London, UK

Wangzhao Song and Albert J. Suurmeijer
Department of Pathology and Medical Biology, University Medical Center Groningen, University of Groningen, RB Groningen, The Netherlands

Eva van den Berg
Department of Genetics, University Medical Center Groningen, University of Groningen, 9700 RB Groningen, The Netherlands

Thomas C. Kwee
Department of Radiology, Nuclear Medicine and Molecular Imaging, University Medical Center Groningen, University of Groningen, RB Groningen, The Netherlands

Paul C. Jutte
Department of Orthopedic Surgery, University Medical Center Groningen, University of Groningen, RB Groningen, The Netherlands

Anne-Marie   Cleton-Jansen   and   Judith V. M. G. Bovée
Department of Pathology, Leiden University Medical Center, Leiden, The Netherlands

Sergio Sandrucci and Claudio Gianotti
Visceral Sarcoma Unit, University of Turin, Cso Dogliotti 14, 10126 Turin, Italy

Agostino Ponzetti, Patrizia Lista and Marinella Mistrangelo
Medical Oncology 1 Division, Città della Salute e della Scienza, Turin, Italy

Baudolino Mussa
Department of Surgical Sciences, University of Turin, Turin, Italy

Giovanni Grignani
Department of Medical Oncology, Candiolo Cancer Institute-FPO, IRCCS, Candiolo, Italy

Oscar Bertetto
Regional Oncologic Network Department, Turin, Italy

Daniela Di Cuonzo and Giovannino Ciccone
Cancer Epidemiology Unit, Città della Salute e della Scienza, Turin, Italy

Anne McTiernan and Jessica Bate
Department of Oncology, University College Hospitals London NHS Foundation Trust, 250 Euston Road, London NW1 2PG, UK

Jeremy Whelan
Department of Oncology, University College Hospitals London NHS Foundation Trust, 250 Euston Road, London NW1 2PG, UK
Children's Cancer and Leukaemia Group Data Centre, Cancer Studies and Molecular Medicine, University of Leicester, Leicester, UK

Allan Hackshaw
Cancer Research UK and UCL Clinical Trials Centre, University College London, London, UK

Alan Craft
Children's Cancer and Leukaemia Group Data Centre, Cancer Studies and Molecular Medicine, University of Leicester, Leicester, UK
Northern Institute for Cancer Research, Newcastle University, Newcastle upon Tyne, UK

Ian Lewis
Children's Cancer and Leukaemia Group Data Centre, Cancer Studies and Molecular Medicine, University of Leicester, Leicester, UK
University of Leeds and Leeds Community Healthcare Trust, Leeds, UK

Robert Grimer
The Royal Orthopaedic Hospital, Birmingham, UK

David Spooner
Queen Elizabeth II Hospital, Birmingham, UK

Andreas Ranft
University Hospital Essen, Essen, Germany

Michael Paulussen
Vestische Kinder- und Jugendklinik Datteln, University Witten/Herdecke, Datteln, Germany

Herbert Juergens
Department of Pediatric Hematology and Oncology, University Children's Hospital Münster, Münster, Germany

Emilien Billon and Audrey Monneur
INSERM UMR1068, CNRS UMR725, Department of Medical Oncology, Centrede Recherche en Cancérologie de Marseille (CRCM), Institut Paoli-Calmettes, 232 Bd de Sainte-Marguerite, 13009 Marseille, France

François Bertucci
INSERM UMR1068, CNRS UMR725, Department of Medical Oncology, Centrede Recherche en Cancérologie de Marseille (CRCM), Institut Paoli-Calmettes, 232 Bd de Sainte-Marguerite, 13009 Marseille, France
Faculty of Medicine, Aix-Marseille University, Marseille, France
French Sarcoma Group, Paris, France

Delphine Perrot
INSERM UMR1068, CNRS UMR725, Department of Medical Oncology, Centrede Recherche en Cancérologie de Marseille (CRCM), Institut Paoli-Calmettes, 232 Bd de Sainte-Marguerite, 13009 Marseille, France
French Sarcoma Group, Paris, France

Anne-Marie Stoppa
Department of Hematology,Institut Paoli-Calmettes, Marseille, France

Lena Mescam
Department of Pathology,Institut Paoli-Calmettes, Marseille, France

Massimo Bocci
Department of Digestive Endoscopy Centre Hospitalier Edmond Garcin, Aubagne, France

Victor M. Villalobos
University of Colorado Anschutz Medical Campus, 1665 Aurora Ct ACP 5329 Mail Stop F704 Aurora, Denver, CO 80045, USA

Stacey DaCosta Byfield and Oluwakayode Adejoro
Optum, MN101-E300, 11000 Optum Circle, Eden Prairie, MN 55344, USA

Sameer R. Ghate
Novartis, One Health Plaza 345/5130B, East Hanover, NJ 07936, USA

Jennifer M. Brown, Afsie Sabokbar, Udo Oppermann, A. Bass Hassan and Nick Athanasou
Nuffield Department of Orthopaedics, Rheumatology and Musculoskeletal and Sciences, Nuffield Orthopaedic Centre, University of Oxford, Oxford OX3 7HE, UK

Akiro Mantoku and Akiro Kudo
Department of Biological Information, Tokyo Institute of Technology, Yokohama 226-8501, Japan

Ruth E. Macpherson and Kevin M. Bradley
Oxford Sarcoma Service (OxSarc), Oxford University Hospitals FoundationTrust, Oxford OX3 7LE, UK
Department of Radiology, Oxford University Hospitals Foundation Trust, Oxford OX3 7LE, UK

Sarah Pratap and Sally Trent
Oxford Sarcoma Service (OxSarc), Oxford University Hospitals FoundationTrust, Oxford OX3 7LE, UK
Department of Oncology, Churchill Hospital, Oxford University Hospitals Foundation Trust, Oxford OX3 7LE, UK

A. Bassim Hassan
Oxford Sarcoma Service (OxSarc), Oxford University Hospitals FoundationTrust, Oxford OX3 7LE, UK
Department of Oncology, Churchill Hospital, Oxford University Hospitals Foundation Trust, Oxford OX3 7LE, UK
NIHR Musculoskeletal Biomedical Research Unit (Sarcoma Theme), Sarcoma and TYA Unit of the NHS Oncology Department, and Sir William Dunn School of Pathology, University of Oxford, South Parks Road, Oxford OX1 3RE, UK

Max Gibbons, Duncan Whitwell, Henk Giele, Paul Critchley and Lucy Cogswell
Oxford Sarcoma Service (OxSarc), Oxford University Hospitals FoundationTrust, Oxford OX3 7LE, UK
Nuffield Orthopaedic Centre, Oxford University Hospitals Foundation Trust, Oxford OX3 7LE, UK

Nick Athanasou
Oxford Sarcoma Service (OxSarc), Oxford University Hospitals FoundationTrust, Oxford OX3 7LE, UK
Nuffield Orthopaedic Centre, Oxford University Hospitals Foundation Trust, Oxford OX3 7LE, UK
NIHR Musculoskeletal Biomedical Research Unit (Sarcoma Theme), Sarcoma and TYA Unit of the NHS Oncology Department, and Sir William Dunn School of Pathology, University of Oxford, South Parks Road, Oxford OX1 3RE, UK

Shaun Wilson
Oxford Sarcoma Service (OxSarc), Oxford University Hospitals FoundationTrust, Oxford OX3 7LE, UK Department of Paediatric Oncology, Oxford University Hospitals Foundation Trust, Oxford OX3 7LE, UK

Mehrdad Khonsari
Department of Radiology, Oxford University Hospitals Foundation Trust, Oxford OX3 7LE, UK

Helen Tyrrell
Department of Oncology, Churchill Hospital, Oxford University Hospitals Foundation Trust, Oxford OX3 7LE, UK

Panagiotis Tsagozis and Otte Brosjö
Department of Orthopaedic Surgery, Karolinska University Hospital, Solna, Sweden Department of Molecular Medicine and Surgery, Karolinska Institutet, Stockholm, Sweden

Index

www.ingramcontent.com/pod-product-compliance
Lightning Source LLC
Chambersburg PA
CBHW061251190326
41458CB00011B/3639